全国高等中医药院校中药学类专业双语规划教材

Bilingual Planned Textbooks for Chinese Materia Medica Majors in TCM Colleges and Universities

中药药理学

Chinese Medicinal Pharmacology

（供中药学类专业使用）

(For Chinese Materia Medica Majors)

主　编　唐民科　徐海波

副主编　方　芳　李红艳　屈　飞　汪　宁

编　者（以姓氏笔画为序）

马秉亮（上海中医药大学）	王　斌（陕西中医药大学）
王艳艳（黑龙江中医药大学）	方　芳（北京中医药大学）
方晓艳（河南中医药大学）	华永庆（南京中医药大学）
刘　娟（成都中医药大学）	杨　柯（广西中医药大学）
李冰涛（江西中医药大学）	李红艳（辽宁中医药大学）
肖洪贺（辽宁中医药大学）	汪　宁（安徽中医药大学）
陈　怡（西南大学药学院·中医药学院）	陈艳芬（广东药科大学）
屈　飞（江西中医药大学）	贺龙刚（福建中医药大学）
徐海波（成都中医药大学）	唐民科（北京中医药大学）
黄莉莉（黑龙江中医药大学）	曹惠慧（南方医科大学）
董世芬（北京中医药大学）	韩　岚（安徽中医药大学）

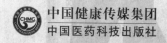

中国健康传媒集团

中国医药科技出版社

内 容 提 要

本教材是"全国高等中医药院校中药学类专业双语规划教材"之一。内容主要包括总论和各论。总论重点讲述中药药理学的学科特色、中药药性理论的现代研究、影响中药药理作用的因素等内容；各论部分按照中药学传统分类顺序，收录中药100味，重点介绍中药的基源、化学成分、传统功效、药理作用、不良反应等。本教材为书网融合教材，即纸质教材有机融合电子教材、教学配套资源（PPT、微课、视频、图片等）、题库系统、数字化教学服务（在线教学、在线作业、在线考试），使教学资源更加多样化、立体化。

本教材供全国高等医药院校中药学类专业使用，也可供从事中药研究、生产、销售工作的人员参考。

图书在版编目（CIP）数据

中药药理学：汉英对照 / 唐民科，徐海波主编 . —北京：中国医药科技出版社，2020.8
全国高等中医药院校中药学类专业双语规划教材
ISBN 978-7-5214-1872-9

Ⅰ.①中… Ⅱ.①唐…②徐… Ⅲ.①中药学－药理学－双语教学－中医学院－教材－汉、英 Ⅳ.①R285

中国版本图书馆 CIP 数据核字（2020）第 097421 号

美术编辑　陈君杞
版式设计　辰轩文化

出版　**中国健康传媒集团** | 中国医药科技出版社
地址　北京市海淀区文慧园北路甲 22 号
邮编　100082
电话　发行：010-62227427　邮购：010-62236938
网址　www.cmstp.com
规格　889×1194 mm ¹⁄₁₆
印张　20½
字数　527 千字
版次　2020 年 8 月第 1 版
印次　2020 年 8 月第 1 次印刷
印刷　三河市万龙印装有限公司
经销　全国各地新华书店
书号　ISBN 978-7-5214-1872-9
定价　66.00 元

获取新书信息、投稿、
为图书纠错，请扫码
联系我们。

近些年随着世界范围的中医药热潮的涌动，来中国学习中医药学的留学生逐年增多，走出国门的中医药学人才也在增加。为了适应中医药国际交流与合作的需要，加快中医药国际化进程，提高来中国留学生和国际班学生的教学质量，满足双语教学的需要和中医药对外交流需求，培养优秀的国际化中医药人才，进一步推动中医药国际化进程，根据教育部、国家中医药管理局、国家药品监督管理局等部门的有关精神，在本套教材建设指导委员会主任委员成都中医药大学彭成教授等专家的指导和顶层设计下，中国医药科技出版社组织全国50余所高等中医药院校及附属医疗机构约420名专家、教师精心编撰了全国高等中医药院校中药学类专业双语规划教材，该套教材即将付梓出版。

本套教材共计23门，主要供全国高等中医药院校中药学类专业教学使用。本套教材定位清晰、特色鲜明，主要体现在以下方面。

一、立足双语教学实际，培养复合应用型人才

本套教材以高校双语教学课程建设要求为依据，以满足国内医药院校开展留学生教学和双语教学的需求为目标，突出中医药文化特色鲜明、中医药专业术语规范的特点，注重培养中医药技能、反映中医药传承和现代研究成果，旨在优化教育质量，培养优秀的国际化中医药人才，推进中医药对外交流。

本套教材建设围绕目前中医药院校本科教育教学改革方向对教材体系进行科学规划、合理设计，坚持以培养创新型和复合型人才为宗旨，以社会需求为导向，以培养适应中药开发、利用、管理、服务等各个领域需求的高素质应用型人才为目标的教材建设思路与原则。

二、遵循教材编写规律，整体优化，紧跟学科发展步伐

本套教材的编写遵循"三基、五性、三特定"的教材编写规律；以"必需、够用"为度；坚持与时俱进，注意吸收新技术和新方法，适当拓展知识面，为学生后续发展奠定必要的基础。实验教材密切结合主干教材内容，体现理实一体，注重培养学生实践技能训练的同时，按照教育部相关精神，增加设计性实验部分，以现实问题作为驱动力来培养学生自主获取和应用新知识的能力，从而培养学生独立思考能力、实验设计能力、实践操作能力和可持续发展能力，满足培养应用型和复合型人才的要求。强调全套教材内容的整体优化，并注重不同教材内容的联系与衔接，避免遗漏和不必要的交叉重复。

三、对接职业资格考试，"教考""理实"密切融合

本套教材的内容和结构设计紧密对接国家执业中药师职业资格考试大纲要求，实现教学与考试、理论与实践的密切融合，并且在教材编写过程中，吸收具有丰富实践经验的企业人员参与教材的编写，确保教材的内容密切结合应用，更加体现高等教育的实践性和开放性，为学生参加考试和实践工作打下坚实基础。

四、创新教材呈现形式，书网融合，使教与学更便捷更轻松

全套教材为书网融合教材，即纸质教材与数字教材、配套教学资源、题库系统、数字化教学服务有机融合。通过"一书一码"的强关联，为读者提供全免费增值服务。按教材封底的提示激活教材后，读者可通过 PC、手机阅读电子教材和配套课程资源（PPT、微课、视频等），并可在线进行同步练习，实时收到答案反馈和解析。同时，读者也可以直接扫描书中二维码，阅读与教材内容关联的课程资源，从而丰富学习体验，使学习更便捷。教师可通过 PC 在线创建课程，与学生互动，开展在线课程内容定制、布置和批改作业、在线组织考试、讨论与答疑等教学活动，学生通过 PC、手机均可实现在线作业、在线考试，提升学习效率，使教与学更轻松。此外，平台尚有数据分析、教学诊断等功能，可为教学研究与管理提供技术和数据支撑。需要特殊说明的是，有些专业基础课程，例如《药理学》等 9 种教材，起源于西方医学，因篇幅所限，在本次双语教材建设中纸质教材以英语为主，仅将专业词汇对照了中文翻译，同时在中国医药科技出版社数字平台"医药大学堂"上配套了中文电子教材供学生学习参考。

编写出版本套高质量教材，得到了全国知名专家的精心指导和各有关院校领导与编者的大力支持，在此一并表示衷心感谢。希望广大师生在教学中积极使用本套教材和提出宝贵意见，以便修订完善，共同打造精品教材，为促进我国高等中医药院校中药学类专业教育教学改革和人才培养做出积极贡献。

全国高等中医药院校中药学类专业双语规划教材
建设指导委员会

数字化教材编委会

前　言

中药药理学是以中医药理论为指导，运用现代科学方法，研究中药与机体相互作用、作用规律的一门学科。从本质上看，它是利用现代科学知识，对中药的特性、功效和毒性等进行全面科学的再认识。中药药理学既是中药学科的重要组成部分，也是药理学科的重要分支，它是连接传统中药学与现代药理学之间的桥梁。开展中药药理研究，可以更好地理解中药的科学内涵。随着中医药的国际化发展，在世界范围内使用中药的人群不断扩大，学习和掌握中药药理学知识，对于指导临床安全合理地使用中药、确保广大民众健康、促进中医药事业可持续发展具有重要意义。

本教材内容主要包括总论和各论。总论重点讲述中药药理学的学科特色、中药药性理论的现代研究、影响中药药理作用的因素等内容；各论部分按照中药学传统分类顺序，收录中药100味，重点介绍中药的药物基源、化学成分、传统功效、药理作用、不良反应等。本教材以中文和英文两种语言对照编写，主要适合作为境内、境外本专科层次，中药学类专业的中药药理学教学的基础参考教材。

本教材在编写过程中，依据现有《中药药理学》教材的主要框架，参考各教材的主要内容，在以下几方面做了尝试和创新。

1. 规范内容　严格按照中药药理学的学科规范，对相关内容重新整理，不符合科学规范的内容不再录入本教材，以使学生对所学知识有清晰的理解。

2. 突出实用　本教材围绕教学及学习过程，在每章开始设置学习目标，突出学习重点，便于教师和学生的教学互动。

3. 书网融合　本教材为书网融合教材，即纸质教材有机融合电子教材、教学配套资源（PPT、微课、视频、图片等）、题库系统、数字化教学服务（在线教学、在线作业、在线考试），使教学资源更加多样化、立体化。

本教材在编写过程中虽力臻完善，但难免存在不足与疏漏之处，提请广大师生批评指正，以便不断完善与修订。

编　者
2020 年 4 月

Foreword

Chinese Medicinal Pharmacology is a discipline that focuses on the interaction of traditional Chinese medicine and the body. Essentially, it is a re-understanding of the characteristics, the traditional efficacy, and the toxicity of traditional Chinese medicine by using modern scientific measures. Chinese Medicinal Pharmacology is not only an important part of the discipline of traditional Chinese medicine, but also an important sub-discipline of pharmacology. It is a bridge between traditional Chinese medicine and modern pharmacology. Research on Chinese Medicinal Pharmacology can enable us to better understand the scientific connotation of traditional Chinese medicine. With the international development of traditional Chinese medicine, the number of people who use Chinese medicine worldwide is expanding. Learning and understanding the knowledge of Chinese Medicinal Pharmacology can guide the clinicians to use traditional Chinese medicine safely and reasonably, ensuring the safety of the general public, and promoting the sustainable development of traditional Chinese medicine worldwide.

The contents of this textbook mainly include general principles and medicinal materials monographs. The general thesis focuses on the disciplinary characteristics of Chinese Medicinal Pharmacology, modern research on the theory of traditional Chinese medicine properties, and factors affecting the pharmacological effects of traditional Chinese medicine. The monographs include 100 Chinese medicinal materials in accordance with the traditional classification order of traditional Chinese medicine. Information about the source, chemical composition, traditional efficacy, pharmacological effect, and adverse effect are included in the medicinal monographs.

In compiling this textbook, the framework and main contents of existing textbooks had been referred. In addition, this textbook made innovations in the following aspects. ①Re-evaluating the research findings: all research findings related with the medicinal materials in the text book had been strictly re-evaluated in accordance with the scientific standard of pharmacological research. Research that does not meet scientific standard is not included in this textbook so that students can have a clear understanding of the knowledge. ②Focusing on practicality: the entire textbook revolves around the teaching and learning activity. Learning objectives, highlights summary, and questions, are set up respectively at the beginning of the textbook to facilitate the teaching and learning. ③The textbook includes both traditional paper-based textbooks, as well as electronic textbooks, teaching supporting resources (PPT, micro-classes, videos, pictures, etc.), examination questions, digital teaching services (online teaching, online homework, online examination) etc. All above make the teaching resources more diverse and three-dimensional.

Although this textbook pursues perfection in translating and editing, it is inevitable that there are deficiencies and omissions. The teachers and students are invited to criticize and correct them so that they can be continuously improved and revised.

The Editors
April, 2020

目录 | Contents

上篇 总论
Part I Pandect

下篇　各论
Part II　Systematics

上篇　总论
Part I　Pandect

第一章 绪论

Chapter 1　Introduction

学习目标┊Objectives

1. **掌握** 中药药理学的定义；中药药理学的研究内容和主要任务。
2. **了解** 中药药理学的发展简史。

1. **Must know** The concept of Chinese Medicinal Pharmacology; research contents and main tasks of Chinese Medicinal Pharmacology.

2. **Desirable to know** The development of Chinese Medicinal Pharmacology.

第一节　概述

Section 1　Overview

PPT

微课

中药药理学是中药学的分支学科，也是药理学的分支学科，它将两者跨学科联系起来。中药药理学为中医临床实践、中西医结合临床实践提供科学指导。中药药理学知识体系既包含传统中医药内容，也涉及现代医学及生命科学研究前沿。发展中药药理学对于传统中医药体系的建设与发展具有重要意义。

Chinese medicinal pharmacology is a sub-discipline of Chinese medicine and a sub-discipline of pharmacology, which is the interdisciplinary connection of the two. Chinese medicinal pharmacology provides scientific instruction for clinical practice of traditional Chinese medicine and clinical practice of integrated traditional Chinese and western medicine. From the perspective of knowledge scope, Chinese medicinal pharmacology contains both traditional Chinese medicine knowledge and the frontier of biomedical sciences and life sciences. The development of the Chinese medicinal pharmacology is of great significance to the construction and development of the whole Chinese medicine system.

一、基本概念与研究内容
1. Basic concepts and main contents

中药药理学是以中医药理论为指导，运用现代科学方法，研究中药与机体相互作用、作用规律的一门学科。其中，中药是指按照中医药理论，用来预防、诊断、治疗疾病的药物，包括植物

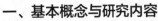

药、动物药、矿物药。机体主要指人体、动物体、病原体，可能涉及器官、组织、细胞、分子等不同层面。

Chinese medicinal pharmacology is a scientific discipline that uses the basic theory of traditional Chinese medicine as a guide and uses modern scientific methods to study the interaction of traditional Chinese medicine with the body. Here Chinese medicine refers to a medicine that prevents, diagnoses, and treats diseases according to the theory of Chinese medicine, including botanical medicine, animal medicine, and mineral medicine. The body mainly refers to human body, animal body, pathogens, which may involve tissues, organs, cells, molecules.

中药药理学研究的内容包括中药效应动力学（简称中药药效学）、中药代谢动力学（简称中药药动学）以及中药毒理学。中药药效学研究中药对机体的影响，即用现代科学理论和方法研究中药对机体的作用及作用规律。中药药动学研究机体对中药的影响，即中药进入机体，通常主要指人体，在体内吸收、分布、代谢、排泄的动态变化过程及规律。中药毒理学旨在研究中药对人体的有害影响及其规律。

The Chinese medicinal pharmacological research includes three aspects: pharmacodynamics, pharmacokinetics, and toxicology. The pharmacodynamics of Chinese medicine is to use modern scientific theories and methods to study the effects of Chinese medicine on the body and the mechanisms of its action. The pharmacokinetics of Chinese medicine is to study the influence of the body, usually refers to the human body, on Chinese medicine, that is the dynamic process of the medicine absorption, distribution, metabolism and excretion. Toxicology of Chinese medicine aims to study the harmful effects of Chinese medicine on the human body and its mechanisms.

二、学科特征与主要任务
2. The characteristics and tasks

中药药理学与天然药物药理学的区别，主要体现在它们的理论基础不同。中药药理学虽然也采用现代科学方法，但是强调以中医药理论为指导开展研究，而天然药物药理学采用现代科学理论体系为指导进行研究。中药药理学有时也会研究单体化合物、单个药用植物，但是总体来看，中药药理学的研究重心是多个中药组成的复方制剂，更多关注多个中药共同产生的综合作用。

The difference between Chinese medicinal pharmacology and natural medicine pharmacology is mainly reflected in their different theoretical basis. Although Chinese medicinal pharmacology also uses modern scientific methods, it emphasizes the use of traditional Chinese medicine theory as a guide to carry out these studies, while natural medicine pharmacology uses modern scientific theoretical system as foundations for research. Traditional Chinese medicine pharmacology sometimes studies chemical compounds and single medicinal plant, but overall, the research focus of Chinese medicinal pharmacology is formula preparations composed of multiple Chinese medicinal materials, especially the comprehensive effects of multiple medicinal materials.

中药药理学的主要任务是：认识和理解中药理论的内涵，阐明中药的药性、功效及中药应用的科学依据；指导中药的新药开发研究及安全性评价；指导临床合理用药，提高中药的临床疗效，减少不良反应事件发生；推动中药现代化、产业化，促进中医药体系的进步和发展。

The main tasks of Chinese medicinal pharmacology are to understand the connotation of traditional Chinese medicine theory, and to reveal the scientific basis of traditional Chinese medicine properties, traditional Chinese medicine efficacy and the application of Chinese medicines; to support the new drug development and safety evaluation of Chinese medicine; to instruct the clinical application of Chinese medicine to improving the clinical efficacy and reducing the occurrence of adverse events; to promote the modernization and industrialization of Chinese medicine, and promote the development of the Chinese medicine system as a whole.

第二节　中药药理学发展简史
Section 2　A brief history

PPT

中药应用于临床已有数千年的历史，关于中药的知识是人们在生产实践和医疗实践过程中逐渐积累起来的。随着自然科学的发展和社会生产力的提升，关于中药的知识也不断丰富完善。中药药理学作为一门新兴学科，它是在传统中药学以及现代药理学基础上发展起来的分支学科。中药药理学的发展经历了思想萌芽、现代发展两个重要阶段。

Traditional Chinese medicine has been used in clinic for thousands of years. The knowledge about traditional Chinese medicine is gradually accumulated in the process of production and medical practice. With the development of natural science and the improvement of social productivity, the knowledge about traditional Chinese medicine has also been constantly enriched and improved. Chinese medicinal pharmacology, as an emerging discipline, is developed on the basis of traditional Chinese medicine and modern pharmacology. The development of Chinese medicinal pharmacology has experienced two important stages of initial exploration and modern development.

一、思想萌芽
1. Initial exploration

中药药理学蕴含古人丰富的用药经验。古人在反复实践的过程中，逐步掌握中药的特性及作用，并利用中药的这些特性和作用治疗各种疾病。从这个角度理解，很早以前人们用中药来治疗疾病时，就为中药药理学发展奠定了基础。

The traditional Chinese medicine contains rich clinical experiences of our ancestors. In the process of repeated clinical observation, they gradually mastered the characteristics and functions of traditional Chinese medicine, and used these characteristics and functions to treat various diseases. From this perspective, long time ago when people used traditional Chinese medicine to treat diseases, they laid the foundation for the development of Chinese medicinal pharmacology.

《神农本草经》约成书于东汉时期，是目前最早的中药专著，书中记载中药的临床应用及作用原理，还记载了中药的四气、五味、有毒无毒等性能。在南北朝时期，陶弘景在《神农本草经》的基础上，编著了《本草经集注》，对药物的性味、功能、主治做了补充，同时完善了中药的产地、采收时期及加工处理方法。"药理"这个词汇，也是最早出现在《本草经集注》中。唐显庆四年（公元 659 年），苏敬等 23 人编撰《唐本草》（又名《新修本草》），该书图文并茂，是中国第一部官修本草，也可算得上世界上第一本药典，对世界中医药发展做出重要贡献。北宋后期，唐慎微编撰《经史证类备急本草》（简称《证类本草》），整理收录了当时各类药物书籍的主要内容，是现存文献学价值最高的本草学著作。北宋末期宋徽宗赵佶编著的《圣济经》中专门设有"药理篇"，是中医药学术著作中最早的药理专论。

Shen Nong's Classic of Materia Medica was written in the Eastern Han dynasty. It is the earliest monograph on Chinese materia medica. It records the clinical application and principle of action of Chinese medicine, and also records the four properties, five flavors, and toxicity of the drugs. In the Northern and Southern dynasties, Tao Hongjing compiled the Collective Commentaries on Classics of Materia Medica on the basis of the Shen Nong's Classic of Materia Medica, which supplemented the property and functional indications of medicines, and at the same time listed the origin, harvest time and processing methods of the medicines. The term "pharmacology" also first appeared in the Collective Commentaries on Classics of Materia Medica. In 659 AD in Tang dynasty, Su Jing and 23 other experts compiled the Tang Materia Medica (also known as Xin Xiu Materia Medica). The book is well illustrated with both description and pictures. It is the first official compendium of Chinese herbal medicine and the first pharmacopoeia in the world, making important contributions to the development of Chinese medicine. In the later period of the Northern Song dynasty, Tang Shenwei compiled the Materia Medica Arranged According to Pattern, which collected the main contents of various medicine books at that time, and was the most valuable medicinal classic book in existence. In the late Northern Song dynasty, Emperor Zhao Ji's Classic of Holy Benevolence specially set up "pharmacology" chapter, which is the earliest monograph on pharmacology in Chinese medicine academic works.

金元时期医药学家的主要工作是搜寻各种药物品种并对其基源进行考证，收集各种方药资料进行整理汇集。在此基础上，利用阴阳五行、气血运行等理论，以药物的形、色、气、味、体等元素，补充中药归经、升降浮沉等药性理论，使中医药理论进一步丰富和完善。

The main contribution of the pharmacists in the Jin and Yuan dynasties was to search for various Chinese materia medica and verify their origins and species, collect various prescription recipes. Also during this period, the Chinse medicinal theory has been greatly enriched and improved. For example, based on the features of the medicine, such as shape, color, smell, taste, and texture, the theory of the five elements, Yin and Yang, and the qi and blood, were used to supplement the medicinal properties of Chinese materia medica including meridian, descending and ascending, etc.

明清时期最有代表性的中药专著是李时珍编写的《本草纲目》，全书共 52 卷，收录中药 1892 种。书中零星出现药理学思想的雏形，例如，在中药"淫羊藿"项下，引用陶弘景的描述"西川北部有淫羊，一日百遍合，盖食此藿所致"。至今淫羊藿作为补肾阳中药常被用于临床治疗性功能障碍。这些描述蕴含药理学思想，对于指导中药药理学研究具有重要意义。

The most representative of the Ming and Qing dynasties is the Compendium of Materia Medica written by Li Shizhen. The book consists of 52 volumes and contains 1892 kinds of Chinese medicine. The prototype of pharmacological thoughts occasionally appeared in the book. For example, regarding the description of a Chinese medicine Yín yáng huò, the author Li Shizhen quoted Tao Hongjing's words, "In the north of this valley, there are some sheep who have strong sexual ability and can mate hundreds of times a day because of the reason for taking this medicine". Until today, Yín yáng huò is often used as a traditional Chinese medicine for the treatment of sexual dysfunction. All these descriptions contain pharmacological ideas, which are of great significance for guiding the research of Chinese medicinal pharmacology today.

中国古代医药学家，既研究中药的功效，也思考和探究其中的机理，这其中就有现代药理学研究的思想萌芽。例如，春秋时期《国语》中就有关于用犬测试乌头毒性的描述；东汉王充编著的《论衡》中阐述了密闭环境对机体的影响；唐代陈藏器编著的《本草拾遗》记载了用黍米、糯米饲养动物，使动物足部出现屈伸障碍的现象；宋代寇宗奭编著的《本草衍义》记载，给骨折的大雁喂服自然铜，可以使骨折康复；宋代苏颂《本草图经》记载，采用临床观察的方法，鉴别人参真假；明代冯梦龙编著的《智囊全集》记载用动物实验来验证荆花的毒性。从这些记载中不难看出，在很早的时候，人们就开始进行药物作用和毒性研究的尝试，有些研究采用动物实验，有些研究采用临床观察，有些研究中甚至已经出现了现代药理学动物模型的概念。这些探索为今天的药理学发展奠定了重要的基础。

Ancient Chinese medical scientists not only studied the efficacy of traditional Chinese medicine, but also explored the underlying rationales for its action. Among them, the idea of modern pharmacology research was sprouting. For example, there is a description of using dogs to test the toxicity of aconite in the book of *Guoyu*; The influence of confined environment on the body appeared in the book *Lunheng* by Wang Chong in the Eastern Han dynasty; The *Supplement to Materia Medica* edited by Chen Zangqi of the Tang dynasty recorded the use of millet and glutinous rice to raise animals, which caused animals foot dysflexion; *Amplification on Materia Medica* by Kou Zongshi in the Song dynasty records that feeding natural copper to the fractured geese can recover the fracture; The Song dynasty Su Song's *The Sketch of Materia Medica* records that clinical observation is used to identify the authenticity of ginseng; The *Complete Works of Think Tank* edited by Feng Menglong in the Ming dynasty records the use of animal experiments to verify the toxicity of the flower from Cercis chinensis. It is not difficult to see from these records that at early times, people began to conduct drug effects and toxicity studies, some studies used animal experiments, some studies used clinical observation, and even some studies have come up with animal model concept. Obviously, these explorations have laid an important foundation for the development of pharmacology today.

二、现代发展
2. Modern development

中药药理学的现代发展可以分为 3 个时期：20 世纪 20 年代起步，20 世纪 50 年代发展，20 世纪 90 年代以后进入高潮期。

The modern development of Chinese medicinal pharmacology can be divided into three periods, which can be summarized as the beginning in the 1920s, the development in the 1950s, and the climax in the 1990s.

20 世纪 20 年代前，国内对中药药理作用的研究较少。随着西方医药体系的引入，药学家开始采用西医理论、技术和方法开展对中药的作用、作用机制及产生作用的物质基础的研究，即用现代药理学方法来研究中药的药效。随着现代药学各学科的建立和发展，逐步开展了对中药的生药学、化学和药理学的研究，使中药从本草走向了与现代药学相结合的新阶段。我国学者袁淑范，比较研究了何首乌浸膏与何首乌蒽醌衍生物对动物肠管运动的影响，认为何首乌在机体中发挥药理作用的部分原因是何首乌中含有蒽醌类衍生物，这是现代最早的中药药理学实验。后续，以陈克恢教授对麻黄素的提取和药理学研究为先导，国内学者相继对川芎、人参、当归、延胡索、黄连、黄柏、柴胡、乌头、蟾酥、仙鹤草、防己、贝母、使君子、常山、鸦胆子等数十种常用中药进行了化学和药理研究，并逐渐形成了一种延续至今的中药药理研究思路，即从天然药材中提取其化学成分，筛选研究其药效，再进行相关药理毒理研究。有些研究成果如麻黄、当归等化学成分和药理作用的研究论文发表后，在世界范围内产生了巨大的反响，从此揭开了中药药理研究的新篇章。在 20 世纪二三十年代共对 50 多味中药的药理作用及化学成分进行了研究。在这一时期，中药药理研究主要集中在对单味药的初步研究。

Before the 1920s, there were few studies on the pharmacological effects of Chinese medicine in China. With the introduction of western medicine system, scientists began to use western medicine theories, technologies and methods to carry out research on the role, mechanism and material basis of the effects of traditional Chinese medicine. With the establishment and development of various disciplines of modern pharmacy, research on pharmacognosy, chemistry and pharmacology of traditional Chinese medicine has been gradually carried out, which has enabled traditional Chinese medicine to switch from a folk medicine to a new stage of modern medicine. Chinese scholar Yuan Shufan has comparatively studied the effects of *Hé shǒu wū* extract and *Hé shǒu wū* anthraquinone derivatives on animal bowel movements, and believes that part of the reason why *Hé shǒu wū* has pharmacological effect on the body is because of anthraquinone derivatives in *Hé shǒu wū*. This is the earliest modern Chinese medicine pharmacology experiment. After the success of professor Chen Kehui's pharmacological research on ephedrine, domestic scholars have successively conducted chemical and pharmacological research on dozens of commonly used traditional Chinese medicines, such as *Chūan xiōng, Rén shēn, Dāng guī, Yán hú suǒ, Huáng lián, Huáng bó, Chái hú, Wū tóu, Chán chú, Xiān hè cǎo, Fáng jǐ, Bèi mǔ, Shǐ jūn zǐ, Cháng shān, Yā dǎn zǐ*. All above gradually formed a research idea of traditional Chinese medicine pharmacology, that is, extracting its chemical components from natural medicinal materials, screening and studying their efficacy related pharmacological and toxicological effects. Some research results such as *Má huáng, Dāng guī* and other chemical constituents and pharmacological effects have been published, which have attracted attentions worldwide, and since then a new chapter in Chinese medicine pharmacology has been opened. In the 1920s and 1930s, a total of more than 50 Chinese medicinal materials were studied for their pharmacological effects and chemical composition. During this period, the pharmacological research of traditional Chinese medicine mainly focused on the preliminary research of individual medicinal material.

新中国成立以后，政府高度重视中医药的研究和发展，要求做好继承、发扬中医中药的工作，中药药理学研究进入了新阶段。在 20 世纪 60 年代，开展了一系列围绕西医相关系统疾病的中药疗效研究，从抗肿瘤、解热、利尿、抗高血压、防治血吸虫病、强心、抗炎、镇痛等方面进行了大量的药物筛选，筛选上千种抗肿瘤、抗菌药物。这段时间还开展了对中药复方的研究，特别是在中药复方防治慢性病、肿瘤等方面做了大量工作，逐步形成了以中医药理论为指导的药理研究。随着中药药理研究不断深入，中药药理学也逐渐发展成为一门既有中药学特色，又具有药理学特色的独特学科，学者们也逐渐着手编写中药药理学教材。1953 年，牟鸿彝编译《国药的药理学》；1954 年，牛颜编著《中药的药理与应用》，张绍昌编著《中药的现代研究》；1978 年，在周金黄教授的指导下，开始了大型专著《中药药理学》的编写，该书首次以中医传统功能分类，对中药药理作用进行了概括和论述。20 世纪 70 年代后期，中药药理学快速发展，此时的中药研究注重以中医药理论为指导，强调辨证论治和整体观念。科学家们采用中医药理论，结合临床研究，逐渐开始中医证候的动物模型探索。在此基础上，开展中药配伍机制、药性理论等药理研究。新技术的引入促使中药药理学的内容不断完善，使研究层次从整体、器官水平提高到了细胞、分子水平，中药药理学体系基本形成。20 世纪 80 年代初，国家中医药管理局正式将中药药理学课程纳入高等教育，标志着中药药理学学科体系已经形成。

Since the establishment of the People's Republic of China, the government has attached great importance to the research and development of traditional Chinese medicine. Chinese medicinal pharmacology has entered a new stage. In the 1950s and 1960s, a series of in-depth studies on the pharmacological effects of traditional Chinese medicine were carried out. More than thousands of Chinese medicine were investigated for the activities of anti-tumor, antipyretic, diuretic, anti-hypertensive, schistosomiasis prevention, cardiotonic, anti-inflammatory, and analgesic. In addition, during this period, research on traditional Chinese medicine formulas has been carried out, and pharmacological research guided by the traditional Chinese medicine theory gradually has been established. With the continuous research development, Chinese medicinal pharmacology has gradually developed into a unique discipline with both Chinese materia medica characteristics and pharmacological characteristics, and scholars have gradually begun to compile teaching materials and books of Chinese medicinal pharmacology. In 1953, Mou Hongyi compiled *Chinese Medicinal Pharmacology*; in 1954, Niu Yan edited *Pharmacology and Application of Traditional Chinese Medicine*; Zhang Shaochang edited *Modern Research on Traditional Chinese Medicine*. In 1978, under the guidance of Professor Zhou Jinhuang, his team began to compile a large-scale monograph, *Traditional Chinese Medicine Pharmacology*, which for the first time summarized and discussed the pharmacological effects of traditional Chinese medicine according to their traditional Chinese medicine function. In the late 1970s, traditional Chinese medicine research focused on the instruction of traditional Chinese medicine theory, emphasizing the Chinese medicine syndrome differentiation and holistic concept. Scientists have adopted traditional medicine theory and combined with clinical research to gradually begin exploring animal models of syndromes. By using the syndrome models, the scientific foundations of Chinese medicine property theory were also investigated. The introduction of new technologies promoted the continuous improvement of Chinese medicinal pharmacology research from the system and organ levels to the cellular and molecular levels, and the Chinese medicinal pharmacology system was basically formed. In the early 1980s, the State Administration of Traditional Chinese Medicine formally incorporated the course of Chinese medicine pharmacology into higher education, marking the formation of the discipline of Chinese medicinal pharmacology.

1985 年随着《中华人民共和国药品管理法》及《新药审批办法》的颁布，中药药理研究进入了新阶段，从纯理论研究转向新药创制。20 世纪末中药药理研究以中药有效部位、有效单体为主要研究对象，采用血清药理学、动物模型、现代分子生物技术等方法，开展中药代谢动力学、中药安全性评价等研究，研究层次从整体深入到组织器官和分子乃至基因层面。中药的药理作用，特别是中药复方的药理作用，其多层次、多靶点的特点，也逐渐被大家认识。

With the promulgation of the *Drug Administration Law of the People's Republic of China* and the *Measures for the Administration of Drug Registration* in 1985, the research of Chinese medicine pharmacology welcomed a booming period, shifting from pure theoretical research to new drug development. At the end of the 20th century, the research of traditional Chinese medicine pharmacology focused on the active fractions and active compound. By using many pharmacological approaches, such as animal models, serum pharmacology, molecular biology, and other methods, the pharmacokinetic and safety are all investigated and evaluated. The Chinese medicinal pharmacological research level during this period has also gradually evolved from the system level to the cellular level, molecular level, and genetic level. The multi-level and multi-target pharmacological effects of traditional Chinese medicine, especially Chinese herbal formulas, are gradually recognized and accepted.

中药药理学是一门新兴学科，随着学科的不断发展，它必将为传统中医药知识体系与现代生命科学体系构建起科学的桥梁，也必将为具有上千年历史的中医药学科发展带来更大的生机。

题库

Chinese medicinal pharmacology is an emerging discipline. With the continuous development of this discipline, it will surely build a scientific bridge between the traditional Chinese medicine knowledge system and the modern life sciences system. It will also bring greater vitality to the development of the discipline of traditional Chinese medicine.

（徐海波）

第二章 中药药性理论的现代研究

Chapter 2 Scientific research on medicinal property theory of Chinese materia medica

 学习目标 | Objectives

1. **掌握** 中药药性的基本概念；四气的现代研究进展。
2. **了解** 五味的现代研究进展。
1. **Must know** The basic concepts of Chinese medicine's medicinal property; the research advances of four properties.
2. **Desirable to know** Research advances of five flavors.

微课

中药药性是根据机体对药物的反应，对中药作用的基本性质和特征的高度概括。中药药性理论是中药理论的核心，也是中药区别于天然药物、化学药物的重要标志。中药药性的主要内容有四气、五味、归经、升降浮沉和毒性等。近几十年来，学者们围绕中药药性理论开展了一系列的现代科学研究工作，在理论探讨、实验研究、临床应用等方面取得一定的成果，对中药药性理论的发展具有现实意义，为药性理论的深入研究奠定了基础。

The medicinal property of Chinese materia medica is a high-level summary of the basic natures and characteristics of traditional Chinese medicinal materials. All the summaries are based on the body's response to medicine treatment. The medicinal property of Chinese materia medica is the core of traditional Chinese medicine theory, and it is also an important feature of traditional Chinese medicine different from natural medicine and western medicine. The main contents of the medicinal property of Chinese materia medica include four properties, five flavors, channels, ascending and descending, and toxicity. In recent decades, many scholars have carried out a series of scientific studies on the theory of traditional Chinese medicine with certain achievements. The scientific research covers theoretical discussion, experimental research, clinical application, etc. All advance in this area have extended our understanding of traditional Chinese medicine and laid a foundation for the in-depth study of the theory of traditional Chinese medicine.

医药大学堂
WWW.YIYAODXT.COM

第一节 中药四气的现代研究

Section 1 Research advances of four properties

中药的四气包括寒、热、温、凉，可以分为两大类，即寒凉与温热。现代研究主要从中枢神经系统、自主神经系统、内分泌系统、能量代谢等方面探讨四气的本质。

The four properties of Chinese material medica include chill, cold, warm, and heat, which can be divided into two categories, namely cold class and warm class. Scientific research about the four properties mainly focus on central nervous system, autonomic nervous system, endocrine system, basal metabolic rate and other aspects.

一、对中枢神经系统功能的影响

1. Central nervous system function

多数寒凉药对中枢神经系统具有抑制性作用。寒凉药可使大鼠脑内多巴胺 β– 羟化酶活性降低，多巴胺、肾上腺素等神经递质含量下降。相反，多数温热药则对中枢神经系统呈现兴奋性作用，可使大鼠脑内多巴胺 β– 羟化酶活性增强，多巴胺、肾上腺素等神经递质的含量增加，且维持在较高水平。

Most cold medicines have inhibitory effects on the central nervous system. Cold drugs can inhibit the activity of dopamine β-hydroxylase in the rat brain, and reduce the content of dopamine, epinephrine and other neurotransmitters. On the contrary, most of the warm drugs show excitatory effects on the central nervous system. Warm drugs can increase the activity of dopamine β-hydroxylase in the rat brain, increase the content of dopamine and epinephrine, and maintain the excitatory neurotransmitters at a high level.

二、对自主神经系统功能的影响

2. Autonomic nervous system function

多数寒凉药能抑制自主神经系统功能，降低自主神经平衡指数，使交感神经活性、肾上腺皮质功能降低。多数温热药则能增强自主神经功能，升高自主神经平衡指数，提高交感神经活性、增强肾上腺皮质功能。

Most cold medicines can inhibit the function of autonomic nervous system, reduce autonomic balance index (indicating the overall performance of autonomic nervous system), and especially reduce sympathetic nerve activity and adrenal gland function. Most warm medicines can enhance autonomic nerve function, increase autonomic balance index, improve sympathetic nerve activity, and enhance adrenal gland function.

三、对内分泌系统功能与基础代谢率的影响
3. Endocrine system and basal metabolic rate

温热药对内分泌功能具有兴奋作用，而寒凉药具有抑制作用。大鼠长期给予温热药，其甲状腺、卵巢、肾上腺皮质等内分泌系统功能增强，血清及垂体内促甲状腺激素（TSH）、黄体生成素（LH）升高，肾上腺皮质激素含量升高，肾上腺皮质激素的代谢产物17-羟皮质类固醇（17-OHCS）从尿液中排出增加。寒凉药则抑制内分泌系统功能，使大鼠血清及垂体内 TSH 下降，下丘脑促甲状腺激素释放激素（TRH）释放减少，肾上腺皮质激素含量降低，大鼠的动情周期延长。另外，温热药通常使机体的基础代谢率增加，而寒凉药通常使机体的基础代谢率降低。

Most warm medicines have exciting effects on endocrine function, while cold medicines have inhibitory effects. When rats are administered with warm medicine for a long time, their thyroid weight, adrenal cortex weight, ovary weight increase, serum and pituitary thyroid stimulating hormone (TSH) and luteinizing hormone (LH) increase, serum adrenocortical hormone increases, and urine 17-hydroxycorticosteroids (17-OHCS) excretion increases. The cold medicines usually have inhibitory effects on the function of the endocrine system, resulting in TSH decrease both in serum and pituitary, thyrotropin-releasing hormone (TRH) decrease in the hypothalamus, the adrenocortical hormone content decreases, and the estrous cycle prolongs. In addition, warm medicines usually enhance the body's basal metabolism, while cold medicines usually weaken the body's basal metabolism.

综上所述，中药的四气是在长期的临床实践过程中，人们根据药物对机体的影响，即通过观察用药前后人体的变化，总结出来的药物特性。这种总结来源于临床实践，是药物与人体相互作用的结果，对于理解中药、研究中药、安全有效地使用中药具有重要意义。

In summary, the four properties are the natures of Chinese materia medica that the practitioners have summarized according to the influence of medicines on the body. The four properties come from clinical practice and are the result of the interaction between drugs and the human body. It is of great significance for us to understand Chinese medicine, study Chinese medicine, and use Chinese medicine safely and effectively.

第二节　中药五味的现代研究
Section 2　Research advances of five flavors

PPT

中药的五味也是中药的重要特性，是中医临床用药的重要依据。现代研究发现，中药的五味与药物所含的化学成分有一定关联性，每一种药味所对应的中药，其所含有的化学成分有一定的规律性。

The five flavors of traditional Chinese medicine are also important characteristics of traditional Chinese medicine and an important basis for the clinical use of traditional Chinese medicine. Scientific research has found that the five flavors of traditional Chinese medicine have a certain correlation with the chemical ingredients contained in the medicine. Medicines with same flavor often contain similar chemical ingredients.

一、辛味中药
1. The acrid medicines

辛味中药主要含挥发油类成分，其次是生物碱、苷类等成分。挥发油是辛味中药发挥作用的主要物质基础。辛味中药主要见于芳香化湿药、开窍药、温里药、解表药、祛风湿药、理气药。辛味中药主要具有扩张血管、改善微循环、发汗、解热、抗炎、抗病原微生物、调节肠道平滑肌运动等药理作用。

The acrid medicines mainly contain volatile oil, followed by alkaloids, glycosides and other components. Volatile oil is the main active material basis for its function. The acrid medicines are mainly distributed in aromatic dampness resolving medicines, astringent medicines, interior-warming medicines, exterior releasing medicines, wind and dampness dispelling medicines, and Qi-regulating medicines. The acrid medicine shows the pharmacological effects of dilating blood vessels, improving microcirculation, sweating, antipyretic, anti-inflammatory, anti-pathogenic microorganisms, regulating intestinal smooth muscle movement, and so on.

二、甘味中药
2. The sweet medicines

甘味中药多含糖类、苷类、蛋白质、氨基酸、维生素等成分。甘味中药主要见于补虚药、消食药、安神药、利水渗湿药。甘味中药具有增强机体抗病能力、抗菌、解热、降血脂、降血压、降血糖、利尿等作用。

Sweet medicines contain sugars, glycosides, proteins, amino acids, vitamins and other ingredients. Sweet medicines are mainly distributed in tonic medicines, digestive medicines, tranquilizing medicines, and damp-draining medicines. Sweet medicine has the effects of enhancing the body's disease resistance, antibacteria, antipyretics, lowering blood lipid, lowering blood pressure, lowering blood sugar, and diuretic.

三、酸味中药
3. The sour medicines

酸味中药多含有机酸和鞣质。酸味中药主要见于收涩药、止血药。酸味中药主要表现抗病原微生物、凝固、吸附等作用。

Most sour medicines contain organic acids and tannins. They are mainly distributed in astringent medicines and hemostatic medicines. Sour medicine mainly shows anti-pathogenic microorganisms, coagulation, physical adsorption and other effects.

四、苦味中药
4. The bitter medicines

苦味中药多含生物碱、苷类、挥发油、黄酮、鞣质。苦味中药主要见于泻下药、理气药、清热药、活血药、祛风湿药。苦味中药主要有抗炎、抗菌等作用。

Bitter medicines mostly contain alkaloids, glycosides, volatile oils, flavonoids, tannins. Bitter medicines are mainly distributed in purgative medicines, Qi-regulating medicines, heat-clearing medicines, blood invigorating and stasis dissolving medicines, wind and dampness dispelling medicines. Bitter medicines have anti-inflammatory and antibacterial effects.

五、咸味中药
5. The salty medicines

咸味中药主要含无机盐成分。咸味中药主要见于化痰药、温里药。咸味中药具有抗肿瘤、抗炎、抗菌、致泻等药理作用。

Salty medicines mainly contain inorganic salts, and are mainly distributed in phlegm medicines and interior-warming medicines. Salty medicine has anti-tumor, anti-inflammatory, antibacterial, diarrhea and other pharmacological effects.

综上所述，中药的五味不一定是真实的味道，更主要反映的是药物作用的特性。不同的化学成分可能是中药五味的物质基础。

In summary, the five flavors of Chinese materia medica are not necessarily actual tastes, but mainly reflect the characteristics of drugs. Different chemical components are the material basis of the Chinese medicine's acrid, sweet, sour, bitter, and salty flavors.

第三节　中药其他药性的现代研究
Section 3　Research advances on other properties of Chinese materia medica

PPT

中药除了四气、五味，还有归经、升降沉浮、有毒无毒等药性，关于这些药性的研究也有一些发现，主要介绍如下。

In addition to the four properties and five flavors, traditional Chinese medicine also has the properties of channel, ascending and descending, and toxicity. There are also some discoveries about these properties. The main research are as follows.

一、中药的归经与升降沉浮
1. Channel, ascending and descending

中药的归经是药物的作用以及其产生的效应的定向与定位，是药物功效与药理作用的综合体现。现代研究发现，有些中药的归经与其药理作用选择性相关；有些中药的归经与其所含有的主要化学成分在体内的分布靶器官相关；有些中药的归经与其所含的微量元素在体内的富集组织相关。可见，中药的归经实质是中药功效的宏观定向与定位，不同类别、不同功效的中药，其功效定位都有一定的规律性，客观、科学地揭示这种规律性，对于更好地利用中药，具有重要意义。

The channel of traditional Chinese medicine is the orientation and positioning of the role of drugs and the effects they produce. It is a comprehensive manifestation of drug efficacy and pharmacological effects. Scientific research has found that the channel of traditional Chinese medicines is sometimes related with their pharmacological effects selectivity, some are related to their target distribution organ in the body, and also some are related to the enrichment location of the trace elements in the medicines.

从现代科学的角度对中药的升降沉浮认识还比较局限。已有的研究主要集中在挖掘药理作用与升降沉浮特性的内在关系等方面。

At present, our understanding of the ascending and descending of Chinese medicine is still relatively limited, and the relevant research carried out mainly focuses on the correlation of pharmacological effects and the characteristics of ascending and descending.

二、中药的有毒与无毒
2. The "Du" and toxicity

中药的毒性与现代毒理学中药物的毒性，都表达药物可能给机体造成不适甚至伤害的特性。但是中药的毒性还有另一层含义，那就是药物作用的偏性，而这个偏性是很多中药发挥作用的基础。

The "Du" of Chinese materia medica and the toxicity of drugs both indicate the characteristics of a drug that may cause discomfort or even damage to the body. However, the "Du" of Chinese medicine has more broad meanings in addition to toxicity itself. The "Du" in Chinese medicine sometimes indicate the partiality of the action of the drug, and this partiality is the efficacy basis of many traditional Chinese medicines.

题库

（唐民科）

第三章 影响中药药理作用的因素
Chapter 3 Factors that influence the pharmacological effects of Chinese medicine

学习目标 | Objectives

1. **掌握** 影响中药药理作用的药物因素。
2. **熟悉** 影响中药药理作用的机体因素和环境因素。

1. Must know The medicinal factors that influence the pharmacological effects of Chinese medicine.

2. Familiar with The organism factors and environmental factors that influence the pharmacological effects of Chinese medicine.

PPT

第一节 药物因素
Section 1 Medicinal factors

影响中药药理作用的药物因素包括药材的品种、产地、炮制方法、药物剂型与煎煮方法、给药剂量及配伍禁忌等。

The medicinal factors that affect the pharmacological effects of Chinese medicine include species, origin, harvesting and storage, processing methods, pharmaceutical forms and decoction methods, dosages, combination and contraindication.

一、品种
1. Species

中药资源丰富，品种繁多。据统计，现有中药种类约 12 800 种。由于中药来源广泛，同名异物和同物异名的现象十分普遍。另外，某些药物因外观非常相似难于辨识，导致误用，影响药材质量及临床疗效。中药品种混淆现象时有存在，如中药五加皮与香加皮易被混淆，含有抗疟活性成分青蒿素的黄花蒿很容易与没有青蒿素成分的青蒿混淆。石斛有 20 多种植物来源，多为兰科石斛属植物的茎，但也有用同科金石斛属植物。中药大黄包括掌叶大黄和唐古特大黄，二者均含有丰富的结合型蒽醌，该活性成分具有清除肠道的作用；然而，源自华北和天山的非正品大黄中结合型蒽醌含量较低，药理作用较弱。有实验研究表明，正品大黄的半数有效量（ED_{50}）为326~1072mg/kg，而非正品大黄的 ED_{50} 则高于3500mg/kg。由此可见，不同来源、不同品种的中药其化学成分和药理作用存在较大差异。因此，临床用药时准确辨识中药对于疾病治疗至关重要。

Chinese materia medica resources are abundant. According to statistics, there are about 12 800 species in Chinese medicine. It is quite common that one medicinal material has lots of species and several names, and that one nomenclature is incorrectly assigned to different material species. In addition, the appearance of some medicinal plant is very similar, which often leads to misuse in clinical practice. For instance, *Wŭ jiā pí* is usually confused with *Xiāng jiā pí*. *Huáng huā hāo* , which has anti-malaria activity, is easy to be confused with *Qīng hāo*, which doesn't have anti-malaria activity. In the case of *Shí hú*, there are more than twenty species, most of which are from Dendrobium genus of Orchidaceous family, while a few of which go to Flickingeria Hawkes genus. *Dà huáng*, including *Zhǎng yè dà huáng* and *Táng gǔ tè dà huáng*, have rich combined anthraquinones which are biologically active ingredients to clear the intestine. However, non-genuine *Dà huáng* originated from Northern China and Tianshan contain low level of combined anthraquinones, showing weaker pharmacological effects. It is reported that genuine *Dà huáng* has an ED_{50} of 326-1072mg/kg, while it is 3500mg/kg for non-genuine *Dà huáng*. It is obvious that there are large differences in the chemical composition and pharmacological effects of different varieties of traditional Chinese medicine. Therefore, it is very important to use appropriate species for disease treatment.

二、产地
2. Origin

中药产地与其品质密切相关。产地的土壤、天气和环境通过影响药材生长而影响药物质量，使其药理作用发生改变。土壤酸碱度会对中药质量产生尤为重要的影响。为使药物产生最佳疗效，临床常用质量稳定、疗效好的“道地药材”，如甘肃的当归、宁夏的枸杞、四川的黄连和附子、内蒙古的甘草、吉林的人参、山西的黄芪和党参、河南的牛膝和地黄、江苏的苍术、云南的三七等。已有研究表明，道地药材的活性成分含量明显高于非道地药材，中药活性成分的含量及组成的差异可导致药理作用和临床疗效的差异。随着药材需求增加，道地药材的产量已远不能满足临床需要。为此，中药引种栽培成为解决道地药材不足的重要途径。目前认为，在药材生产时应在道地药材的原产地进行种植，以保证药材质量。总之，在使用中药时，必须高度重视药材产地因素。

The origin of Chinese medicine is closely related to the quality of Chinese medicine. The soil, weather and environment at the place of origin affect the growth of the medicinal materials, and then affect the quality of the medicine, which influences its pharmacological effects. The soil pH will have a particularly important impact on the quality of Chinese medicine. In order to make the drug have the best effect, it is often suggested that the authentic medicinal materials should be used clinically, such as *Dāng guī* of Ganshu province, *Gǒu qí* of Ningxia province, *Huáng lián* and *Fù zǐ* of Sichuan province, *Gān cǎo* of Inner Mongolia, *Rén shēn* of Jilin province, *Huáng qí* and *Dǎng shēn* of Shanxi province, *Niú xī* and *Dì huáng* of Henan province, *Cāng zhú* of Jiangsu province, *Sān qī* of Yunnan province, etc. Studies have shown that the content of active ingredients in authentic medicinal herbs is significantly higher than that of inauthentic herbs. Differences in the content and composition of active ingredients in Chinese medicines will lead to differences in pharmacological effects and clinical efficacy. Unfortunately, with the increase in demand for medicinal materials, the output of authentic medicinal materials is far from meeting clinical needs. For this reason, the modern cultivation of Chinese medicine have become an important way to solve the shortage of authentic medicinal materials. It is believed that even for the modern cultivation, the medicinal materials should be arranged to grow in the original place of authentic medicinal materials to ensure the quality of medicinal materials. In short, the origin of the medicine has great influence on its medicinal efficacy.

三、采收和贮存
3. Harvesting and storage

不同药用植物的根、茎、叶、花、果实、种子或全草都有一定的成熟期，由于中药的化学成分在不同生长周期中变化很大，因此，最好在有效成分达到峰值水平时采收中药，以期带来最佳的临床效果。研究表明，在第四季度采收的丹参中活性成分丹参酮 II$_A$ 和丹参酮 I 含量比其他季度高出 2~3 倍。人参皂苷成分在 8 月后含量最高，应在 8~9 月采收人参。薄荷在开花盛期采收者其挥发油含量最高。黄花蒿中的活性成分青蒿素在开花前盛叶期最高，可达到 0.6%，开花后青蒿素含量下降。金银花中具有抗菌作用的有效成分绿原酸在花蕾期的含量较开花期高，因此金银花的最佳采收时期为花蕾期。以全体植株或地上部分入药的草本植物常在枝叶茂盛期采收。以叶为入药部位的药材（如侧柏叶）应在开花至花盛时采收。花类药材应在药材处于花期时采收。以果实入药的药材通常在果实成熟时采收。根或根茎类药材一般在早春或晚秋时采挖；相反，树皮类药材（如厚朴）常在清明至夏至时剥取。为避免中药在长期储存的过程中活性成分含量降低，在储存药物时常选择干燥、通风、避免日光直射的场所。如刺五加在高温、高湿、日光直射的环境下贮存 6 个月，其中的丁香苷几乎消失殆尽，如果将刺五加放在标准环境下，可保存 3 年以上。为避免中药在贮存时发生变质、发霉和虫蛀等现象，中药须贮存在适宜条件下。

The roots, stems, leaves, flowers, fruits, seeds, and whole grass of different medicinal plants have certain maturity periods. Because the chemical composition of Chinese medicines varies greatly in different growth cycles, it is best to harvest Chinese medicines when the active ingredients reach peak levels so as to bring the best clinical results. Studies have shown that the content of tanshinone II$_A$ and tanshinone I in *Dān shēn* collected in the fourth season of a year is 2 to 3 times higher than in other seasons. The content of ginsenoside in *Rén shēn* is highest after August, so *Rén shēn* should be harvested from August to September. The volatile oil content of *Bò he* is highest during flowering. Arteannuin, the active ingredient in *Huáng huā hāo*, rises to the peak level at 0.6% (w/w) before flowering, and the arteannuin decreased afterwards. In contrast, the content of chlorogenic acid, an active ingredient with antibacterial action in *Jīn yín huā*, is higher in the bud, so the best harvest time for *Jīn yín huā* is in the budding stage. Chinese herbs whose whole plants or above ground parts are used for medication are often collected during the lush foliage period. Medicinal materials, such as *Cè bǎi yè* whose leaves are used as pharmaceutical part, should be harvested prior to or during flowering. In general, flower herbs should be picked, in the flowering period. Fruit medicinal herbs are usually harvested when they are ripe. The roots or rhizomes are usually excavated in early spring or late autumn. In contrast, bark medicinal materials, such as *Hòu pò* are often stripped in early summer to midsummer. In order to avoid the decrease of active ingredients in Chinese materia medica during the long-term storage, the place where the medicine is stored is often protected from direct sunlight, and kept in dry and ventilated condition. For example, if *Cì wǔ jiā* is stored under hot, damp, and direct sunlight circumstance for 6 months, then its active ingredients, the syringin, will almost disappear. However, if it is stored in a standard milieu, its shelf life could be more than 3 years. Since most Chinese medicines come from plant, it should be stored under appropriate conditions to avoid deteriorate, mold and worms.

四、中药炮制
4. Processing methods

中药炮制会影响中药的成分，从而影响其药理作用和临床疗效。在临床实践中，使用中药之前，通常需要加工，以减少或降低药物的毒性或副作用、增强疗效、稳定药物质量、改变药物性能与功效。炮制对中药药理作用的影响体现在以下几方面。

Processing has influence on Chinese medicine ingredients, thus affecting pharmacological effects and clinical efficacy. Prior to clinical application, Chinese medicines usually need to be processed to reduce the toxicity or side effect, enhance the efficacy, stabilize the quality, and change the performance and efficacy of the medicine.

（一）降低毒性或副作用
4.1 Reduction of toxicity or side effect

附子中的乌头碱具有心脏毒性，可致心律失常甚至心室纤颤。附子经浸漂、煎煮等炮制过程后，乌头碱成分被破坏，与生品相比炮制品的心脏毒性降低。芍药中所含的安息酸对胃有刺激性作用，将芍药炒制后可降低安息酸含量，减轻对胃的刺激性。在渗漉液灌服小鼠的研究中发现，制品首乌的半数致死量（LD_{50}）比生品高 20 倍以上；在小鼠腹腔注射渗漉液的研究中发现，制首乌的 LD_{50} 比生品高出数十倍。

Aconitine contained in *Fù zǐ* is cardiotoxic and can cause arrhythmia and even fibrillation of the heart. After *Fù zǐ* is processed by dipping, decocting, etc., most of the aconitine is destroyed and the processed products have lower cardiotoxicity than the raw products. The benzoic acid contained in *Sháo yào* has an irritating effect on the stomach, and the content of benzoic acid can be reduced after the *Sháo yào* is parched, and the side effects of *Sháo yào* decreases subsequently. Another example is about *Shǒu wū*. With oral administration to mice, it was found that the LD_{50} of processed *Shǒu wū* was more than 20 times higher than that of raw products. When intraperitoneal injection into mice, it was found that the LD_{50} of processed *Shǒu wū* was dozens of times higher than unprocessed one.

（二）增强疗效和稳定药效
4.2 Enhancement of effectiveness and shelf life extension

中药经炮制后可增强疗效。延胡索中的游离生物碱如延胡索甲素、四氢帕马丁等难溶于水，水煎液溶出量少。醋炒后，游离生物碱与醋酸结合形成易溶于水的醋酸盐，水煎液中生物碱的溶出量增加，镇痛作用增强。许多有效成分为苷类化合物的中药，也含有能分解苷类的酶。若这些中药不加炮制，苷类在酶的作用下将被分解影响药效。如苦杏仁中的苦杏仁苷具有不稳定性，在贮藏时因温度、湿度的影响，易被苦杏仁中的酶分解，含量降低。采取适当的炮制方法，可破坏酶活性，保证药材的质量。

The effects of Chinese medicinal materials can be improved after processing. Free alkaloids in *Yán hú suǒ*, such as corydalis A and corydalis B, are hardly soluble in water and the alkaloids in water decoction is very small. After vinegar frying, free alkaloids and acetic acid are combined to form water-soluble acetate salts. The amount of alkaloids in the decoction increased and the analgesic effect is enhanced. Many Chinese medicinal plant whose active ingredients are glycoside compounds normally also contain enzymes that can decompose glycosides. If these Chinese medicinal materials are not processed, the glycosides will be broken down under the action of enzymes so that the pharmacological affects will be reduced. For example, in a condition with high temperature and humidity, amygdaloside, the active ingredient in *Kǔ xìng rén*, is easily decomposed by *Kǔ xìng rén* contained synaptase. Adopting appropriate processing methods can destroy enzyme activity and ensure the quality and efficacy of medicinal materials.

（三）改变药物性能与功效

4.3 Alteration of property and efficacy

炮制后中药的性能及功效也可能发生改变。如生晒参炮制为红参后，会产生新的化学成分，如人参炔三醇、人参皂苷 Rh$_1$、人参皂苷 Rh$_2$、人参皂苷 Rg$_2$ 和人参皂苷 Rg$_3$ 等，其中，人参皂苷 Rg$_2$ 对癌细胞有抑制作用。

The property and efficacy of Chinese materia medica can be changed after processing. For instance, after the *Shēng shài shēn* is processed into *Hóng shēn*, new chemical components such as panaxytiol, panaxsaponin Rh$_1$, Rh$_2$, Rg$_2$ and Rg$_3$ will be produced. Rg$_2$, as a new ingredient, has an inhibitory effect on cancer cells.

五、中药剂型及煎煮
5. Pharmaceutical forms and boiling methods

中药约有 30 种剂型，包括汤剂、丸剂、片剂、注射剂、胶囊剂、散剂、糊剂、提取物颗粒、控释制剂和缓释剂型等。由于不同的剂型制造工艺和给药方式不同，中药的吸收和血药浓度受到影响，导致药理作用的强度和性质发生变化。例如，口服枳实和青皮的汤剂对血压没有影响，但注射可以使血压升高。

There are about thirty Chinese medicine pharmaceutical forms, including decoctions, pills, tablets, injections, capsules, powders, pastes, extract granules, tinctures, controlled-release preparations and sustained-release dosage forms. Due to different manufacturing processes and different dosage forms, the absorption and blood concentration of the Chinese materia medica are affected, resulting in changes in the strength and properties of pharmacological action. For instance, *Zhǐ shí* and *Qīng pí* decoction have no effect on blood pressure, but it can elevate blood pressure when injected intravenously.

汤剂是指将药物用煎煮或浸泡后去渣取汁的方法制成的液体剂型，是目前应用最广泛的中药剂型。由于煎煮方法与汤剂中有效成分的溶出密切相关，因此中药煎煮时讲究"先煎、后入""文火、武火"。如中药复方中有大黄时应后下，避免煎煮时间过长蒽醌类化合物被分解，泻下作用减弱。大黄煎煮时间越长，鞣质释出越多，泻下作用减弱。通常，含挥发油成分较多的中药、茎叶类中药，需煎煮火力强，时间短；相反，籽实类、矿物类中药，需煎煮火力温和，时间长。

Decoction is the most widely used dosage form at present. The decoction is a liquid dosage form prepared by boiling medicinal materials in water. As the decoction method is closely related to the dissolution of the active ingredients, some Chinese medicine materials may need decocting in advance, while others may need to be put into the decoction sometime later depending on the active ingredients. For instance, *Dà huáng* in Chinese herbal formula is commonly put into the boiling pot a short time before stop boiling to prevent the anthraquinones being decomposed. In addition, the longer the boiling time, the more tannin release from *Dà huáng*, which can lead to a decreased diarrhea effect of *Dà huáng*. In general, Chinese medicines containing abundant volatile oil, such as herbal leaves and stems, should be shortly decocted with strong fire. In contrast, the tonics, minerals and fruits should be boiled with soft fire for longer time.

六、药物配伍和禁忌
6. Combination and contraindication

（一）配伍
6.1　Combination

中药常以配伍形式用于临床，以达到增强疗效、减轻毒性和副作用的目的。中医所说的"七情"配伍，是指单行、相须、相使、相畏、相杀、相恶、相反。①单行：指一味中药单独使用，通常使用针对性较强的药物治疗较单一的病情，疗效显著。②相须：指功效相近的两种药物配伍使用以助长疗效。如石膏可从根本上去火，但作用弱、维持时间短；知母可长期退热，作用强而持久。两者合用，退热作用显著。③相使：指两种功效不同的中药合用时，辅药可提高主药功效。如大黄与黄芩联用时，大黄可提高黄芩清热泻火的功效。④相畏：指两种药物配伍时，一种药物的毒性或副作用能被另一种药物减轻或消除。如生半夏、天南星与生姜配伍时，其毒性可被生姜减轻或消除，即生半夏、天南星畏生姜。⑤相杀：指一种药物能消除另一种药物的毒性或副作用。如生姜能减轻生半夏、天南星的毒性，即生姜杀生半夏和天南星。相畏、相杀是同一配伍关系的正反两种说法。⑥相恶：指两种药物联用后能相互牵制使作用抵消或药效消失。如人参和莱菔子联用时，莱菔子会拮抗人参补气的作用。一般而言，相恶是中药配伍的禁忌。⑦相反：指两种药物配伍使用会产生毒性或副作用。如甘草和甘遂配伍时，甘草中的皂苷会增加甘遂中毒性萜类物质的溶出，使药液毒性增加，即甘草反甘遂。

Chinese materia medica is often used clinically in the form of combination to achieve the purpose of enhancing efficacy and reducing toxic and side effects. Traditionally, herbs are combined in seven different patterns, named "the Seven Features", including single action, synergism, enhancement, counter drive, suppression, antagonism, incompatibility. ①Single action literally means the single use of Chinese medicine. Usually using powerful function medicines to treat simple conditions, and the effect is usually significant. ②Synergism literally means the compatibility of two drugs with similar efficacy to promote the efficacy of each other. Such as *Shí gāo* can eliminates the Fire radically and briefly, but the effect is weak and the duration is short. *Zhī mǔ* can gently diminishes the Heat for a long time, and the effect is strong and long-lasting. When they are in combination, the Fire and Heat are drastically abrogated for a long duration. ③Enhancement literally means that when two Chinese medicines with different function are combined, the adjuvant can improve the efficacy of the primary herb. For instance, *Dà huáng* is used in combination with *Huáng qín*, *Dà huáng* can improve the effectiveness of *Huáng qín* in relieving heat and fire. ④Counter drive literally means when two Chinese medicines are combined, the toxic or side effects of one Chinese medicine can be reduced or eliminated by the other. For instance, the toxic effects of *Bàn xià* and *Tiān nán xīng* are counteracted by *Shēng jiāng*. In other words, *Bàn xià* and *Tiān nán xīng* fears *Shēng jiāng*. ⑤Suppression refers to the Chinese medicine eliminates toxic or side effects of another in the formula. Counter drive and suppression are two different ways of describing the same thing. ⑥Antagonism means one Chinese medicines can neutralize the effects of the other. For instance, *Lái fú*

zǐ antagonizes the ability of *Rén shēn* to tonify Qi, relieve hypoxia and fatigue. Generally, Antagonism should be avoided in Chinese herbal combination. ⑦ Incompatibility means that there will be some toxic and side effects produced when two Chinese medicines combined. For instance, following combination of *Gān cǎo* and *Gān suì* in decoction, the glycyrrhizin of *Gān cǎo* can promote the dissolution of the toxic terpene of *Gān suì*, resulting in undesired toxicity to patients.

临床用药时，为增强药物疗效并降低毒性和副作用，获得最大的药理及临床效果，处方配伍时应充分利用相须、相使配伍，避免相恶、相反配伍。

In clinical use, in order to enhance the efficacy of the Chinese medicines and reduce the toxic and side effects, so as to obtain the maximum pharmacological and clinical responses, it is necessary to utilize the combination of synergism and enhancement in the prescription, to avoid antagonism and incompatibility.

（二）禁忌

6.2 Contraindication

禁忌主要是指药物配伍的不相容和妊娠禁忌。传统意义上，药物组合禁忌是指相恶和相反的组合，但是随着药理学研究进展，现在还包括一些新的研究发现，如鞣质在煎剂中可能会沉淀生物碱，导致功效降低，因此建议不要将含生物碱的中药与含鞣质的中药混合使用，如黄连和黄柏不能与地榆及五倍子联合使用。

The contraindications mainly refer to combinational incompatibility and pregnancy contraindications. Traditionally, combinational incompatibility means the combination of antagonism and incompatibility. However, now it also include some new research findings, such as the alkaloid may be precipitated by tannin in decoction, leading to reduced efficacy of herbs, it is recommended that alkaloid containing herbs should not be combined with tannin rich herbs, such as *Huáng lián* and *Huáng bó*, should not be used with *Dì yú* and *Wǔ bèi zǐ*.

妊娠禁忌指某些中药对胎儿有害，甚至可能导致流产，临床用药时根据药物对孕妇和胎儿的危害程度，将药物分为禁用和慎用两类。禁用药是指毒性高、药性猛的中药，妊娠期间禁用，如川乌、草乌、水蛭、虻虫、三棱、莪术、巴豆、大戟、芫花、麝香、斑蝥等。慎用药包括活血化瘀药如桃仁、温里药如细辛、行气药如沉香等，这些中药在妊娠期间慎用。

Contraindication for pregnancy means some Chinese materia medica are harmful to the fetus and even lead possibly to miscarriage. On the basis of the toxicity of Chinese materia medica, contraindication for pregnancy is classified into two categories involving prohibition and prudence. Prohibition medicines include Chinese materia medica with high toxicity and powerful potency, such as *Chuān wū*, *Cǎo wū*, *Shuǐ zhì*, *Méng chóng*, *Sān léng*, *É zhú*, *Bā dòu*, *Dà jǐ*, *Yuán huā*, *Shè xiāng* and *Bān máo*. These herbs are prohibited for clinical use during pregnancy. Prudent Chinese materia medica include the blood-invigorating and stasis-resolving medicines, such as *Táo rén*, the interior-warming medicines, such as *Xì xīn*, and the Qi-regulating medicines, such as *Chén xiāng*.

用药期间有些食物不宜食用。如服用发汗药时禁食生冷食品，服用调理脾胃药时禁食油腻、辛辣刺激性食物。总之，一般建议用药期间，患者应饮食清淡、营养平衡。

There are some dietary contraindications for pharmaceutical therapeutics. For instance, the raw and cold food and drink should be prohibited when the exterior-releasing herbs are taken. The greasy and spicy food should be banned when the herbs are mediating the functions of spleen and stomach of the patient. In a word, a light diet with balanced nutrition and high energy is generally recommended for the patient taking Chinese herbal medication.

第二节 机体因素
Section 2 Patients factors

PPT

一、生理状况
1. Physiological condition

中药药效受年龄、性别、种族、身体状况和精神状态等机体因素的影响。年龄和种族的差异可能导致个体用药方案的差异。通常来说，正在发育阶段的少儿、肝肾功能减退的老年人应适当减少药量。依据中医用药原则，婴幼儿属稚阳之体，不宜服用强效补阳药物；老年人器官功能低下，不宜服用攻泄驱邪的药物。

The effectiveness of Chinese medicine are influenced by the host factors including age, gender, ethnicity, physical condition and mental state. Differences in age and ethnicity may lead to differences in individual drug-dosage regimens. Generally, the dose to children and the elderly should be reduced appropriately. According to the principle of Chinese medicine, infants and young children are rich in infantile Yang, and it is not suitable to take powerful herbs to tonify Yang. In contrast, the elderly due to reduced biological functions are not suitable to take much herbs draining downwards and dispersing evil Qi.

妊娠、母乳喂养、雌激素水平等因素都会影响女性对药物的敏感度。益母草常用于治疗痛经并促进子宫修复。红花、大戟、麝香等中药可兴奋子宫。莪术、水蛭、姜黄等会影响孕激素水平。芫花、甘遂等药物不仅会损害子宫内膜功能，还会影响胎儿发育。

Factors such as pregnancy, breastfeeding, and estrogen levels can affect female's sensitivity to Chinese medicine. *Yì mǔ cǎo* is often used to treat dysmenorrhea and promote the involution of uterus. *Hóng huā*, *Dà jǐ* and *Shè xiāng* and other Chinese medicine can excite the uterus. *É zhú*, *Shuǐ zhì* and *Jiāng huáng*, etc., can influence progesterone levels. Herbs such as *Yuán huā* and *Gān suì* not only damage endometrial function, but also affect embryo development.

体重、身高、脂肪含量会影响药物进入人体后的分布容积和血药浓度。很多中药含有脂溶性成分，这些脂溶性成分会分布在脂肪组织中，暂时储存并发挥作用，药效缓慢而温和。瘦弱、脂肪含量少的患者用药时药效快、作用时间短。

Weight, height, and the amount of adipose will affect the volume of distribution and blood concentration of the herb after it enters the body. A lot of Chinese materia medica contain liposoluble ingredients. These constituents are distributed in adipose tissue for temporarily storage and later action, and the effects are slow and mild. While patients who are emaciated and have less adipose may show fast and shorter response.

精神状态也是影响药效的另一个重要因素。与悲观患者相比，情绪乐观的患者治疗效果更好。安慰剂是一种不含药物，但可以调节精神状态、增强药效的物质。据报道，安慰剂对某些慢性病，如高血压、头痛、心绞痛等的有效率可在 30% 以上。在对中药新药临床评价时，常采用双盲法和安慰剂对照法排除安慰剂的作用。

Mental state is another vital factor that affects the effectiveness of the Chinese materia medica.

Generally, compared with pessimistic patients, optimistic individuals have better treatment results. The placebo is a substance that does not contain medicines, but can regulate mental state and enhance the consequence of the medicine. It has been reported that placebo has an effective rate of more than 30% for certain chronic diseases such as hypertension, headache, and angina pectoris. In the clinical evaluation of new Chinese medicines, double-blind and placebo-controlled trials are often used to rule out the effect of placebo.

二、病理状态
2. Pathological condition

中药药效常受病理状态的影响。肝肾功能障碍的患者药效作用时间较长，毒性或副作用可能会增加。例如，黄芩和穿心莲可用于退热，但对正常体温没有影响；麻黄汤对发热患者起到发汗作用，而对体温正常者不起作用。此外，与健康人相比，五苓散对肾功能不全的患者利尿作用更明显。

The actions of Chinese medicine is often affected by pathological conditions. Patients with liver and kidney dysfunction have longer pharmacodynamic effects and may increase toxic and side effects. *Huáng qín* and *Chuān xīn lián* can relieve fever, while they have no effect on normal body temperature. *Má Huáng Tāng* exerts the diaphoresis function on the patient with a fever, but it does not on the healthy individual with normal body temperature. Also, *Wǔ Líng Sǎn* is a more powerful diuretic to the hydropic patient with renal dysfunction, in comparison to healthy people.

三、肠道内微生态环境
3. Intestinal microorganisms

机体肠道内寄居多种微生物。肠道菌群与机体保持动态平衡以维持正常的机体功能。多数中药口服后经肠道菌群转化，最终影响中药在体内的吸收和功效。有些药物经肠道菌群中的酶分解转化后，分子质量减小，极性降低，促进吸收，药效增强。例如，甘草中的甘草酸只有经肠道菌群分解为甘草次酸后，才能被机体吸收显示药理活性。大黄和番泻叶中的成分番泻苷本身没有泻下作用，只有经肠道菌群分解为大黄酸蒽酮才能发挥泻下的药理作用。滥用抗生素会引起肠道菌群紊乱，从而导致番泻苷在肠道的转化减少，药物泻下作用减弱。可见，肠道菌群对中药的作用有重要影响。

There are many microorganisms in the intestine of the body. A balanced relationship between the intestinal microorganisms and the body is important to maintain the normal physical function. Most of the Chinese medicines are transformed by the intestinal microorganisms after oral administration, which ultimately affects the absorption and efficacy of Chinese medicines. In general, after the Chinese materia medica transformed by the enzymes in the intestinal microorganisms, the molecular weight and polarity are reduced, it is easier to be absorbed, and the effect is better. For instance, Glycyrrhizic acid in *Gān cǎo* can be absorbed by the body after it is decomposed into glycyrrhetic acid by the intestinal microorganisms to show its pharmacological effectiveness. The ingredient anthraglucosennin in *Dà huáng* does not have a draining downwards effect, and only through decomposition by the intestinal microorganisms into anthraquinone can it play its biologically activity. The alteration of intestinal flora, usually incurred by abuse of antibiotics, may diminish

Chinese herbal transformations and reduce the activity of the medicine. Therefore, intestinal microogranisms have great influence on Chinese medicines.

第三节　环境因素
Section 3　Environmental factors

一、气候因素
1. Weather

气候因素是影响药效的重要因素之一。环境改变尤其是气候变化会导致中药作用出现明显差异。如麻黄在温热环境中，发汗效果更明显。

Weather factors are one of the important factors affecting the efficacy of medicines. Environmental changes, especially weather change, can lead to differences in of Chinese medicine response. Such as *Má Huáng* exerts stronger potency of diaphoresis in damp and hot environment, compared to in standard environment.

二、昼夜节律
2. Circadian rhythm

药物在机体的吸收受昼夜节律变化的影响。例如，采用大鼠观察天麻素的作用，结果显示，20:00 给药时药效强、作用快；8:00 给药时药效差，血药浓度达峰值（T_0）最迟；2:00 给药血药浓度–时间曲线下面积（AUC）最小，生物利用度最低。再如，开展附子、乌头中乌头碱急性毒性研究，结果显示，12:00 给药小鼠死亡率最高，达 66.7%，同剂量 20:00 给药，小鼠死亡率最低，只有 13.3%。

Herbs absorption in the body is affected by changes in circadian rhythm. For example, in the study of the efficacy of gastrodin on rats, it was found that the efficacy of taking medicine at 20:00 was strong and the effect was fast; the action was poor when taken at 8:00, and the blood drug peaked at the latest; The the area under the curve (AUC) is the smallest and the bioavailability is the lowest when given at 2:00. Another case is the study on the acute toxicity of aconitine in *Fù zǐ* and *Chuān wū*. The mortality rate of mice administered at 12:00 was the highest, reaching 66.7%, and the mortality rate of mice at the same dose was the lowest, around 13.3% when administrated at 20:00.

三、医疗环境
3. Medical conditions

医护人员的言行与技能操作、医院设施、用药支出等医疗环境均能影响中药的药理作用及药效。积极的医疗环境无疑有利于患者的预后和康复，因此应为患者营造最佳的医疗环境，以达到最佳的治疗效果。

Other factors such as the talks and attitude of medical staff, the operation of nurse, and medication cost, can all influence the pharmacological effects and efficacy of Chinese medicine. The positive medical environment is undoubtedly conducive to the prognosis and rehabilitation of patients, so it is recommended to create the best medical environment for patients to achieve the best treatment results.

（徐海波）

下篇　各论

Part II　Systematics

第四章　解表药
Chapter 4　Exterior releasing medicines

 学习目标 | Objectives

1.**掌握**　解表药的主要药理作用；麻黄、柴胡与功效相关的药理作用、药效物质基础；麻黄的不良反应。

2.**了解**　桂枝、葛根的主要药理作用和药效物质基础。

1. **Must know**　The main pharmacological effects of exterior releasing medicines; the main pharmacological effects related to the traditional efficacies, mechanisms of action, and key active components of *Má huáng* and *Chái hú*; the adverse effects of *Má huáng*.

2. **Desirable to know**　The main pharmacological effects and key active components of *Guì zhī* and *Gě gēn*.

第一节　概述
Section 1　Overview

PPT

　　凡以发散表邪，解除表证为主要功效的药物称为解表药。本类药多味辛，质轻扬，主入肺、膀胱经，偏行肌表。解表药主要具有发汗的作用，通过发汗发散表邪，解除表证，防止表邪入里，控制疾病的发展。部分解表药还兼有止咳平喘、利水消肿、解肌透疹、祛风除湿等作用，可用于咳喘、水肿、荨麻疹、风疹、风湿痹痛、皮肤瘙痒、外科疮疡等。

　　Chinese materia medica that can remove exterior evil and relieve exterior syndrome are regarded as exterior releasing medicines. Most medicines in this category are pungent in flavor, and enter the meridians of lung and bladder. They mainly induce sweating to remove exterior evil, relieve the exterior syndrome, and then prevent diseases progression. Some of them have efficacies on relieving the tussis and asthma, alleviating edema, diuresis, releasing flesh and promoting eruption, dispelling wind and removing dampness, etc., which can be used for treating cough and asthma, edema, urticaria, rubella, rheumatic arthralgia, skin itching, sore and ulcer, etc.

　　表证是指六淫外邪（外界的各种致病因素）侵犯人体的浅表部位（皮肤、肌肉、经络）引起的证候。恶寒是表证的核心症状，所谓"有一分恶寒，便有一分表证"。中医认为恶寒是外邪郁遏卫阳，卫气不能"温分肉，肥腠理"所致；西医学研究认为恶寒是皮肤血管收缩，皮肤血流量

医药大学堂
WWW.YIYAODXT.COM

减少，肌表温度下降刺激冷觉感受器，信息传入中枢引起。

Exterior syndrome is caused by exterior evil (external pathogenic factors) attack the body surface (skin, muscle, or meridians). Aversion to cold is the key symptom, and also is the most important diagnosis gist of exterior syndrome. Traditional Chinese medicine believes that aversion to cold is caused by external obstruct defensive Yang and defensive Qi can't "warm the muscle, nourish the body". Modern medical science believes that aversion to cold is attributed to excessive cold exposure, which may induce the constriction of skin vessel, reduce the skin blood flow, and further decrease the skin temperature and stimulate the temperature regulating center.

西医学认为表证的产生是机体抵抗力下降，细菌病毒等感染所致，临床可见恶寒（或恶风）、发热、头身痛、关节痛、无汗（或有汗）、鼻塞、咳嗽等证，同时伴有炎症反应。因此，中医学表证与西医学中上呼吸道感染（感冒、流感等）、多种传染病和急性感染性疾病初期的症状表现相似。现代药理研究表明，解表药治疗表证的作用与下列药理作用有关。

From the point of modern medicine, reduced body immune function and pathogenic microbial infection are considered as the major causes of exterior syndrome. The manifestations of exterior syndrome include aversion to cold (or aversion to wind), fever, headache and body pain, joint pain, sweating or absence of sweating, stuffy nose, cough, etc., accompanied by inflammation, which is similar to upper respiratory tract infection (common cold, influenza, etc.) and other infectious diseases at the early stage. The exterior clearing function is related to the following pharmacological effects.

1. **发汗**　《黄帝内经》云"在皮者汗而发之""因其轻而扬之"。汗法是中医治疗表证的重要治法。解表药均有不同程度的发汗作用。一般而言，辛温解表药（如麻黄、桂枝等）的发汗作用强于辛凉解表药（如柴胡、葛根等）。解表药引起的发汗多属温热性发汗，外界温度对其发汗作用有较大的影响。此外，中枢神经系统（CNS）功能亦与发汗密切相关。解表药发汗涉及多个环节，如兴奋汗腺、扩血管和促进血液循环等。

(1) Diaphoresis　*Huangdi's Internal Classic* recorded that "treating superficial syndrome with sweating therapy", and "treating mild disease with dissipating therapy". Diaphoresis (sweating) is the most important therapeutic method for treating exterior syndrome in Chinese medicine. Most exterior releasing medicines exert diaphoretic effect, and the effect of pungent-warm exterior releasing medicines, such as *Má huáng* and *Guì zhī*, is usually stronger than that of pungent-cool exterior releasing medicines, including *Chái hú*, *Gě gēn*, etc. This effect can be affected by environmental temperature that higher environmental temperature is beneficial to sweating. Central nervous system (CNS) function also affects the diaphoretic effect of exterior releasing medicines. The mechanisms underlying this effect may include increasing the sweat gland secretion, promoting vessel dilation, or improving the blood circulation.

2. **解热**　解表药大多有不同程度的解热作用，可使实验性发热动物体温降低，如柴胡、桂枝、荆芥、防风、葛根等，以柴胡的解热作用最为显著。部分药物还能使正常动物的体温下降。一般而言，辛凉解表药的解热作用强于辛温解表药。某些解表药对体温有双向调节作用，不仅能降低发热动物的体温，且能使低体温动物的体温恢复至正常水平，如桂枝。解表药的解热作用具有起效快、维持时间短的特点，与清热药不同。解表药的解热作用除与抑制病理性发热的多个环节有关外，还与发汗和扩张血管促进散热、拮抗炎症反应、抑制病原微生物等作用有关。

(2) Antipyresis　Most of the exterior releasing medicines are capable of reducing the body temperature of fever animals, and exert antipyretic activity, such as *Chái hú*, *Guì zhī*, *Jīng jiè*, *Fáng fēng*, and *Gě gēn*. Among them, *Chái hú* has the strongest antipyretic activity. Some exterior releasing medicines can reduce the normal body temperature of animals. Generally speaking, the antipyretic activity of pungent-cool exterior releasing medicines is more powerful than pungent-warm exterior releasing medicines. Some medicines in this category have the bi-directional thermo-regulation effect, like *Guì zhī*. It not only can downregulate the body temperature in fevered experimental animals, but also have the ability to raise the body temperature of hypothermic animals. The antipyretic effect of exterior releasing medicines is quick and short time,which is different from that of heat-clearing medicines. The underlying mechanisms of antipyresis include promoting diaphoresis and vessel dilation to help heat dissipation, anti-inflammation, anti-pathogenic microorganism, and etc., besides inhibiting the links of pathological fever.

3. 镇痛、镇静 头痛、周身痛和关节痛是表证的常见症状。大多数解表药具有镇痛作用，可以有效缓解临床疼痛症状，对多种动物的实验性疼痛具有镇痛效果，使痛阈提高，如柴胡、桂枝、防风、荆芥、白芷、羌活、细辛等。一般来说，辛温解表药的镇痛作用较辛凉解表药的镇痛作用强。解表药多属于外周性镇痛药，主要通过影响外周致痛物质的合成和释放发挥作用，部分可通过作用于中枢发挥镇痛作用，如细辛。

(3) Analgesia and sedation Headache, body and joint pain are the most common symptoms of exterior syndrome. Many exterior releasing medicines, such as *Chái hú*, *Guì zhī*, *Fáng fēng*, *Jīng jiè*, *Bái zhǐ*, *Qiāng huó*, and *Xì xīn*, can relieve pain and increase pain threshold in experimental animals, which indicate the analgesic effect. Pungent-warm exterior releasing medicines usually show stronger analgesic activity than pungent-cool exterior releasing medicines. The analgesic activity is mainly through the regulation of the synthesis and releasing of algogenic substances in nervous system, with the exception of a few medicines, such as *Xì xīn*, which directly acting on CNS to exert analgesic activity.

外感风寒患者常因表证困扰而烦躁不安。除麻黄外，大部分解表药有一定的镇静作用，能降低小动物自主活动数，或协同巴比妥类药物起催眠作用。

Patients suffering from external wind-cold are usually dysphoria because of exterior syndrome. Except *Má huáng*, most exterior releasing medicines have sedative activity. They can lower the spontaneous motor activity and enhance sedative-hypnotic effect of barbiturates in animal models.

4. 抗炎 呼吸道炎症是表证的常见症状，也是贯穿表证始终的一个基本病理过程。大部分解表药有抗炎作用，对急性炎症作用较为明显，如麻黄、桂枝、柴胡、生姜、辛夷、细辛、羌活等。一般而言，辛凉解表药抗炎作用优于辛温解表药。解表药抗炎机制与兴奋下丘脑-垂体-肾上腺皮质功能、抑制花生四烯酸代谢、抑制炎症介质生成和释放、抑制炎症反应信号通路等有关。

(4) Anti-inflammation Respiratory inflammation is the common symptom of exterior syndrome, and inflammation is the most important pathological process of exterior syndrome. Exterior releasing medicines usually exert prominent anti-inflammatory activity. It is reported that *Má huáng*, *Guì zhī*, and *Chái hú*, *Shēng jiāng*, *Xīn yí*, *Xì xīn*, and *Qiāng huó*, all can inhibit inflammation on several inflammatory animal models, especially on acute inflammation models. The anti-inflammatory activity of pungent-cool exterior releasing medicines is usually stronger than pungent-warm exterior releasing medicines. The underlying mechanisms are probably attributed to stimulating hypothalamus-pituitary-adrenal axis, inhibiting arachidonic acid metabolism, decreased the generation and releasing of inflammatory mediators, and attenuating some inflammatory signaling pathways.

5. 抗病原微生物 表证是外邪客表所致，细菌、病毒等均可视为外邪。体内、外试验表明大多数解表药有一定的抗菌、抗病毒作用，部分药物体外虽无明确的抗病原微生物作用，但体内却有一定的拮抗效应，这可能与诱导内源性抗病原微生物物质生成有关，如诱导内源性干扰素生成。

(5) Anti-pathogenic microorganism　Pathogenic microbial infection is one of the main disease causes of exterior syndrome. Most exterior releasing medicines have anti-bacterial or anti-virus activities in *in vivo* and *in vitro* experiment models. Some medicines have anti-infective activity *in vivo* although they have no specific anti-pathogenic microorganisms *in vitro*, which may be related to inducing the production of endogenous substances with anti-pathogenic microorganisms, such as endogenous interferon.

6. 影响免疫功能　大多数解表药具有增强机体免疫功能或促进内毒素抗体生成作用，部分药物还有一定的免疫抑制作用，为其临床治疗过敏性疾病提供了药理学基础。

(6) Regulating immune system　Most exterior releasing medicines can enhance the immune system function or stimulate the production of endotoxin antibodies, and some medicines have the immunosuppressive action.

常用解表药的主要药理作用见表 4-1。

The main pharmacological effects of commonly used exterior releasing medicines are summarized in Table 4-1.

表 4-1　常用解表药的主要药理作用

类别	药物	发汗	解热	抗菌	抗病毒	镇痛	镇静	抗炎	抗过敏	其他
辛温解表药	麻黄	+	+	+	+	+	−	+	+	平喘、利尿、升血压、兴奋中枢、镇咳、祛痰、降血糖
	桂枝	+	+	+	+	+	+	+	+	利尿、强心、扩血管、利胆、抗肿瘤
	细辛	−	+	+	+	+	+	+	−	平喘、祛痰、强心、升血压、抗衰老
	生姜	+	+	+	+	+	−	+	+	镇吐、促消化液分泌、抗溃疡、抗氧化、抗肿瘤、降血脂
	荆芥	−	+	+	+	+	+	+	+	止血、抗氧化、平喘、抗肿瘤
	防风	−	+	+	+	−	−	+	+	促进免疫功能、抗凝血、抗肿瘤
	紫苏	−	+	+	+	+	+	+	+	镇咳、祛痰、平喘、止血、降血脂、抗氧化
	白芷	−	+	+	−	+	−	−	+	光敏作用、抗肿瘤
	苍耳子	−	+	+	+	−	−	−	+	细胞毒作用
辛凉解表药	柴胡	−	+	+	+	+	+	+	+	保肝、利胆、降血脂、抗抑郁、抗肿瘤、抗溃疡
	葛根	−	+	−	−	−	−	−	−	抗心肌缺血、改善微循环、抗心律失常、改善血液流变学、抗血栓、降血压、降血脂、降血糖、抗肿瘤
	薄荷	+	+	+	+	−	+	−	−	保肝、利胆、溶石排石、抗氧化
	桑叶	−	+	+	+	+	−	−	−	镇咳、祛痰
	菊花	−	+	+	+	−	−	+	−	降血压、降血脂、抗氧化、抗肿瘤
	牛蒡子	−	+	+	+	−	−	−	−	降压
	升麻	−	+	+	+	+	−	+	+	抗肿瘤、抗骨质疏松

注："+"表示有明确作用；"−"表示无作用，或未查阅到相关研究文献

第二节　常用药物

Section 2　Commonly used medicines

PPT

| 麻黄 | *Má huáng*（Herba Ephedrae） |

【来源 / Origin】

本品为麻黄科植物草麻黄（*Ephedra sinica* Stapf.）、中麻黄（*Ephedra intermedia* Schrenk et C. A. Mey.）或木贼麻黄（*Ephedra equisetina* Bge.）的干燥草质茎。主要分布于东北、西北、华北地区。秋季采收，草质茎晒干生用、蜜炙或捣绒用。

Má huáng is the dried herbaceous stem of *Ephedra sinica* Stapf., *Ephedra intermedia* Schrenk et C. A. Mey. or *Ephedra equisetina* Bge., family of *Ephedraceae*. The plant is widely cultivated in northeast, northwest, and north China. In autumn, the herbaceous stem is harvested and sun-dried. Crude *Má huáng*, honey-fried *Má huáng*, or *Má huáng* that pound to a floss are usually used as Chinese medicine.

【化学成分 / Chemical ingredients】

主要含生物碱和挥发油。生物碱多为苯丙胺类生物碱，其中主要有效成分为左旋麻黄碱（*L*-ephedrine），占生物碱总量的80%~85%，以及右旋伪麻黄碱（*D*-pseudoephedrine）、去甲基麻黄碱（nor-ephedrine）、去甲基伪麻黄碱（nor-pseudoephedrine）、左旋甲基麻黄碱（*L*-methyl-ephedrine）、右旋甲基伪麻黄碱（*D*-methyl-pseudoephedrine）。挥发油中含2,3,5,6–四甲基吡嗪（2,3,5,6-tetramethylpyrazine）、*L*-α–萜品烯醇（*L*-α-terpineol）等。此外尚含有鞣质、黄酮、多糖、有机酸等成分。

Má huáng mainly contains alkaloids and volatile oils. Alkaloids are the key active components, the content of amphetamines alkaloids ranks top among all the alkaloids, including about 80% to 85% *L*-ephedrine, *D*-pseudoephedrine, nor-ephedrine, nor-pseudoephedrine, *L*-methyl-ephedrine, *D*-methyl-pseudoephedrine, and etc. Volatile oils of *Má huáng* consist of *L*-α-terpineol, 2,3,5,6-tetramethylpyrazine, and so on. Besides, *Má huáng* also contains tannin, flavonoids, polysaccharide, organic acid, etc.

【药性与功效 / Chinese medicine properties】

味辛、微苦，性温，归肺、膀胱经。具有发汗解表、宣肺平喘、利水消肿的功效。用于治疗风寒感冒、胸闷喘咳、风水水肿等证。

In Chinese medicine theory, *Má huáng* is pungent, slightly bitter in flavor, and warm in nature, and it can enter the meridians tropism of lung and bladder. *Má huáng* can induce sweating and release exterior, ventilate lung and relieve dyspnea, alleviate edema and promote diuresis. Clinically it can be used for common cold, chest oppression, cough, asthma, and wind edema.

【药理作用 / Pharmacological effects】

1. 发汗　麻黄发汗作用明显，但不同炮制品、不同活性成分发汗作用强度不同。生品麻黄的发汗作用强于蜜炙麻黄和清炒麻黄，麻黄挥发油、左旋甲基麻黄碱发汗作用较强。此外，环境温度升高增加麻黄的发汗作用，而机体在麻醉状态下麻黄的发汗作用明显减弱，提示外界环境温度以及中枢神经系统功能状态对麻黄的发汗作用也有影响。麻黄发汗机制与兴奋体温调节中枢、增强散热，兴奋外周 α 受体，抑制汗腺导管对钠离子的重吸收、增加汗液分泌有关。麻黄挥发油是其发汗的主要物质基础。

(1) Diaphoresis *Má huáng* has significant diaphoretic effect. Different processed products and ingredients exhibit different intensity of diaphoretic effect. Crude *Má huáng* has better diaphoretic effect than honey-fried and plain stir-fried products. The diaphoretic effect of volatile oils and *L*-methylephedrine is stronger. The diaphoretic effect of *Má huáng* is stronger when used in warm environment, and significantly impaired in anesthetic conditions, which indicate that environmental temperature and CNS function also impact this effect. The underlying mechanisms can be attributed to stimulating thermoregulator center and promoting heat dissipation, exciting α receptor, preventing the reabsorption of sodium ions by sweat ducts and increasing sweat gland secretion. Volatile oils are suggested to be the main active ingredients for diaphoresis.

2. 平喘　麻黄、麻黄挥发油、麻黄碱、伪麻黄碱均有平喘作用。近年来又从草麻黄中分离出两种新的平喘成分：2,3,5,6- 四甲基吡嗪及 *L*-α- 萜品烯醇。蜜炙麻黄平喘作用最强，其次是生品麻黄，清炒麻黄作用最弱。麻黄碱平喘作用机制如下。①麻黄碱化学结构与肾上腺素相似，可以直接兴奋 $β_2$ 和 $α_1$ 肾上腺素受体。兴奋支气管平滑肌上的 $β_2$ 受体，可松弛支气管平滑肌；兴奋肥大细胞上的 $β_2$ 受体，可阻止过敏介质，如组胺（His）、5- 羟色胺（5-HT）、白三烯（LTs）等的释放；兴奋支气管黏膜血管平滑肌上的 $α_1$ 受体，使末梢血管收缩，减轻支气管黏膜肿胀。②促进肾上腺素能神经和肾上腺髓质嗜铬细胞释放去甲肾上腺素和肾上腺素，从而间接发挥拟肾上腺素作用。③促进肺部前列腺素 E（PGE）的释放，直接活化腺苷酸环化酶或抑制该酶的分解，使细胞内环磷酸腺苷（cAMP）含量增加而起到松弛支气管平滑肌的作用。④抑制抗体的产生。⑤抑制炎症介质的生成和释放。麻黄碱性质稳定，其平喘作用与肾上腺素相比显效较慢，作用温和、持久，且可口服。

(2) Relieving asthma *Má huáng* and its active components such as ephedrine, pseudoephedrine and volatile oils can relieve asthma. 2,3,5,6-tetramethylpyrazine and *L*-α-terpilenol from *Ephedra sinica* Stapf. are the new components which have anti-asthmatic action. The anti-asthmatic effect for different processed *Má huáng* is different, the best is honey-fried *Má huáng*, and then is crude and plain stir-fried products respectively. The mechanisms of relieving asthma by ephedrine are as follows. ①Ephedrine and adrenaline (Adr) are similar in chemical structure, so ephedrine can excite $β_2$ adrenoceptor and $α_1$ adrenoceptor directly. Activation of $β_2$ adrenoceptor results in the relaxation of bronchial smooth muscle, and prevent the release of allergic media from mast cells, including histamine (His), 5-hydroxytryptamine (5-HT), leukotrienes (LTs), etc. Activation of $α_1$ adrenoceptor causes the constriction of peripheral vessel and relieves the swollen of bronchial mucosa. ②Ephedrine induces the secretion of noradrenaline and adrenaline from adrenergic nerve and adrenal medullary chromaffin cells. ③Ephedrine stimulates the secretion of lung prostaglandin E (PGE), directly activates the adenylate cyclase or inhibits the degradation of the adenylate cyclase to increase the contents of cyclic adenosine monophosphate (cAMP), and finally relaxes bronchial smooth muscle. ④Ephedrine inhibits the production of antibodies. ⑤Ephedrine suppresses the expression and release of inflammatory mediators. Ephedrine has stable chemical properties, and its anti-asthmatic effect is slow, moderate, lasting and orally-available compared with Adr.

3. 利尿　麻黄利水消肿的功效与其利尿作用有关，以右旋伪麻黄碱的利尿作用最显著。利尿作用机制与其扩张肾血管使肾血流增加和阻碍肾小管对钠离子的重吸收有关。

(3) Promoting diuresis The effect of *Má huáng* on eliminating edema is related to its diuretic effect, *D*-pseudoephedrine has the most significant diuretic effect. The mechanism may be related to

33

increasing renal blood flow by dilating renal vessels, and inhibiting reabsorption of sodium ion by nephric tubule.

4. 抗病原微生物　麻黄挥发油对金黄色葡萄球菌、甲型和乙型溶血链球菌、流感嗜血杆菌、肺炎链球菌、炭疽杆菌、白喉棒状杆菌、大肠埃希菌、奈瑟菌等均有不同程度的体外抑制作用。麻黄挥发油对甲型流感病毒 PR_8 株感染的小鼠有治疗作用。

(4) Anti-pathogenic microorganism　*Má huáng* volatile oils have certain inhibitory effects on *Staphylococcus aureus*, *Hemolytic streptococcal* A and B, *Haemophilus influenzae*, *Diplococcus pneumoniae*, *Bacillus anthracis*, *Corynebacterium diphtheriae*, *Escherichia coli* and *Neisser's diplococcus* in different degrees *in vitro*. The volatile oils of *Má huáng* can be used to treat mouse infection caused by influenza A virus PR_8 strain.

5. 抗炎　麻黄水提物、醇提物对多种炎症动物模型都表现出抗炎作用，可以抑制炎症早期水肿和后期肉芽组织生成。伪麻黄碱的抗炎作用最强，甲基麻黄碱、麻黄碱次之。麻黄碱的抗炎作用与其抑制花生四烯酸的释放和代谢有关。

(5) Anti-inflammation　Both aqueous and ethanol extracts of *Má huáng* can inhibit inflammation in various inflammatory models, including inhibit the edema at the early stage of inflammation and depress the granuloma formation at the late stage of inflammation. Pseudoephedrine has the strongest anti-inflammatory effect, followed by methyl-ephedrine and ephedrine. The mechanism is associated with inhibition on the secretion and metabolism of arachidonic acid.

6. 强心、升高血压　麻黄碱有拟肾上腺素样作用，可直接兴奋心肌 β_1 受体和血管平滑肌 α_1 受体而呈现正性肌力、正性频率作用，并能使血管收缩，外周阻力增加而使血压升高。其升压特点是作用缓慢、温和、持久，反复应用易产生快速耐受性。

(6) Cardiotonic action and elevating blood pressure　Ephedrine has adrenergic activity. It can activate β_1 adrenoceptor of heart and α_1 adrenoceptor on vascular smooth muscle, which causes positive inotropic and positive frequency effect, constricted blood vessels, increased peripheral resistance, resulting in a slow, moderate, and lasting blood pressure elevation. The tolerance may occur if ephedrine is repeatedly used within a short period.

7. 兴奋中枢　麻黄碱脂溶性强，易通过血脑屏障（BBB）。治疗剂量麻黄碱能兴奋大脑皮质和皮质下中枢，引起精神兴奋、失眠等症状，亦能兴奋中脑、延髓呼吸中枢和血管运动中枢。

(7) Stimulating CNS　Ephedrine is highly lipid soluble and readily penetrates the Blood-Brain-Barrier (BBB). At therapeutic dosage, ephedrine may stimulate cerebral cortex and subcortical center to cause mental excitement and insomnia. It can also excite mesencephalon, medullary respiratory center and vasomotor center.

8. 其他作用　麻黄还有解热、镇痛、抗过敏、镇咳、化痰等作用。

(8) Other effects　*Má huáng* also has the effects on antipyresis, analgesic, antianaphylaxis, resolving phlegm, and relieving cough.

【不良反应 / Adverse effects 】

人口服过量麻黄碱可引起中毒，出现头晕、耳鸣、烦躁不安、心悸、血压升高、瞳孔散大、排尿困难等症状，甚至出现心肌梗死、心律失常或死亡，亦有引起肝损害的报告。

Orally administrated with overdose of ephedrine may cause poisoning, such as dizziness, tinnitus dysphoria, palpitations, hypertension, mydriasis, dysuria, and even myocardial infarction, arrhythmia, or death. It has also been reported that irrational use of ephedrine induced liver injury in clinical.

桂枝 ┆ *Guì zhī* (Ramulus Cinnamomi)

【来源 / Origin】

本品是樟科植物肉桂（*Cinnamomun cassia* Presl.）的干燥嫩枝。主产于广东、广西及云南等地。春、夏二季采收，除去叶，晒干，生用。

Guì zhī is the dried twigs of *Cinnamomun cassia* Presl., which is widely cultivated in Guangxi, Guangdong, and Yunnan province in China. In summer and autumn, the branchlet is harvested and sun-dried for the use of Chinese medicine.

【化学成分 / Chemical ingredients】

有效成分为挥发油，含量为 0.43%~1.35%。挥发油中主要成分是桂皮醛（cinnamaldehyde），其含量为 62.29%~78.75%；另有桂皮酸（cinnamic acid）及少量乙酸桂皮酯（cinnamyl acetate）、乙酸苯丙酯（phenylpropy acetate）、桂皮醇（cinnamyl alcohol）等。此外，尚含有香豆素（coumarin）、原儿茶酸（protocatechuic acid）等。

Guì zhī contains about 0.43% to 1.35% volatile oil, and cinnamaldehyde (about 62.29% to 78.75%) is the most abundant volatile oil in *Guì zhī*. Besides, *Guì zhī* also contains cinnamic acid, cinnamyl acetate, phenylpropy acetate, cinnamyl alcohol, coumarin and protocatechuic acid, etc.

【药性与功效 / Chinese medicine properties】

味辛、甘，性温，归心、肺、膀胱经。具有发汗解肌、温通经脉、助阳化气、平冲降气的功效。主治风寒感冒、脘腹冷痛、血寒经闭、关节痹痛、痰饮、水肿、心悸。

In Chinese medicine theory, *Guì zhī* has the nature of pungent, sweet, and warm, and it can enter the meridian of heart, lung, and bladder. *Guì zhī* can induce sweating, release flesh, warm and activate meridians, assist yang to transform Qi, and descend adverse-rising Qi. Clinically it can be used for treating common cold, abdominal cold-pain blood cold and amenorrhea, arthralgia, phlegm, fluid retention, edema and palpitations.

【药理作用 / Pharmacological effects】

1. **发汗**　桂枝单用发汗力弱，若与麻黄配伍，则发汗力增强。桂枝发汗作用与桂皮油扩张血管，改善血液循环，促使血液流向体表有关。

(1) Diaphoresis　The diaphoretic activity of *Guì zhī* is not strong. However, when combined with *Má huáng*, the diaphoretic effect can be improved remarkably. The underlying mechanisms are attributed to promoting vessel dilation, improving the blood circulation, and increasing blood flow to body surface.

2. **解热、镇痛**　桂枝对体温有双向调节作用。桂枝水煎剂及其有效成分桂皮醛、桂皮酸可使伤寒杆菌、副伤寒杆菌菌苗致热的家兔体温降低，能使正常小鼠的体温和皮肤温度下降；水煎液对酵母所致发热大鼠亦有解热作用，但对安痛定所致低体温大鼠有升温作用。其解热作用可能与扩张皮肤血管，促进发汗使散热增加有关。桂枝水煎剂、醇提液、挥发油或桂皮醛对小鼠热刺激、醋酸致痛均有抑制作用。

(2) Antipyresis and analgesia　*Guì zhī* have the bi-directional thermo-regulation effect. *Guì zhī* decoction, cinnamaldehyde and cinnamic acid show anti-pyretic effect in experimental pyretic animal models caused by typhoid vaccine, and paratlyphoid vaccine, or yeast solution. They also can lower the body and skin temperature of healthy animals. *Guì zhī* also can raise the body temperature of hypothermic animals that caused by antondine injection, indicating its bi-directional thermo-regulation effect. The mechanisms can be attributed to dilating skin blood vessel, promoting diaphoresis, and dissipating heat. *Guì zhī* decoction, ethanol extract, volatile oil and cinnamaldehyde can relieve pain caused by thermal stimulation or acetic acid in mice.

3. 抗炎、抗过敏　桂枝挥发油对急慢性及免疫性炎症均有效，能明显抑制二甲苯引起的小鼠耳郭肿胀；减轻角叉菜胶引起的大鼠足趾肿胀；减少醋酸引起的小鼠腹腔伊文思蓝染料渗出；抑制小鼠棉球肉芽肿；抑制脂多糖（LPS）引起的大鼠血液中白细胞数目增加和炎症细胞聚集；对大鼠佐剂型关节炎也有抑制作用。桂枝还能抑制 IgE 所致的肥大细胞脱颗粒及释放介质，抑制补体活性，表现为抗过敏作用。

(3) Anti-inflammation and anti-anaphylaxis　*Guì zhī* volatile oil can inhibit acute, chronic, and immune inflammation. Experiments show the volatile oils from *Guì zhī* alleviate ear swelling in mice and foot swelling in rats induced by dimethylbenzene and carrageenan respectively. Volatile oils also inhibit the acetic acid induced abdominal vascular hyper-permeability and inhibit cotton ball granuloma in mice. In lipopolysaccharide (LPS) induced pneumonia in rats, volatile oils decrease the white blood cell count and inhibit the inflammatory cells migrating towards the infected sites. Volatile oils also have inhibitory effect on adjuvant arthritis in rats. Besides, *Guì zhī* can suppress mast cell degranulation caused by IgE and restrains the alexin activity.

4. 镇静、抗惊厥　桂枝的水提物、总挥发油及其有效成分桂皮醛可使小鼠自主活动减少，使巴比妥类催眠药的催眠作用增强，可对抗苯丙胺所致的 CNS 过度兴奋，并能延长士的宁所致强直性惊厥的死亡时间，减少烟碱引起的强直性惊厥及死亡的发生率，可以抑制小鼠的听源性惊厥等。

(4) Sedation and anti-convulsion　*Guì zhī* water extract, volatile oil, and cinnamaldehyde can reduce the spontaneous motor activity of mice, synergize the hypnotic effect of barbiturates, counteract the CNS overexcitement that caused by benzedrine, prolong the death time and decrease death rate of tonic convulsion induced by strychnine or nicotine, and inhibit audiogenic seizures in animal models, etc.

5. 抗病原微生物　桂枝挥发油、桂皮醛在体外对多种致病细菌、病毒都有抑制作用。如金黄色葡萄球菌、伤寒杆菌、白色葡萄球菌、铜绿假单胞菌、变形杆菌、甲型链球菌、乙型链球菌、大肠埃希菌、白念珠菌、枯草芽孢杆菌、肺炎球菌、炭疽杆菌、霍乱弧菌、结核分枝杆菌、流感病毒亚洲甲型京科 68-1 株、埃可病毒（ECHO11）等。

(5) Anti-pathogenic microorganism　*Guì zhī* volatile oil and cinnamaldehyde can inhibit several bacteria and viruses *in vitro*, including *Staphylococcus aureus*, *Salmonella typhi*, *Staphylococcus albus*, *Pseudomonas aeruginosa*, *Proteus species*, alpha *Streptococcus*, beta *Streptococcus*, *Escherichia coli*, *Candida albicans*, *Bacillus subtilis*, *Streptococcus pneumoniae*, *Bacillus anthracis*, *Vibrio cholera*, *Proteusbacillus vulgaris*, *Mycobacterium tuberculosis*, Asian influenza virus 68-1strain, enteric cytopathogenic human orphan virus 11 (ECHO11), etc.

6. 其他作用　桂枝还有扩张血管、改善血液循环、抗氧化、抗焦虑、抗抑郁、利尿等作用。

(6) Other effects　*Guì zhī* also has the activities of vasodilation, improvement of microcirculation, anti-oxidation, antianxiety, anti-depression, and diuresis.

柴胡 ¦ *Chái hú (Radix Bupleuri)*

【来源 / Origin】

本品为伞形科植物柴胡（*Bupleurum chinense* DC.）或狭叶柴胡（*Bupleurum scorzonerifolium* Willd.）的干燥根。前者习称"北柴胡"，主产于河南、河北、辽宁等省；后者习称"南柴胡"，主产于湖北、江苏、四川等省。春、秋二季采挖，除去茎叶，干燥，生用或醋炙用。

Chái hú is the dried root of *Bupleurum chinense* DC. or *Bupleurum scorzonerifolium* Willd., family of *Umbelliferae*. The former is called North *Chái hú*, which is widely cultivated in Henan, Hebei, and

Liaoning province in China, and the latter is called South *Chái hú*, and is widely cultivated in Hubei, Jiangsu, and Sichuan province in China. In spring and autumn, the root is harvested and sun-dried. Crude *Chái hú* or vinegar-baked *Chái hú* are used as Chinese medicine.

【化学成分 / Chemical ingredients】

主要含皂苷类、甾醇类、挥发油、黄酮类、多糖等。皂苷类主要成分有柴胡皂苷（saikoside A，B，C，D)；甾醇类主要为 α– 菠菜甾醇（α-spinasterol)，尚有豆甾醇（stigmasterol）等；挥发油主要有柴胡醇（bupleurumol)、丁香酚（eugenol)、己酸（hexanoic acid)、γ– 十一酸内酯（γ-undecanolactone)、对–甲氧基苯二酮（4'-methoxyacetophenone）等。此外，尚含有生物碱、氨基酸、木脂素类、香豆素类等。

Chái hú mainly contains saponins, sterols, volatile oils, flavonoids, polysaccharides, etc. Saponins include saikoside A, B, C, D. Sterols include α-spinasterol, stigmasterol, etc. Volatile oils include bupleurumol, eugenol, hexanoic acid, γ-undecanolactone, 4'-methoxyacetophenone, etc. *Chái hú* also contains alkaloids, amino acids, lignans, coumarins, etc.

【药性与功效 / Chinese medicine properties】

味辛、苦，性微寒，归肝、胆经。具有疏散退热、疏肝解郁、升举阳气的功效。用于感冒发热、寒热往来、胸胁胀痛、月经不调、子宫脱垂、脱肛等证。

In Chinese medicine theory, *Chái hú* is pungent and bitter in flavor, slightly cold in nature, and it can enter the meridian of liver and gallbladder. *Chái hú* has the efficacies of dispersing heat and reducing fever, soothing liver and relieving depression, raising Yang Qi. Clinically it can be used for cold fever, alternating of chills and fever, chest and hypochondrium pain, menstrual irregularities, prolapse of uterus, rectocele, etc.

【药理作用 / Pharmacological effects】

1. 解热 柴胡为解热的要药。柴胡煎剂、注射液、醇浸膏、挥发油、粗皂苷、皂苷元等对多种原因（伤寒、副伤寒疫苗、大肠埃希菌液、发酵牛奶、酵母液及内生致热原等）引起的动物实验性发热，均有明显的解热作用，且能使正常动物的体温降低。柴胡皂苷、皂苷元 A 和挥发油是其解热的主要成分。丁香酚、己酸、γ– 十一酸内酯和对–甲氧基苯二酮等是挥发油解热作用的主要成分。与柴胡皂苷相比，挥发油的解热作用具有用量小、作用强和毒性小的特点。柴胡挥发油解热的部位可能为下丘脑体温调节中枢，通过抑制该部位神经元内 cAMP 的产生或释放，抑制体温调定点上移，使体温降低。此外，柴胡对病原微生物的抑制和杀灭作用也是其解热的作用环节之一。

(1) **Antipyresis** *Chái hú* has apparent antipyretic effect. *Chái hú* decoction, injection, ethanol extract, volatile oils, crude saponins and sapogenin all show anti-pyretic effect in experimental pyretic animal models that caused by typhoid vaccine, paratyphoid vaccine, *Escherichia coli*, fermented milk, yeast solution or endogenous pyrogen. They can even lower the body temperature of healthy animals. Saikosides, saikogenin A and volatile oils are regarded as the main active ingredients of antipyretic effects, while eugenol, hexanoic acid, γ-undecanolactone and 4'-methoxyacetophenone are the main antipyretic ingredient in volatile oils. Compared to saikoside, the antipyretic effect of volatile oils has the merits of small dosage, low toxicity and high efficiency. Volatile oils of *Chái hú* act on the hypothalamus thermo-regulator center, inhibit the production and release of cAMP in neurons, and suppress the up shift of the body temperature regulation point to decrease body temperature. Besides, the anti-pathogenic microorganism activity of *Chái hú* also contributes to its antipyretic effect.

2. 抗炎 柴胡煎液、柴胡皂苷和柴胡挥发油均有抗炎作用，对多种实验性炎症模型有效。柴胡抗炎的主要成分为柴胡皂苷和挥发油。柴胡的抗炎作用可能与以下环节有关。①柴胡皂苷能兴奋腺垂体分泌促肾上腺皮质激素（ACTH），刺激肾上腺引起皮质激素的合成和分泌。②柴胡皂苷D是血小板活化因子（PAF）的抑制剂，通过抑制PAF达到抗炎作用。③抑制炎症反应的多个环节（如渗出、毛细血管通透性增加、炎症介质的释放、白细胞游走、结缔组织增生）等。

(2) Anti-inflammation *Chái hú* decoction, saikoside and volatile oils all exert anti-inflammatory activity in several inflammatory animal models. Saikosides and volatile oils are the main active ingredients of anti-inflammation. The mechanisms are as follows. ①Saikosides stimulate adenohypophysis to secrete adrenocorticotropic hormone (ACTH), which further stimulate adrenal gland to promote the synthesis and release of adrenal cortical hormone. ②Saikoside D is an inhibitor of platelet activating factor (PAF), it may exert anti-inflammatory activity by PAF inhibition. ③Saikosides and volatile oils inhibit several aspects of inflammatory process, including restraining inflammatory exudation, decreasing capillary permeability, impeding inflammatory mediator release, leukocyte migration and connective tissue hyperplasia.

3. 抗病原微生物　柴胡具有抗菌、抗病毒作用。柴胡体外对金黄色葡萄球菌、溶血性链球菌、霍乱弧菌、结核分枝杆菌、钩端螺旋体有一定的抑制作用；对流感病毒、柯萨奇病毒、呼吸道合胞病毒、肝炎病毒、单纯疱疹病毒、牛痘病毒、人乳头瘤病毒等均具有较强的抑制作用，还能对抗 I 型脊髓灰质炎病毒导致的细胞突变。柴胡对鸡胚内流感病毒有显著的抑制作用，能显著降低鼠肺炎病毒所致的小鼠肺指数增高，阻止肺组织渗出性变性，降低肺炎病毒所致小鼠的死亡率。柴胡抗病毒的主要成分为皂苷类成分，作用机制与其抑制 Na^+-K^+-ATP 酶而引起能量和水盐代谢变化有关。

(3) Anti-pathogenic microorganism *Chái hú* preparations inhibit the growth of several types of bacteria, including *Staphylococcus aureus*, *Haemolytic streptococcus*, *Vibrio cholerae*, *Mycobacterium tuberculosis*, Leptospira, and strongly suppress the replication of influenza virus, coxsackie virus, respiratory syncytial virus, hepatitis virus, herpes simplex virus, human papilloma virus and cowpox virus *in vitro*. Furthermore, *Chái hú* can resist the cell mutation induced by type I polio virus, inhibit the proliferation of influenza virus in chicken embryo, and decrease the mortality and pulmonary weight index, prevent exudative degeneration of lung in mice attacked by pneumovirus. Saikosides are regarded as the main active ingredients. The underlying mechanisms are attributed to changes of energy, water and salt metabolism that caused by Na^+-K^+-ATPase inhibition.

4. 镇痛、镇静、抗癫痫　柴胡煎剂、柴胡皂苷可提高实验动物的痛阈，对多种实验性疼痛模型动物（小鼠尾压刺激法、电击鼠尾法/热板法、醋酸扭体法等）呈现镇痛作用，柴胡皂苷镇痛作用可部分被纳洛酮和阿托品所拮抗。

(4) Analgesia, sedation and anti-epilepsy *Chái hú* decoction and saikosides can relieve pain and increase pain threshold in mice that cause by tail pressure, tail shock, hot plate or acetic acid. The analgesic effect of saikosides can be partially antagonized by naloxone or atropine.

柴胡煎剂、总皂苷对 CNS 有明显的抑制作用，可使实验动物自发活动减少，条件反射抑制，延长巴比妥类药物的睡眠时间，拮抗兴奋剂（苯丙胺、咖啡因、去氧麻黄碱等）诱导的中枢兴奋作用。

Chái hú decoction and saponins exhibit significant inhibitory activity on CNS. They can reduce the spontaneous motor activity of mice, suppress conditioned reflex, synergize the hypnotic effect of barbiturates, counteract benzedrine, caffeine, or metamfetaminum-mediated excitation of CNS.

柴胡皂苷和挥发油腹腔注射给药可降低小鼠戊四氮发作阈值模型（MSTT）和最大电休克模

型（MES）的惊厥发生率，还可拮抗癫痫强直阵挛发作。柴胡注射液能抑制毛果芸香碱致家兔和大鼠癫痫模型的脑电活动。柴胡皂苷和挥发油是其主要的物质基础。

Chái hú volatile oils and saikosides have antiepileptic effect. They can decrease the incidence of convulsion on metrazol seizure threshold test (MSTT) or maximal electroshock seizure (MES) mice, and inhibit generalized tonic-clonic seizures in animal models, etc. *Chái hú* injection can prevent brain electrical activity of pilocarpine-induced acute epilepsy on rabbits and rats. *Chái hú* volatile oils and saikosides are the main active ingredients.

5. 增强免疫　柴胡多糖可提高巨噬细胞、自然杀伤（NK）细胞的功能，且能增加库普弗（Kupffer）细胞的吞噬功能，提高淋巴细胞转化率，提高病毒特异性抗体滴度，抑制迟发型超敏反应等。柴胡果胶多糖可促进脾细胞 IgG 生成，柴胡皂苷能提高 T 淋巴细胞、B 淋巴细胞的活性和 IL-2 的分泌。柴胡多糖和柴胡皂苷是增强免疫功能的主要药效物质。

(5) Enhancing immunity　*Chái hú* can strengthen the immune function. *Chái hú* polysaccharides enhance the function of Kupffer cells, natural killer (NK) cells and macrophage, increase lymphocyte transformation rate and specific antibody titer of virus, and suppress delayed type hypersensitivity, etc. *Chái hú* pectic polysaccharides promote the generation of IgG in spleen cells. Saikosides enhance the activity of T and B cells and the secretion of IL-2. *Chái hú* polysaccharides and saikosides are the main active ingredients.

6. 保肝、利胆、降血脂　柴胡、醋炙柴胡、柴胡皂苷对多种原因（四氯化碳、乙醇、伤寒疫苗、霉米、D-半乳糖等）所致动物实验性肝损伤有一定的保护作用，能使血清谷丙转氨酶（ALT）、谷草转氨酶（AST）的活性降低，肝糖原和肝蛋白含量增加，肝细胞的损伤减轻，能促进肝功能恢复。柴胡的保肝机制与多环节有关，具体如下。①柴胡皂苷对生物膜（如线粒体膜）有直接保护作用。②柴胡皂苷能促进脑垂体分泌 ACTH，升高血浆皮质醇，能拮抗外源性甾体激素对肾上腺的萎缩作用，提高机体对非特异性刺激的抵抗力。③降低细胞色素 P450 活性，减少肝细胞坏死，促进肝细胞再生。④活化巨噬细胞，促进抗体、干扰素的产生。⑤增强 NK 细胞和淋巴因子激活的杀伤（LAK）细胞的活性。⑥促进蛋白质和肝糖原合成，降低过氧化脂质含量。此外，柴胡具有防止肝纤维化的作用，主要有效成分为柴胡皂苷，其作用机制如下：通过清除自由基和抑制脂质过氧化等作用保护肝细胞；抑制肝星状细胞分泌胶原蛋白，进而抑制细胞增殖；合成肝内细胞外基质。

(6) Hepatoprotective, choleretic and anti-hyperlipidemia effects　*Chái hú*, vinegar-baked *Chái hú* and saikosides all show therapeutic effects on liver damage induced by carbon tetrachloride, ethanol, typhus vaccine, mouldy rice or D-galactosamine in experimental animals, indicated by decreasing activities of serum alanine aminotransferase (ALT) and aspartate aminotransferase (AST), increasing levels of hepatic glycogen and hepatic protein, relieving liver cell damage, and promoting the recovery of liver function. The hepatoprotective mechanisms of *Chái hú* saponins are related to the followings. ①Direct protective effect on bio-membrane, such as mitochondrial membrane. ② Stimulating pituitary-adrenal cortical system and increasing the secretion of glucocorticoid to promote the anti-stress ability of the cells. ③Inhibiting the enzymatic activity of cytochrome P450, decreasing hepatocyte necrosis, and promoting hepatocyte regeneration. ④ Activating macrophage and increasing the production of antibodies and interferon. ⑤ Improving the activity of NK and lymphokine activated killer (LAK) cells. ⑥ Promoting the synthesis of hepatic glycogen and protein, decreasing the levels of lipid peroxidase. Moreover, saikosides have anti-hepatic fibrosis action, which can be attributed to scavenging free radicals and inhibiting lipid peroxide production, suppressing the secretion of collagen by hepatic stellate cell and cell proliferation, and promoting the synthesis of intrahepatic extracellular matrix.

柴胡水浸剂和煎剂有明显的利胆作用，能使实验动物胆汁排出量增加，使胆汁中的胆酸、胆色素和胆固醇浓度降低。醋炙柴胡利胆作用最强。利胆作用的物质基础是黄酮类物质。

Chái hú decoction and water extract increase the bile flow of model animals and decrease the concentrations of cholic acid, bile pigment and cholesterol in the bile. Vinegar-baked *Chái hú* has the strongest choleretic effect, and flavonoids are suggested as the active ingredients.

柴胡皂苷能使实验性高脂血症动物的胆固醇、甘油三酯和磷脂水平降低，其中以甘油三酯的降低尤为显著。柴胡降血脂作用可抑制脂肪肝的形成和发展。柴胡能加速 ^{14}C-胆固醇及其代谢产物从粪便排泄，可能是影响脂质代谢的主要环节。皂苷 A、皂苷 D，皂苷元 A、皂苷元 D 及柴胡醇被认为是影响脂质代谢的主要成分。

Saikosides are capable of reducing levels of cholesterol, triglyceride, and phospholipid in experimental hyperlipidemia animal, and the reduction of triglyceride is more significant. Therefore, *Chái hú* has the ability to preventing the formation and development of fatty liver. *Chái hú* can accelerate the excretion of ^{14}C-cholestrol an its metabolites from feces,which maybe the main mechanism affecting lipid metabolism.Saponins A and D,sapogenin A and D,and bupleurumol are considered as the main ingredients.

7. 抗抑郁 柴胡对慢性应激抑郁模型、不可预见性刺激加孤养诱发的抑郁症模型、四肢束缚的抑郁模型具有良好的拮抗效应，能够改善其行为学异常，调节神经递质的紊乱。柴胡皂苷 A 是其抗抑郁的药效物质基础，作用机制与调节脑内单胺类神经递质代谢和抗氧化有关。

(7) Anti-depression *Chaí hú* improves the abnormal state of behavior and neurotransmitters in several depression animal models provoked by chronic stress, solitary feeding plus unpredictable stimulus, or restriction of four limbs. Saikosides A is suggested to be the main active ingredients. The mechanism is related to regulating the metabolism of monoamine neurotransmitters and resisting oxidation in CNS.

8. 其他作用 柴胡升举阳气，对肠平滑肌和子宫平滑肌有收缩作用。柴胡粗皂苷、柴胡多糖对乙醇、吲哚美辛、盐酸等诱导的多种实验性胃黏膜损伤模型有保护作用。柴胡水提物和柴胡皂苷有抗肿瘤作用。柴胡皂苷可以影响物质代谢，促进动物体内蛋白质合成，使肝糖原合成增加，促进葡萄糖利用，抑制脂肪的分解。

(8) Other effects *Chái hú* can induce intestine and uterine smooth muscle contraction. Total *Chái hú* saponins and *Chái hú* polysaccharose exert protective function on experimental gastric mucosal injury induced by ethanol, indomethacin, hydrochloric acid, etc. *Chái hú* water extracts and saponins have anti-tumor activity. Saikosides also affect substance metabolism, including promoting the synthesis of protein and glycogen, promoting glucose metabolism, and inhibiting steatolysis.

【不良反应 / Adverse effects 】

本品毒性较小。口服较大剂量可出现嗜睡、工作效率降低、食欲减退、腹泻等表现。柴胡注射液不良反应主要有晕厥、呕吐、过敏，严重者可见过敏性休克。

Oral contraception of large dose of *Chái hú* may cause central inhibition, such as hypersomnia, low work efficiency, anorexia and diarrhea, etc. The adverse reactions caused by *Chái hú* injections occasionally include dizziness, vomiting, anaphylactic reaction, and even anaphylactic shock, etc.

葛根 ┊ *Gě gēn (Radix Puerariae lobatae)*

【来源 / Origin】

本品为豆科植物野葛 [*Pueraria lobata* (Willd.) Ohwi] 的干燥根。主产于河南、湖南、浙江、四川。秋、冬二季采挖。生用，或煨用。

Gě gēn is the root of *Pueraria lobate* (Willd.) Ohwi., which is widely cultivated in Henan, Hunan, Zhejiang, and Sichuan province in China. In autumn and winter, the root is harvested and sun-dried for the use of Chinese medicine.

【化学成分 / Chemical ingredients】

主要含有黄酮类成分，含量为 0.06%~12.30%，包括葛根素（puerarin）、大豆苷（daidzin）、大豆苷元（daidzein）等。此外，还含有香豆素类、葛根苷类、三萜皂苷及生物碱类成分。

Gě gēn contains about 0.06% to 12.30% flavonoids, including puerarin, daidzin, daidzein, etc. Besides, *Gě gēn* also contains coumarins, glycosides, triterpenoid saponin and alkaloids, etc.

【药性与功效 / Chinese medicine properties】

味甘、辛，性凉，归脾、胃经。具有解肌退热、生津止渴、透疹、升阳止泻、通经活络、解酒毒的功效。主治外感发热头痛、项背强痛、口渴、消渴、麻疹不透、热痢、泄泻、眩晕头痛、中风偏瘫、胸痹心痛、酒毒伤中等证。

In Chinese medicine theory, *Gě gēn* is pungent and sweet in flavor, cold in nature, and meridian tropism in spleen and stomach. *Gě gēn* has the efficacies of releasing flesh and reducing fever, promoting fluid production to quench thirst, promoting eruption, raising Yang and checking diarrhea, dredging channels and activating collaterals, relieve alcoholism. Clinically it can be used for external-contraction fever and headache, severe pain of nape and back, thirst, consumptive thirst, measles without adeqrate eruption, heat dysentery, diarrhea, headache and dizziness, apoplectic hemiplegia, chest impediment and heart pain, alcoholism.

【药理作用 / Pharmacological effects】

1. **解热**　葛根煎剂、乙醇浸膏、葛根素、葛根粉等对实验性发热动物（伤寒混合菌苗、2,4-二硝基苯酚、蛋白胨等）均有解热作用。葛根素是其解热的药效物质之一。葛根解热的机制可能与扩张皮肤血管，促进血液循环和加强呼吸运动而增加散热有关，亦与葛根素阻断中枢部位的 β 受体而使 cAMP 生成减少有关。

(1) **Antipyresis**　*Gě gēn* decoction, ethanol extract, and puerarin show anti-pyretic effect in experimental pyretic animals that caused by typhoid and paratyphoid vaccine, 2,4-dinitrophenol, and peptone, etc. Puerarin is the main active ingredients. The mechanisms are attributed to dilating skin vessel, promoting superficial blood circulation and respiratory movement to release heat. The inhibitory effect of puerarin on central β receptor and decreasing cAMP level are also contribute to the anti-pyretic effect.

2. **降血糖**　葛根煎剂和葛根醇提物均能降低大鼠空腹血糖，提高胰岛素敏感指数，醇提物对地塞米松造成的胰岛素抵抗具有改善作用。葛根素为葛根降血糖作用的主要有效成分，可使四氧嘧啶性高血糖小鼠的血糖明显下降，血清胆固醇含量减少，并能改善糖耐量。葛根素可调节 β 内啡肽水平，降低糖尿病大鼠血清中晚期糖基化终末产物（AGEs）和单核细胞趋化蛋白（MCP）水平，减轻心肌的病变程度；还可通过激活 α_{1A} 肾上腺素受体，增加葡萄糖摄取从而改善胰岛素抵抗。

(2) **Hypoglycemic action**　*Gě gēn* decoction and ethanol extracts reduce the fasting blood-

glucose level and elevate insulin sensitivity index in diabetic rats. *Gě gēn* ethanol extracts improve dexamethasone-induced insulin resistance in rats. Puerarin is suggested to be the main active ingredient. It can lower the blood glucose, reduce serum cholesterol content, and improve glucose tolerance of hyperglycemic mice induced by alloxan. The mechanism may be related to regulating the synthesis of β-endorphin, downregulating the levels of serum advanced glycosylation end products (AGEs) and monocyte chemoattractant protein (MCP), relieving cardiomyopathy, and alleviating insulin resistance by activating $α_{1A}$ adrenergic receptor and promoting the uptake and utilization of glucose.

3. 抗心肌缺血 葛根水煎剂、醇浸膏、葛根总黄酮、葛根素和大豆苷元能对抗垂体后叶素引起的大鼠心肌缺血。葛根抗心肌缺血的主要有效成分为葛根素，有类似β受体阻断剂作用。其抗心肌缺血与以下环节有关。①抑制心肌细胞河豚毒素不敏感型（TTxr）钠内流和 I_{KI} 瞬间电流。②改善微循环，减少血栓素 A_2（TXA_2）生成，改善缺血区血液供应。③减少缺血引起的心肌乳酸的生成，降低缺血与再灌注时心肌的耗氧量和心肌含水量，改善缺血再灌注后心肌超微结构。④抑制心肌组织丙二醛（MDA）和髓过氧化物酶（MPO）的生成，减轻氧化应激损伤。⑤减少心钠素和血管紧张素 II 的释放。

(3) Anti-myocardial ischemia *Gě gēn* decoction, ethanol extract, total flavonoids, puerarin, and daidzein all prevent myocardial ischemia induced by pituitrin. Puerarin is the main active ingredient with effects similar to β receptor blockers. The mechanisms are as follows. ①Inhibiting tetrodotoxin-resistance (TTxr) sodium influx and instantaneous current of I_{KI}. ② Improving microcirculation, decreasing thromboxane A_2 (TXA_2) level, and promoting blood supply in ischemic areas. ③Reducing lactate production, diminishing oxygen consumption and liquid water content of myocardium during ischemia and reperfusion, improving the myocardium ultrastructure. ④ Reducing malondialdehyde (MDA) and myeloperoxidase (MPO) levels in myocardial tissue, preventing oxidative stress injury. ⑤ Inhibiting the release of atrial natriuretic factor (ANF) and angiotensin II.

4. 抗心律失常 葛根乙醇提取物、葛根黄酮、葛根素和大豆苷元灌胃后能明显对抗氯化钡、乌头碱、氯化钙、氯仿-肾上腺素和急性心肌缺血等所致的大鼠心律失常。葛根素静脉注射能明显对抗乌头碱、氯化钡所致的心律失常，能延长心肌动作电位时程，抑制延迟整流钾电流。其机制可能为通过影响心肌细胞膜对 K^+，Na^+，Ca^{2+} 的通透性，延长心肌细胞的动作电位时程，降低心肌兴奋性、自律性及传导性等。

(4) Anti-arrhythmia *Gě gēn* ethanol extract, total flavonoids, puerarin, and daidzein inhibit the arrhythimia caused by barium chloride, aconitine, calcium chloride, chloroform-epinephrine and acute myocardial ischemia in rats. Puerarin injection prolongs cardiac action potential duration, and suppresses the delayed rectification potassium current in barium chloride or aconitine induced arrhythimia in rats. The underlying mechanisms of puerarin are related to its regulatory effects on myocardial cellular membrane permeability for K^+, Na^+, Ca^{2+}, which prolong the action potential duration of cardiomyocytes and further reduce the excitability, auto rhythmicity, and conductivity of myocardium.

5. 扩张外周血管、降低血压 葛根水煎剂、总黄酮、葛根素可扩张高血压动物外周血管，有降压作用。葛根素呈现内皮依赖性舒血管效应，该作用与一氧化氮（NO）系统及三磷酸腺苷（ATP）敏感的钾通道有关。葛根素、大豆苷元能降低血浆肾素和血管紧张素水平，减少血浆儿茶酚胺含量。降压机制可能与β受体阻断效应和抑制肾素-血管紧张素-醛固酮系统（RAA）有关。

(5) Dilating peripheral vascular vessel and anti-hypertension *Gě gēn* water extract, total flavonoids, and puerarin have effects of dilating blood vessel and reducing blood pressure on hypertensive animal models. Puerarin presents endothelium-dependent vasodilatation that correlated with NO system and ATP-sensitive potassium channel. Puerarin and daidzein decrease the levels of plasma renin, angiotensin and catecholamine. The hypotensive mechanisms of *Gě gēn* are attributed to its inhibitory effects on β-receptors and renin-angiotensin-aldosterone (RAA) system.

6. 抗血栓、改善血液流变性　葛根素能抑制二磷酸腺苷（ADP）与 5-HT 联合诱导的家兔、绵羊及正常人血小板聚集，大鼠灌服葛根总黄酮能降低全血黏度和血小板黏附率。葛根还可改善不稳定型心绞痛和糖尿病患者血液流变性，降低血黏度。

(6) Antithrombosis and improving hemorheology　Puerarin restrains the platelet aggregation of rabbits, sheep and normal volunteers induced by adenosine diphosphate (ADP) combined with 5-HT *in vitro*. Oral administration of total flavonoids reduces blood viscosity and platelet adhesion in rats. *Gě gēn* also improves hemorheology and lowers the blood viscosity of patients with diabetes or unstable angina pectoris.

7. 其他作用　葛根素有改善学习记忆和抗痴呆的作用，这与其减轻胆碱能神经元损伤，增加乙酰胆碱转移酶活性和功能，催化乙酰胆碱合成有关。此外，葛根尚具有降血脂、抗氧化、抗肿瘤、保肝、解酒等作用。

(7) Other effects　Puerarin improves the learning and memory ability of dementia animals by alleviating the cholinergic neuron impairment, improving the activity of choline acetyltransferase, and promoting the synthesis of acetylcholine. *Gě gēn* also possesses anti-hyperlipidemic, anti-oxidative, anti-tumor, hepatoprotective, and anti-alcoholic activities.

【 不良反应 / Adverse effects 】

葛根素注射液偶尔可引起药物热、过敏性药疹、过敏性休克、速发性喉头水肿、消化道出血、溶血、肾绞痛、血红蛋白尿、丙氨酸转氨酶升高、心脏骤停、窦房结抑制等不良反应。

Puerarin injection may occasionally cause adverse reactions, such as fever, allergic drug eruption, anaphylactic shock, laryngeal edema, digestive bleeding, hemolysis, renal colic, hemoglobinuria, elevation of the activity of blood alanine aminotransferase, sudden cardiac arrest, and sinus node block.

题库

（曹惠慧　方　芳）

第五章　清热药

Chapter 5　Heat-clearing medicines

学习目标｜Objectives

1. **掌握**　清热药的主要药理作用；黄芩、黄连、苦参、穿心莲与功效相关的药理作用、药效物质基础。

2. **了解**　金银花、大青叶与板蓝根、鱼腥草、知母、栀子、牡丹皮、牛黄、青蒿的主要药理作用和药效物质基础。

1. **Must know**　The main pharmacological effects of heat-clearing medicines; the efficacy related pharmacological effects, mechanism, and material basis of *Huáng qín, Huáng lián, Kǔ shēn, Chuān xīn lián*.

2. **Desirable to know**　The main pharmacological effects and material basis of *Jīn yín huā, Dà qīng yè* and *Bǎn lán gēn, Yú xīng cǎo, Zhī mǔ, Zhī zǐ, Mǔ dān pí, Niú huáng*, and *Qīng hāo*.

第一节　概述

Section 1　Overview

凡以清解里热为主要功效，用以治疗里热证的药物，称为清热药。本类药物主要归肺、胃、心、肝、大肠经，药性寒凉，味多苦、辛。寒凉泻热、苦寒清解、作用偏里，故本类药物根据其主要功效分为清热解毒药、清热泻火药、清热燥湿药、清热凉血药和清虚热药五类。

All Chinese materia medical that are mainly used to clear and treat the interior heat and its syndromes are classified as heat-clearing medicines. These medicines are traditionally used to clear heat-syndrome of the interior. They majorly enter the meridians of lung, stomach, heart, liver and large intestine. They mainly have cool and cold nature, usually bitter and acrid flavor. Cool and cold can expel the heat, bitter and cold can eliminate the heat, and internal effect. Depending on their major functions, these drugs are divided into five categories: heat-clearing and detoxifying drugs; heat-clearing and fire-purging drugs; heat-clearing and damp-drying drugs; heat-clearing and blood-cooling drugs; and deficient heat-clearing drugs.

里热证主要是外邪内传、入里化热，或内郁化热所致的证候。因热伤津液，故面红身热、口渴冷饮、小便黄赤、大便干结；因热属阳，阳主动，故躁动不安而多言。里热证多见于西医学中多种感染性疾病的发热期，也见于一些非感染性疾病，如某些变态反应性疾病、出血性疾病和肿瘤等。现代药理研究表明，清热药治疗里热证与下列药理作用有关。

The interior heat syndrome is mainly caused by the internal transmission of external evil, or the internal depression transformated into heat. The syndromes include red face, body heat, thirsty, cold drink, yellow-red urine, and dry stool because of heat injury body fluids. In addition, because the heat belongs to Yang and Yang takes the initiative, so restless and talkative are also the common syndromes. The interior heat syndrome is similar to the syndromes of fever period of various infectious diseases in western medicine which include some non-infectious diseases, such as some allergic diseases, hemorrhagic diseases and tumors. The heat-cleaning function is related to the following pharmacological effects.

1. 抗病原微生物　体外试验证实，黄连、金银花、穿心莲、栀子、知母、青蒿等对革兰阳性菌和革兰阴性菌都有抑制作用；黄连、黄芩等对幽门螺杆菌有抑制作用；黄连、黄芩、金银花等对多种皮肤真菌也有抑制作用。体内、外试验证实，黄连、金银花、穿心莲、知母、栀子等对流感病毒、疱疹病毒和乙型肝炎病毒等均有抑制作用；黄连、苦参等对阿米巴原虫有抑制作用；青蒿等对红细胞内期疟原虫有直接杀灭作用。

(1) **Anti-pathogenic microorganisms**　*In vitro*, most of heat-clearing medicines, such as *Huáng lián*, *Jīn yín huā*, *Chuān xīn lián*, *Zhī zǐ*, *Zhī mǔ*, *Qīng hāo*, can inhibit the activity of Gram-positive and Gram-negative bacteria; *Huáng lián* and *Huáng qín* can inhibit *Helicobacter pylori*; *Huáng lián*, *Huáng qín* and *Jīn yín huā* also have inhibitory effects on multiple dermatophytes. *Huáng lián*, *Jīn yín huā*, *Chuān xīn lián*, *Zhī mǔ*, *Zhī zǐ* can inhibit influenza virus, herpes virus and hepatitis B virus *in vivo* and *in vitro*; *Huáng lián* and *Kǔ shēn* can inhibit amoeba; *Qīng hāo* can directly kill Plasmodium in the erythrocytic stage.

2. 抗细菌毒素、降低细菌毒力　黄连、金银花、板蓝根等能中和、降解内毒素或破坏其正常结构，并抑制内毒素诱导的炎症介质合成与过度释放，降低死亡率；黄连等具有抗外毒素作用，且在无抑菌作用浓度就能抑制金黄色葡萄球菌凝固酶的形成。

(2) **Anti-bacterial toxin, reducing bacterial virulence**　Some of heat-clearing medicines, such as *Huáng lián*, *Jīn yín huā*, *Bǎn lán gēn* can neutralize or degrade endotoxin or destroy its structure, inhibit the synthesis and excess release of inflammatory mediators induced by endotoxin, and reduce mortality; *Huáng lián* has the effect of anti-exotoxin, it can inhibit the formation of *Staphylococcus aureus* coagulase at the concentration which has no antibacterial effect.

3. 抗炎　大多数清热药对实验性炎症的各个环节均有一定的抑制作用，其抗炎作用机制主要有兴奋垂体–肾上腺皮质系统，抑制炎症反应；抑制各种炎症介质的合成与释放。

(3) **Anti-inflammation**　Most of heat-clearing medicines have certain inhibitory effects on all aspects of experimental inflammation. The anti-inflammatory mechanism mainly includes: exciting pituitary- adrenal cortex system；inhibiting the synthesis and release of various inflammatory mediators.

4. 解热　大多数清热药具有明显的解热作用，与解表药不同的是，清热药退热多不伴有明显的发汗，其解热作用机制与抗病原微生物、中和及降解内毒素、抑制内生致热原生成等有关。

(4) **Antipyretic effects**　Most of heat-clearing medicines have obvious antipyretic effect. Different from the exterior-releasing medicines, heat-clearing medicines exert antipyretic effects without obvious sweating. The antipyretic mechanism is related to anti-pathogenic microorganisms, neutralization and degradation of endotoxin, inhibition of endogenous pyrogen formation, etc.

5. 抗肿瘤　清热药，尤其是清热解毒药如黄连、苦参、穿心莲、青蒿、青黛等具有较强的抗肿瘤作用，可控制肿瘤及周围的炎症水肿，减轻症状。

(5) **Anti-tumor**　Heat-clearing medicines, especially clearing heat and detoxifying drugs such as *Huáng lián*, *Kǔ shēn*, *Chuān xīn lián*, *Qīng hāo*, *Qīng dài* have strong anti-tumor effects. They can control

inflammation and edema in tumor and the surrounding and alleviate symptoms.

6. **影响免疫功能** 金银花、黄连、青蒿等可增强机体免疫能力，能促进单核巨噬细胞系统（MPS）的吞噬活性、增强细胞免疫及体液免疫等。黄芩、苦参又可抑制多种类型的变态反应，能抑制肥大细胞脱颗粒，抑制过敏介质释放；穿心莲、苦参能抑制迟发型超敏反应。

(6) Effects on immune function *Jīn yín huā*, *Huáng lián*, *Qīng hāo* can enhance the immune function, which promote the phagocytosis of mononuclear phagocyte system (MPS), enhance cell immunity and humoral immunity. *Huáng qín* and *Kǔ shēn* can inhibit many kinds of allergic reactions, degranulation of mast cells and release of allergic mediators. *Chuān xīn lián* and *Kǔ shēn* can inhibit delayed-type hypersensitivity.

7. **其他作用** 清热药通常还有降血压、降血糖、降血脂、抗血小板聚集、抗氧化、保肝、镇静、抗生育等作用。

(7) Other effects The heat-clearing medicines have other effects of reducing blood pressure, blood glucose and blood lipid, Inhibiting platelet aggregation, anti-oxidation, hepatoprotection, sedation, anti-fertility, etc.

常用清热药的主要药理作用见表 5-1。

The main pharmacological effects of commonly used heat-cleaning medicines are summarized in Table 5-1.

表 5-1　常用清热药主要药理作用

类别	药物	解热	抗炎	抗毒素	抗菌	抗真菌	抗病毒	抗肿瘤	调节免疫	其他
清热泻火药	知母	+	+	−	+	+	+	+	−	抑制交感神经功能、降血糖、改善学习记忆能力等
	石膏	+	+	−	−	−	−	−	+	抗凝、利尿
	栀子	+	+	−	+	+	+	−	−	镇静催眠、保肝、利胆、降血压等
清热燥湿药	黄芩	+	+	+	+	+	+	+	+	保肝、利胆、降血压、调血脂等
	黄连	+	+	+	+	+	+	+	+	抗血小板聚集、抗心律失常、抗溃疡、降血糖等
	黄柏	−	+	−	+	+	+	+	+	抗溃疡、调节胃肠运动、抗心律失常、降血压等
	苦参	+	+	−	+	+	+	+	+	抗心律失常、抗心肌缺血、抗肝纤维化、平喘等
清热解毒药	金银花	+	+	+	+	−	+	+	+	利胆、降血压、调血脂、止血、抗氧化等
	连翘	+	+	+	+	+	+	−	+	保肝、镇吐等
	大青叶	+	+	+	+	+	+	−	+	保肝、抑制肠蠕动等
	板蓝根	+	+	+	+	+	+	−	+	保肝、抗血小板聚集、降血脂等
	鱼腥草	+	+	+	+	+	+	+	+	胃保护作用
	蒲公英	−	−	+	+	−	+	+	+	抗溃疡、利胆、保肝等
	穿心莲	+	+	+	+	+	+	+	+	抗血小板聚集、抗心律失常、抗心肌缺血等
	山豆根	+	+	+	+	+	+	+	+	保肝、抗心律失常、抗溃疡等
	牛黄	+	+	+	+	−	+	−	−	镇静、抗惊厥、抗血小板聚集、降血压等

续表

类别	药物	解热	抗炎	抗毒素	抗病原微生物			抗肿瘤	调节免疫	其他
					抗菌	抗真菌	抗病毒			
清热凉血药	生地黄	−	−	−	−	−	−	−	+	抑制交感神经功能、降血糖、促进造血等
	牡丹皮	+	+		+	+	+	+	+	镇静、抗惊厥、保肝、降血糖、抗血小板聚集等
	紫草	+	+		+	+	+	+	+	止血、降血糖等
清虚热药	青蒿	+	+		+	+	+	+	+	抗疟原虫、抑制心脏等
	地骨皮	+	+		+				+	降血糖、调血脂、降血压等

注："+"表示有明确作用；"−"表示无作用，或未查阅到相关研究文献

第二节 常用药物

Section 2 Commonly used medicines

PPT

知母 ┆ *Zhī mǔ* (*Rhizoma Anemarrhenae*)

【来源 / Origin】

本品为百合科植物知母（*Anemarrhena asphodeloides* Bge.）的干燥根茎。主产于河北、山西、广东等地。春秋二季采收，除去地上部分及须根，洗净，晒干。

Zhī mǔ is the dry root of *Anemarrhena asphodeloides* Bge. *Zhī mǔ* is widely cultivated in Hebei, Shanxi, and Guangdong province in China. It is harvested in spring and autumn. The sun dried root without the ground and fibrous roots is used for Chinese medicinal preparation.

【化学成分 / Chemical ingredients】

主要含知母皂苷（timosaponin）A-I、知母皂苷 A-II、知母皂苷 A-III、知母皂苷 A-IV、知母皂苷 B-I 及知母皂苷 B-II 等多种甾体皂苷。皂苷元主要为菝葜皂苷元（sarsasapogenin）。此外，还含有芒果苷（mangiferin）、异芒果苷（isomangiferin）和知母多糖（anemaran）。

Zhī mǔ contains a variety of steroidal saponins such as timosaponin A-I, A-II, A-III, A-IV, B-I and B-II. Sapogenins are mainly sarsasapogenin. In addition, it contains mangiferin, isomangiferin and anemaran.

【药性与功效 / Chinese medicine properties】

味苦、甘，性寒，归肺、胃、肾经。具有清热泻火、生津润燥的功效。主治外感热病，高热烦渴，肺热燥咳，骨蒸潮热，内热消渴，肠燥便秘。

In Chinese medicine theory, *Zhī mǔ* has the nature of bitter, sweet and cold. It can enter the meridians of lung, stomach, and kidney. *Zhī mǔ* can clear heat and purge fire, promote liquid production to moisten dryness. Clinically, it can be used for exogenous fever, polydipsia due to hyperpyrexia, cough due to lung heat, steaming bone fever, consumptive thirsty due to interior heat, and constipation due to intestinal dryness.

医药大学堂
WWW.YIYAODXT.COM

【药理作用 / Pharmacological effects】

1. 抗病原微生物　知母水煎液体外对结核分枝杆菌、伤寒杆菌、志贺菌属、白喉棒状杆菌、金黄色葡萄球菌、肺炎链球菌有抑制作用。芒果苷是其抗结核分枝杆菌的有效成分之一。异芒果苷及芒果苷均具有抗单纯疱疹病毒作用。知母对某些致病性皮肤真菌及白念珠菌也有抑制作用。

(1) Anti-pathogenic microorganisms　*Zhī mǔ* water decoction has inhibitory effects on *Mycobacterium tuberculosis, Typhoid bacillus, Shigella., Diphtheria bacillus, Staphylococcus aureus* and *Diplococcus pneumoniae in vitro*. Mangiferin is suggested to be the effective ingredients against *Mycobacterium tuberculosis*. Both isomangiferin and mangiferin can inhibit herpes simplex virus. *Zhī mǔ* can also inhibit certain pathogenic *Dermatophyte* and *Candida albicans*.

2. 解热　知母水提物对大肠埃希菌所致的家兔高热有预防和治疗作用，其解热特点为慢而持久，机制与抑制产热过程有关，通过抑制与产热有关的细胞膜上的 Na^+-K^+-ATP 酶，使产热减少。知母解热的主要有效成分是芒果苷、菝葜皂苷元、知母皂苷。

(2) Antipyretic effect　*Zhī mǔ* water extract have preventive and therapeutic effects on hyperthermia of rabbits caused by *E. coli*. Its antipyretic characteristics are slow and persistent. The mechanism is related to the inhibition of the heat production process through inhibiting the Na^+-K^+-ATPase on the cell membrane. Mangiferin, sarsasapogenin and timosaponins are suggested to be the main active ingredient for antipyretic effect.

3. 抗炎　知母中的芒果苷和总多糖具有显著的抗炎作用。知母能抑制二甲苯致小鼠耳郭肿胀和醋酸致腹腔毛细血管通透性增加。知母总多糖具有抗炎活性，通过促进肾上腺分泌糖皮质激素及抑制炎症组织 PGE 的合成或释放而发挥抗炎作用。

(3) Anti-inflammatory effect　Mangiferin and anemaran have significant anti-inflammatory effects. *Zhī mǔ* could inhibit xylene-induced auricular swelling and acetic acid induced permeability of intraperitoneal capillary in mice. Anemaran has anti-inflammatory activities through promoting the release of adrenocortical hormone and inhibiting the synthesis or release of PGE from tissues.

4. 影响交感神经和 β 受体功能　知母及其皂苷元能降低血、脑、肾上腺中多巴胺-β 羟化酶活性，减少 NE 合成和释放。可使阴虚模型动物脑、肾中 β 受体功能下降，从而降低交感神经功能。

(4) Effects on the function of the sympathetic nerve and β receptor　*Zhī mǔ* and its sapogenins can reduce the activity of dopamine-β-hydroxylase in blood, brain and adrenal gland, and the synthesis and release of NE. It can inhibit the function of β receptor in brain and kidney of Yin-deficiency model animals, to reduce the function of sympathetic nerve.

5. 降血糖　知母皂苷具有抑制 α 葡糖苷酶的作用，能降低四氧嘧啶诱发的糖尿病小鼠血糖。知母多糖能降低正常小鼠和高血糖大鼠的血糖、增加肝糖原含量、增强骨骼肌对葡萄糖摄取能力。

(5) Lowering blood glucose effect　Timosaponins can inhibit α-glucosidase and reduce blood glucose of diabetic mice induced by alloxan. Anemarans can reduce blood glucose in normal mice and hyperglycemic rats, increase glycogen content in liver, and enhance the uptake of glucose by skeletal muscle.

6. 改善学习记忆能力　知母皂苷能有效促进东莨菪碱、亚硝酸钠和乙醇记忆障碍模型小鼠的学习记忆能力，并且能提高血管性痴呆大鼠的学习记忆能力，对脑缺血后神经元损伤、炎症损伤具有一定的保护作用。

(6) Improving learning and memory function　Timosaponins can improve the learning and memory ability of scopolamine, sodium nitrite and ethanol induced memory impairment in mice. Meanwhile, timosaponins can improve the learning and memory ability of rats with vascular dementia, reduce the neuronal injury and inflammation induced by cerebral ischemia.

7. 其他作用　知母皂苷尚有抗肿瘤、抗骨质疏松、抗血小板聚集、降血脂作用。芒果苷有明显利胆作用。

(7) Other effects　Timosaponins have other pharmacological effects, such as anti-tumor, anti-osteoporosis, inhibition of platelet aggregation, hypolipidemia. Mangiferin has obvious choleretic effect.

栀子 ┊ *Zhī zǐ* (*Gardenia Jasminoides*)

【来源 / Origin】

本品为茜草科植物栀子（*Gardenia jasminoides* Ellis.）的干燥成熟果实。主产于长江以南各省。秋冬二季采收，晒干生用。

Zhī zǐ is the dried ripe fruits of *Gardenia jasminoides* Ellis. The plant is widely cultivated in provinces to the south of Yangtze River. It is harvested in autumn and winner. The sun dried fruits is used for Chinese medicinal preparation.

【化学成分 / Chemical ingredients】

主要有效成分为环烯醚萜苷类，如栀子苷（Gardenia jasminoides），京尼平苷（geniposide）及其水解产物京尼平（genipin）和山栀苷（shanzhiside）等。此外，尚含有 D- 甘露醇，β- 谷甾醇、熊果酸、齐墩果酸和豆甾醇。

The main effective ingredients of *Zhī zǐ* are iridoid glycosides, such as Gardenia jasminoides, geniposide and its hydrolysates genipin and shanzhiside. *Zhī zǐ* also contains D-mannitol, β-sitosterol, ursolic acid, oleanolic acid, stigmasterol.

【药性与功效 / Chinese medicine properties】

味苦，性寒，归心、肺、三焦经。具有泻火除烦、清热利尿、凉血解毒的功效。主治热病心烦，黄疸尿赤，血淋涩痛，血热吐衄，目赤肿痛，火毒疮疡；外治扭挫伤痛。

In Chinese medicine theory, *Zhī zǐ* has the nature of bitter, cold. It can enter the meridians of heart, lung, and triple energizer. *Zhī zǐ* can purge fire and relieve fidgetiness, clear heat and promote urination, cool the blood and remove toxin. Clinically, it can be used for vexation due to pyreticosis, jaundice, reddish urine, hematuria, blood-heat, hematemesis, epistaxis, conjunctival congestion, swelling and pain of eyes and throat, fire-toxicity syndrome, sore and ulcer on skin, etc. It can also treat sprain and bruising for external application.

【药理作用 / Pharmacological effects】

1. 镇静催眠　栀子生品及各种炮制品均有一定的镇静作用，可延长小鼠睡眠时间，减少自发活动，且经炒焦、炒炭后镇静作用明显增强。栀子可增强戊巴比妥钠的催眠作用，使小鼠睡眠时间显著延长。

(1) Sedative and hypnotic effects　The raw *Zhī zǐ* and various processed products have certain sedative effect, which can prolong the sleep time of mice and reduce spontaneous activity, and the sedative effect is obviously enhanced after fried burnt or fried charcoal. *Zhī zǐ* can also enhance the hypnotic effect of sodium pentobarbital which significantly prolong the sleep time of mice.

2. 解热抗炎　栀子生品及各种炮制品的乙醇提取物对酵母所致发热大鼠具有解热作用，生品作用强于炮制品。栀子水提物和栀子总苷对二甲苯所致耳郭肿胀、醋酸所致小鼠腹腔毛细血管通透性增高、甲醛及角叉菜胶所致大鼠足肿胀、大鼠棉球肉芽组织增生均有明显的抑制作用，生品强于各种炮制品。京尼平苷是其抗炎的主要物质基础。

(2) Antipyretic and anti-inflammatory effects　The ethanol extract of raw *Zhī zǐ* and various processed products have antipyretic effect on febrile rats caused by yeast, and the antipyretic effect of raw *Zhī zǐ* is stronger than that of processed products. The water extracts of *Zhī zǐ* and total *Zhī zǐ* glycosides also have significant inhibitory effects on xylene-induced auricular swelling, acetic acid-induced the increase of peritoneal capillary permeability in mice, formaldehyde and carrageenan-induced foot swelling in rats, and cotton ball-induced granulation tissue hyperplasia in rats. The anti-inflammatory effects of raw products are stronger than that of processed products. Geniposide is suggested to be the main active ingredient for anti-inflammation.

3. 保肝利胆　栀子不同炮制品的水提物和醇提物对四氯化碳所致小鼠急性肝损伤有保护作用，以生品作用为强，炒炭无效。栀子苷、京尼平苷能减轻四氯化碳、半乳糖胺引起的肝损害，可使大鼠急性黄疸模型血清胆红素、谷丙转氨酶（ALT）、谷草转氨酶（AST）明显降低。栀子有效成分栀子苷、京尼平苷均可促进胆汁分泌。栀子苷、京尼平苷是其利胆、保肝的物质基础，其中，京尼平苷是通过水解生成京尼平而发挥利胆作用的。

(3) Hepatoprotection and cholagogic effects　The water extract and ethanol extract from different processed products of *Zhī zǐ* have a protective effect on carbon tetrachloride-induced acute liver injury in mice, of which the raw material shows the strongest effect and the fried charcoal is invalid. Gardenia jasminoides and geniposide can alleviate liver damage caused by carbon tetrachloride and galactosamine, and significantly reduce serum bilirubin, ALT and AST in acute jaundice rats. Gardenia jasminoides and geniposide of *Zhī zǐ* can promote bile secretion. Gardenia jasminoides and geniposide are suggested to be the main effective ingredients for hepatoprotection and cholagogic effects. Geniposide exerts cholagogic effects by hydrolyzing to genipin.

4. 保护胰腺　栀子总苷能促进大鼠胰腺分泌，降低胰酶活性，对胰腺细胞膜、线粒体膜、溶酶体膜均有稳定作用，有减轻胰腺炎作用。促进胰腺分泌作用以京尼平作用最强，降低胰酶活性以京尼平苷作用最显著。

(4) Pancreatic protection　Total *Zhī zǐ* glycosides can promote pancreatic secretion and reduce pancreatic enzyme activity in rats. It has a membrane stabilizing effect on pancreatic cell membrane, mitochondrial membrane and lysosomal membrane, and can alleviate pancreatitis. Genipin had the strongest effect in promoting pancreatic secretion and geniposide had the most significant effect in reducing pancreatic enzyme activity.

5. 其他作用　栀子水煎液对多种细菌、皮肤癣菌和病毒具有抑制作用。栀子水煎液和醇提物无论口服或注射给药均具有持久降压作用。此外，栀子还有降血脂、抗内毒素、保护神经细胞、调节胃肠运动作用。

(5) Other effects　*Zhī zǐ* water decoction has inhibitory effects on a variety of bacteria, dermatophytes and viruses. Whether orally or injected, the water decoction and ethanol extract of *Zhī zǐ* both have enduring anti-hypertensive effects. In addition, *Zhī zǐ* has some other pharmacological effects, such as hypolipidemic, anti-endotoxin, protection of nerve cells, regulation of gastrointestinal motility.

【不良反应 / Adverse effects】

栀子及其有效成分对肝脏有一定毒性作用。

Zhī zǐ and its active ingredients have a certain toxic effect on the liver.

黄芩 ┊ *Huáng qín (Radix Scutellariae)*

【来源 / Origin】

本品为唇形科草本植物黄芩（*Scutellaria baicalensis* Georgi.）的干燥根。主产于河北、山西、内蒙古、河南及陕西。春、秋二季采收，除去残茎、须根，晒干。

Huáng qín is the dried root of *Scutellaria baicalensis* Georgi. The plant is mainly cultivated in Hebei province, Shanxi province, Inner Mongolia Autonomous region, Henan province and Shaanxi province in China. It is harvested in spring and autumn. After stubble and fibrous root are removed, the sun dried roots are used for Chinese medicinal preparation.

【化学成分 / Chemical ingredients】

有效成分为黄酮类，包括黄芩苷（baicalin）、黄芩素（baicalein）、汉黄芩苷（wogonoside）、汉黄芩素（wogonin）、千层纸素 A(oroxylin A)、黄芩新素 I (skullcapfavone I)、黄芩新素 II（skullcapfavone II）。此外，尚含有 β–谷甾醇、葡萄糖醛酸和多种微量元素等。

The main chemical ingredients of *Huáng qín* are flavonoids, including baicalin, baicalein, wogonoside, wogonin, oroxylin A, skullcapfavone I and skullcapflavone II. In addition, it also contains β-sitosterol, glucuronic acid and many trace elements.

【药性与功效 / Chinese medicine properties】

味苦，性寒，归肺、胆、胃、小肠和大肠经。具有清热燥湿、泻火解毒、止血安胎的功效。主治湿热泻痢、肺热咳嗽、热病烦渴、黄疸、目赤肿痛、积热吐血、胎动不安、痈肿疮疖等。

In Chinese medicine theory, *Huáng qín* has the nature of bitter and cold. It can enter the meridians of lung, gallbladder, stomach and large intestine. *Huáng qín* can clear heat, dry damp, purge fire and remove toxin, hemostasis and prevent miscarriage. Clinically it can be used for damp-heat diarrhea, cough due to lung-heat, polydipsia due to fever, jaundice, swelling and pain in the eyes, haematemesis due to accumulation of heat, threatened abortion, abscess and furuncle, etc.

【药理作用 / Pharmacological effects】

1. 抗菌 黄芩体外对耐药大肠埃希菌、产超广谱 β–内酰胺酶大肠埃希菌、表皮葡萄球菌、痤疮丙酸杆菌、金黄色葡萄球菌、耐甲氧西林金黄色葡萄球菌、铜绿假单胞菌、幽门螺杆菌、肠炎沙门菌、耐氟康唑白念珠菌和都柏林念珠菌具有抑制作用。

(1) Anti-bacterial effects *Huáng qín* has bacteriostatic effect *in vitro*. It has inhibitory effects on resistant *Escherichia coli*, extended spectrum β-lactamase producing *Escherichia coli*, *Staphylococcus epidermidis*, *Propionibacterium acnes*, *Staphylococcus aureus*, methicillin-resistant *Staphylococcus aureus*, *Pseudomonas aeruginosa*, *Helicobacter pylori*, *Salmonella enteritidis*, fluconazole resistant *Candida albicans* and *Candida Dublin*.

2. 解热、抗炎 黄芩茎叶总黄酮灌胃和腹腔注射均能降低干酵母引起的发热大鼠体温。

(2) Antipyretic, anti-inflammatory effects Oral administration and intraperitoneal injection of total flavonoids of *Huáng qín* can reduce the temperature of rats with fever caused by dry yeast.

黄芩水提取物能抑制多种诱导因素引起的各期炎症反应。对鲜蛋清、角叉菜胶致大鼠足肿胀，醋酸致小鼠腹腔毛细血管通透性增高，二甲苯致小鼠耳郭肿胀，脂多糖（LPS）致大鼠急性肺损伤的水肿程度等急性炎症均有抑制作用；具有抑制亚急性炎症作用，可减少小鼠羧甲基纤维素囊中的白细胞数目，抑制大鼠巴豆油性气囊肿的形成。

The aqueous extract of *Huáng qín* can inhibit the inflammatory response caused by various inducers. It can inhibit acute inflammation such as foot swelling of rats caused by fresh egg white and carrageenan, increased capillary permeability of mice caused by acetic acid, ear swelling of mice caused by xylene, and edema caused by lipopolysaccharides (LPS) in rats with acute lung injury. It can inhibit subacute inflammation which reduce the chemotaxis of leukocytes induced by carboxymethylcellulose and the formation of gas cyst caused by croton oil in rats.

3. 调节免疫、抗过敏　黄芩对机体免疫功能具有双向调节作用。黄芩醇提物能减少大鼠腹腔肥大细胞释放组胺，抑制大鼠皮肤过敏反应。

(3) Immune regulation and anti-allergy effects　*Huáng qín* has a dual regulation effect on immune function. Alcohol extract of *Huáng qín* can reduce histamine release from peritoneal mast cells and inhibit cutaneous anaphylaxis in rats.

（1）免疫抑制　黄芩抗Ⅰ型变态反应（过敏反应）作用显著。能抑制 N-Fomyl-Met-Leu-Phe (FMLP) 和酵母多糖（OZ）激活的中性粒细胞（PMN）和单核细胞（MNC），也能抑制 PHA 诱导的淋巴细胞增殖。黄芩免疫抑制作用的环节如下。①稳定肥大细胞膜，减少炎症介质释放。②影响花生四烯酸代谢，抑制炎症介质的生成。其免疫抑制作用主要有效成分为黄芩苷、黄芩素等。

1) Immunosuppression　*Huáng qín* has a significant inhibitory effect on type Ⅰ allergy (anaphylaxis). It can inhibit the release of polymorphonuclear neutrophils(PMN) and Monocyte(MNC) activated by N-Fomyl-Met-Leu-Phe (FMLP) and yeast polysaccharide, and can also inhibit lymphocyte proliferation induced by PHA. The mechanisms of immunosuppressive effect of *Huáng qín* include the followings. ①Stabilizing the mast cell membrane and reducing the release of inflammatory mediators. ②Affecting the metabolism of arachidonic acid and inhibiting the formation of inflammatory mediators. Baicalin and baicalein are suggested to be the main effective components of immunosuppression.

（2）免疫增强　黄芩苷在 10～320μg/ml 浓度范围可增强 NK 细胞活性，当浓度大于 640μg/ml 时，NK 细胞活性明显降低。黄芩苷及黄芩素均能抑制免疫缺陷病毒 –1（HIV-1）及免疫缺陷病毒反转录酶（HIV-1 RT）的活性，黄芩素作用强于黄芩苷。

2) Immune enhancement　Baicalin can enhance NK cell activity in the concentration range of 10-320μg/ml, When the concentration is higher than 640μg/ml, the activity of NK cells is decreased significantly. Baicalin and baicalin can inhibit the activity of immunodeficiency virus (HIV-1) and HIV-1 reverse transcriptase, and baicalin has a stronger effect than baicalin.

4. 保肝、利胆　黄芩对半乳糖胺、四氯化碳、士的宁诱导的肝损伤有保护作用。其保肝作用与抗氧自由基损伤有关，可增加小鼠肝匀浆中谷胱甘肽过氧化物酶（GSH-Px）的活性，降低过氧化脂质（LPO）的含量，可抑制氯化亚铁和抗坏血酸的混合物激活的小鼠肝脏脂质过氧化。保肝主要有效成分是黄芩苷和黄芩素。黄芩及黄芩素等可增加胆汁排泄。

(4) Hepatoprotection and cholagogic effects　*Huáng qín* can protect liver injury induced by galactosamine, carbon tetrachloride and strychnine. The hepatoprotection of *Huáng qín* is related to preventing the damage induced by oxygen free radical, which can increase the activity of glutathione peroxidase (GSH-Px), and reduce the content of lipid peroxide (LPO) in liver of mice. It can also inhibit the lipid peroxidation of liver activated by the mixture of ferrous chloride and ascorbic acid in mice. Baicalin and baicalein are suggested to be the main effective ingredients of hepatoprotection. *Huáng qín* and baicalein can increase bile secretion.

5. 抗凝血　黄芩素、汉黄芩素、千层纸素 A、黄芩新素Ⅱ等通过抑制凝血酶诱导的纤维蛋白原转化为纤维蛋白，对抗胶原、ADP、花生四烯酸诱导的血小板聚集，产生抗凝血作用。

(5) Anticoagulation　Baicalein, wogonin, oroxylin A, skullcapfavone Ⅱ can inhibit the conversion of fibrinogen to fibrin induced by thrombin. It can resist the platelet aggregation induced by collagen,

ADP and arachidonic acid, which shows anticoagulant effect.

6. 降血脂、抗动脉粥样硬化　黄芩具有改善脂质代谢、抗动脉粥样硬化作用。汉黄芩素、黄芩新素Ⅱ可升高高脂血症大鼠血清中高密度脂蛋白胆固醇（HDL-C）水平，降低血清总胆固醇（TC）水平；黄芩苷、黄芩素能降低血清甘油三酯（TG）含量。

(6) Antilipidemic and antiatherogenic effects　*Huáng qín* can improve lipid metabolism and resist atherosclerosis. Wogonin and skullcapflavone Ⅱ can increase high density lipoprotein cholesterol (HDL-C) level and reduce total cholesterol (TC) level in serum of experimental hyperlipidemia rats. Baicalein and baicalein can reduce the content of serum triglyceride (TG).

7. 影响心血管系统

(7) Effects on cardiovascular system

（1）扩张血管　黄芩苷可对抗 NE 和 KCl 及 $CaCl_2$ 所致的大鼠离体主动脉条收缩；黄芩茎叶总黄酮能对抗垂体后叶素致大鼠心肌缺血，并可增加离体豚鼠的冠脉血流量。其扩血管作用与阻滞钙通道有关。

1) Vasodilation Baicalin has vasodilatory effect　It can resist the contraction of aortic strips of rat induced by NE, KCl and $CaCl_2$ *in vitro*. The total flavones of *Huáng qín* can antagonize the myocardial ischemia induced by pituitrin in rats and increase the coronary blood flow of guinea pigs. Its vasodilatory effect is related to the blocking of calcium ion channels.

（2）抑制心肌收缩　黄芩苷可抑制心肌收缩，降低心肌耗氧量。

2) Inhibiting myocardial contractility　Baicalin can inhibit myocardial contraction and reduce myocardial oxygen consumption.

（3）抗心律失常　黄芩苷对乌头碱及冠脉结扎复灌性诱发大鼠心律失常、毒毛花苷 G 诱发豚鼠心律失常及电刺激家兔心脏诱发室颤均有明显的对抗作用。

3) Artiarrhthmia　Baicalin has antiarrhythmic effect. It has obvious antagonistic effect on arrhythmia induced by aconitine or coronary ligation and reperfusion in rats, arrhythmia induced by ouabain in guinea pigs and ventricular fibrillation induced by electrical stimulation in rabbits.

8. 其他作用　黄芩中黄酮类化合物还具有抗脂质过氧化作用、利尿作用等。

(8) Other effects　The flavonoids in *Huáng qín* also have anti-lipid peroxidation and diuretic effects.

【**不良反应 / Adverse effects**】

黄芩水煎剂口服不良反应较少，犬口服浸剂每日 15g/kg，连续 8 周，除可见粪便稀软外，未见其他明显毒性。

Oral administration of *Huáng qín* decoction has little adverse reaction. Dogs orally administered *Huáng qín* decoction 15g/kg daily for 8 weeks, no obvious toxicity was found except visible soft feces.

黄连 ┊ *Huáng lián* (*Rhizoma Coptidis*)

【**来源 / Origin**】

本品为毛茛科植物黄连 *Cogtis chinensis* Franch.、三角叶黄连 *Coptis deltoidea* G. Y. Cheng et. Hsian.，或云连 *Coptic teata* Wall. 的干燥根茎。主产于中国中部及南部各省。秋季采收 5~7 年的植株，除去苗叶、须根，干燥，生用。

Huáng lián is the dried rhizome of *Cogtis chinensis* Franch., *Coptis deltoidea* G. Y. Cheng et. Hsian., and *Coptic teata* Wall. The plant is mainly cultivated in central and southern provinces of China. 5~7 years old *huáng lián* is harvested in autumn. After shoot, leaf and fibrous root are removed, the sun dried roots are used for Chinese medicinal preparation.

【化学成分 / Chemical ingredients 】

黄连根茎含有多种生物碱，包括小檗碱（berberine，又称黄连素）、黄连碱（coptisine），掌叶防己碱（palmatine，又称巴马亭）、药根碱（jatrorrhizine）、表小檗碱（epiberberine）、甲基黄连碱（worenine）、非洲防己碱（columbamine）、木兰花碱（magnoflorine）等。其中以小檗碱含量最高，黄连、三角叶黄连及云连中含量均超过 4%。此外，尚含有阿魏酸（ferulic acid）和绿原酸（chlorogenic acid）等。

The main chemical ingredients of *Huáng lián* are alkaloids, including berberine, coptisine, palmatine, jatrorrhizine, epiberberine, worenine, columbamine and magnoflorine, etc. The content of berberine is the highest, there is more than 4% in *Coptis chinensis*, *Coptis deltoides* and *Coptis teata*. In addition, it also contains ferulic acid and chlorogenic acid.

【药性与功效 / Chinese medicine properties 】

味苦，性寒，归心、脾、胃、肝、胆、大肠经。具有清热燥湿、泻火解毒之功效。主治湿热痞满、呕吐、泻痢、黄疸、高热神昏、心火亢盛、心烦不寐、血热吐衄、目赤吞酸、牙痛、消渴、痈肿疔疮，外用可治疗湿疹、湿疮。

In Chinese medicine theory, *Huáng lián* has the nature of bitter and cold. It can enter the meridians of heart, spleen, stomach, liver, gallbladder, and large intestine. *Huáng lián* can clear heat, dry damp, purge fire and remove toxin. Clinically it can be used for stuffiness and fullness due to damp-heat, emesis, diarrhea, jaundice, hyperthermia and coma, heart-fire hyperactivity, vexation and insomnia, vomiting and epistaxis due to blood heat, red eyes and acid swallow, toothache, consumptive thirsty, abscess and furuncle; it can be used externally to treat eczema.

【药理作用 / Pharmacological effects 】

1. 抗病原微生物　黄连体外对多种细菌、真菌等有抑制或杀灭作用，黄连及小檗碱能提高机体对细菌内毒素的耐受能力。黄连煎液及小檗碱在体外及体内均有抗阿米巴原虫作用；小檗碱对多种流感病毒有抑制作用。其抗菌机制主要如下。①抑制菌体核酸的功能。②抑制菌体功能蛋白酶的活性。③抑制菌体分裂。④降低细菌致病性等。

(1) Anti-pathogenic microorganisms　*Huáng lián* can inhibit or kill many kinds of bacteria and fungi *in vitro*. *Huáng lián* and berberine can improve the tolerance to bacterial endotoxin. *Huáng lián* decoction and berberine can resist amoeba *in vitro* and *in vivo*. Berberine has inhibitory effect on a variety of flu virus. Its antibacterial mechanisms mainly includes the followings. ①Inhibiting the function of bacterial nucleic acid. ②Inhibiting the activity of bacterial functional protease. ③Inhibiting the division of bacteria. ④ Reducing the pathogenicity of bacteria, etc.

2. 止泻　黄连及小檗碱能对抗大肠埃希菌、霍乱毒素所致的腹泻及蓖麻油、番泻叶引起的非感染性腹泻，减轻小肠绒毛水肿、分泌亢进等炎症反应，降低动物死亡率。

(2) Antidiarrheal effects　*Huáng lián* and berberine can resist diarrhea caused by *E. coli* or cholera toxin and non-infectious diarrhea caused by castor oil or senna leaf. It can reduce the edema and hypersecretion of intestinal villi, and reduce the mortality of animals.

3. 抗炎、解热　黄连对急、慢性炎症均有抑制作用。皮下注射小檗碱对二甲苯致小鼠耳肿胀、醋酸致小鼠腹腔毛细血管通透性增加、组胺致大鼠皮肤毛细血管通透性增加、角叉菜胶致大鼠足跖肿胀等急性炎症及棉球肉芽肿等慢性炎症均有抑制作用。小檗碱抗炎机制包括如下几方面。①抑制趋化因子 ZAP 诱导的中性粒细胞趋化，抑制酵母多糖诱导的多形核白细胞活化。②降低中性粒细胞中磷脂酶 A_2（PLA_2）的活性，减少炎症介质的生成。③减少炎症组织中前列腺素

E_2（PGE_2）生成。黄连抗炎作用的主要活性成分是小檗碱、药根碱及黄连碱。黄连注射液通过抑制中枢发热介质 cAMP 的生成或释放，降低白细胞致热原所致发热家兔的体温。

(3) Anti-inflammation and antipyresis *Huáng lián* can inhibit acute and chronic inflammation. Subcutaneous injection of berberine can inhibit acute inflammation, such as xylene-induced ear swelling in mice, acetic acid-induced increase of capillary permeability in abdominal cavity of mice, histamine-induced increase of capillary permeability in rat skin, carrageenan-induced foot swelling of rats, and chronic inflammation of cotton ball granuloma. The anti-inflammatory mechanism of berberine includes the followings. ①Inhibiting neutrophil chemotaxis induced by chemokine ZAP, inhibiting the activation of polymorphonuclear leukocytes induced by yeast polysaccharide. ②Reducing the activity of phospholipase A_2 (PLA_2) in neutrophils, reducing the production of inflammatory mediators. ③Reducing the production of prostaglandin E_2 (PGE_2) in inflammatory tissue. Berberine, jatrorrhizine and coptisine are suggested to be the main anti-inflammatory components of *Huáng lián*. *Huáng lián* can reduce the body temperature of rabbits caused by leukocyte pyrogen by inhibiting the production and release of cAMP in CNS.

4. 抗消化性溃疡　黄连及小檗碱具有抗实验性胃溃疡作用。对应激性溃疡及阿司匹林–乙醇、盐酸–乙醇所致大鼠胃黏膜损伤有保护作用，并可促进溃疡面愈合。小檗碱抗溃疡作用与其抑制胃酸分泌和抗幽门螺杆菌作用有关。

(4) Anti-peptic ulcer effects　*Huáng lián* and berberine have anti-gastrohelcosis effect. It has protective effect against ulcer induced by stress and gastric mucosal injury induced by aspirin-ethanol and hydrochloric acid-ethanol, and can promote the healing of ulcer surface. The anti-ulcer effect of berberine is related to its inhibition of gastric acid secretion and anti-*helicobacter pylori* effect.

5. 降血糖　黄连水煎液及小檗碱口服可降低正常小鼠的血糖。小檗碱可降低葡萄糖和肾上腺素引起的血糖升高，对自发性糖尿病 KK 小鼠及四氧嘧啶性糖尿病小鼠也有降血糖作用，并能改善 KK 小鼠的糖耐量。小檗碱降血糖的同时改善糖尿病性并发症，通过提高机体抗氧化及清除自由基能力，防止糖尿病肾病及血管病变。小檗碱降血糖作用机制主要是抑制肝脏糖异生和（或）促进外周组织的葡萄糖酵解。

(5) Hypoglycemic effects　Orally administered *Huáng lián* decoction and berberine can reduce the blood glucose of normal mice. Berberine can treat hyperglycemia caused by glucose and adrenaline, and also has hypoglycemic effect on spontaneous diabetic KK mice and alloxan-induced diabetic mice, and can improve the glucose tolerance of KK mice. Berberine can improve diabetic complications while lowing blood sugar. The diabetic nephropathy and angiopathy can be prevented by improving the ability of antioxidation and scavenging free radicals. The hypoglycemic mechanism of berberine is mainly to inhibit glycogenesis of liver and (or) to promote glycolysis of peripheral tissues.

6. 抗肿瘤　黄连中小檗碱对裸鼠鼻咽肿瘤移植瘤有抑制作用。小檗碱对艾氏腹水癌及淋巴瘤 NK/LY 细胞有抑制作用。黄连抗肿瘤作用主要表现为细胞毒作用，还与促进癌细胞分化，抑制癌细胞呼吸，阻碍癌细胞嘌呤和核酸的合成，干扰癌细胞代谢等途径有关。

(6) Antitumor effects　*Huáng lián* has inhibitory effect on transplanted tumor of nasopharynx in nude mice. Berberine can inhibit the proliferation of Ehrlich ascites carcinoma and lymphoma natural killer cell/ lymphocyte (NK/ LY) cells *in vitro*. The anti-tumor effect of *Huáng lián* is cytotoxic effect. In addition, promoting the differentiation of cancer cells, inhibiting the respiration, the synthesis of purine and nucleic acid of cancer cells, and interfering with the metabolism of cancer cells are involved in the anti-tumor effects of *Huáng lián*.

7. 影响心血管系统

(7) Effects on the cardiovascular system

（1）正性肌力　小檗碱在 0.1~300μmol/L 的浓度范围内剂量依赖性地对动物离体及整体心脏产生正性肌力作用，加快衰竭心脏的左心室内压变化最大速率，增加心输出量，降低左室舒张末压，减慢心率，有抗心力衰竭作用。其作用与增加心肌细胞内 Ca^{2+} 浓度有关。但用量过大则阻滞钙通道，导致心肌收缩力下降。

1) Positive inotropic action　Berberine in the concentration range of 0.1-300μmol/L has a positive inotropic effect on the heart in a dose-dependent manner *in vivo* and *in vitro*. For heart failure, it can accelerate the maximum rate of change of left ventricular internal pressure, increase cardiac output, reduce left ventricular end diastolic pressure, and slow heart rate. Its effect is related to the increase of Ca^{2+} concentration in cardiomyocytes. However, if the dosage is too large, the calcium channel will be blocked, resulting in the decrease of myocardial contractility.

（2）抗心律失常　小檗碱静脉注射可使清醒大鼠心率先加快而后缓慢持久地减慢，小檗碱能防治 $CaCl_2$、乌头碱、$BaCl_2$、肾上腺素、电刺激及冠状动脉结扎所致的心律失常（室性期前收缩、心室颤动）。小檗碱抗心律失常作用与抑制心肌 Na^+ 内流，阻滞 Ca^{2+} 通道，从而降低心肌自律性、延长动作电位时程及有效不应期，消除折返冲动等有关。

2) Antiarrhythmia　Berberine can make the heart rate of conscious rats speed up first and then slow down slowly and persistently. Berberine can prevent and treat arrhythmia (ventricular premature beat, ventricular fibrillation) caused by $CaCl_2$, aconitine, $BaCl_2$, adrenaline, electrical stimulation and coronary artery ligation. The antiarrhythmic effect is related to the inhibition of myocardial Na^+ influx, the blocking of Ca^{2+} channel, the reduction of myocardial automaticity, the prolongation of action potential duration and effective refractory period, and the elimination of reentry impulse.

（3）降压　小檗碱对清醒和麻醉动物有降血压作用，这与小檗碱竞争性拮抗 α 受体有关。黄连所含的巴马亭、药根碱、木兰花碱等也有降血压作用。

3) Hypotensive effect　Because of the competitive antagonism of α receptor, berberine has hypotensive effect on conscious and anesthetized animals. Palmatine, jatrorrhizine and magnoflorine also have hypotensive effect.

8. 其他作用　黄连和小檗碱还具有抗心肌缺血、抗脑缺血、抗血小板聚集、镇静、催眠作用。

(8) Other effects　*Huáng lián* and berberine also have the effects of anti-myocardial ischemia, anti-cerebral ischemia, anti-platelet aggregation, sedation and hypnosis.

【不良反应 / Adverse effects】

黄连粗提取物小鼠灌胃的 LD_{50} 为 2.95g/kg。黄连总生物碱的小鼠急性毒性远大于黄连粗提取物，0.28g/kg 即可引起所有受试小鼠死亡。黄连中小檗碱、黄连碱、掌叶防己碱和药根碱是黄连引起毒性的主要成分，其中以小檗碱毒性最强。

The LD_{50} of *Huáng lián* extract was 2.95g/kg by intragastric administration in mice. The acute toxicity of total alkaloid of *Huáng lián* is much greater than that of *Huáng lián* extract. Total alkaloid (0.28g/kg) could cause all mice to die. Berberine, coptisine, palmatine and jatrorrhizine are suggested to be the main toxic components, among which berberine is the most toxic.

苦参　┆　*Kǔ shēn (Radix Sophorae Flavescentis)*

【来源 / Origin】

本品为豆科植物苦参 *Sophora flavescens* Ait. 的干燥根。中国各地均产。春秋二季采收，去除芦头、须根，洗净，切片，晒干，生用。

Kǔ shēn is the dried root of *Sophora flavescens* Ait.. The plant is mainly cultivated in all over China. It is harvested in spring and autumn. After stem and fibrous root are removed, the sun dried roots are used for Chinese medicinal preparation.

【化学成分 / Chemical ingredients】

主要成分为生物碱和黄酮类，具有药理活性的生物碱主要是苦参碱（matrine）、氧化苦参碱（oxymatrine）、槐果碱（sophocarpine）、槐胺碱（sophoramine）及槐定碱（sophoridine）。黄酮类成分有苦参醇（kurarinol）、苦参素（kusherin）等。此外，尚含有三萜皂苷、二烷基色原酮、氨基酸、脂肪酸、蔗糖等。

The main chemical ingredients of *Kǔ shēn* are alkaloids and flavonoids, and its main pharmacological components in alkaloids are matrine, oxymatrine, sophocarpine, sophoramine and sophoridine. The flavonoids are kurarinol, kusherin and so on. In addition, it also contains triterpenoid saponins, dialkyl chromones, amino acids, fatty acids, sucrose, etc.

【药性与功效 / Chinese medicine properties】

味苦、性寒，归心、肝、胃、大肠、膀胱经。具有清热燥湿、杀虫、利尿的功效。主治热痢便血、黄疸、尿闭、赤白带下、阴肿阴痒、湿疹、皮肤瘙痒、疥癣麻风。

In Chinese medicine theory, *kǔ shēn* has the nature of bitter and cold. It can enter the meridians of heart, liver, stomach, large intestine, and bladder. *Kǔ shēn* can clear heat, dry damp, kill insects and increase urination. Clinically it can be used for hematochezia due to heat dysentery, jaundice, anuresis, leukorrheal diseases, pudendal swelling and itching, eczema, skin itching, scabies and leprosy.

【药理作用 / Pharmacological effects】

1. 抗病毒　苦参总碱在体内外均有抗柯萨奇 B_3 型病毒的作用。体外可减轻该病毒引起的细胞病变，体内可抑制病毒在心肌中增殖，延长感染小鼠存活时间，其抗病毒机制与抑制蛋白质合成有关。

(1) **Antiviral effect**　Total alkaloids of *Kǔ shēn* have antiviral effect on Coxsackie B_3 virus *in vitro* and *in vivo*, which can alleviate the cytopathy caused by the virus *in vitro*, and inhibit the proliferation of the virus in myocardium and prolong the survival time of infected mice. The antiviral mechanism is related to the inhibition of protein synthesis.

2. 抗炎、解热　苦参水煎液及苦参生物碱均有抗炎作用，能抑制大鼠蛋清性足肿胀。苦参碱及氧化苦参碱对正常小鼠和摘除肾上腺小鼠，均能抑制巴豆油和冰醋酸诱发的炎症，其抗炎作用不依赖垂体–肾上腺系统。苦参注射给药可降低正常大鼠体温和四联菌苗引起的家兔体温升高。

(2) **Anti-inflammatory and antipyretic effects**　*Kǔ shēn* decoction and alkaloids have anti-inflammatory effect, which can inhibit egg white-induced foot swelling in rat. Matrine and oxymatrine can inhibit the inflammation induced by croton oil and glacial acetic acid in normal and adrenalectomized mouse. Its anti-inflammatory effect does not depend on the pituitary-adrenal system. Injection of *Kǔ shēn* can low the body temperature of normal rats and the fervescence of rabbits caused by tetralogy vaccine.

3. 免疫抑制　苦参生物碱具有免疫抑制作用。体外能抑制小鼠脾脏 T 淋巴细胞增殖及白细胞介素 2（IL-2）的生成或释放。体内可抑制小鼠腹腔巨噬细胞的吞噬能力，降低马血清致豚鼠过敏性休克的死亡率。苦参碱的作用比槐果碱强。

(3) **Immunosuppression effects**　Alkaloids of *Kǔ shēn* have immunosuppressive effect, which can inhibit the proliferation of spleen T cells and the production or release of IL-2 *in vitro*, and can also inhibit the phagocytosis of mouse peritoneal macrophages and reduce the mortality of anaphylactic shock

in guinea pigs caused by horse serum *in vivo*. Immunosuppressive effect of matrine is stronger than that of sophocarpine.

4. 抗肿瘤 苦参生物碱具有对抗小鼠移植性肿瘤作用，能延长艾氏腹水癌小鼠生存时间。对小鼠肉瘤 S_{180}、小鼠实体性宫颈癌（U_{14}）也有抑制作用。其抗肿瘤作用机制如下。①诱导癌细胞凋亡。②促进癌细胞分化。③抑制癌细胞 DNA 合成。④直接细胞毒作用。

(4) Antitumor effects Alkaloids of *Kǔ shēn* have antitumor effects on transplanted tumor mice, which can prolong the survival time of mice with Ehrlich ascites carcinoma, and also can inhibit sarcoma S_{180} and substantive cervical cancer (U_{14}) in mice. Its antitumor mechanism includes the followings. ①Inducing apoptosis of cancer cells. ②Increasing differentiation of cancer cells. ③Inhibiting synthesis of cell DNA. ④Direct cytotoxic effects.

5. 抗心律失常 苦参能对抗乌头碱、毒毛花苷 G、儿茶酚胺类药物、氯化钡及结扎冠脉诱发的大鼠心律失常。苦参生物碱抗心律失常作用的电生理学基础包括降低异位节律点自律性、消除折返冲动（减慢传导）及 β 受体阻断作用等。

(5) Antiarrhythmic effects *Kǔ shēn* has antiarrhythmic effect in rat induced by aconitine, ouabain, catecholamine, barium chloride and ligation coronary. The electrophysiological basis of the antiarrhythmic effect of alkaloids of *Kǔ shēn* includes reducing the self-regulation of heterotopic rhythm points, eliminating the reentry impulse (slowing down conduction) and β receptor blocking effect.

6. 抗心肌缺血 苦参能减轻垂体后叶素引起的急性心肌缺血，抑制 T 波低平等心电图缺血性变化。苦参抗心肌缺血作用与其扩张冠脉及外周血管，增加心肌血氧供应和降低心肌耗氧量有关。

(6) Anti-myocardial ischemia effects *Kǔ shēn* can alleviate the acute myocardial ischemia caused by pituitrin and inhibit the ischemic changes of ECG like low T wave. The anti-myocardial ischemia effect of *Kǔ shēn* is related to the dilation of coronary and peripheral vessels, the increase of myocardial oxygen supply and the decrease of myocardial oxygen consumption.

7. 其他作用 苦参还有平喘、抗溃疡、镇静和保肝的作用。

(7) Other effects *Kǔ shēn* has anti-asthmatic effect, anti-ulcer effect, sedative effect and hepatoprotective effect.

【不良反应 / Adverse effects】

苦参总碱 0.5~1.82g/kg 灌胃，小鼠出现间歇性抖动和痉挛，进而呼吸抑制甚至死亡，LD_{50} 为 586.2 ± 80.46mg/kg；小鼠腹腔注射 LD_{50} 为 147.2 ± 14.8mg/kg。苦参碱小鼠肌内注射 LD_{50} 为 74.15 ± 6.14mg/kg；氧化苦参碱小鼠肌内注射 LD_{50} 为 256.74 ± 57.36mg/kg；苦参总黄酮小鼠静脉注射的 LD_{50} 为 103.1 ± 7.66g/kg。

After gavaging total alkaloids of *Kǔ shēn* in the range of 0.5-1.82g/kg, mice show intermittent shaking and spasm, and then respiratory depression or even death, its LD_{50} is 586.2 ± 80.46mg/kg. The LD_{50} of intraperitoneal injection of total alkaloids of *Kǔ shēn* is 147.2 ± 14.8mg/kg. The LD_{50} of intramuscular administration of matrine is 74.15 ± 6.14mg/kg. The LD_{50} of intramuscular administration of oxymatrine is 256.74 ± 57.36mg/kg. The LD_{50} of intravenous injection of total flavonoids of *Kǔ shēn* is 103.1 ± 7.66g/kg.

金银花 ┊ *Jīn yín huā* (*Flos Lonicerae*)

【来源 / Origin】

本品为忍冬科木质藤本植物忍冬（*Lonicera japonica* Thunb.）的花蕾。中国各地均有分布。夏初花含苞未开时采收，阴干，生用。

Jīn yín huā is the dry flower bud of *Lonicera japonica* Thunb. The plant is distributed throughout China. At the beginning of summer, it is harvested when they are still in bud. The sun dried flowers in the shade is used for Chinese medicinal preparation.

【化学成分 / Chemical ingredients】

主要活性成分为绿原酸类化合物，如绿原酸（chlorogenic acid）和异绿原酸（isochlorogenic acid）。此外，尚含有机酸类、黄酮类如木犀草素（luteolin）、三萜皂苷类如忍冬苷（loniceoside）和无机元素。

Main active components of *Jīn yín huā* are chlorogenic acid compounds, such as chlorogenic acid and isochlorogenic acid. In addition, it also contains organic acid, flavonoids (e.g., luteolin), triterpene saponins（e. g., loniceoside）and inorganic elements.

【药性与功效 / Chinese medicine properties】

味甘，性寒，归肺、心、胃经。具有清热解毒的功效。主治外感发热、疮痈疖肿、热毒泻痢。

In Chinese medicine theory, *Jīn yín huā* is sweet in taste and cold in nature, and attributive to lung, stomach and large intestine channels. *Jīn yín huā* can clear heat and remove toxin. Clinically, it can be used for fever due to exogenous infection, sores, furuncle, diarrhea due to heat toxin.

【药理作用 / Pharmacological effects】

1. 抗病原微生物 金银花煎剂对溶血性链球菌、大肠埃希菌、志贺菌属、铜绿假单胞菌、伤寒杆菌、副伤寒杆菌、霍乱弧菌、肺炎链球菌、脑膜炎奈瑟菌、百日咳鲍特菌等常见致病菌均有一定的抑菌作用。绿原酸和异绿原酸是金银花主要抗菌成分。金银花水提物还具有抵抗呼吸道合胞病毒、H1N1甲型流感病毒、疱疹病毒、腺病毒的作用，其作用机制与直接灭活、阻止病毒吸附和抑制生物合成等有关。

(1) **Anti-pathogenic microorganisms** *Jīn yín huā* water decoction has various degrees of antibacterial effect on a variety of common pathogenic bacteria such as *Hemolytic streptococcus*, *Escherichia coli*, *Shigella genera*, *Pseudomonas aeruginosa*, *Salmonella typhi*, *Salmonella paratyphi*, *Vibrio cholerae*, *Diplococcus pneumoniae*, *Neisseria meningitidis* and *Bordetella pertussis in vitro*. Chlorogenic acid and isochlorogenic acid are suggested to be the main antibacterial components of *Jīn yín huā*. *Jīn yín huā* water extract also has antiviral effect on respiratory syncytial virus, H1N1 influenza A virus, herpes virus, adenovirus. Its mechanism is related to direct inactivation of the virus, preventing virus adsorption and inhibiting virus biosynthesis.

2. 抗内毒素 金银花提取物绿原酸可减少内毒素引起的小鼠死亡数，对内毒素引起的发热有解热作用，并加速内毒素从血中清除。

(2) **Anti-endotoxin** Chlorogenic acid can reduce mortality of mice induced by endotoxin. It can alleviate the febrile reaction induced by endotoxin, accelerate the clearance of endotoxin from the blood.

3. 解热、抗炎 金银花煎剂对不同致热原所致发热有显著的解热效果。此外，金银花水提取物有明显的抗炎作用，对蛋清、角叉菜胶、二甲苯所致足跖水肿均具有抑制作用。

(3) **Antipyretic and anti-inflammatory effects** *Jīn yín huā* water decoction has significant antipyretic effects caused by different pyrogens. In addition, *Jīn yín huā* water extract has obvious anti-inflammatory effect which can inhibit the foot edema caused by egg white, carrageenan and xylene.

4. 增强免疫功能 金银花煎剂能促进白细胞、炎症细胞的吞噬功能，降低中性粒细胞体外分泌功能，恢复巨噬细胞的吞噬功能，提高淋巴细胞转化率（LTR），其作用与绿原酸有关。

(4) **Improve immune function** *Jīn yín huā* water decoction can promote the phagocytosis of leukocytes and inflammatory cells, reduce the secretion of neutrophils *in vitro*, restore the phagocytosis

of macrophages, and enhance the lymphocyte transformation rate (LTR). Chlorogenic acid is suggested to be the active ingredient for the enhancement of immune function.

5. 保肝、利胆　金银花中忍冬总皂苷通过加强对乙酰氨基酚在体内的解毒代谢，对其所致小鼠肝损伤有明显的保护作用，可减轻肝病理损伤。此外，金银花中的绿原酸类化合物具有显著的利胆作用，可增加小鼠的胆汁分泌。

(5) Hepatoprotection and cholagogic effects　The total saponins of *Jīn yín huā* can enhance the detoxification and metabolism of paracetamol *in vivo*, and can allieviate liver pathological injury it in mice. In addition, chlorogenic acid compounds in *Jīn yín huā* have a significant cholagogic effect, which can increase the bile secretion of mice.

6. 抗氧化　金银花的黄酮类成分具有明显的抗氧化活性。绿原酸成分具有还原铁离子、清除羟自由基的能力，也是其抗氧化作用的物质基础。金银花能修复自由基引起的损害，延缓细胞衰老，促进新陈代谢。

(6) Antioxidation　The flavonoids of *Jīn yín huā* have obvious antioxidative activity. Chlorogenic acid has the ability of reducing iron ions and scavenging hydroxyl radicals, which is also suggested to be the material basis for the antioxidation. *Jīn yín huā* can repair the damage caused by free radicals, delay cell aging and promote metabolism.

7. 其他作用　金银花尚具有抗肿瘤、抗血小板聚集、降血脂、抗早孕作用。

(7) Other effects　*Jīn yín huā* has some other pharmacological effects, such as anti-tumor, inhibition of platelet aggregation, hypolipidemia, abortifacient effect.

【不良反应 / Adverse effects】

金银花不良反应较少，水煎液口服无明显毒性。但含金银花的注射剂可引起过敏反应，甚至过敏性休克。

Jīn yín huā has less adverse reactions. The decoction of *Jīn yín huā* had no obvious toxicity. *Jīn yín huā* injection can cause allergic reaction, even anaphylactic shock.

大青叶与板蓝根 ┊ *Dà qīng yè and Bǎn lán gēn (Folium Isatidis and Radix Isatidis)*

【来源 / Origin】

大青叶为十字花科植物菘蓝（*Isatis indigotica* Fort.）的干燥叶；板蓝根为菘蓝的根。中国各地均有分布。夏秋二季采收叶片和根，晒干，生用。

Dà qīng yè is the dry leaves of *Isatis indigotica* Fort.; dry root of *Isatis indigotica* Fort. is called *Bǎn lán gēn*. The plant is distributed throughout the China. It is harvested in summer and autumn. The sun dried leaves and root are used for Chinese medicinal preparation.

【化学成分 / Chemical ingredients】

二者的主要化学成分有菘蓝苷（isatan B，又称大青素 B）、靛蓝（indigo）、靛玉红（indirubin）、多糖。菘蓝苷经弱碱水解生成吲哚醇，继而转化成靛蓝和果糖酮酸。

The main chemical ingredients of *Dà qīng yè* and *Bǎn lán gēn* are isatan B, indigo, indirubin, and polysaccharide, etc. Isatan B can be hydrolyzed by weak base to produce indole alcohol, which is then converted into indigo and fructone acid.

【药性与功效 / Chinese medicine properties】

味苦，性寒，归心、胃经。具有清热解毒、凉血消斑的功效。主治热毒入血，发斑神昏，咽喉肿痛，丹毒口疮。

In Chinese medicine theory, *Dà qīng yè* and *Bǎn lán gēn* have the nature of bitter and cold. They can enter the meridians of heart and stomach. Their functions include heat-clearing, detoxification, blood-cooling and removing ecchymosis, which cure toxic heat into the blood, coma, swollen sore throat, erysipelas and aphtha.

【药理作用 / Pharmacological effects】

1. 抗病原微生物　大青叶和板蓝根煎液具有广谱抗菌作用，对金黄色葡萄球菌、溶血性链球菌、大肠埃希菌、志贺菌属、流感嗜血杆菌、伤寒杆菌、肺炎链球菌、脑膜炎奈瑟菌、白喉棒状杆菌等常见致病菌有一定的抑制作用；还具有杀灭钩端螺旋体的作用。大青叶和板蓝根抗病毒作用确切，对H1N1甲型流感病毒、流行性乙型脑炎病毒、腮腺炎病毒、单纯疱疹病毒、H5N1禽流感病毒和柯萨奇病毒均有抑制作用。靛蓝、靛玉红是其抗病原微生物的有效成分。

(1) **Anti-pathogenic microorganisms** *Dà qīng yè* and *Bǎn lán gēn* water decoctions have an inhibitory effect on various bacteria, such as *Staphylococcus aureus*, *hemolytic streptococcus*, *Escherichia coli*, *Shigella spp.*, *Haemophilus influenzae*, *typhoid bacilli*, *diplococcus pneumoniae*, *Neisseria meningitidis* and *diphtheria bacilli*. *Dà qīng yè* and *Bǎn lán gēn* also have bactericidal action on Leptospira. The antiviral effect of *Dà qīng yè* and *Bǎn lán gēn* is definite, and they can inhibit H1N1 influenza A virus, epidemic encephalitis B virus, mumps virus, herpes simplex virus, H5N1 avian influenza virus and Coxsackie virus. Indigo and indirubin are suggested to be the effective components of anti-pathogenic microorganism.

2. 提高机体免疫功能　板蓝根多糖对特异性和非特异性免疫功能均有一定的增强作用，可增加正常小鼠脾脏重量；增加正常小鼠外周血白细胞、淋巴细胞数；提高单核巨噬细胞系统的吞噬能力，促进碳粒廓清；促进溶血素抗体生成。

(2) **Improving immune function** *Bǎn lán gēn* polysaccharide can improve the specific and non-specific immune function. It can increase the spleen weight of normal mice. It also can improve the amount of peripheral blood leukocytes and lymphocytes. It can enhance the phagocytosis of the reticuloendothelial system to promote the clearance of carbon particles. It can promote production of hemolysin antibody.

3. 抗内毒素　大青叶和板蓝根煎液可抑制内毒素所致实验动物发热及相关炎症介质和细胞因子释放，降低致死率。

(3) **Anti-endotoxin** *Dà qīng yè* and *Bǎn lán gēn* water decoctions can inhibit endotoxin-induced fever and release of related inflammatory mediators and cytokines, and reduce the mortality in animals.

4. 保肝　大青叶与板蓝根煎液具有保肝作用，靛蓝灌胃对四氯化碳引起的动物肝损伤有保护作用。

(4) **Hepatoprotection** *Dà qīng yè* and *Bǎn lán gēn* water decoctions have hepatoprotective effect. Indigo can protect against liver injury caused by carbon tetrachloride.

5. 其他作用　大青叶和板蓝根尚具有抗白血病、降血脂、抑制血小板聚集作用。

(5) **Other effects** *Dà qīng yè* and *Bǎn lán gēn* have some other pharmacological effects, such as anti-leukemia, hypolipidemia, inhibition of platelet aggregation.

【不良反应 / Adverse effects】

大青叶与板蓝根口服偶有胃肠道反应，如恶心、呕吐、食欲下降等。板蓝根注射液可引起过敏反应，如荨麻疹、多形红斑、过敏性皮炎、多发性肉芽肿、过敏性休克，甚至死亡。

Oral administration of *Dà qīng yè* and *Bǎn lán gēn* occasionally has gastrointestinal reactions, such as nausea, vomiting, loss of appetite, etc. *Bǎn lán gēn* injection can cause allergic reactions, such as urticaria, pleomorphic erythema, allergic dermatitis, multiple granuloma, anaphylactic shock, and even death.

鱼腥草 ┊ Yú xīng cǎo (Houttuynia Cordata)

【来源 / Origin】

本品为三白草科植物蕺菜（Houttuynia cordata Thunb.）的全草。分布于长江以南各省。夏秋二季采收，洗净，晒干，生用。

Yú xīng cǎo is the whole herb of Houttuynia cordata Thunb. The plant is mainly produced in provinces south of Yangtze River. It is harvested in summer and autumn. The sun dried the whole herb after washing is used for Chinese medicinal preparation.

【化学成分 / Chemical ingredients】

主要化学成分为挥发油。挥发油成分含癸酰乙醛（decanoylacetaldehyde，又称鱼腥草素）及月桂醛（lauraldehyde）等，鱼腥草的特殊气味与癸酰乙醛有关。此外，鱼腥草中还含有大量黄酮、钾盐、绿原酸（chlorogenic acid）。

Its main chemical compositions are volatile oil. Volatile oil components contain decanoylacetaldehyde and lauraldehyde, etc. The special odor of Yú xīng cǎo is related to decanoylacetaldehyde. In addition, it also contains flavonoids, potassium salts and chlorogenic acid.

【药性与功效 / Chinese medicine properties】

味辛，性微寒，归肺经。具有清热解毒、消痈排脓、利尿通淋的功效。主治肺痈咳吐脓血，肺热咳嗽，热毒疮疡，热淋。

In Chinese medicine theory, Yú xīng cǎo has the nature of acrid and cold. It can enter the meridian of lung channel. Yú xīng cǎo can clear heat and remove toxin, dissolve carbuncle and apocenosis, promote diuresis and relieve stranguria, which cure lung carbuncle-induced spitting pus and blood, lung-heat cough, heat toxin-induced ulcer and gonorrhea.

【药理作用 / Pharmacological effects】

1. 抗病原微生物　鱼腥草水提物体外对金黄色葡萄球菌、溶血性链球菌、肺炎链球菌、白喉棒状杆菌、流感杆菌、志贺菌属、大肠埃希菌均有抑制作用。鱼腥草抗菌主要活性成分为癸酰乙醛，因其化学性质不稳定，故鱼腥草鲜品抗菌作用优于干品。另外，鱼腥草水提物对结核分枝杆菌、单纯疱疹病毒、H1N1甲型流感病毒、埃可病毒具有抑制作用。

(1) Anti-pathogenic microorganisms　Yú xīng cǎo water extract has inhibitory effects on Staphylococcus aureus, Hemolytic streptococcus, Diphtheria bacillus, Haemophilus influenzae, Shigella genera and Escherichia. coli in vitro. The main antimicrobial active ingredient of Yú xīng cǎo is decanoylacetaldehyde. Because its chemical properties are unstable, the antimicrobial effect of fresh Yú xīng cǎo is better than that of dry products. In addition, Yú xīng cǎo water extract has inhibitory effects on Mycobacterium tuberculosis, herpes simplex virus, H1N1 influenza virus, and ECHO virus.

2. 解热、抗炎　鱼腥草注射液对酵母致大鼠发热及大肠埃希菌内毒素致家兔发热均有解热作用。鱼腥草水提物能抑制大鼠甲醛性足跖肿胀、巴豆油和二甲苯引起的小鼠耳肿胀及皮肤毛细血管通透性增加，以及醋酸致小鼠腹腔毛细血管通透性增加。

(2) Antipyretic and anti-inflammatory effects　Yú xīng cǎo injection has antipyretic effects on yeast-induced fever in rats and Escherichia. coli endotoxin-induced fever in rabbits. Yú xīng cǎo water extract can inhibit foot swelling induced by formaldehyde in rats, ear swelling and the increase of skin capillary permeability induced by croton oil and xylene in mice, and the increase of peritoneal capillary permeability induced by acetic acid in mice.

3. **影响免疫功能** 鱼腥草水提物体外可增强白细胞吞噬能力，对 X 线和环磷酰胺所致白细胞减少有调节作用。

(3) The effects on the immune function *Yú xīng cǎo* water extract can enhance the phagocytosis of leukocytes, protect against leukopenia induced by X-ray and cyclophosphamide.

4. **止咳、平喘** 鱼腥草水煎液对氨水引起的小鼠咳嗽有镇咳作用。鱼腥草挥发油有平喘作用，对卵白蛋白、慢反应物质（SRA-A）、乙酰胆碱（ACh）致敏豚鼠离体气管平滑肌有舒张作用。

(4) Antitussive and antiasthmatic effect *Yú xīng cǎo* water decoction has antitussive effect on ammonia-induced cough in mice. The volatile oil of *Yú xīng cǎo* has antiasthmatic effect, which can relax the isolated bronchial smooth muscle of guinea pigs sensitized by ovalbumin, slow reactive substance (SRA-A) and acetylcholine (ACh).

5. **利尿** 鱼腥草水煎液具有一定的利尿作用，能使毛细血管扩张，肾血流量增加，增加尿量，具有肾脏保护作用。

(5) Diuretic effects *Yú xīng cǎo* water decoction has a certain diuretic effect, which can make capillaries expand, increase renal blood flow, increase urine volume, and has renal protective effect.

6. **其他作用** 鱼腥草尚有抗内毒素、抗癌作用。

(6) Other effects *Yú xīng cǎo* has other pharmacological effects, such as anti-endotoxin and anti-tumor effects.

【不良反应 / Adverse effects】

鱼腥草毒性较小，口服有鱼腥臭味，肌内注射有刺激性，可引起疼痛。鱼腥草注射液可引起过敏反应，如皮疹、过敏性紫癜、恶寒、发热、胸闷、心悸、呼吸困难、肺水肿，甚至过敏性休克。

Yú xīng cǎo has less adverse effects. Orally administered *yú xīng cǎo* has fishy taste, and intramuscular injection with *Yú xīng cǎo* has irritation which can cause pain. *Yú xīng cǎo* injection can cause allergic reactions, such as rash, allergic purpura, aversion to cold, fever, chest tightness, palpitation, dyspnea, pulmonary edema, and even anaphylactic shock.

穿心莲 ┊ *Chuān xīn lián (Herba Andrographis)*

【来源 / Origin】

本品为爵床科植物穿心莲 [*Andrographis paniculata* (Burm. f.)Nees] 的全草。主产于中国华南、华东及西南各省。秋初刚开花时采收，切段，晒干，生用。

Chuān xīn lián is the whole herb of *Andrographis paniculata* (Burm. f.) Nees. The plant is mainly produced in south, east and southwest of China. It is harvested at the beginning of the autumn. The sun dried whole herb is used for Chinese medicinal preparation.

【化学成分 / Chemical ingredients】

主要有效成分为内酯类，内酯类化合物主要存在于穿心莲叶中，包括穿心莲内酯（andrographolide，又称乙素）、去氧穿心莲内酯（deoxy andrographolidc，又称甲素）、新穿心莲内酯（neoandrographolide，又称丙素）、脱水穿心莲内酯（dehydroandrogrepholide）。此外，尚含有黄酮类化合物，系多甲氧基黄酮（polymethoxy flavonoids），主要存在于穿心莲根中。

The main chemical compositions of *Chuān xīn lián* are lactones mainly contained in the leaf, including andrographolide, deoxy andrographolidc, neoandrographolide and dehydroandrogrepholide. In addition, *Chuān xīn lián* contains flavones, which are polymethoxy flavonoids, mainly contained in the root.

【药性与功效 / Chinese medicine properties】

味苦，性寒，归肺、胃、大肠、小肠经。具有清热解毒、燥湿的功效。主治发热头痛、肺热喘咳、咽喉肿痛，以及湿热泻痢、热淋、湿疹。

In Chinese medicine theory, *Chuān xīn lián* has the nature of bitter and cold. It can enter the meridians of lung, stomach, large intestine and small intestine. *Chuān xīn lián* can clear heat and remove toxin, dry dampness. Clinically, it can be used for fever, headache, cough and asthma due to lung-heat, sore throat, diarrhea, gonorrhea and eczema due to damp-heat.

【药理作用 / Pharmacological effects】

1. 抗病原微生物　穿心莲内酯类成分体外可抑制金黄色葡萄球菌和肺炎链球菌，对呼吸道合胞病毒、流感病毒也具有抑制作用。

(1) **Anti-pathogenic microorganisms**　Andrographolides can inhibit *Staphylococcus aureus* and *Diplococcus pneumoniae in vitro*. It also can inhibit respiratory syncytial virus and H1N1 influenza A virus.

2. 解热、抗炎　穿心莲内酯类成分可抑制伤寒、副伤寒杆菌引起的发热。此外，穿心莲内酯类成分对蛋清及角叉菜胶足跖注射致炎症大鼠模型均有抗炎作用。

(2) **Antipyretic and anti-inflammatory effects**　Andrographolides can inhibit the fever caused by *typhoid bacilli* and *paratyphoid bacilli*. In addition, andrographolides have anti-inflammatory effect on the inflammatory rat model induced by egg white and carrageenan.

3. 影响免疫功能　穿心莲内酯是一种具有调节机体非特异性免疫功能的免疫刺激剂。穿心莲内酯及黄酮类化合物肌内注射能增强 NK 细胞、单核巨噬细胞吞噬能力，并提高外周血溶菌酶活性，增强机体非特异性免疫功能。但穿心莲内酯灌胃给药能抑制单核巨噬细胞的吞噬功能，并使小鼠胸腺萎缩，显示免疫抑制作用。说明不同给药途径穿心莲对免疫功能影响也不同。

(3) **Effects on immunity function**　Andrographolide is a kind of immunostimulant which can enhance the non-specific immune function of body. Intramuscular injection of andrographolide and flavonoids can enhance the phagocytic capacity of NK cells and monocyte macrophages, and enhance the lysozyme activity in peripheral blood to enhance the non-specific immune function of the body. However, andrographolide orally administered can inhibit the phagocytic function of monocyte macrophages and atrophy the thymus of mice, showing immunosuppressive effects. This indicates that different administration of *Chuān xīn lián* has different effects on immune function.

4. 抗心肌缺血　穿心莲内酯能明显改善垂体后叶素所致实验性大鼠心肌缺血状态。同时对心肌缺血再灌注损伤具有保护作用，能降低心肌细胞内 Na^+ 和 Ca^{2+} 含量，降低 K^+ 和 Mg^{2+} 含量，减少心律失常发生，其机制与减轻氧自由基损害，改善心肌缺血再灌注过程中的离子紊乱有关。

(4) **Anti-myocardial ischemia**　Andrographolide can significantly improve the myocardial ischemia induced by pituitrin in rats. It also can protect myocardial ischemia-reperfusion injury, which can reduce the content of Na^+, Ca^{2+}, K^+, Mg^{2+} in cardiomyocytes, and reduce the occurrence of arrhythmias. Its mechanism is related to the reduction of oxygen free radical damage and improving the ion disorder during myocardial ischemia-reperfusion.

5. 抗肿瘤　穿心莲内酯对多种实验性移植性肿瘤有抑制作用，穿心莲黄酮本身虽无抗肿瘤作用，但能增强环磷酰胺的抗肿瘤作用。

(5) **Antitumor effect**　Andrographolide has an inhibitory effect on a variety of experimental transplanted tumor. The flavonoids of *Chuān xīn lián* have no antitumor effect, but they can enhance the antitumor effect of cyclophosphamide.

6. 保肝、利胆　穿心莲内酯能对抗四氯化碳所致的大鼠肝损伤，提高肝细胞存活率，降低血清中谷草转氨酶（AST）和谷丙转氨酶（ALT）水平。穿心莲内酯能明显促进大鼠和豚鼠胆汁分泌，增加胆酸和胆盐排泄。

(6) Hepatoprotection and cholagogic effects Andrographolide can resist the liver injury caused by carbon tetrachloride in rats, improve the survival rate of hepatocytes, and reduce the levels of glutamic oxalacetic transaminase (AST) and glutamic-pyruvic transaminase (ALT) in serum. Andrographolide also can significantly promote bile secretion in rats and guinea pigs, and increase bile acid and bile salt excretion

7. 其他作用 穿心莲尚具有抗氧化、拟胆碱样作用、终止妊娠等作用。

(7) Other effects *Chuān xīn lián* has the effects of antioxidation, cholinergic action-like and pregnancy termination effects.

【不良反应 / Adverse effects】

穿心莲口服可引起胃部不适、食欲减退等症状。含穿心莲注射液可引起过敏反应，严重者可引起过敏性休克。

Oral administration of *Chuān xīn lián* can cause stomach discomfort, anorexia and other symptoms. The injections containing *Chuān xīn lián* can cause allergic reactions, even cause anaphylactic shock in severe cases.

牛黄 ┊ *Niú huáng* (*Calculus Bovis*)

【来源 / Origin】

本品为牛科动物黄牛（*Bos taurus domesticus* Gmelin）的胆囊结石。由牛胆汁或猪胆汁经提取加工而成的称人工牛黄，用作天然牛黄的代用品。

Niú huáng is the gallstone of *Bos taurus domesticus* Gmelin. If it is made from bovine bile or pig bile by extracting and processing, it is then called artificial Calculus bovis, which is used as a substitute for natural Calculus bovis.

【化学成分 / Chemical ingredients】

天然牛黄的主要化学成分包括胆红素（bilirubin）及其钙盐、胆酸（cholicacid）、去氧胆酸（deoxycholicacid）及其盐类、胆甾醇（cholesterol）、麦角甾醇（ergosterd）、卵磷脂（lecithin）、脂肪酸（fatty acid）、维生素 D，以及无机元素钙、钠、铁、钾、铜、镁、磷等，其中胆红素含量高达 40% 以上。尚含类胡萝卜素及丙氨酸（alanine）、甘氨酸（glycine）、牛磺酸（taurine）、天冬氨酸（aspartic acid）、精氨酸（arginine）、亮氨酸（leucine）、蛋氨酸（methionine）等多种氨基酸及两种酸性肽类成分 SMC-S2 和 SMC-F。

The main chemical components of *Niú huáng* are bilirubin and its calcium salt, cholicacid, deoxycholicacid and its salts, cholesterol, ergosterd, lecithin, fatty acid, vitamin D, inorganic elements calcium, sodium, iron, potassium, copper, magnesium, phosphorus, etc., of which bilirubin content is over 40%. It also contains many amino acids such as carotenoid, alanine, glycine, taurine, aspartic acid, arginine, leucine, methionine and two acidic peptide components: SMC-S2 and SMC-F.

【药性与功效 / Chinese medicine properties】

味苦，性凉，归肝、心经。具有清热解毒、息风止痉、化痰开窍的功效。主治温热病及小儿惊风、壮热神昏、痉挛抽搐；痰热阻闭心窍所致神昏；热毒郁结所致咽喉肿痛、口舌生疮、痈疽疔毒证。

In Chinese medicine theory, *Niú huáng* has the nature of bitter, and cool. It can enter the meridians of liver and heart. *Niú huáng* can clear heat and remove toxin, stop wind to relieve convulsion, resolve phlegm for resuscitation. Clinically, it can be used for warm heat diseases and infantile convulsion, febrile unconsciousness, cramp and twitch; coma due to phlegm-heat blocking heart; swelling and pain in throat, sore in mouth and tongue, carbuncle and deep-rooted carbuncle due to heat-poison stagnation, etc.

【药理作用 / Pharmacological effects】

1. 抗病原微生物 牛黄中胆汁酸对结核分枝杆菌有抑制作用，去氧胆酸对四联球菌、金黄色葡萄球菌、脑膜炎奈瑟菌、溶血性链球菌也有相似的抑制作用。其机制可能与胆汁盐降低细菌细胞膜表面张力，破坏细菌细胞膜，裂解细菌，抑制细菌生长有关。牛黄中多种成分对流行性乙型脑炎病毒有不同程度的灭活作用。实验证明，小鼠皮下感染流行性乙型脑炎病毒，牛黄对感染小鼠有显著的保护作用。其中胆红素的抑制指数最高，去氧胆酸次之，胆酸较低，人工牛黄亦有效果。但牛黄对脑内感染的流行性乙型脑炎病毒无效。

(1) Anti-pathogenic microorganisms   Cholicacid in *Niú huáng* can inhibit *Mycobacterium tuberculosis*, and deoxycholicacid has similar inhibitory effect on *Micrococcus tetragenus*, *Staphylococcus aureus*, *Neisseria meningitidis* and *Streptococcus hemolyticus*. The mechanism may be related with the bile salts which reduce the surface tension of bacterial cell membrane, destroy the bacterial cell membrane and lysate the bacteria, inhibit the growth of bacteria. Various ingredients of *Niú huáng* have different degrees of inactivation of epidemic type B encephalitis virus. The experiment proved that *Niú huáng* had significant protective effect on mice subcutaneously infected with epidemic type B encephalitis virus. Among them, the inhibition index of bilirubin is high, followed by deoxycholicacid, and the cholicacid is low. Artificial Calculus bovis is also effective. However, *Niú huáng* is ineffective against epidemic type B encephalitis virus infection in the brain.

2. 抗炎 牛黄混悬液对实验性急性和慢性炎症均有抑制作用，能减轻二甲苯致小鼠耳肿胀及蛋清致大鼠足跖肿胀，且能降低醋酸所致小鼠腹腔毛细血管通透性增加。人工牛黄的抗炎作用与天然牛黄相似。

(2) Anti-inflammation   The suspension of *Niú huáng* has an inhibitory effect on experimental acute and chronic inflammation, which can reduce xylene-induced ear swelling in mice and egg white-induced foot swelling in rats, and acetic acid-induced the increase of capillary permeability in mice. The anti-inflammatory effect of artificial Calculus bovis is similar to that of natural Calculus bovis.

3. 解热 牛黄中胆酸和去氧胆酸均能降低酵母和 2,4– 二硝基酚所致发热大鼠体温，且能降低正常大鼠体温。牛磺酸是解热作用的主要成分。人工牛黄亦有相似作用。

(3) Antipyresis   Cholicacid and deoxycholicacid in *Niú huáng* can reduce the body temperature of rats with fever induced by yeast or 2,4-dinitrophenolin, and it can also reduce the body temperature of normal rats. Taurine is suggested to be the main active ingredient for antipyretic effect. The artificial Calculus bovis also has similar antipyretic effect.

4. 镇静、抗惊厥 牛黄中的牛磺酸和去氧胆酸具有明显镇静作用，能明显减少小鼠的自主活动次数，能减轻咖啡因引起的中枢兴奋，协同戊巴比妥钠起催眠作用，延长小鼠睡眠时间。牛磺酸可能为抑制性神经递质或神经调节剂（neuromodulator），能对抗印防己毒素、戊四氮等引起的小鼠惊厥，是牛黄抗惊厥作用的主要有效成分。人工牛黄亦有类似的镇静、抗惊厥作用。

(4) Sedation and anticonvulsion   Taurine and deoxycholicacid in *Niú huáng* have obvious sedative effect. It can significantly reduce the number of autonomous activities of mice and inhibit the central excitation caused by caffeine. It has the synergistic effect with the hypnotic effect of pentobarbital sodium, which prolong the sleeping time of mice. Taurine may be an inhibitory neurotransmitter or neuromodulator, which can resist the convulsion caused by picrotoxin (PCT) and pentylenetetrazol (PTZ) in mice, and it is the main active ingredient of *Niú huáng* for anticonvulsion. The artificial Calculus bovis also has similar sedation and anticonvulsion.

5. 其他作用 牛黄还具有强心、降压、镇咳、祛痰、平喘、利胆、解痉等药理作用。

(5) Other effects *Niú huáng* has other pharmacological effects, such as cardiotonic function, lowering blood pressure, antitussive and expectorant effect, relieving asthma, cholagogic effects and spasmolysis.

【不良反应 / Adverse effects 】

牛黄口服一般无毒，人工牛黄过量使用易引起腹泻，严重可导致昏迷而死亡；天然牛黄则很少腹泻。但静脉注射则产生严重的神经系统及心脏抑制，并发生溶血。孕妇慎服。

Oral administration of *Niú huáng* is generally less adverse effects, and the excessive use of artificial Calculus bovis is easy to cause diarrhea, even lead to coma and death; the natural Calculus bovis rarely causes diarrhea. But intravenous injection can produce serious inhibition of nervous system and heart, and hemolysis. Administration of *Niú huáng* should be with caution for pregnant women.

牡丹皮 ┆ *Mǔ dān pí (Cortex Moutan Radicis)*

【来源 / Origin 】

本品为毛茛科植物牡丹（*Paeonia suffruticosa* Andr.）的干燥根皮。主产于安徽、山东等省。秋季采收，去除须根、外皮，趁鲜湿剥去木心，晒干，生用。

Mǔ dān pí is the dried root bark of *Paeonia suffruticosa* Andr. The plant is mainly cultivated in Anhui province and Shandong province in China. It is harvested in autumn. The sun dried root with fibrous root removed and wood core peeled off while it's fresh are used for Chinese medicinal preparation.

【化学成分 / Chemical ingredients 】

主要成分有牡丹酚（paeonol，又称丹皮酚）、牡丹酚苷（paeonoside）、牡丹酚原苷（paeonolide）、芍药苷（paeoniflorin）、苯甲酰芍药苷（benzoylpaeoniflorin）、羟基芍药苷（oxypaeoniflnrin）、苯甲酰羟基芍药苷（benzoyl-oxypaeoniflorin）以及牡丹酚新苷（apiopaeonoside）。另外，尚含有 β– 谷甾醇（β-sitosterol）、胡萝卜苷（daucosterol）、齐墩果酸（oleanic acid）、白桦脂酸（betulic acid）、白桦脂醇（betulin）和挥发油等。

The main chemical ingredients of *Mǔ dān pí* are paeonol, paeonoside, paeonolide, paeoniflorin, benzoylpaeoniflorin, oxypaeoniflnrin, benzoyl-oxypaeoniflorin and apopaeonoside. In addition, it also contains β - sitosterol, daucosterol, oleanic acid, betulin and volatile oil, etc.

【药性与功效 / Chinese medicine properties 】

味苦、辛，性微寒，归心、肝、肾经。具有清热凉血、活血化瘀的功效。主治温毒发斑，吐血衄血，夜热早凉，无汗骨蒸，经闭痛经，痈肿疮毒，跌打伤痛。

In Chinese medicine theory, *Mǔ dān pí* has the nature of bitter, acrid and slightly cold. It can enter the meridians of heart, liver and spleen. *Mǔ dān pí* can clear heat, cool blood, invigorate blood and dissolve stasis. Clinically it can be used for skin rashes caused by virulent heat-evil, hematemesis and hemorrhage, fever in night and cool at dawn, steaming bone fever without sweating, amenorrhea, dysmenorrheal, carbuncle, contusions and traumatic injury.

【药理作用 / Pharmacological effects 】

1. 抗病原微生物 牡丹皮水提物和醇提物以及丹皮酚体外对金黄色葡萄球菌、溶血性链球菌、肺炎球菌、枯草杆菌、大肠埃希菌、伤寒杆菌、副伤寒杆菌、痢疾杆菌、变形杆菌、铜绿假单胞菌、百日咳鲍特菌及霍乱弧菌等有抑制作用，对皮肤真菌也有抑制作用。

(1) Anti-pathogenic microorganisms The water and alcohol extracts of *Mǔ dān pí* and paeonol have an inhibitory effect on *Staphylococcus aureus, Hemolytic streptococcus, Pneumococcus, Bacillus subtilis, Escherichia coli, Salmonella typhi, Salmonella paratyphi, Shigella dysenteriae, Proteusbacillus vulgaris, Pseudomonas aeruginosa, Bordetella pertussis* and *Vibrio cholerae*, as well as skin fungus *in vitro*.

2. 抗炎　牡丹皮水提物和总苷对实验性急性炎症有抑制作用。对弗氏完全佐剂性关节炎大鼠的原发性炎症反应和继发性炎症反应有抑制作用，对去肾上腺大鼠仍有显著的抗炎作用，其抗炎作用不依赖垂体–肾上腺系统功能，与其抑制炎症细胞游走，减少炎症组织前列腺素合成有关。抗炎主要活性成分为丹皮酚。

(2) Anti-inflammation Water extract and total glucosides of *Mǔ dān pí* have inhibitory effects on experimental acute inflammation. It can inhibit the primary inflammatory response and secondary inflammatory response of rats with Freund's complete adjuvant arthritis, and also has significant anti-inflammatory effect on adrenalectomized rats. Its effect does not depend on the pituitary-adrenal system, which is related to its inhibition of inflammatory cell migration and reduction of prostaglandin synthesis in inflammatory tissues. Paeonol is suggested to be the main active ingredient for anti-inflammation.

3. 调节免疫及抗过敏　丹皮酚及总苷具有免疫调节作用。丹皮酚可增强单核巨噬细胞功能，体外可促进刀豆蛋白A（ConA）诱导大鼠T淋巴细胞增殖反应及T淋巴细胞产生IL-2，还可促进脂多糖（LPS）诱导B淋巴细胞增殖反应及巨噬细胞产生IL-1。丹皮酚对特异性免疫功能有抑制作用，能降低脾细胞溶血素抗体水平。丹皮酚腹腔注射能抑制补体经典途径的溶血活性。

(3) Immune regulation and anti-allergy Paeonol and total glucosides have immunoregulatory effects. It can enhance the function of monocyte macrophages, promote the T-lymphocyte proliferation induced by ConA and the production of IL-2 by T-lymphocytes *in vitro*, and promote the B-lymphocyte proliferation and the production of IL-1 by peritoneal macrophages in rats induced by LPS. Meanwhile, it can also inhibit the specific immune function which reduce the level of hemolysin antibody in spleen cells. Intraperitoneal injection of paeonol can inhibit the hemolytic activity of complement in the classical pathway.

丹皮酚对实验性Ⅱ～Ⅳ变态反应均有抑制作用。腹腔注射丹皮酚能对抗大鼠被动皮肤过敏反应（PCA）及豚鼠Forssman皮肤血管炎反应，抑制由牛血清白蛋白（BSA）诱导的大鼠Arthus型足跖肿胀，抑制二硝基氟苯（DNFB）致迟发型小鼠耳郭接触性皮炎。

Paeonol has an inhibitory effect on experimental Ⅱ - Ⅳ allergic reactions. Intraperitoneal injection of paeonol can resist passive cutaneous anaphylaxis (PCA)in rats and the reaction of Forssman cutaneous vasculitis in guinea pig, inhibit the Arthus type plantar swelling induced by bovine serum albumin (BSA) in rats, and inhibit the dinitrofluorobenzene (DNFB) induced delayed auricular contact dermatitis in mice.

4. 对中枢神经系统的作用

(4) Effect on the central nervous system

（1）抗惊厥　丹皮酚对电刺激、戊四氮、士的宁、氨基脲所致小鼠惊厥有对抗作用，并可协同苯巴比妥起抗惊厥作用。

1) Anticonvulsant effects　Paeonol can inhibit convulsions induced by electricity, pentylenetetrazol, strychnine and semicarbazide in mice. There is synergistic effect with phenobarbital in anti-convulsion.

（2）镇痛　丹皮酚可提高热致痛小鼠痛阈，减少醋酸致痛小鼠的扭体反应次数，其镇痛作用无明显耐受现象和药物依赖性，且不被纳洛酮翻转。

2) Analgesic effects　Paeonol can increase the pain threshold in mice induced by heat and reduce the number of writing reactions in mice induced by acetic acid. Its analgesic effect has no obvious

tolerance and drug dependence, and was not reversed by naloxone.

（3）解热 牡丹皮对 2,4- 二硝基苯酚、内毒素、干酵母致大鼠发热有明显解热作用。

3) Antipyretic effects *Mŭ dān pí* has a significant antipyretic effect on fever induced by 2,4-dinitrophenol, endotoxin and dry yeast in rat.

5. 对心脑血管系统的作用

(5) Effect on the cardiovascular and cerebrovascular system

（1）抗血小板聚集 牡丹皮能抑制 ADP、胶原和肾上腺素诱导的健康人血小板聚集，减少血栓素 A_2（TXA_2）的生成。丹皮酚体内外均剂量依赖性地抑制凝血酶诱导的血小板聚集及 5-HT 释放。

1) Anti-platelet aggregation *Mŭ dān pí* can significantly inhibit the platelet aggregation induced by ADP, collagen and adrenaline, and reduce the production of thromboxane A_2 (TXA_2) in healthy persons. Paeonol can inhibit thrombin-induced platelet aggregation and 5-HT release in a dose-dependent manner *in vivo* and *in vitro*.

（2）改善血液流变学 丹皮酚可降低大鼠全血表观黏度，使血细胞比容降低，同时降低红细胞聚集性和血小板黏附性，使红细胞的变形能力显著增强。

2) Improving hemorheology Paeonol can reduce the whole blood apparent viscosity and hematocrit, decrease erythrocyte aggregation and platelet adhesiveness, and significantly enhance the deformability of red blood cells in rats.

（3）抗心肌缺血 牡丹皮可降低缺血心肌组织 MDA 含量和血中 CPK 浓度，增强心肌组织 SOD 活性，保持心肌细胞超微结构完整性。

3) Anti-myocardial ischemia *Mŭ dān pí* can reduce MDA content in ischemic myocardium and CPK concentration in blood, enhance SOD activity in myocardium and maintain the ultrastructural integrity of cardiomyocytes.

（4）抗动脉粥样硬化 丹皮酚可抑制高脂饲料所致实验性动脉粥样硬化斑块形成，可降低血清胆固醇（TC）、甘油三酯（TG）、低密度脂蛋白（LDL）、极低密度脂蛋白（VLDL）等含量，提高高密度脂蛋白（HDL）含量，抑制主动脉脂质斑块形成。

4) Anti-atherosclerosis Paeonol can inhibit the formation of experimental atherosclerotic plaque caused by high fat diet. It can reduce contents of serum cholesterol (TC), triglyceride (TG), low-density lipoprotein (LDL), and very low-density lipoprotein (VLDL), and increase the content of high-density lipoprotein (HDL), thus inhibiting formation of aortic lipid plaque.

（5）抗脑缺血 丹皮酚对大鼠反复性短暂脑缺血再灌注所致炎症反应引起的脑损伤具有保护作用。

5) Anti-cerebral ischemia Paeonol has a protective effect on the brain damage caused by inflammatory response induced by repeated transient cerebral ischemia-reperfusion in rat.

6. 保肝 丹皮总苷对异烟肼和利福平等所致小鼠肝损伤有保护作用，可降低血清 ALT、AST、肝匀浆脂质过氧化产物 MDA 的含量，提高血清和肝脏谷胱甘肽过氧化物酶活力，减轻肝细胞变性和坏死程度，并促进小鼠肝脏糖原合成和提高血清蛋白含量。

(6) Hepatoprotection Total glycosides of *Mŭ dān pí* can protect the liver injury of mice caused by isoniazid and rifampin, reduce the content of serum ALT, AST, and MDA of liver homogenate, improve glutathione peroxidase activity of serum and liver, reduce liver cell degeneration and necrosis, promote the synthesis of glycogen in mouse liver and increase the content of serum protein.

7. 降血糖 丹皮多糖可降低正常小鼠和葡萄糖诱发小鼠高血糖的血糖水平。

(7) Hypoglycemic effects　Polysaccharide of *Mǔ dān pí* can reduce the blood glucose level of normal mice and glucose-induced hyperglycemic mice.

8. 其他作用　牡丹皮还有抗肿瘤、抗早孕、降压、抗心律失常等作用。

(8) Other effects　*Mǔ dān pí* also has antitumor, anti-early pregnancy, hypotensive effect, and antiarrhythmic effect, etc.

【不良反应 / Adverse effects】

丹皮酚 50% 花生油剂小鼠灌胃的 LD_{50} 为 4.9 ± 0.47g/kg，腹腔注射的 LD_{50} 为 735mg/kg。丹皮酚磺酸钠小鼠腹腔注射的 LD_{50} 为 6.9g/kg。丹皮酚磺酸钠大鼠腹腔注射 250mg/kg、500mg/kg、750mg/kg，共 30 日，对肝肾功能均无明显影响，各脏器无异常病理改变，大剂量组胃黏膜出现水肿，但无溃疡发生。未发现该药有致畸作用。

The LD_{50} of 50% paeonol(diluted in peanut oil) is 4.9 ± 0.47g/kg by oral administration, 735mg/kg by intraperitoneal injection. The LD_{50} of paeonol sulfonate is 6.9g/kg by intraperitoneal injection. The rats are intraperitoneally injected with sodium paeonol sulfonate (250mg/kg, 500mg/kg, 750mg/kg) for 30 days, there is no significant effect on liver and kidney function, no abnormal pathological changes in organs. The gastric mucosa in the high dose group shows edema, but no ulcer. No teratogenic effect is found.

青蒿 ¦ *Qīng hāo* (Artemisia Apiacea)

【来源 / Origin】

本品为菊科植物黄花蒿（*Artemisia annua* L.）的干燥地上部分。中国各地均有分布。夏秋二季采收，切段，鲜用或阴干，生用。

Qīng hāo is the dry ground part of *Artemisia annua* L.. The plant is cultivated throughout China and harvested in summer and autumn. Fresh *Qīng hāo* or dry *Qīng hāo* after cutting into section is used for Chinese medicinal preparation.

【化学成分 / Chemical ingredients】

主要含有倍半萜类成分，主要有青蒿素（artemisinin），青蒿甲、乙、丙、丁、戊素（artemisinin Ⅰ ~ Ⅴ），青蒿酸（artemisic acid），青蒿酸甲酯（methyl artemisin），青蒿醇（artemisinol）。此外，尚含有黄酮类及挥发油类成分。

The main chemical compositions of *Qīng hāo* are which mainly contain artemisinin, artemisinin Ⅰ-Ⅴ, artemisic acid, methyl artemisin and artemisinol. In addition, it also contains flalonoids and volatile oils.

【药性与功效 / Chinese medicine properties】

味苦、辛，性寒，归肝、胆经。具有清热解暑、除蒸、截疟的功效。主治暑邪发热，阴虚发热，夜热早凉，骨蒸劳热，疟疾寒热，湿热黄疸。

In Chinese medicine theory, *Qīng hāo* has the nature of bitter, spicy and cold. It can enter the meridians of liver and gallbladder. *Qīng hāo* can clear summer-heat and steaming heat, clearing hectic heat, prevent attack of malaria. Clinically, it can be used for fever due to summer heat or Yin deficiency fever in night and abating at dawn, steaming bone fever and consumptive fever, malaria, jaundice due to damp-heat .

【药理作用 / Pharmacological effects】

1. 抗病原微生物

(1) Anti-pathogenic microorganisms

（1）抗菌　青蒿素及其衍生物对表皮葡萄球菌、卡他球菌、炭疽杆菌、白喉棒状杆菌有较强的抑制作用，对金黄色葡萄球菌、铜绿假单胞菌、志贺菌属、结核分枝杆菌也有一定的抑制作用。

1) Antimicrobial effect　Artemisinin and its derivatives have strong inhibitory effects on *Staphylococcus epidermidis*, *Catarrhal coccus*, *Bacillus anthracis* and *Diphtheria Bacillus*. It also has certain inhibitory effects on *Staphylococcus aureus*, *Pseudomonas aeruginosa*, *Shigella* and *Mycobacterium tuberculosis*.

（2）抗疟原虫　青蒿素是青蒿的抗疟有效成分，具有高效低毒的特点。青蒿素对疟原虫配子体有杀灭作用。青蒿素体内对疟原虫红细胞内期有直接杀灭作用，但对红细胞前期和外期无影响。其抗疟机制主要是影响疟原虫的膜结构，首先是抑制疟原虫表膜、线粒体膜，其次是核膜、内质网膜，对核内染色质也有一定的影响。其作用方式主要是使原虫表膜和线粒体功能紊乱，阻断摄取营养的途径，最终导致原虫死亡。

2) Antimalarial effect　Artemisinin is the effective ingredient of *Qīng hāo* for antimalarial effect, with the characteristic of high efficiency and low toxicity. Artemisinin can kill plasmodium gametophytes. It has a direct killing effect on the erythrocytic stage of plasmodium falciparum, but it has no effect on pre-erythrocytic stage and exo-erythrocytic stage. The antimalarial mechanism is mainly to affect the membrane structure of the plasmodium. Firstly, it can inhibit the surface membrane and mitochondrial membrane of plasmodium falciparum, secondly, it can inhibit the nuclear membrane and endoplasmic reticulum membrane. It also affects the nuclear chromatins. It causes the dysfunction of the plasmodium epimembrane and mitochondria, block the way of nutrition intake, and ultimately leads to plasmodium death.

（3）抗血吸虫　青蒿素及其多种衍生物均有抗血吸虫的作用。青蒿素对幼虫期的血吸虫具有杀灭作用，还能杀灭进入宿主体内的幼虫，用于感染日本血吸虫尾蚴后的早期治疗。其抗血吸虫活性基团是过氧桥，作用机制是抑制虫体的糖代谢。

3) Anti-schistosomiasis　Artemisinin and its derivatives have anti-schistosomiasis effect. Artemisinin can kill the larval stage of schistosomiasis and the larvae entering the host, which can be used in the early treatment of infection with cercariae of Schistosoma japonicum. The active group of artemisinin to resist schistosomiasis is a peroxy bridge which can inhibit the glycometabolism of Schistosoma.

2. **解热、抗炎**　青蒿水提物具有显著解热作用，能使正常动物体温和酵母诱导的实验性发热动物体温下降。青蒿水提物具有抗炎作用，对蛋清、酵母诱导的关节肿胀和二甲苯所致小鼠耳郭肿胀有明显的抑制作用。

(2) **Antipyretic and anti-inflammatory effects**　*Qīng hāo* water extract has a significant antipyretic effect, which can decrease the body temperature of both normal animals and experimental febrile animals induced by yeast. *Qīng hāo* water extract also has anti-inflammatory effects, which significantly inhibit the joint swelling induced by egg white or yeast, and ear swelling induced by xylene in mice.

3. **影响免疫功能**　青蒿素对免疫系统作用较为复杂，目前多认为是抑制作用，可抑制小鼠迟发性变态反应；青蒿琥酯可促进 Ts 细胞增殖，抑制 Th 细胞产生，阻止白细胞介素和各类炎症介质的释放，从而起到免疫调节作用。

(3) **The effects on the immune function**　Artemisinin has a complex effect on the immune system. At present, it is considered as an inhibitory effect, which can inhibit the delayed allergic reaction of mice. Artesunate play an immunomodulatory role, which can promote the proliferation of Ts cells and inhibit the production of Th cells to prevent the release of interleukin and inflammatory mediators.

4. **抗肿瘤**　青蒿素及其衍生物青蒿琥酯和蒿甲醚对多种肿瘤细胞增殖具有抑制作用，其机制涉及抑制血管新生、诱导细胞凋亡、阻滞细胞周期、产生自由基和活性氧破坏肿瘤细胞膜。

(4) Antitumor effects Artemisinin and its derivatives artesunate and artemether have inhibitory effects on the proliferation of a variety of tumor cells. The mechanisms include inhibition of angiogenesis, induction of apoptosis, inhibition of cell cycle, production of free radicals and reactive oxygen species to destroy tumor cell membrane.

5. **其他作用** 青蒿挥发油有镇咳、祛痰、平喘作用；青蒿素尚有抑制心肌收缩力、抗心律失常、抗组织纤维化作用。

(5) Other effects The volatile oil of *Qīng hāo* has antitussive, expectorant and anti-asthmatic effects. Artemisinin also has the effects of inhibiting myocardial contractility, anti-arrhythmia and anti-fibrosis.

【不良反应 / **Adverse effects**】

青蒿具有一定副作用，少数患者口服可出现恶心、呕吐、腹痛、腹泻等消化道症状，但大部分停药后可自行恢复。青蒿注射液偶可引起过敏反应。动物生殖毒性试验显示青蒿素、蒿甲醚及青蒿琥酯均有胚胎毒性作用。

Orally administered *Qīng hāo* can cause gastrointestinal symptoms such as nausea, vomiting, abdominal pain, diarrhea, etc., which can recover after drug withdrawal. *Qīng hāo* injection can occasionally cause allergic reactions. Animal reproductive toxicity experiments showed that artemisinin, artemether and artesunate have embryotoxic effects.

（杨 柯 贺龙刚 方 芳）

题库

第六章 泻下药
Chapter 6 Purgative medicines

学习目标 | Objectives

1. **掌握** 泻下药的主要药理作用；大黄与功效相关的药理作用、药效物质基础和泻下作用机制。

2. **了解** 芒硝、番泻叶、芦荟的主要药理作用和药效物质基础。

1. **Must know** The main pharmacological effects of purgative medicines; the efficacy related pharmacological effects, mechanism of action, and material basis of *dà Huáng*.

2. **Desirable to know** The main pharmacological effects and material basis of *Máng xiāo*, *Fān xiè yè*, *Lú huì*.

第一节 概述
Section 1 Overview

PPT

微课

凡能引起腹泻或滑润大肠、促进排便的药物，称为泻下药。本类药具有泻下通便、消除积滞、通腑泻热、祛除水饮等功效，主要用于热结便秘、寒积便秘、肠胃积滞、实热内结以及水肿停饮等所呈现的里实证候。泻下药药性多苦寒或甘平，多入胃、大肠经。根据泻下药泻下程度不同，大体分为攻下药、润下药、峻下逐水药三类。

All Chinese materia medica that can cause diarrhea or smooth large intestine and promote defecation are called purgative medicines. It can promote defecation or even cause diarrhea, not only for relieving constipation, but also for driving stagnant matter, excessive heat and retained fluid out of the body. It is mainly used for treating constipation due to heat or cold accumulation, gastrointestinal stasis due to excess heat, edema, fluid retention and other internal excess syndromes. Most purgative medicines have the nature of bitter and cold, or sweet and mild, enter the meridians of stomach and large intestin. According to the different characteristics of purgative effects, purgative medicines are classified into three types: offensive purgative, emollient laxative, and drastic hydragogue.

里实证是肠胃实热内结、阴亏津枯，或水饮内停所致的一类证候。从西医学角度看，肠胃实热内结的证候见于急性单纯性肠梗阻、粘连性肠梗阻、蛔虫性肠梗阻、急性胆囊炎、急性胰腺炎、急性阑尾炎等多种急腹症，也见于某些急性感染性疾病，症见高热、腹痛、谵语、神昏、烦躁、惊厥等。阴亏津枯的证候多见于老人、幼儿及产后便秘者，并可见于大病后期及临床各科

73

手术后体质虚弱者，肠推进性蠕动减弱而引起便秘。水饮内停证候与西医学中胸膜炎、肝硬化腹水、右心功能不全的表现相似，主要表现为胸腹部积水。总之，里实证的主要病因是胃肠道蠕动功能减弱、病原微生物感染等，其病理过程包括便秘、发热、腹痛、炎症等。现代药理研究表明，泻下药治疗里实证与下列药理作用有关。

Interior excess pattern refers to any pattern/syndrome resulting from external pathogen transforming into heat and entering the interior to affect the stomach and intestines. From the point of view of modern medicine, excess heat of intestines and stomach can be seen in acute simple intestinal obstruction, adhesive intestinal obstruction, ascaris intestinal obstruction, acute cholecystitis, acute pancreatitis, acute appendicitis and other acute abdominal diseases, as well as in some acute infectious diseases, such as high fever, abdominal pain, delirium, coma, fidgety, convulsion. The syndrome of Yin deficiency and fluid exhaustion is more common in the elderly, children and postpartum constipation, as well as weak patients in the late stage of serious disease and after operation due to the decrease of intestinal propulsive peristalsis induced constipation. The symptoms of water retention are similar to those of pleurisy, cirrhosis ascites and right heart insufficiency in modern medicine, mainly manifested as hydrothorax and ascites. In general, the main causes of internal excess syndrome are the decrease of gastrointestinal peristalsis and with pathogenic microorganism, etc., The pathological characteristics include constipation, fever, pain, inflammation, etc. Purgative medicines can be used to treat the syndromes above mentioned. The purgative function is related to the following pharmacological effects.

1. 泻下　本类药及其复方均能使肠蠕动增加，具有程度不同的泻下作用，根据其作用特点，可分为刺激性泻药、容积性泻药及润滑性泻药。大黄、番泻叶、芦荟等药物的致泻成分均为结合型蒽苷，口服抵达大肠后在细菌酶的作用下水解为苷元，刺激大肠黏膜下神经丛，使肠管蠕动增加而排便，为刺激性泻药。芒硝主要成分为硫酸钠，口服后在肠腔内不能吸收，发挥高渗作用，使肠腔保留大量水分，肠容积增大，刺激肠壁，促进肠蠕动而泻下，为容积性泻药。火麻仁、郁李仁等含有大量脂肪油，使肠道润滑，粪便软化，同时脂肪油在碱性肠液中能分解产生脂肪酸，可对肠壁产生温和的刺激作用，具有润肠通便作用，为润滑性泻药。

(1) Purgative effects　Purgative medicines can increase the peristalsis of intestine and have different degree of purgative effects. According to the characteristics of purgative effects, purgative medicines can be divided into stimulant laxatives, volumetric laxatives and lubricative laxatives. The purgative components of *Dà Huáng, Fān xiè yè, Lú huì* are combined-anthraquinone glycosides, which can be hydrolyzed into aglycones by bacterial enzymes in the large intestine after oral administration. Aglycones stimulate the never fibers in the mucosa of the large intestine to increase the peristalsis of the colon, and promote defecation, which named as stimulant laxatives. The main component of *Máng xiāo* is sodium sulfate, which can not be absorbed in the intestinal cavity after oral administration, but it can retain a large amount of water in the intestinal cavity due to the high osmotic pressure, to increase the intestinal volume, stimulate the intestinal wall, and promote the intestinal peristalsis and defecation, which named as volumetric laxatives. *Huǒ má rén, Yù lǐ rén* contain fat oil, which can lubricate the intestines and soften faeces. In addition, fat oil can be decomposed into fatty acids in alkaline intestinal fluid, which can mildly stimulate the intestinal wall to cause defecation. They are named as lubricative laxatives.

2. 利尿　芫花、甘遂、牵牛子、商陆等均有较强的利尿作用。用芫花煎剂给大鼠灌胃可见尿量明显增加，同时排钠量亦增加。这些药临床应用时，有明显利尿消肿效果。大黄中所含蒽醌亦有轻度利尿作用，其机制与抑制肾小管上皮细胞 Na^+-K^+-ATP 酶有关。

(2) Diuretic effects　*Yuán huā, Gān suì, Qiān niú zǐ* and *Shāng lù* have strong diuretic effect. Orally

adminstered *Yuán huā* decoction significantly increase the urine volume and Na^+ excretion in rats. They also showed obvious diuretic and detumescence effects in clinical application. The anthraquinones of *Dà huáng* also has a mild diuretic effect, which is related to the inhibition of Na^+- K^+- ATPase in renal tubular epithelial cells.

3. 抗病原微生物　大黄、芦荟中所含大黄酸、大黄素、芦荟大黄素，对多种致病菌、某些真菌、病毒及阿米巴原虫有抑制作用。

(3) Anti-pathogenic microorganism　Rhein, emodin and aloe emodin from *Dà huáng* and *Lú huì* can inhibit a variety of pathogens, some fungi, viruses and amoeba.

4. 抗炎　大黄和商陆均有明显的抗炎作用，能抑制炎症早期水肿及后期肉芽组织增生。大黄素可抑制单核巨噬细胞分泌肿瘤坏死因子α（TNF-α）、白细胞介素 1（IL-1）、白细胞介素 6（IL-6）、白细胞介素 8（IL-8）等炎症细胞因子，还能抑制内毒素诱导的上述细胞因子的分泌。商陆皂苷能兴奋垂体–肾上腺皮质系统，从而发挥抗炎作用。大黄的抗炎机制可能与抑制花生四烯酸代谢有关。

(4) Anti-inflammatory effects　*Dà huáng* and *Shāng lù* have obvious anti-inflammatory effects, which can inhibit the edema in the early stage of inflammation and the proliferation of granulation tissue in the later stage. *Dà huáng* can inhibit mononuclear phagocytes to secrete tumor necrosis factor-α (TNF-α), interleukin-1, interleukin-6, interleukin-8 (IL-1, IL-6, IL-8), etc., and also inhibit the secretion of the above cytokines induced by endotoxin. Saponin of *Shāng lù* has anti-inflammatory effect through stimulating the pituitary-adrenal cortex system, while *Dà huáng* exert the anti-inflammatory effect by inhibiting the metabolism of arachidonic acid.

5. 抗肿瘤　大黄、芦荟、商陆、芫花、大戟均有抗肿瘤作用。大黄酸、大黄素及芦荟大黄素能抑制小鼠黑色素瘤、乳腺癌和艾氏腹水癌。商陆对小鼠肉瘤 S_{180} 有抑制作用。抗癌机制可能是抑制肿瘤细胞蛋白质的合成。

(5) Antitumor effects　*Dà huáng*, *Lú huì*, *Shāng lù*, *Yuán huā* and *Dà jǐ* have antitumor effects. Rhein, emodin and aloe emodin can inhibit melanoma, breast cancer and Ehrlich ascites cancer in mice. *Shāng lù* has inhibitory effect on sarcoma S_{180} in mice. The anti-tumor mechanisms may be to inhibit the synthesis of protein in tumor cells.

常用泻下药的主要药理作用见表 6-1。

The main pharmacological effects of commonly used purgative medicines are summarized in Table 6-1.

表 6-1　常用泻下药的主要药理作用

类别	药物	泻下	利尿	抗菌	抗肿瘤	抗炎	调节免疫	其他药理作用
攻下药	大黄	+	+	+	+	+	+	止血、抗溃疡、抗氧化、降血脂、改善肾功能、保肝、利胆、抗病毒
	芒硝	+	+	+	–	–	+	利胆
	番泻叶	+	–	–	–	–	–	止血、肌肉松弛
	芦荟	+	–	+	+	+	+	降血脂、愈创
峻下逐水药	牵牛子	+	+	–	–	–	–	—
	芫花	+	+	+	+	+	+	镇咳、祛痰、致流产、抗早孕
	大戟	+	+	+	+	–	–	镇痛
	商陆	+	+	+	+	+	+	镇咳、祛痰、抗病毒
	巴豆	+	–	+	–	+	–	镇痛
	甘遂	+	+	–	–	–	–	抗生育、抗氧化
润下药	火麻仁	+	–	–	–	–	–	降血脂、抗氧化
	郁李仁	+	–	–	–	–	–	降压

注："+"表示有明确作用；"–"表示无作用，或未查阅到相关研究文献

第二节　常用药物
Section 2　Commonly used medicines

PPT

| 大黄 ┊ *Dà huáng* (*Radix et Rhizoma Rhei*) |

【来源 / Origin】

本品为蓼科植物掌叶大黄（Rheum palmatum L.）、唐古特大黄（Rheum tanguticum Maxim. ex Balf.）或药用大黄（Rheum officinale Baill.）的干燥根及根茎。主产于青海、甘肃、四川等地。秋末茎叶枯萎或次春发芽前采挖，除去细根，刮去外皮，切瓣或段，干燥后使用。

Dà huáng is the dried root and rhizome of Rheum palmatum L., Rheum tanguticum Maxim. ex Balf. and Rheum officinale Baill. The plant is widely cultivated in Qinghai province, Gansu province and Sichuan province in China. It is harvested in the late autumn while the stems and leaves are withered or before germination in spring, then removed the small roots, scraped off the skin, cut into segments. The dried root and rhizome are used for Chinese medicinal preparation.

【化学成分 / Chemical ingredients】

主要含蒽醌衍生物和二蒽酮类。蒽醌类成分以结合型和游离型两种形式存在。大部分为结合型蒽醌苷，少部分为游离型苷元，如大黄酸、大黄酚、大黄素、芦荟大黄素和大黄素甲醚。此外，大黄还含有大量鞣质，如 d–儿茶素、没食子酸以及多糖等。结合型蒽醌苷和二蒽酮苷为大黄主要泻下成分，其中二蒽酮苷中的番泻苷 A、番泻苷 B、番泻苷 C、番泻苷 D、番泻苷 E、番泻苷 F 泻下作用最强。

Dà huáng contains anthraquinone derivatives and dianthrones. Anthraquinones from *Dà huáng* exist in the form of combination and free. Most of them are conjugated anthraquinone glycosides. A few are free aglycones, such as rhein, chrysophanol, emodin, aloe emodin and emodin methyl ether. In addition, *Dà huáng* also contains a lot of tannins, such as d-catechin, gallic acid and polysaccharides. Conjugated anthracyside and dianthrone glycosides are the main purgative components of *Dà huáng*, among which sennoside A, sennoside B, sennoside C, sennoside D, sennoside E and sennoside F had the strongest purgative effect.

【药性与功效 / Chinese medicine properties】

味苦，性寒，归脾、胃、大肠、肝、心包经。具有泻下攻积、清热泻火、凉血解毒、逐瘀通经、利湿退黄之功效。用于实热积滞便秘、血热吐衄、目赤咽肿、痈肿疔疮、肠痈腹痛、瘀血经闭、产后瘀阻、跌打损伤、湿热痢疾、黄疸尿赤、淋证、水肿，外治烧烫伤。酒大黄善清上焦血分热毒，用于目赤咽肿及牙龈肿痛；熟大黄泻下力缓，泻火解毒，用于火毒疮疡；大黄炭凉血化瘀止血，用于血热有瘀出血证。

In Chinese medicine theory, *Dà huáng* has the nature of bitter, cold. It can enter the meridians of the spleen, stomach, large intestine, liver and pericardium. *Dà huáng* can induce purgation and defecation clear heat and purge fire, cool the blood and expell toxin, expelling stasis and dredge channels, drain dampness and anti-icterus. Clinically it can be used for constipation with excess heat, abdominal pain due to stagnation, hematemesis and epistaxis due to blood heat, red eyes, throat swelling, intestinal carbuncle, furuncle, carbuncle, blood stasis amenorrhea, postpartumstagnation, traumatic injury, dysentery and jaundice due to damp-heat, stranguria, edema, etc. It can also externally used for burns and scalds *Dà huáng* processed by wine is good at clearing blood heat and toxin in upper energizer which can be used for red eye, swollen pharynx and gingivitis. Fried *Dà huáng* has mild purgative effect which can purge fire and detoxification, and be used for sores due to fire toxin. *Dà huáng* charcoal can cool blood, remove blood stasis and stop bleeding which can be used for hemorrhage sydrome with blood heat and stasis.

【药理作用 / Pharmacological effects】

1. 泻下　大黄具有明显的泻下作用。其致泻主要成分为结合型蒽苷，以番泻苷 A 和大黄酸苷为主，其中以番泻苷 A 作用最强，大黄素亦具有使肠推进性蠕动增加而利于排便的作用。大黄泻下作用机制与以下环节相关。①口服后，结合型蒽苷大部分未经小肠吸收而抵达大肠，被肠道细菌酶（主要为 β 葡糖苷酶）水解成大黄酸蒽酮而刺激肠黏膜及肠壁肌层内神经丛，促进肠蠕动而致泻。②大黄酸蒽酮、大黄素具有胆碱样作用，可兴奋平滑肌上 M 胆碱受体，加快肠蠕动。③大黄酸蒽酮可抑制肠细胞膜上 Na^+-K^+-ATP 酶，阻碍 Na^+ 使肠道内渗透压升高，肠道容积增大，机械性刺激肠壁，使肠蠕动加快。

(1) **Purgative effects**　*Dà huáng* has an obvious purgative effect. Conjugated anthraquinones, especial sennoside A and rheinoside, are suggested to be the main components for purgative effect, and the purgative effect of sennoside A is the strongest. Emodin also enhance intestinal propulsive peristalsis to promote defecation. The mechanism of purgative effects may attribute to the following aspects. ①After oral administration, most of the combined anthraquinone glycosides reach the large intestine without absorption by the small intestine, and is hydrolyzed by the intestinal bacterial enzyme (mainly β-glucosidase) to rhein anthrone, which stimulates the intestinal mucosa and the nerve plexus in the muscular layer of the intestinal wall, promotes the intestinal peristalsis and diarrhea. ②Rhein anthrone and emodin have cholinergic effect, which can stimulate M choline receptor on smooth muscle and accelerate intestinal peristalsis. ③*Dà huáng* can inhibit the Na^+-K^+-ATPase in the intestinal smooth muscle, prevent the transport of Na^+ from the intestinal lumen to the cell, lead to the increase of intestinal lumen osmotic pressure and volume of intestinal cavity, and then stimulate mechanically the intestinal wall to accelerate intestinal peristalsis.

通常认为大黄属于刺激性泻药，其致泻作用部位在大肠，大黄对结肠电活动有兴奋作用。大黄素对小肠运动亦具有明显的增强作用，通过炭末推进法和木糖吸收实验表明，大黄素灌胃给药可以明显刺激肠壁，反射性地使肠壁推进性蠕动幅度增大，利于排便。

It is generally believed that *Dà huáng* is an irritant, the site of diarrhea caused by *Dà huáng* is the large intestine, and *Dà huáng* has an excitatory effect on colonic electrical activity. Emodin can also significantly enhance the movement of the small intestine. The carbon dust propulsion and xylose absorption experiments show that intragastric administration of emodin can obviously stimulate the intestinal wall, and the reflex increases the amplitude of propulsive peristalsis, which is beneficial to defecation.

煎煮时间与炮制方法可影响大黄泻下作用，经炮制和久煎后，大黄结合型蒽苷易被水解成苷元，番泻苷 A 仅存少量，而苷元在小肠内易被破坏，故泻下作用减弱。另外，久煎后大黄含有的鞣质大量溶出，鞣质对肠蠕动有抑制作用。研究表明生大黄煎煮 10 分钟，蒽苷溶出率最高，泻下作用最强；生大黄比酒炙大黄及醋炙大黄泻下作用强。

Decoction time and processing method can affect the purgative effect of *Dà huáng*. After processing and prolonged decocting, *Dà huáng* combined anthraquinone glycosides are easy to be hydrolyzed into aglycone. Sennoside A is only a small amount, but aglycone is easy to be destroyed in the small intestine, so the purgative effect is weakened. In addition, a large number of tannins in *Dà huáng* were dissolved after decoction for a long time, and tannins had an inhibitory effect on intestinal peristalsis. The results showed that when the raw *Dà huáng* was decocted for 10 minutes, the dissolution rate of combined anthraquinone glycosides was the highest and the purgative effect was the strongest. The purgative effect of raw *Dà huáng* was stronger than that of *Dà huáng* fried with wine and vinegar.

2. 保肝、利胆 大黄对实验性肝损伤具有明显保护作用，可减轻肝细胞肿胀、变性和坏死。大黄通过促进肝细胞 RNA 合成及肝细胞再生；刺激人体产生干扰素，抑制病毒繁殖；促进肝脏血液循环，改善微循环等途径，产生保肝作用。大黄能疏通肝内毛细胆管，促进胆汁分泌，因而改善胆小管内胆汁淤积，增加胆红素排泄。大黄还能促进胆囊收缩，松弛胆囊奥迪括约肌，使胆汁排出量增加。

(2) Hepatoprotection and choleretic effects *Dà huáng* has a significant protective effect on experimental liver injury, which can reduce the swelling, degeneration and necrosis of liver cells. *Dà huáng* can protect the liver by promoting the synthesis of RNA and the regeneration of liver cells, stimulating the production of interferon, inhibiting the propagation of virus, promoting the blood circulation of liver and improving microcirculation. *Dà huáng* can dredge the bile duct capillary in the liver, promote bile secretion, thus improving bile stasis in the bile duct and increasing bilirubin excretion. *Dà huáng* can also promote gallbladder contraction and relax the gallbladder Oddi sphincter to increase bile output.

3. 保护黏膜 大黄能促进胃黏膜 PGE 生成，增强胃肠黏膜屏障功能；大黄鞣质可减少实验性胃溃疡大鼠胃液分泌量，降低胃液游离酸度；大黄素、芦荟大黄素、大黄酚、大黄酸等对幽门螺杆菌均有抑制作用。

(3) Protective effect of gastric mucosa *Dà huáng* has a protective effect on gastric mucosa, which can promote the generation of PGE in gastric mucosa and enhance the barrier function of gastrointestinal mucosa; the tannin of *Dà huáng* can reduce the secretion of gastric juice and the free acidity of gastric juice in experimental gastric ulcer rats; emodin, aloe emodin, chrysophanol and rhein can inhibit *Helicobacter pylori*.

4. 抗急性胰腺炎 大黄所含大黄素、芦荟大黄素、大黄酸能抑制胰蛋白酶、胰脂肪酶等胰酶的分泌，改善胰腺微循环，松弛奥迪括约肌，减轻胰管压力，其中大黄素抑制作用较强。大黄能促进急性胰腺炎模型动物病理损伤的修复，通过抑制胰酶的活性可以抑制急性胰腺炎的始动环节。抑制胰酶活性主要用制大黄，其中醋炒大黄明显抑制胰蛋白酶活性，酒炒大黄对胰蛋白酶抑制作用较强，而大黄炭和酒炖大黄则能抑制脂肪酶活性。

(4) Anti acute pancreatitis Emodin, aloe emodin and rhein can inhibit the secretion of trypsin, pancreatic lipase and other pancreatic enzymes, improve the microcirculation of the pancreas, relax the biliary sphincter, and reduce the pressure of the pancreatic duct. The inhibitory effect of emodin is stronger. *Dà huáng* can promote the repair of pathological injury in acute pancreatitis model, which inhibit the acute pancreatitis by inhibiting the activity of pancreatin. Among them, vinegar-frying *Dà huáng* obviously inhibited trypsin activity, wine-frying *Dà huáng* had a strong inhibition on trypsin activity, while *Dà huáng* charcoal and wine stewed *Dà huáng* could inhibit lipase activity.

5. 利尿、改善肾功能 大黄素、大黄酸、芦荟大黄素灌胃给药有明显的利尿作用，尿中 Na^+ 和 K^+ 排出增加，给药后 2~4 小时利尿作用达高峰，且竞争性抑制 Na^+-K^+-ATP 酶活性。故大黄利尿作用与大黄蒽醌衍生物抑制肾髓质 Na^+-K^+-ATP 酶，使 Na^+ 重吸收减少、排出增加有关。大黄煎服后能明显降低血中尿素氮和肌酐水平，延缓慢性肾衰的发展，这一作用已在临床广泛用于治疗氮质血症。用腺嘌呤饲喂大鼠导致血尿素氮和肌酐含量增加，给大黄后可使其明显降低，尿中排出量显著增多。

(5) Diuresis and improvement of renal function Emodin, rhein and aloe emodin administered orally has obvious diuretic effect, they can promote the excretion of Na^+ and K^+ in urine, and the diuretic effect reached the peak 2 to 4 hours after administration. Emodin, rhein and aloe emodin showed a strong competitive inhibition on $Na^+ - K^+$-ATPase activities. The diuresis of *Dà huáng* may attribute to the inhibition of *Dà huáng* anthraquinone derivatives on Na^+-K^+-ATPase in renal medulla, which can reduce the reabsorption and increase the excretion of Na^+. *Dà huáng* decoction can significantly reduce the level of blood urea nitrogen (BUN) and creatinine in blood and delay the development of chronic renal failure, which has been widely used for azotaemia in clinical practice. *Dà huáng* administered orally can prevent the increase of urea nitrogen and creatinine in the blood of rats fed with adenine and promote the excretion from urine.

6. 对血液系统的作用

(6) Effect on blood system

（1）止血 大黄能缩短出血时间，作用确切，见效快。所含d–儿茶素、没食子酸为其有效成分。止血作用环节为：促进血小板的黏附和聚集功能；增加血小板数和纤维蛋白原含量，缩短凝血时间；降低抗凝血酶Ⅲ活性；收缩损伤局部血管，降低毛细血管通透性。大黄炒炭止血效果好。

1) Hemostasis *Dà huáng* can shorten the bleeding time, which is exact and rapid. d-catechin and gallic acid are suggested to be the effective components. The hemostasis may attribute to the following aspects: promoting the adhesion and aggregation of platelets; increasing the number of platelets and the content of fibrinogen, shortening the clotting time; reducing the activity of antithrombin Ⅲ; increasing the contraction of the damaged blood vessels, and reducing the permeability of capillaries. Hemostasis of *Dà huáng* charcoal is better.

（2）改善血液流变性 与大黄降低血脂、血液黏度及血细胞比容有关。此外，大黄能降低血管脆性，改善微循环障碍。

2) Improving hemorheology *Dà huáng* can improve hemorheology, which is related to the reduction of blood lipid, blood viscosity and hematocrit. In addition, *Dà huáng* can reduce vascular brittleness, improve the microcirculation disturbance.

（3）降血脂 大黄可降低血清中总胆固醇、甘油三酯、低密度脂蛋白、极低密度脂蛋白含量。其降脂作用可能是减少胆固醇吸收，促进胆固醇类物质排出。

3) Lowering blood lipid *Dà huáng* can lower the content of total cholesterol, triglyceride, low density lipoprotein and very low density lipoprotein in serum. The lowering blood lipid effect maybe attribute to inhibiting the absorption of cholesterol and promoting the excretion of cholesterol.

7. 抗病原微生物 大黄具有广泛的抗细菌、抗真菌、抗病毒、抗原虫等作用，抗菌的有效成分是游离苷元，其中以大黄酸、大黄素和芦荟大黄素的抗菌作用最强。对葡萄球菌、链球菌、淋球菌最敏感，其次为白喉棒状杆菌、炭疽杆菌、伤寒杆菌、痢疾杆菌。大黄抗菌作用的机制主要是抑制细菌核酸和蛋白质合成以及糖代谢。

(7) Antipathogenic microorganism *Dà huáng* has the effects of anti-bacteria, anti-fungus, anti-virus, anti-protozoon, etc. Free aglycones are suggested to be the active ingredient of anti-bacterial effects, among which rhein, emodin and aloe emodin have the strongest anti-bacterial effect. It is most sensitive to *Staphylococcus aureus*, *Streptococcus* and *Neisseria gonorrhoeae*, followed by *Corgnebacterium diphtheria*, *Bacillus anthrax*, *Salmonella typhi* and *Shigella dysentery*. The anti-bacterial mechanism of *Dà huáng* is mainly related to inhibiting synthesis of bacterial nucleic acid and protein, and the metabolism of glucose.

8. 抗炎　大黄对多种实验性炎症模型表现出明显的抗炎作用，对炎症早期的渗出、水肿和炎症后期的结缔组织增生均有明显的抑制作用。对切除双侧肾上腺大鼠仍有抗炎作用，说明大黄抗炎作用可能与垂体–肾上腺系统无关。目前认为大黄抗炎作用机制主要是抑制环氧化酶，使 PGE 合成减少，并抑制白三烯 B_4 的合成，还可能与抑制 NF-κB 信号活化有关。

(8) Anti-inflammatory effects　*Dà huáng* has obvious anti-inflammatory effect on a variety of experimental inflammatory models, which can alleviate exudation and edema in the early stage of inflammation and connective tissue proliferation in the later stage of inflammation. The anti-inflammatory effect of *Dà huáng* on rats with bilateral adrenal gland resection is still observed, indicating that the anti-inflammation is not dependent on the pituitary-adrenal system. At present, the anti-inflammatory mechanism of *Dà huáng* is mainly considered to inhibit cyclooxygenase, reduce the synthesis of PGE, and inhibit the synthesis of leukotriene B_4. In addition, it may be related to the inhibition of NF-κB signal activation.

9. 抗肿瘤　大黄蒽酮衍生物、大黄酸、大黄素和芦荟大黄素都具有明显抗肿瘤作用，对小鼠黑色素瘤、乳腺癌、艾氏腹水癌均有抑制作用，d–儿茶素能抑制淋巴肉瘤的生长。抗肿瘤机制是影响癌细胞代谢的多个环节，既能抑制癌细胞的呼吸及氨基酸、糖代谢中间产物的氧化和脱氢过程，又能抑制 DNA 和 RNA 及蛋白质的生物合成，但对宿主正常组织无明显影响。

(9) Antitumor activity　*Dà huáng* anthrone derivatives, rhein, emodin and aloe emodin all have obvious antitumor effects, which can inhibit the mouse melanoma, breast cancer and Ehrlich ascites cancer, d-catechin can inhibit the growth of lymphosarcoma. The anti-tumor effect is mainly attribute to affecting multiple aspects of cancer cell metabolism. It can inhibit the respiration of cancer cells, the oxidation and dehydrogenation of amino acids and sugar metabolites, and the biosynthesis of DNA, RNA and protein, however, it can not affect the normal tissues of the host.

【不良反应 / Adverse effects】

大黄中含鞣酸及其他成分，具有收敛止泻的作用。久服大黄可致肠壁神经感受细胞应激性降低，不能产生正常蠕动和排便反射，形成不服大黄就不能排便的泻剂依赖性便秘。另外，大黄使用过量可造成小鼠肝损伤和肾损伤。

Dà huáng contains tannic acid and other components, which has the efficacy of astringency and checking diarrhea. Taking *Dà huáng* for a long time decrease sensitivity of the nerve receptors in the intestinal wall, inhibit the normal peristalsis and defecation reflex, and cause the constipation with the laxative dependence, that means you cannot defecate without *Dà huáng*. In addition, overdose of *Dà huáng* can cause liver damage and kidney damage in mice.

芒硝 | *Máng xiāo (Natrii Sulfas)*

【来源 / Origin】

本品是含硫酸盐类矿物芒硝族芒硝，经加工精制而成的结晶体。

Máng xiāo is a crystal of mirabilite minerals containing sulfate, which is formed by processing and refining.

【化学成分 / Chemical ingredients】

主要含有含水硫酸钠（$Na_2SO_4 \cdot 10H_2O$），占 96%~98%，尚含少量硫酸镁、硫酸钙和氯化钠等。

The main component of *Máng xiāo* is sodium sulfate ($Na_2SO_4 \cdot 10 H_2O$, about 96%-98%), containing a small amount of magnesium sulfate, calcium sulfate and sodium chloride.

【药性与功效 / Chinese medicine properties 】

味咸、苦，性寒，归胃、大肠经。具有泻下通便、润燥软坚、清火消肿之功效。用于实热积滞，腹满胀痛，大便燥结，肠痈肿痛；外治乳痈、痔疮肿痛。

In Chinese medicine theory *Máng xiāo* has the nature of salty, bitter and cold . It can enter the meridians of stomach and large intestine. *Máng xiāo* can remove accumulation with purgation, moisten dryness and soften hard mass, clear away fire and alleviate edema. Clinically it can be used for stagnation due to excess heat, abdominal fullness and distending pain, constipation, swelling and pain due to intestinal abscess, etc. External application of *Máng xiāo* can treat acute mastitis, swelling and pain due to haemorrhoids.

【药理作用 / Pharmacological effects 】

1. 泻下　芒硝口服后，硫酸钠水解产生大量硫酸根离子，不易被肠壁吸收，使肠内渗透压升高，阻止肠腔内水分吸收，致肠容积扩大，肠腔扩张，刺激肠壁引起肠蠕动增加而致泻。同时硫酸钠本身对肠壁也有刺激作用。芒硝泻下作用速度与饮水量有关，饮水量多，泻下作用出现快，反之则较慢。

(1) Purgative effects　Oral administration of *Máng xiāo containing* sodium sulfate is hydrolyzed to produce a lot of sulfate ions which is not easy to be absorbed by the intestinal wall, lead to the increase of intestinal osmotic pressure and the decrease of the water absorption in intestinal cavity, expand intestinal volume and stimulate intestinal wall, promote intestinal peristalsis to induce defecation. At the same time, sodium sulfate itself has a stimulating effect on the intestinal wall. The purgative effects of *Máng xiāo* is related to the amount of water intake, the amount of drinking water is more, the purgative effect is faster, otherwise it is slower.

2. 抗肿瘤　玄明粉（主要成分为无水硫酸钠）可使致癌剂促癌和诱癌率明显下降。抗癌机制可能与酸化肠内环境，减少脱氧胆酸含量，抑制肠上皮细胞 DNA 合成，降低对致癌物的敏感性有关。

(2) Anti-tumor effects　*Xuán míng powder* (mainly composed of anhydrous sodium sulfate) can obviously reduce cancer-promoting rate and the inducing-cancer rate of carcinogenic agent. The mechanisms of anti-cancer effect may be related to acidifying intestinal environment, reducing the content of deoxycholate, inhibiting the synthesis of DNA in intestinal epithelial cells, and reducing the susceptibility to carcinogens.

3. 抗炎　10%~25% 硫酸钠外敷于感染性创面，可加快淋巴循环，增强单核巨噬细胞的吞噬功能，具有抗炎作用。

(3) Anti-inflammatory effects　External application of 10%-25% sodium sulfate can inhibit inflammation by accelerating lymph circulation, and enhancing the phagocytic function of reticuloendothelial cells.

4. 利胆　芒硝小剂量口服，可刺激小肠壶腹部，反射性地引起胆囊收缩、胆道括约肌松弛，故能促进胆汁排出。

(4) Cholagogic effects　small dose of *Máng xiāo* administered orally can promote bile excretion by stimulating the ampulla of small intestine to cause reflexively gallbladder contraction and the relaxation of sphincter muscle of bile duct.

5. 利尿　4.3% 无菌硫酸钠静脉注射有利尿作用。

(5) Diuretic effects　Intravenous injection of 4.3% sterile sodium sulfate has diuretic effect.

【不良反应 / Adverse effects】

口服芒硝时，浓度过高可引起幽门痉挛，产生胃不适感，影响胃排空。芒硝含钠离子多，故水肿患者慎用。孕妇忌用。

When taking *Máng xiāo* orally with the high concentration, which can cause pyloric spasm, produce gastric discomfort and affect gastric emptying. *Máng xiāo* contains more sodium ions, so patients with edema should be careful. Pregnant women should not use it.

番泻叶 ┊ *Fān xiè yè (Folium Sennae)*

【来源 / Origin】

本品是豆科植物狭叶番泻（Cassia angustifolia Vahl）或尖叶番泻（Cassia acutifolia Delile）的干燥小叶。前者主产于印度、埃及和苏丹；后者主产于埃及，我国广东、广西及云南亦有栽培。通常于 9 月采收，晒干，生用。

Fān xiè yè is the dried leaflets of Cassia angustifolia Vahl or Cassia acutifolia Delile of legume. Cassia angustifolia Vahl is mainly produced in India, Egypt and Sudan. Cassia acutifolia Delile is mainly produced in Egypt while it also cultivated in Guangdong province, Guangxi province and Yunnan province in China. It is usually harvested in September. The sun dried leaf is used for Chinese medicinal preparation.

【化学成分 / Chemical ingredients】

主要含有蒽醌衍生物及二蒽酮类衍生物，约含 1.5%，主要成分为番泻苷 A~F。此外，还含有大黄酸、大黄酚、大黄素、芦荟大黄素、黄酮类成分、蔗糖等。

Fān xiè yè mainly contains 1.5% anthraquinone derivatives and dianthraone derivatives, including sennoside A, B, C, D, E, F. *Fān xiè yè* also contains rhein, chrysophanol, emodin, and aloe emodin.

【药性与功效 / Chinese medicine properties】

味甘、苦，性寒，归大肠经。具有泻热行滞、通便、利水之功效。用于热结积滞、便秘腹痛、水肿胀满等证。

In Chinese medicine theory, *Fān xiè yè* has the nature of sweet, bitter, and cold. It can enter the meridians of the large intestine. *Fān xiè yè* can purge heat and remove stagnation, promote defecation and diuresis. Clinically it can be used for stagnation due to heat accumulation, constipation, fluid retention and abdominal distends.

【药理作用 / Pharmacological effects】

1. 泻下　本品含蒽醌衍生物，其泻下作用及刺激性较含蒽醌类其他泻药更强，主要有效成分为番泻苷 A、番泻苷 B，作用机制同大黄。

(1) Purgative effects　*Fān xiè yè* contains anthraquinone derivatives, whose purgative effect and irritation are stronger than that of other anthraquinone laxatives. sennoside A and B are suggested to be the main active components for purgation. Purgative mechanism of *Fān xiè yè* is the same as *Dà huáng*.

2. 抗菌　番泻叶破坏番茄晚疫病菌菌体细胞膜的通透性发挥抑菌作用，大黄素是其有效成分之一。

(2) Antibacterial effects　Emodin is one of the effective components of *Fān xiè yè*, which destroys the permeability of cell membrane of Phytophthora infestans.

3. 止血　番泻叶口服可增加血小板及纤维蛋白原，缩短凝血时间、血浆复钙时间、凝血活酶时间及血块收缩时间，有助于止血。

(3) Hemostasis effects　*Fān xiè yè* administered orally can increase the content of platelet and fibrinogen. It can shorten blood clotting time, plasma recalcification time, thromboplastin time and clot contraction time, which is helpful for hemostasis.

【不良反应 / Adverse effects】

少数患者大剂量服用后可出现腹痛，但排便后自行缓解。本品可刺激盆神经，并使盆腔器官充血，故月经期及妊娠妇女慎用或忌用。

A small number of patients may have abdominal pain after taking a large dose of *Fān xiè yè*, but it can be relieved spontaneously after defecation. *Fān xiè yè* can stimulate the pelvic nerve and make the pelvic organs congested, so menstrual period and pregnant women should be cautious or avoid using it.

芦荟 ┃ *Lú huì (Aloe)*

【来源 / Origin】

本品为百合科植物库拉索芦荟（Aloe barbadensis Miller.）、好望角芦荟（Aloe ferox Miller.）或其他同属植物叶的汁液浓缩干燥物。全年可采，一般鲜用，或割取叶片收集流出的液汁蒸发至适当浓度，逐渐冷却凝固而得。

Lú huì is dry and concentrated juice from the leaf of Aloe barbadensis Miller., Aloe ferox Miller. or other plants of the same genus. It is harvested all year round. Generally fresh used, or cut the leaves to collect the juice and evaporate to the appropriate concentration, and gradually coagulate.

【化学成分 / Chemical ingredients】

主要含有蒽醌及其苷，包括芦荟大黄素（aloe emodin）、芦荟大黄素苷（aloin barbaloin）、芦荟皂苷（aloesaponarin）、芦荟苦素（aloesin）、高塔尔芦荟素（homonataloin）等。此外，还含有萘酮、树脂、有机酸、单糖、多糖、蛋白质、草酸钙、纤维等。

Lú huì contains anthraquinone and its glucoside, including aloe emodin, aloin barbaloin, aloesaponarin, aloesin, and homataloin. In addition, it also contains naphthalenone, resin, organic acid, monosaccharide, polysaccharide, protein, calcium oxalate, fiber, etc.

【药性与功效 / Chinese medicine properties】

味苦，性寒，归肝、胃、大肠经。具有清肝热、通便之功效。主治热结便秘，惊痫抽搐。

In Chinese medicine theory, *Lú huì* has the nature of bitter and cold. It can enter the meridians of liver, stomach, and large intestine. *Lú huì* can clear liver heat and promote defecation. Clinically it can be used for constipation due to heat accumulation, epilepsy and convulsion.

【药理作用 / Pharmacological effects】

1. 泻下　芦荟中所含蒽醌衍化物，尤其是芦荟苷，能在肠道中释放出大黄素等发挥刺激性泻下作用。对离体小肠无促进蠕动作用，其泻下的主要作用部位在大肠。

(1) **Purgative effects**　The anthraquinone derivatives of *Lú huì*, especially barbaloin, can release emodin in intestine to cause stimulating diarrhea. The main action site of *Lú huì* is large intestine because it has no effect on peristalsis of isolated small intestine.

2. 保肝　芦荟总苷对动物实验性肝损伤有保护作用，能降低 CCL_4 或硫代乙酰胺引起的 ALT 升高，其作用强度接近于联苯双酯。

(2) **Hepatoprotective effects**　Total glycosides of *Lú huì* has protective effect on experimental liver injury in animals, which can reduce the increased ALT caused by CCl_4 or thioacetamide. The intensity of hepatoprotection is close to that of biphenyl diester.

3. 愈创　给予人工结膜水肿家兔 10% 的芦荟水浸液，可缩短愈合天数；对人工创伤的鼠背有轻度的促愈合作用。近几年发现芦荟中多聚糖醛酸酯有促进肉芽生长的作用，以芦荟叶浆制成的含多糖类的凝胶制剂可用于皮肤或其他组织创伤及烧伤。

(3) Healing wound effects   The 10% aqueous extract of *Lú huì* can shorten the healing days in rabbits with artificial conjunctival edema, and can slightly promote the healing of rat back with artificial trauma, the polysaccharide aldehydes from *Lú huì* can promote the growth of granulation. Polysaccharide gel made from leaves of *Lú huì* can be used for trauma and burns in the skin or other tissues.

4. 抗肿瘤、抗菌   芦荟中蒽醌衍生物具有高效杀伤肿瘤细胞的能力，0.3μg/ml 浓度对 L_{929} 细胞杀伤活性达 50% 以上，对 GM_{803} 和 MethA 在 2.5μg/ml 时杀伤活性达 50% 以上。芦荟苷是芦荟叶皮中的主要抗菌活性成分，能够有效地抑制测试菌的生长，对革兰阳性菌的抗性略高于革兰阴性菌，抗菌活性明显高于芦荟大黄素。

(4) Anti-tumor, antibacterial effects   The anthraquinone derivatives from *Lú huì* have high efficiency of killing tumor cells. Anthraquinone derivatives can kill more than 50% L_{929} cells at the concentration of 0.3μg/ml; and kill more than 50% GM_{803} and MethA cells at the concentration of 2.5μg/ml. Aloin is the main antibacterial active component in *Lú huì* leaf-skin, which can effectively inhibit the growth of bacteria. Its resistance to Gram-positive bacteria is slightly higher than that to Gram-negative bacteria, and its antibacterial activity is significantly higher than that of aloe emodin.

5. 其他作用   芦荟还具有美容、抗衰老、镇痛、促智、抗胃溃疡、促进睡眠以及止血等多方面作用。

(5) Other effects   *Lú huì* also has many functions, such as cosmetology, anti-aging, analgesia, reinforcing intelligence, anti-gastric ulcer, promoting sleep and hemostasis.

【不良反应 / Adverse effects】

人食用后可能出现腹痛、腹泻、呕吐、肾炎、结肠黑变等不良反应。

Taking *Lú huì* may lead to abdominal pain, diarrhea, vomiting, nephritis, melanosis coli and other adverse reactions.

（王 斌 方 芳）

题库

医药大学堂
WWW.YIYAODXT.COM

第七章 祛风湿药
Chapter 7 Wind-damp-dispelling medicines

 学习目标 | Objectives

1.**掌握** 祛风湿药的主要药理作用；秦艽、独活、防己、五加皮、雷公藤与功效相关的药理作用、作用机制及药效物质基础；雷公藤的不良反应。

2.**了解** 痹证的临床表现；秦艽、独活、防己的不良反应。

1. Must know The main pharmacological effects of wind-damp-dispelling medicines; the pharmacological effects related to efficacies, and material basis of *Qín jiāo, Dú huó, Fáng jǐ, Wǔ jiā pí, Léi gōng téng* and the adverse effects of *Léi gōng téng*.

2. Desirable to know The clinical symptoms of Bì syndrome; the adverse effects of *Qín jiāo, Dú huó, Fáng jǐ.*

第一节 概述
Section 1 Overview

PPT

　　凡以祛除风寒湿邪、解除痹痛为主要功效的药物称为祛风湿药。本类药按其功效分为祛风湿散寒药、祛风湿清热药和祛风湿强筋骨药三类。本类药物大多味苦、辛，性温，归肝、脾、肾经。中医理论认为辛能祛风、苦能燥湿、温以散寒，故本类药物具有祛风散寒除湿之功效，部分药物还能舒经活络、止痛、强筋骨，临床主要用于治疗痹证。

Any Chinese materia medica that can remove pathogenic wind, cold and damp from the muscles, sinews, joints and bones, alleviate painful obstruction in order to relieve arthromyodynia(Bì syndrome), is known as wind-damp-dispelling medicines. According to the various characteristics and effects, these medicines in this chapter usually are classified into three types: wind-damp-cold dispelling medicines; wind-damp-heat dispelling medicines; wind-damp-dispelling and sinew-bone strengthening medicines. These medicines are mostly pungent and bitter in flavor, warm in nature, and entering liver, spleen and kidney meridians. According to the theory of Chinese medicine, pungent flavor is prone to removing wind, bitter is apt to dry damp, and warm tends to dissipate cold, so medicines of this chapter have the efficacies of dispelling wind, expelling dampness, eliminating cold, and some of them have the efficacies in dredging channels and activating collaterals, stopping pain, and strengthening sinew and bone.

Therefore, they are usually used in treating arthromyodynia.

痹证可因机体正气不足时感受风寒湿邪，流注经络关节发病，也可因感受风湿热之邪或风寒湿之邪郁久化热，以致风湿热邪闭阻经络关节而发病。痹证的主要临床表现有骨、关节、韧带、滑囊等疼痛、酸楚、麻木、重着、灼热，甚或关节肿胀、运动障碍，其临床特征类似于西医学中风湿热、风湿、类风湿关节炎及多种结缔组织病等。祛风湿药治疗痹证主要与下列药理作用有关。

Arthromyodynia is attributed to stagnation of pathogenic wind, cold and damp in joints, meridians and collaterals when Qi is weak. Arthromyodynia is also attributed to stagnation of pathogenic wind, damp, heat, or pathogenic wind, cold and damp transform into heat in joints, meridians and collaterals. The clinical symptoms of arthromyodynia are local pain, soreness, numbness, heaviness, or hotness of bone, joints, lagament, bursa, even articular swelling and movement disorders. These clinical characteristics are similar to rheumatic fever, rheumatism, rheumatoid arthritis and connective tissue diseases, etc. The wind-damp dispelling function is related to the following pharmacological effects.

1. **抗炎** 炎症是痹证的主要病理之一。祛风湿药中的大多数药物具有抗炎作用，对多种急慢性实验性炎症模型均有不同程度的拮抗作用，表现为减轻炎症局部的基本病理变化，缓解局部组织红、肿、热、痛症状。如秦艽、独活、雷公藤、五加皮、防己可抑制大鼠急性足跖肿胀和小鼠急性耳郭肿胀。雷公藤、五加皮等可抑制大鼠棉球肉芽增生及佐剂性关节炎。其抗炎作用机制与兴奋下丘脑–垂体–肾上腺皮质系统功能及抑制炎症介质的释放有关。

微课

(1) Anti-inflammation Inflammation is the main pathological characteristic of arthromyodynia. Most wind-damp-dispelling medicines have anti-inflammatory effects, which can relieve the symptoms of acute and chronic experimental inflammations, such as redness, swelling, heat and pain. For example, *Qín jiāo*, *Dú huó*, *Léi gōng téng*, *Wǔ jiā pí*, *Fáng jǐ* can inhibit acute inflammations of footpad swelling in rats and ear swelling in mouse. *Léi gōng téng*, *Wǔ jiā pí* can restrain chronic inflammations of cotton pellet granuloma and adjuvant arthritis in rats. The mechanism of anti-inflammation may be related to activating hypothalamus-pituitary-adrenalaxis (HPA) and inhibiting the release of inflammation mediators.

2. **镇痛** 疼痛是痹证的临床症状之一，常见骨、关节、肌肉疼痛。祛风湿药中的秦艽、防己、青风藤、五加皮等均有镇痛作用，可显著提高实验动物的痛阈。青风藤碱、粉防己碱等具有显著的镇痛作用，其镇痛作用分别为吗啡的 1/10 和 1/8。

(2) Analgesia Pain is one of the clinical symptoms of arthromyodynia, especially bone, joint and muscle pain is common. Wind-damp-dispelling medicines have the analgesic effect which can enhance the threshold of pain, such as *Qín jiāo*, *Fáng jǐ*, *Qīng fēng téng*, *Wǔ jiā pí*, etc. Sinoacutine and tetrandrine exhibit the analgesic potency equal to 1/10 and 1/8 that of morphine, respectively.

3. **影响免疫功能** 风湿性疾病的发病大部分与机体的免疫功能异常密切相关。风湿性疾病患者常伴有体液免疫功能和细胞免疫功能异常。本类药物祛风湿功效与其抑制机体过强的免疫功能有密切关系。例如，雷公藤所含的多种活性成分如雷公藤总苷、雷公藤甲素、雷公藤红素等能明显抑制溶血素抗体的形成，且对移植物抗宿主反应和迟发型超敏反应均有明显的抑制作用。

(3) Regulating immune function Most rheumatic diseases are closely related to the disorder of immune function. The efficacies of wind-damp-dispelling medicines are concerned with the inhibition on the disordered immune function. Many active ingredients of *Léi gōng téng*, for example, tripterygium glycosides, triptolide, celastrol can inhibit the formation of hemolysin antibody, and also inhibit host versus graft reaction and delayed hypersensitivity reaction.

另外，部分祛风湿药对免疫功能有促进作用，如五加皮总皂苷和多糖可提高小鼠单核巨噬细胞系统的吞噬功能和小鼠血清抗体的滴度。

医药大学堂
WWW.YIYAODXT.COM

Otherwise, some wind-damp-dispelling medicines can promote immune function. For example, the total saponins and polysaccharide of *Wǔ jiā pí* can improve the phagocytosis of reticuloendothelial system and the titer of serum antibody in mice.

4. **其他作用**　雷公藤、防己等有一定抗肿瘤作用；防己、秦艽、独活、青风藤等有一定降血压作用。

(4) Other effects　*Léi gōng téng* and *Fáng jǐ* show certain anti-tumor effect. *Fáng jǐ*, *Qín jiāo*, *Dú huó* and *Qīng fēng téng* show a certain effect on lowering blood pressure.

常用祛风湿药的主要药理作用见表 7-1。

The main pharmacological effects of commonly used wind-damp-dispelling medicines are shown in table 7-1.

表 7-1　常用祛风湿药的主要药理作用

类别	药物	抗炎	镇痛	对免疫功能的影响	其他药理作用
祛风湿散寒药	独活	+	+	+	镇静、降血压、抗心律失常、抑制血小板聚集、抗肿瘤
	川乌	+	+	+	强心、升血压、降血糖
	威灵仙	+	+	–	抗心肌缺血、抗病原微生物、抗疟、利胆
	木瓜	+	+	–	抗肿瘤、抗病原微生物
	青风藤	+	+	+	镇静、降血压、兴奋胃肠平滑肌
祛风湿清热药	秦艽	+	+	–	镇静、解热、保肝利胆、升血糖、降血压、利尿、抗病原微生物
	防己	+	+	+	降血压、抗心律失常、抗心肌缺血、抑制血小板聚集、抗纤维化、抗肿瘤、抗病原微生物
	豨莶草	+	+	+	扩张血管、降血压、抗血栓形成、改善微循环、抗病原微生物、抗疟
	雷公藤	+	+	+	改善血液流变学、杀虫、抗病原微生物、抗生育、抗肿瘤
	臭梧桐	+	+	–	镇静、降血压
祛风湿强筋骨药	五加皮	+	+	+	镇静、抗利尿、抗应激、性激素样作用、降血糖、抗溃疡

注："+"表示有明确作用；"–"表示无作用，或未查阅到相关研究文献

第二节　常用药物

Section 2　Commonly used medicines

PPT

秦艽 ┊ *Qín jiāo (Radix Gentianae Macrophyllae)*

【来源 / Origin】

本品为龙胆科植物秦艽（*Gentiana macrophylla* Pall.）、麻花秦艽（*Gentiana straminea* Maxim.）、

粗茎秦艽（*Gentiana crassicaulis* Duthie ex Burk.）或小秦艽（*Gentiama dahurica* Fisch.）的干燥根。主产于陕西、甘肃、内蒙古、四川等地。春、秋二季采挖，除去泥沙，晒干。

Qín jiāo is the dry root of *Gentiana macrophylla* Pall., *Gentiana straminea* Maxim., *Gentiana. crassicaulis* Duthie ex Burk. and *Gentiana dahurica* Fisch., family of Gentianaceae. *Qín jiāo* is widely cultivated in Shaanxi province, Gansu province, inner Mongolia autonomous region and Sichuan province, etc. The raw materials are harvested in the spring and autumn, then dried in the sun after the silt is removed.

【化学成分 / Chemical ingredients】

主要含有龙胆苦苷（含量为 0.2%~1.5%），在提取过程中使用氨液可使化学性质不稳定的龙胆苦苷转变为生物碱秦艽碱甲（即龙胆碱）、秦艽碱乙（即龙胆次碱）、秦艽碱丙。此外还含有挥发油和糖类等。

Qín jiāo contains 0.2%~1.5% gentiopicroside. when ammonia solution is used in the extraction and separation, it reacts with gentiopicroside to generate gentianine, gentianidine and gential. Additionally, *Qín jiāo* contains polysaccharide and volatile oil as well.

【药性与功效 / Chinese medicine properties】

味辛、苦，性平，归胃、肝、胆经。具有祛风湿、清湿热、止痹痛、退虚热的功效。主治风湿痹痛、中风半身不遂、筋脉拘挛、骨节酸痛、湿热黄疸、骨蒸潮热、小儿疳积发热等证。

In Chinese medicine theory, *Qín jiāo* has the nature of pungent, bitter and neutral. It can enter the meridians of stomach, liver and gallbladder. *Qín jiāo* can dispel wind and damp, clear damp-heat, relieve impediment pain and retreat deficiency-heat. Clinically, it can be used for arthralgia, apoplectic hemiplegia, hepertonicity of the sinews, generalized joint aching pain, damp-heat jaundice, steaming bone tidal fever, gan accumulation with heat effusion in children, etc.

【药理作用 / Pharmacological effects】

1. 抗炎　秦艽有明显的抗炎作用。粗茎秦艽的水提物和醇提物对巴豆油引起的小鼠耳郭肿胀和角叉菜胶引起的大鼠足跖肿胀均有明显的抑制作用。抗炎主要有效成分为秦艽碱甲。抗炎作用机制可能是通过兴奋下丘脑–垂体–肾上腺皮质轴，使促肾上腺皮质激素（ACTH）分泌增加，从而增强肾上腺皮质功能。

(1) Anti-inflammation　*Qín jiāo* has anti-inflammatory effect. The water and ethanol extract of *Qín jiāo* can inhibit ear swelling induced by croton oil in mice and the foot swelling induced by carrageenan in rats. The major active ingredient is gentiopicroside. The mechanism of anti-inflammation is involved in activating hypothalamus-pituitary-adrenal axis to increase adrenocorticotropic hormone (ACTH) secretion and enhance adrenocortical function.

2. 镇痛　秦艽水提物、醇提物和秦艽碱甲可抑制醋酸所致的小鼠扭体反应，减轻热板或光热刺激所致小鼠和大鼠的疼痛反应，但作用持续时间短，与延胡索和草乌配伍可增强其镇痛作用。

(2) Analgesia　*Qín jiāo* exhibit analgesic effect. The water and ethanol extract of *Qín jiāo* can inhibit writhing response induced by acetic acid in mice, and also reduce the pain response of mice and rats induced by hot plate or photothermal stimulation, but the analgesic effect lasted for a short time. The analgesic effect can be enhanced combination with *Yán hú suǒ* and *Cǎo wū*.

3. 抑制免疫功能　秦艽水煎液能明显抑制绵羊红细胞（SRBC）所致的小鼠迟发型超敏反应（DTH），明显降低小鼠的胸腺指数。秦艽醇提物对小鼠胸腺淋巴细胞和脾脏淋巴细胞的增殖有抑制作用。

(3) Immunosuppression　The water extract of *Qín jiāo* can restrain delayed type hypersensitivity (DTH) induced by sheep red blood cell (SRBC), and reduce the weight index of thymus in mice. Ehanol extract of *Qín*

jiāo can suppress the proliferation of thymus and spleen lymphocytes in mice.

4. 保肝、利胆　龙胆苦苷对 CCL_4 所致小鼠急性肝损伤模型有保护作用，能降低谷丙转氨酶（ALT）和谷草转氨酶（AST）活性，增加肝组织中谷胱甘肽过氧化物酶（GSH-Px）活力。此外，龙胆苦苷能增加大鼠胆汁分泌，促进胆囊收缩，具有利胆作用。

(4) Hepatoprotection and cholagogic effects　Gentiopicroside can protect the liver from acute injury induced by CCl_4, decrease the activity of serum alanine aminotransferase (ALT), aspartate aminotransferase (AST), and increase the activity of liver glutathione peroxidase (GSH-Px). In addition, gentiopicroside increases the bile flow and gallbladder contraction in rats, which exhibits cholagogic effect as well.

5. 其他作用　秦艽还有利尿、促进尿酸排泄、镇静、升血糖等作用。

(5) Other effects　*Qín jiāo* has other pharmocological effects, such as diuresis, promoting the excretion of uric acid, sedation and increasing blood glucose.

【不良反应 / Adverse effects】
常用剂量秦艽水煎服可能引起胃不适，剂量过大有引起恶心、呕吐、腹泻的个案病例报告。

Qín jiāo decoction may cause gastrointestinal discomfort in the normal dosage, while large dosage of *Qín jiāo* maybe cause nausea, vomiting, diarrhea in some individuals.

独活 ┊ *Dú huó (Radix Angelicae Pubescentis)*

【来源 / Origin】
本品为伞形科植物重齿毛当归（*Angelica pubescens* Maxim. f. *biserrata* Shan et Yuan）的干燥根。主产于湖北、四川及江西等地。春初或秋末采挖，除去须根和泥沙，烘干。

Dú huó is the dried root of *Angelica pubescens* Maxim. f. *biserrata* Shan et Yuan, family of Umbelliferae. The plant is widely cultivated in Hubei province, Sichuan province and Jiangxi province in China. The raw materials are harvested in the early spring and late autumn, then heated and dried after fibrous roots and silt are removed.

【化学成分 / Chemical ingredients】
主要含有挥发油和香豆素类成分。挥发油主要含单萜类及其衍生物，占总挥发油的 22.23%；倍半萜类及其衍生物，占总挥发油的 17.26%。香豆素化合物主要为东莨菪素、二氢欧山芹醇、二氢欧山芹醇乙酸酯、甲氧基欧芹酚、毛当归醇、当归醇、花椒毒素、佛手柑内酯、伞形花内酯、异欧前胡素等。此外还含有植物甾醇、有机酸和糖类化合物。

Dú huó contains volatile oils and coumarins. 22.23% of volatile oil is monoterpenoids and its derivatives. 17.26% of volatile oil is sesquiterpenes and its derivatives. Coumarins include scopoletin, columbianetin, columbianetin acetate, osthole, anpubesol, pubesol, xanthotoxin, bergapten, umbelliferone, isoimperatorin. Moreover, *Dú huó* also contains phytosterol, organic acid, carbohydrate, etc.

【药性与功效 / Chinese medicine properties】
味辛、苦，微麻舌，性微温，归肾、膀胱经。具有祛风除湿、通痹止痛之功效。用于风寒湿痹、腰膝疼痛、少阴伏风头痛等证。

In Chinese medicine theory, *Dú huó* has the nature of pungent, bitter and warm, It can enter the meridians of kidney and bladder. *Dú huó* can dispel wind and eliminate dampness, resolve arthromyodynia and relieve pain. Clinically, it can be used for wind-cold-damp impediment, pain in waist and knee, lesser Yin headache, etc.

【药理作用 / Pharmacological effects】

1. 抗炎　独活具有显著的抗炎作用。独活水煎液灌胃对小鼠急性腹膜炎和耳郭肿胀有明显的抑制作用。独活挥发油对大鼠角叉菜胶所致足跖肿胀有明显的抑制作用，作用时间可维持4小时以上。

(1) Anti-inflammation　The decoction of *Dú huó* can inhibit the inflammation of acute peritonitis and ear swelling in mice. The volatile oils of *Dú huó* restrain the foot swelling of rats induced by carrageenan, which can sustain more than 4 h after a single administration.

2. 镇痛　独活水煎液灌胃对小鼠醋酸扭体有明显减轻作用。独活提取物灌胃给药能提高小鼠热刺激的痛阈。

(2) Analgesia　The decoction of *Dú huó* alleviates the pain of mice induced by intraperitoneal injection of acetic acid. Moreover, oral administration with the extract of *Dú huó* elevate the pain threshold induced by heat stimulation.

3. 抑制免疫功能　独活对晶体牛血清白蛋白（BSA）引起的Ⅲ型超敏反应和2,4-二硝基氯苯所致的迟发型超敏反应有显著抑制作用。独活提取物可显著减少BSA所致家兔急性血清病（Ⅲ型超敏反应）的尿蛋白排出量，并对2,4-二硝基氯苯所致小鼠迟发型超敏反应的耳郭肿胀有显著的抑制作用。

(3) Immunosuppression　*Dú huó* can suppress delayed type hypersensitivity induced by 2,4-dinitrochlorobenzene and type Ⅲ hypersensitivity induced by bovine serum albumin(BSA). After 10-day oral administration, the extract of *Dú huó* decrease the excretion of urine protein in rabbits with acute serum sickness (type Ⅲ hypersensitivity) induced by BSA. It also attenuates the ear swelling in mice induced by 2,4-dinitrochlorobenzene.

4. 其他作用　独活还有抗血小板聚集、降血压、抗心律失常、抗肿瘤等药理作用。

(4) Other effects　*Dú huó* also has other effects, such as antiplatelet aggregation, antihypertension, antiarrhythmia, and anti-tumor effects, etc.

【不良反应 / Adverse effects】

独活中的佛手柑内酯、花椒毒素和异欧前胡素等呋喃香豆素类化合物为光活性物质，可引起日光性皮炎，使皮肤红肿、色素增加，甚至表皮增厚等。

Furocoumarins (xanthotoxin, bergapten, and isoimperatorin) in *Dú huó* are photoactive substances which may cause sunlight dermatitis, leading to redness and swelling, pigmentation, even the epidermis thickening of the skin.

防己 ┊ *Fáng jǐ (Radix Stephaniae Tetrandrae)*

【来源 / Origin】

本品为防己科植物粉防己（*Stephania tetrandra* S. Moore）的干燥根。主产于安徽、浙江、江西、福建等省。秋季采挖，洗净，除去粗皮，晒干。

Fáng jǐ is the dried root of *Stephania tetrandra* S. Moore, family of Menispermaceae. The plant is widely cultivated in Anhui province, Zhejiang province, Jiangxi province, Fujian province in China. The raw materials are harvested in the autumn, then dried in the sun after the rough outer bark is removed.

【化学成分 / Chemical ingredients】

含多种生物碱，主要有粉防己碱（汉防己甲素），含量约为1%，防己诺林碱（汉防己乙素），含量约0.5%，其余为轮环藤酚碱、汉防己丙素、汉防己B_6、氧化防己碱和防己菲碱。此外，尚含有黄酮苷、多糖、酚类、有机酸、挥发油等。

Fáng jǐ contains various alkaloids, including about 1% tetrandrine, 0.5% demethyltetrandrine and other alkaloids, such as cyclanoline, hanfangchin C, hanfangchin B₆, oxofangchirine, stephanthrine, etc. *Fáng jǐ* also contains flavonoid glycosides, polysaccharide, phenols, organic acids, and volatile oils.

【药性与功效 / Chinese medicine properties】

味苦，性寒，归膀胱、肺经。具有祛风止痛、利水消肿之功效。用于风湿痹痛、脚气水肿，小便不利、湿疹疮毒。

In Chinese medicine theory, *Fáng jǐ* has the nature of bitter and cold. It can enter the meridians of lung and bladder. *Fáng jǐ* can dispel wind, relieve pain, increase secretion of urine and alleviate edema. Clinically, it can be used for wind-damp impediment pain, barbiers, dropsy, disuria, eczema and sore-toxin, etc.

【药理作用 / Pharmacological effects】

1. 抗炎 粉防己及粉防己碱具有抗炎作用。粉防己碱对多种炎症反应的各个环节均有不同程度的抑制作用，可抑制急性炎症时毛细血管通透性的升高，抑制中性粒细胞的黏附、趋化和吞噬及白细胞介素–1（IL-1）和肿瘤坏死因子（TNF-α）等细胞因子的产生。粉防己碱可增强肾上腺皮质功能而抗炎。

(1) Anti-inflammation *Fáng jǐ* and tetrandrine can suppressed almost all phases of various inflammatory reactions. Tetrandrine decreases the capillary permeability, impedes the adhesion, migration and phagocytosis of the neutrophils, and also inhibits the production of cytokines (IL-1, TNF-α, etc.) in acute inflammation. In addition, tetrandrine can enhance the function of adrenal cortex to achieve anti-inflammation.

2. 抑制免疫 粉防己及粉防己碱具有抑制免疫功能作用。粉防己醇提取物对小鼠脾脏和胸腺淋巴细胞增殖均有抑制作用。粉防己碱可选择性抑制 T 细胞依赖性免疫反应，尤其是淋巴细胞增殖和分化，还可抑制迟发型超敏反应和抗体生成，并能抑制小鼠移植心脏的排异反应，延长其存活时间。

(2) Immunosupression *Fáng jǐ* and tetrandrine have the immunosuppressive effect. Ethanol extract of *Fáng jǐ* inhibits the proliferation of lymphocyte of spleen and thymus in mice. Tetrandrine selectively suppresses T cell dependent immune response, especially inhibits lymphocyte proliferation and differentiation, attenuates delayed hypersensitivity reaction and the formation of antibodies. It can also inhibit the rejection of transplanted mouse heart and prolong the survival time.

3. 对心血管系统的作用

(3) Effects on cardiovascular system

(1) 降血压 汉防己甲素有降血压作用。静脉注射粉防己碱即刻引起舒张压和平均动脉压下降，而心率和收缩压不变。降压作用与阻滞 Ca^{2+} 内流、扩张外周血管有关。

1) Antihypertensive effects Tetrandrine can reduce blood pressure. Intravenous injection of tetrandrine reduces the diastolic pressure and mean arterial pressure quickly, and keeps the heart rate and systolic pressure unchanged. The mechanism is related to blocking calcium influx and dilating the peripheral blood vessels.

(2) 抗心肌缺血及再灌注损伤 粉防己碱能抗心肌缺血及再灌注损伤，尤以对心肌舒张功能及冠脉循环的保护作用更为明显，可降低冠状动脉左前降支结扎心肌梗死模型犬的心肌梗死面积，抑制心电图 S-T 段抬高，降低血中磷酸激酶活性。

2) Resisting myocardial ischemic and reperfusion injury Tetrandrine protects the myocardial from ischemic reperfusion injury, especially protects the diastolic function and coronary circulation. It reduces

the myocardial infarction area induced by ligation of left anterior descending coronary branch artery in dogs, decreases the S-T segment elevation of ECG, and diminishes the activity of serum phosphokinase.

（3）抗心律失常　粉防己碱对多种原因引起的心律失常都有抑制作用，可以减少室速和室颤的发生率。

3) Anti-arrhythmia　Tetrandrine can inhibit arrhythmia induced by various causes, which can reduce the incidence of ventricular tachycardia and fibrillation.

（4）阻滞 Ca^{2+} 通道　粉防己碱具有阻滞 Ca^{2+} 通道的作用，是一种天然可逆性 L 型钙通道阻滞剂。

4) Blocking Ca^{2+} channel　Tetrandrine is a natural reversible L-type calcium channel blocker, which can block the Ca^{2+} channel.

4. 抑制胶原增生及组织纤维化　粉防己碱能显著抑制组织纤维及胶原增生。粉防己碱能抑制肝纤维化的形成，其作用机制可能与抑制储脂细胞的增殖分化，减少Ⅳ型胶原在肝组织中的沉积有关。

(4) Resisting collagen hyperplasia and tissue fibrosis　Tetrandrine can inhibit the proliferation of fiber and collagen. It can reduce the formation of hepatic fibrosis, and the mechanism is related to inhibiting the proliferation of fat-storing cells and decreasing the deposition of type Ⅳ collagen in the liver.

5. 抗硅沉着病　粉防己碱具有抗硅沉着病作用，能抑制硅沉着病组织中Ⅰ型胶原基因、Ⅲ型胶原基因的转录，降低硅沉着病变中胶原蛋白的合成；并能使硅沉着病胶原纤维松散、降解，阻止前胶原转化，抑制肺纤维化。

(5) Anti-silicosis　Tetrandrine has anti-silicosis effect. It restrains the gene transcription of type Ⅰ, Ⅲ collagen, decrease the synthesis of collagen protein in silicosis pathological tissues. Moreover, tetrandrine can make silicosis collagen fiber loosen and degraded, and also prevent procollagen transformation to restrain pulmonary fibrosis.

6. 其他作用　粉防己还有抗脑缺血、抗肿瘤、抑制血小板聚集等作用。

(6) Other effects　Tetrandrine has other effects, such as anti-cerebral ischemia, anti-tumor, resisting platelets aggregation, etc.

【不良反应 / Adverse effects】

部分患者口服粉防己碱后会出现轻度嗜睡、乏力、恶心、上腹部不适，长期口服可能会引起面部色素沉着，停服药后可消退。大剂量注射给药可出现血红蛋白尿及轻度贫血、头昏、恶心、呕吐、寒战、呼吸紧迫和窒息，甚至出现急性肾小球坏死。

Some patients have mild drowsiness, fatigue, nausea and epigastric discomfort after taking tetrandrine. Long-term oral administration tetrandrine may cause pigmentation on face, which can fade after withdrawal it. High-dose tetrandrine injection may lead to hemoglobinuria, mild anemia, dizziness, nausea, vomiting, chills, respiratory distress and asphyxia, and even acute glomerular necrosis.

五加皮 ｜ *Wŭ jiā pí* (*Cortex Acanthopanax Radicis*)

【来源 / Origin】

本品为五加科植物细柱五加（*Acanthopanax gracilistylus* W. W. Smith）的干燥根皮。主产于湖北、河南、安徽、四川等地。夏、秋二季采挖，剥取根皮，晒干。

Wŭ jiā pí is the dried root bark of *Acanthopanax gracilistylus* W. W. Smith, family of Araliaceae. The plant is widely cultivated in Hubei province, Henan province, Anhui province, Sichuan province in China. The raw materials are harvested in the summer and autumn, then dried in the sun after the root bark is removed.

【化学成分 / Chemical ingredients】

主要含有刺五加苷 B（即紫丁香苷）、刺五加苷 B1、棕榈酸、右旋芝麻素、16α- 羟基 -(-)- 贝壳松 -19- 酸、β- 谷甾醇、β- 谷甾醇葡萄糖苷、亚油酸及维生素 A、维生素 B 等。

Wǔ jiā pí contains eleutheroside B, eleutheroside B1, palmitic acid, sesamin, 16α-hydroxy-(-)-kauran-19-oic acid, β-sitosterol, β-sitosterol glucoside, linolenic acid and vitamin A, vitamin B, etc.

【药性与功效 / Chinese medicine properties】

味辛、苦，性温，归肝、肾经。具有祛风除湿、补益肝肾、强筋壮骨、利水消肿之功效。用于治疗风湿痹痛、筋骨痿软、小儿行迟、体虚乏力、水肿、脚气等证。

In Chinese medicine theory, *Wǔ jiā pí* has the nature of pungent, bitter and warm, It can enter the meridians of liver and kidney. *Wǔ jiā pí* can dispel wind and eliminate dampness, supplement liver and kidney, strengthen sinew and bone, excrete water and alleviate swelling. Clinically, it is used for wind-damp impediment pain, flaccidity of extremities, retardation of walking in children, weakness and lack of strength, edema, beriberil, etc.

【药理作用 / Pharmacological effects】

1. 抗炎　五加皮的乙醇提取液对大鼠蛋清性及甲醛性关节炎有抑制作用。体外与体内试验研究结果表明，五加皮醇提物对环氧化酶 -1（COX-1）和环氧化酶 -2（COX-2）均有抑制作用，在相同剂量时，对 COX-2 的抑制率大于 COX-1。抑制环氧化酶可能是五加皮抗炎作用的机制之一。

(1) Anti-inflammation　Ethanol extract of *Wǔ jiā pí* can restrain the inflammation of arthritis in rats induced by egg white and formaldehyde. Ethanol extract of *Wǔ jiā pí* can inhibit the activities of cyclooxygenase-1 (COX-1) and COX-2 *in vivo* and *in vitro*, and its inhibition on COX-2 is stronger than its inhibition on COX-1 at the same dose. The anti-inflammation mechanism of *Wǔ jiā pí* may be related to inhibition of cyclooxygenase.

2. 免疫调节　细柱五加皮水煎醇沉液对免疫功能有抑制作用，可明显降低小鼠腹腔巨噬细胞的吞噬百分率和吞噬指数，抑制小鼠脾脏抗体形成。乳鼠半心移植实验证明细柱五加皮有一定抗排异作用，可使移植心肌平均存活时间显著延长。五加皮总苷和多糖有提高机体体液免疫功能的作用，能促进小鼠单核巨噬细胞系统的吞噬功能，使血清炭末廓清率明显提高，并增加小鼠血清抗体的浓度。

(2) Regulating immune function　Ethanol deposit solution of *Wǔ jiā pí* can suppress the immune function, which is shown in reducing the phagocytic percentage and phagocytic index of peritoneal macrophages, and inhibiting spleen antibody forming in mice. The experiment of half heart transplantation in sucking mice shows that *Wǔ jiā pí* can significantly prolong the average survival time of transplanted myocardium, indicating that it has anti-rejection effects. The total glucosides and polysaccharides of *Wǔ jiā pí* can improve the humoral immune function of mice, which is shown in promoting the phagocytosis of reticuloendothelial system, increasing the clearance rate of serum carbon, and increasing the concentration of serum antibody.

3. 其他作用　五加皮还有抗肿瘤、抗疲劳、抗应激、降血糖等药理作用。

(3) Other effects　*Wǔ jiā pí* has other effects, such as anti-tumor, anti-fatigue, anti-stress, and hypoglycemic activity, etc.

雷公藤 | *Léi gōng téng* (*Radix Folium seu Flos Tripterygii Wilfordii*)

【来源 / Origin】

本品为卫矛科植物雷公藤（*Tripterygium wilfordii* Hook. f.）的干燥根。主产于福建、浙江、安徽、河南等地。秋季采挖，晒干。

Léi gōng téng is the dried root of *Tripterygium wilfordii* Hook. f., family of Celastraceae. The plant is widely cultivated in Fujian province, Zhejiang province, Anhui province, Henan province in china. It is harvested in autumn and dried in the sun.

【化学成分 / Chemical ingredients】

主要含有生物碱类、二萜类、三萜类、倍半萜类等成分。生物碱类有雷公藤碱、雷公藤次碱、雷公藤新碱、雷公藤戊碱、雷公藤碱乙等；二萜类化合物有雷公藤甲素（雷公藤内酯醇）、雷公藤乙素、雷公藤氯内醇酯等；三萜内酯类有雷公藤内酯甲、雷公藤内酯乙、雷公藤三萜酸、雷公藤红素等；倍半萜类有雷藤素、萨拉子酸等。

Léi gōng téng contains alkaloids, diterpenoids, triterpenoids and sesquiterpenoids. The essential components of alkaloids are Wilfordine, wilforine, uonine, wilforidine and wilforgine. The main components of diterpenoids are triptolide, tripdiolide and tripchlorolide. The main components of triterpenoids are wilforlide A, wilforlide B and triptotriterpenic acid and celastrol. The main components of sesquiterpenoids are wilformide and salaspermicacid, etc.

【药性与功效 / Chinese medicine properties】

味辛、苦，性寒，有毒，归肝、肾经。具有祛风除湿、活血通络、消肿定痛、杀虫解毒之功效。用于类风湿关节炎、风湿性关节炎、跌打损伤等。

In Chinese medicine theory, *Léi gōng téng* has the nature of bitter and cold, with strong toxicity. It can enter the meridians of heart and liver. *Léi gōng téng* can dispel wind and eliminate dampness, invigorate blood and activate collaterals, disperse swelling and relieve pain, kill worms and relieve toxin. Clinically, it was used for rheumatoid arthritis, rheumatic arthritis, traumatic injury, etc.

【药理作用 / Pharmacological effects】

1. 免疫抑制 雷公藤及其多种成分对体液免疫与细胞免疫均有明显的抑制作用。雷公藤及其提取物能使大鼠胸腺、脾脏等淋巴器官萎缩，血液白细胞数减少，淋巴细胞总数减少，中性粒细胞与单核细胞相对增加；抑制 T 细胞的增殖和活性；抑制 B 细胞增殖和抗体生成。

(1) Immunosupression *Léi gōng téng* and its ingredients can inhibit humoral immunity and cellular immunity. *Léi gōng téng* and its extracts can induce thymus and spleen atropy, decrease the number of leukocytes and lymphocytes, and increase the number of neutrophils and monocytes relatively; *Léi gōng téng* can also inhibit the proliferation of T and B cells, and the production of antibody.

2. 抗炎 雷公藤对急慢性炎症均有抑制作用。对炎症早期的血管通透性增加、炎症细胞趋化、炎症介质的产生和释放及炎症后期纤维增生等具有明显的抑制作用。雷公藤多苷是雷公藤抗炎作用的主要有效成分之一。雷公藤的抗炎作用机制与抑制炎症介质的产生和释放有关，并通过兴奋下丘脑-垂体-肾上腺皮质系统，促进肾上腺皮质激素释放。

(2) Anti-inflammation *Léi gōng téng* can inhibit the acute and chronic inflammation. *Léi gōng téng* may decrease the capillary permeability, chemotaxis of inflammatory cells, production of inflammatory mediators in the early stage of inflammation and the fibroplasia in the late stage of inflammation. Tripterysium glycosides is one of the major components of anti-inflammation of *Léi gōng téng*. The mechanism is involved in decreasing the production release of inflammatory mediators.

Moreover, *Léi gōng téng* activates hypothalamus-pituitary-adrenal axis, enhances the function of adrenal cortex, and promotes the synthesis of adrenocortical hormone to inhibit the inflammation.

3. 镇痛　雷公藤有镇痛作用。雷公藤流浸膏对醋酸所致小鼠扭体反应和热板法所致疼痛均有显著的抑制作用。

(3) Analgesia　*Léi gōng téng* has the analgesic effect. *Léi gōng téng* extract can inhibit writhing response induced by acetic acid and pain induced by hot plate in mice.

4. 改善血液流变学　雷公藤乙酸乙酯提取物能降低佐剂关节炎大鼠全血和血浆黏度、纤维蛋白原含量，减少血细胞比容，降低血小板最大聚集率，改善佐剂关节炎大鼠的血液流变学。

(4) Improving hemorheology　Ethyl acetate extract of *Léi gōng téng* can reduce the whole blood viscosity, plasma viscosity and fibrinogen content, and can also decrease hematocrit and maximum platelet aggregation rate to improve hemorheology in rats with adjuvant arthritis.

5. 抗菌、抗病毒、杀虫　雷公藤对金黄色葡萄球菌、607 分枝杆菌、枯草杆菌有明显抑制作用；对真菌尤其是皮肤白念珠菌等抑制作用最强，对革兰阴性菌也有一定效果；雷公藤红素是其主要抑菌成分。萨拉子酸还可抵抗人类免疫缺陷病毒活性。雷公藤水浸剂、醇浸液及醚提物还能杀虫、蛆、蝇等。

(5) Anti-bacteria, anti-virus, insecticidal effects　*Léi gōng téng* can inhibit the growth of *staphylococcus aureus*, *607 mycobacteria*, *bacillus subtilis*, and fungus, especially has the strongest inhibition on candida albicans. In addition, *Léi gōng téng* exhibit certain inhibitory effect on gram negative bacteria as well. The key ingredient of antibacterial effect is tripterine. Salaspermicacid also has anti-HIV activity. Water, alcohol, and ether extract of *Léi gōng téng* can also kill insects, maggots, flies, etc.

6. 其他作用

(6) Other effects

（1）抗生育　雷公藤制剂及其多种成分具有抑制生育的作用。成年雄性大鼠灌服雷公藤多苷 10mg/kg，8 周后全部失去生育能力，作用的靶细胞主要是精母细胞和精子细胞，能降低初级精母细胞核内 DNA 含量，也可抑制精子的变形和成熟。雷公藤氯内酯醇具有更强的抗生育作用，可致大鼠附睾尾精子存活率和密度明显下降而不育。雷公藤多苷片可使育龄女性月经减少甚至闭经，阴道上皮细胞不同程度地萎缩；使雌性大鼠的动情周期不规则，子宫重量减轻。雷公藤抗生育作用具有可逆性，停止给药后 6~8 个月生育功能可以恢复。

1) Anti-fertility　*Léi gōng téng* preparations and its various components have anti-fertility effect. All of the male rats treated with 10mg/kg tripterygium glycosides daily for 8 weeks, lose the ability of fertility. The target cells of *Léi gōng téng* are spermatocytes and sperms which can reduce the DNA content in the nucleus of primary spermatocytes, inhibit sperm motility and maturation. Tripchlorolide has the stronger antifertility effect, which can decreased sperm survival rate and density of cauda epididymidis of rats and lead to infertility. Tripterysium glycosides tablets can induce hypomenorrhea, even amenorrhoea in fertile women, and cause vaginal epithelial cells to atrophy. Tripterysium glycosides tablets can also cause irregular estrous cycle and decrease uterine weight in female rats. The anti-fertility effect of *Léi gōng téng* is reversible, and the fertility function can be restored after stopping the medicine for 6-8 months.

（2）抗肿瘤　雷公藤及其提取物有抑制肿瘤的作用，雷公藤甲素、乙素和雷公藤内酯有抗肿瘤作用，对多种瘤株都有抑制作用。

2) Anti-tumor　*Léi gōng téng* and its extract posses the anti-tumor effect. Triptolide, tripdiolide and triterpenoids are active anti-tumor components, which can inhibit various tumor strains.

【不良反应 / Adverse effects】

1. **消化系统损害** 雷公藤致消化系统不良反应发生频率高，且在正常剂量范围内就可发生，主要表现为恶心、呕吐、胃部不适、腹痛、腹鸣、腹泻、便血、食欲减退、口干、食管下部灼烧感等。约有 1/3 的患者服用雷公藤后会导致 ALT 升高，严重者出现黄疸、肝大、肝脏出血及肝坏死，多发生在用药后 2~4 周。

(1) Digestive system *Léi gōng téng* cause the adverse reactions in the digestive system with high incidence, and may occur in the normal dose range. The main symptoms include nausea, vomiting, stomach discomfort, stomachache, borborygmi, diarrhea, hematochezia, loss of appetite, dry mouth, burning sensation in the lower esophagus, etc. *Léi gōng téng* also causes liver damage with increased activity of glutamic-pyruvic transaminase (ALT), jaundice, hepatomegaly, bleeding and liver necrosis, which usually occur 2~4 weeks after treatment.

2. **皮肤黏膜损害** 引起色素沉着、黄褐斑、红斑、口腔及唇糜烂、指（趾）甲变薄及软化、脱发等。

(2) Skin and mucous damage Symptoms include pigmentation, yellow brown spots, erythema, mouth and lip erosion, fingernail (toenail) thinning and softening, alopecia, etc.

3. **骨髓抑制** 雷公藤对骨髓有抑制作用，可引起白细胞、红细胞、血小板及血细胞减少、弥散性小血管内凝血、再生障碍性贫血、类白血病反应和继发性白血病。

(3) Bone marrow suppression *Léi gōng téng* has the inhibitory effect on bone marrow, which leads to a decrease in white blood cells, red blood cells and platelets, as well as diffuse intravascular coagulation and regeneration barrier anemia, leukemoid reaction and secondary leukemia.

4. **生殖系统毒性** 男性表现为精子数量显著减少、活动力下降、畸形率增加，造成生育能力下降或不育，长期用药可造成性欲减退、睾丸萎缩、男性乳房增大。男性儿童可因药物致青春期性腺发育障碍而发生生殖器发育不良；女性因卵巢功能受抑制而表现为月经紊乱如月经增多、减少或闭经，育龄妇女可致不孕。

(4) Reproductive toxicity For men, *Léi gōng téng* can reduce the number and activity of sperm. It also increases deformity rate and leads to reducing fertility or sterility. Long-term administration can cause loss of libido, testicular atrophy, male breast enlargement. It can cause adolescent gonadal development disorder in male children, result in genital dysplasia. In addition, *Léi gōng téng* can reduce the function of ovarian and lead to menstrual disorders and infertility in women.

5. **心血管系统毒性** 主要表现为心悸、胸闷、气短、心律失常及心电图改变，心电图显示房室传导阻滞、室性期前收缩及心肌损害。常发生于超常用量及原有心血管病患者，严重中毒者可出现血压急剧下降，心肌供血不足，甚至出现心源性休克、心力衰竭。

(5) Toxicity in cardiovascular system The main clinical symptoms include palpitation, chest tightness, shortness of breath, arrhythmia and ECG abnormality, such as atrioventricular conduction disturbance, premature ventricular beats and myocardial damage. These symptoms are more common in the patients with original cardiovascular disease or long-term administration. Severe poisoning symptoms include dramatic decrease of blood pressure, myocardial blood deficiency, and even emergence of cardiac shock, and heart failure.

6. **泌尿系统损害** 可引起急性肾衰竭，表现为少尿或无尿、水肿、血尿、蛋白尿、管型尿、腰痛或伴肾区叩击痛、氮质血症、酸中毒，甚至因急性肾衰竭而死亡。

(6) Urinary system lesion Patients with *Léi gōng téng* poisoning may be accompanied with renal damage, mainly acute renal failure. The symptoms include oliguria or anuria, edema, hematuria, proteinuria, cylindruria, lumbago with percussion pain in renal area, azotemia, acidosis, even death due to acute renal failure.

7. 神经系统毒性 可引起神经细胞变性并导致神经系统损害，主要表现为头晕、头痛、乏力、失眠或嗜睡、肌肉疼痛、四肢麻木、抽搐，并可导致听力减退、复视、记忆力减退、周围神经炎、脑水肿等。

(7) Nervous system toxicity *Léi gōng téng* can cause nerve cell degeneration and nervous system damage. Symptoms include dizziness, headache, fatigue, insomnia or drowsiness, muscle pain, numbness of limbs, convulsions, hearing loss, diplopia, memory loss, peripheral neuritis, and cerebral edema, etc.

8. 免疫抑制 治疗量对免疫功能有抑制作用，超量则会引起淋巴器官萎缩和淋巴细胞凋亡。

(8) Immunosuppression *Léi gōng téng* can suppress the immune function with therapeutic dose. Overdose of *Léi gōng téng* leads to atrophy of lymphoid organ and apoptosis of lymphocytes.

题库

（方晓燕　方　芳）

第八章　芳香化湿药

Chapter 8　Aromatic damp-resolving medicines

学习目标｜Objectives

1. **掌握**　芳香化湿药的主要药理作用；苍术、厚朴、广藿香与功效相关的药理作用、作用机制及药效物质基础。

2. **了解**　湿阻中焦证的主要病理表现；厚朴、苍术、广藿香的不良反应。

1. **Must know**　The main pharmacological effects of dampness resolving with aromatic medicines; the pharmacological effects, mechanism, and material base of *Hòu pò*, *Cāng zhú*, and *Guǎng huò xiāng*.

2. **Desirable to know**　Syndrome of dampness obstructing in middle energizer and its main pathological manifestations; the adverse effects of *Hòu pò*, *Cāng zhú*, and *Guǎng huò xiāng*.

第一节　概述

Section 1　Overview

微课

PPT

　　凡气味芳香，以化湿运脾为主要功效的药物称为芳香化湿药。本类药物主入脾、胃、肺经，性温，味苦、辛。温能行气、辛能发散、苦能燥湿，故本类药物一般具有舒畅气机、宣化湿浊、健脾醒胃的功效。临床主要用于治疗湿困脾胃、湿阻中焦证，也可用于治疗湿温、暑湿证。

All Chinese medicines materials that have an aromatic smell and are used to resolve dampness are classified as aromatic damp-resolving medicines. Medicines in this category mainly enter the meridians of the spleen, stomach, and lung. The nature of this class of medicines is warm, bitter and acrid. In theory of traditional Chinese medicine, the medicines with warm nature can move Qi; the medicines with acrid nature have dispersing effect; and the medicines with bitter nature can dry dampness. Therefore, this kind of medicines generally have the effects of relaxing Qi movement and resolving dampness turbidity, invigorating spleen and enlivening stomach. They are mainly used in the syndrome of dampness retention in spleen-stomach, syndrome of dampness obstructing in middle energizer, dampness-warm syndrome, and summerheat-dampness syndrome in clinical practice.

　　湿与水异名同类，湿为水之渐，水为湿之积。脾胃为后天之本，主运化，能够运化水湿。脾运化失司，则水运内停而为湿。内停之湿为异常之湿，称为湿邪。脾喜燥而恶湿，土爱暖而悦芳

医药大学堂
www.yiyaodxt.com

香。湿邪为病，易伤脾胃，脾胃为湿困，则脾阳不升，胃气不降，水湿内聚，气机不畅，可见脘腹痞满、呕吐泛酸、大便溏薄、食少体倦、口甘多涎、舌苔白腻等症状，临床表现为湿阻中焦证。主要病理表现为胃肠动力与水液代谢障碍、肠黏膜屏障破坏、病原微生物异常等，与西医学中消化系统疾病表现相似。芳香化湿药临床主要用于急慢性胃肠炎、痢疾、胃肠过敏、胃溃疡、胃无力、胃下垂、胃肠神经官能症及消化不良等疾病的治疗。

In theory of traditional Chinese medicine, dampness and water are the same substance but have different name. Dampness is the product of gradual development of water, while water is accumulated by dampness. Spleen and stomach are the acquired foundation and govern transportation and transformation, so they can transport and transform the dampness and water. If the function of spleen is abnormal, the water transportation will stop and lead to dampness. The stopped dampness in the body is an abnormal dampness, which is called pathogenic dampness. The spleen prefers dryness and is averse to dampness, while the earth likes warmth and fragrance. As a pathogenic factor, dampness can damage the spleen and stomach. Dampness retaining in spleen and stomach will lead to the failure of spleen Yang to ascend and stomach Qi to descend, accumulation of water and dampness in the body and obstruction of Qi movement, which can induce some symptoms such as abdominal fullness, serious vomiting, soft stool, eating less and tiredness, increased saliva, white and greasy tongue coating, etc. These clinical manifestations are syndrome of dampness obstructing in middle energizer. At present, the following pathological manifestations may be observed in syndrome of dampness obstructing in middle energizer, such as disorder of gastrointestinal movement and water metabolism, destruction of intestinal mucosal barrier, and abnormality of pathogenic microorganism, etc. Generally speaking, the main pathological manifestations of dampness obstructing in middle energizer are similar to digestive system diseases in western medicine, so they can be used for the treatments of acute and chronic gastroenteritis, dysentery, gastrointestinal allergy, gastric ulcer, gastric weakness or gastric ptosis, neurosis, dyspepsia and so on.

"湿淫于内，治宜苦热，佐以酸淡，以苦燥之"。化湿药多辛香苦燥，能够辟秽、宣化湿浊、运化脾胃，改善患者临床症状。挥发油类成分是芳香化湿药的主要药效物质基础，在药材中含量较高。如厚朴挥发油含量约为1%，苍术因产地不同挥发油含量在1%~9%，广藿香挥发油含量约为1.5%。因挥发油具有易挥发的特性，本类药物煎煮时间不宜过长，以免影响临床疗效。

"Excesses of dampness in the body should be cured with medicines with bitter flavor and heat property, supplemented with sourness and blandness." Most of these aromatic medicines for resolving dampness are acrid or bitter in flavor, which can dispel filth and expel the dampness turbidity, transport and transform the spleen and stomach to improve the symptoms of clinic. As the main active substance basis, the content of volatile oils is high in the medicinal materials. There are several examples: the content of volatile oils in *Hòu pò* is about 1%; the content of volatile oils in *Guǎng huò xiāng* is around 1.5%; the concent of volatile oils in *Cāng zhú* varies from 1% to 9% according to different producing areas. Because of the easier vaporization characteristics of volatile oils, the cooking time should not be too long, and excessive cooking time can easily lead to the loss of effective ingredients and decrease the clinical efficiency.

常用的芳香化湿药主要包括厚朴、苍术、广藿香、佩兰、砂仁、白豆蔻、草豆蔻等，具有化湿作用的复方主要有藿香正气散、平胃散、霍胆丸等。芳香化湿药治疗湿阻中焦证主要与下列药理作用有关。

The commonly used aromatic damp-resolving medicines in clinic mainly include *Hòu pò*, *Cāng zhú*, *Guǎng huò xiāng*, *Pèi lán*, *Shā rén*, *Bái dòu kòu*, *Cǎo dòu kòu*, etc. and the formulas with the resolving dampness effect include *Huoxiang Zhengqi San*, *Pingwei San*, *Huodan Wan*, and so on. The treatment of dampness obstructing in middle energizer with aromatic damp-resolving medicines is related to the following pharmacological effects.

1. 调节胃肠运动　芳香化湿药能够调节胃肠运动功能。例如，佩兰能够促进胃肠内容物排空，砂仁可以促进肠管平滑肌运动；厚朴、苍术、广藿香等对乙酰胆碱和氯化钡引起的离体肠肌痉挛有不同程度的解痉作用。

(1) Regulate gastrointestinal movement　This kind of medicines can regulate gastrointestinal movements. For example, *Pèi lán* can promote the emptying of gastrointestinal contents, and *shā rén* can stimulate the smooth muscle movement of the intestine. On the other hand, *Hòu pò*, *Cāng zhú*, *Guǎng huò xiāng* can inhibit isolated intestinal muscle spasm caused by acetylcholine and barium chloride.

2. 保护胃肠黏膜　芳香化湿药能够增加胃黏膜血流量，促进胃黏膜修复，抗实验性溃疡；促进大鼠血清胃泌素分泌，促进消化道黏膜生长。例如，苍术能够提高胃液中前列腺素 E_2（PGE_2）含量，保护胃黏膜免受多种外源性因素的损伤；广藿香挥发油具有肠黏膜保护作用，能显著提高肠黏液分泌量，促进肠上皮细胞紧密连接蛋白 ZO-1 和 Occludin 蛋白表达，提高胃黏膜超氧化物歧化酶（SOD）活性，降低胃黏膜丙二醛（MDA）含量。

(2) Protect gastrointestinal mucosa　Aromatic damp-resolving medicines have effects on increasing the blood flow of gastric mucosa and promoting the repair of injured gastric mucosa, so they were used to treat gastric ulcers. They also can increase the blood flow of gastric mucosa and promote the secretion of serum gastrin which can promote the growth of gastrointestinal mucosa. For example, *Cāng zhú* can elevate the content of prostaglandin E_2 (PGE_2) in gastric juice, which can protect the gastric mucosa from a variety of exogenous factors. Volatile oils in *Guǎng huò xiāng*, which have protective effect on intestinal mucosa can significantly stimulate intestinal mucus secretion, promote expression of tight junction protein ZO-1 and Occludin in intestinal epithelial cells, increase the activity of superoxide dismutase (SOD) and decrease the content of malondialdehyde (MDA) in gastric mucosa.

3. 影响消化液分泌　多数芳香化湿药含有挥发油类成分，能够通过刺激嗅觉、味觉感受器，或刺激局部黏膜，反射性地影响消化腺分泌。例如，厚朴、广藿香、砂仁、白豆蔻、草豆蔻、草果等能够刺激消化液分泌；苍术能够抑制胃酸分泌，临床上用于治疗胃溃疡。

(3) Affect digestive secretion　Most of the aromatic damp-resolving medicines contain volatile oils, which can reflexively affect the secretion of the digestive glands by stimulating receptors of olfactory and taste or local mucosa. Many medicines could stimulate the secretion of digestive fluid, such as *Hòu pò*, *Guǎng huò xiāng*, *Bái dòu kòu*, *Cǎo dòu kòu*, *Cǎo guǒ*; *Cāng zhú* can inhibit the secretion of gastric acid and is used to treat gastric ulcers in clinic.

4. 抗病原微生物　芳香化湿药具有不同程度的抗病原微生物作用。例如，厚朴煎剂对于金黄色葡萄球菌、α- 溶血性链球菌、白喉棒状杆菌、枯草杆菌、痢疾杆菌、伤寒杆菌、副伤寒杆菌、霍乱弧菌、大肠埃希菌、变形菌、铜绿假单胞菌、须毛癣菌、肺炎链球菌、百日咳鲍特菌有体外抑制或杀灭作用；苍术挥发油对于金黄色葡萄球菌、酵母菌、青霉菌、黑曲霉菌、黄曲霉菌、大肠埃希菌、枯草芽孢杆菌等细菌和真菌具有较好的抑制作用，临床上苍术用于医院环境消毒和动植物细菌性疾病的防治。

(4) Anti-microbial effects　Most aromatic damp-resolving medicines have inhibitory effects on pathogenic microbial. *Hòu pò* decoction can inhibit various pathogenic microbial *in vitro*, such as *Staphylococcus aureus*, *α-streptococcus hemolyticus*, *Corynebacterium diphtheriae*, *Bacillus subtilis*,

Shigella dysenteriae, *Salmonella typhi*, *Salmonella paratyphi*, *Vibrio cholerae*, *Escherichia* coli, *Proteus*, *Pseudomonas aeruginosa*, *Trichophyton mentagrophytes*, *Streptococcus pneumoniae*, and *Bordetella pertussis*. Volatile oil of *Cāng zhú* has a good inhibitory effect on *Staphylococcus aureus*, *Saccharomyces*, *Penicillium*, *Aspergillus niger*, *Aspergillus flavus*, *Escherichia coli*, *Bacillus subtilis* and other bacteria and fungi. It is clinically used for disinfection of hospital environment and prevention and treatment of bacterial diseases of animals and plants.

5. **调节水液代谢**　芳香化湿药能够降低湿阻中焦证模型大鼠血清醛固酮（ALD）及肾小管水通道蛋白（AQP_2）水平，升高结肠水通道蛋白（AQP_3）水平。例如，苍术能够降低模型大鼠血清 ALD 和 AQP_2 水平，升高 AQP_3 水平；平胃散能通过调节血清中水液代谢调节激素的平衡，从而调节尿量，使细胞内外电解质达到平衡，同时通过调节肝脏水转运蛋白的表达、含量和磷酸化活性，使人体水液代谢趋于平衡。

(5) Regulate water metabolism　Aromatic damp-resolving medicines can decrease the level of aldosterone (ALD) in serum and aquaporin 2 (AQP_2) in renal tubules, and increase the level of colonic aquaporin 3 (AQP_3) in colon of rats with dampness obstruction in middle energizer. For example, n-butanol extract from *Cāng zhú* can decrease serum ALD and AQP_2 levels and increase the AQP_3 level of model rats with dampness obstruction in middle energizer. *Pingwei San* can regulate hormones in the serum to adjust the amount of urine to maintain the internal and external balance of electrolytes. At the same time, by regulating the expression, content and phosphorylation activity of AQP in liver, *Pingwei san* can balance the entire body's water metabolism.

芳香化湿药还具有不同程度的抗肿瘤、抗过敏、抗炎、抗血栓、抑制血小板聚集、祛痰等药理作用。

Aromatic damp-resolving medicines have other pharmacological effects like anti-tumor, anti-allergy, anti-inflammation, anti-thrombosis, anti-platelet aggregation, and expectorant effect.

常用芳香化湿药的主要药理作用见表8-1。

The main pharmacological effects of commonly used aromatic damp-resolving medicines are summarized in Table 8-1.

表 8-1　常用芳香化湿药的主要药理作用

药物	调节胃肠运动	调节消化液分泌	保护胃肠黏膜	抗病原微生物	其他药理作用
厚朴	+	+	+	+	抗炎、抗氧化、肌肉松弛、中枢抑制、抗肿瘤
苍术	+	+	+	+	保肝利胆、利尿、抗炎镇痛、降血糖
广藿香	+	+	+	+	抗炎镇痛、抗氧化、镇咳、平喘
砂仁	+	–	+	+	抑制血小板聚集、免疫抑制、降血糖、促进胆汁分泌
白豆蔻	+	+	–	+	平喘
草豆蔻	+	+	+	+	平喘、抗脑缺血
草果	–	–	–	+	—
佩兰	+	+	+	–	祛痰、抗肿瘤

备注："+"表示有明确作用；"–"表示无作用，或未查阅到相关研究文献

PPT

第二节　常用药物
Section 2　Commonly used medicines

| 厚朴 ┊ *Hòu pò* (*Magnoliae Officinalis Cortex*) |

【来源 / Origin】

本品为木兰科植物厚朴（*Magnolia officinalis* Rehd. et Wils.）或凹叶厚朴（*Magnolia officinalis* Rehd. et Wils. var. *Biloba* Rehd. et Wils.）的干燥干皮、根皮及枝皮。原产于湖北，现多栽培。4~6 月剥取，根皮和枝皮直接阴干；干皮置沸水中微煮后，堆置阴湿处，"发汗"至内表面呈紫褐色或棕褐色时，蒸软，取出，卷成筒状，干燥。

Hòu Pò is the dried bark of *Magnolia officinalis* Rehd. et Wils. or *Magnolia officinalis* Rehd. et Wils. var. *Biloba* Rehd. et Wils. The plant is native to Hubei province in China, but now most of them are cultivated. The raw materials are collected from April to June, the root bark and branch bark should be dried directly; the trunk barks need to be boiled in boiling water stacked in the damp place until the inner surface becomes purple or brown, then steamed, rolled and dried.

【化学成分 / Chemical ingredients】

主要含挥发油类、木质素类、生物碱类成分。挥发油含量约为 1%，主要是桉叶油醇（eudesmol）、聚伞花素（cymene）。木质素类成分主要有厚朴酚（magnolol）、四氢厚朴酚（tetrahydromagnolol）、异厚朴酚（isomagnolol）、和厚朴酚（honokiol）及冰基厚朴酚（ice-based magnolol）等。生物碱类成分主要有木兰箭毒碱（magnocurarine）、柳叶木兰碱（salicifoline）、番荔枝碱（anonaine）、白兰花碱（michelalbine）等。此外，尚含莰烯（camphene）、α 蒎烯（α pinene）、松油醇（terpineol）等。

The chemical ingredients of *Hòu pò* are mainly divided into three types, namely volatile oil, lignin, and alkaloid. There is about 1% volatile oil, including eudesmol and cymene. Lignins contain magnolol, tetrahydromagnolol, isomagnolol, honokiol and ice-based magnolol. Magnocurarine, salicifoline, anonaine and michelalbine are the key alkaloids. In addition, there is a small amount of camphene, α pinene and terpineol in *Hòu Pò*.

【药性与功效 / Chinese medicine properties】

味苦、辛，性温，归脾、胃、肺、大肠经。具有燥湿消痰、下气除满的功效。用于湿滞伤中、脘痞吐泻、食积气滞、腹胀便秘、痰饮喘咳等证。

In Chinese medicine theory, *Hòu pò* has a warm nature, bitter and acrid. It can enter the meridians of spleen, stomach, lungs, and large intestine. *Hòu pò* can dry dampness to dispel phlegm, down Qi to relieve fullness. It is clinically used in treatment for dampness stagnation damaging middle, gastric stuffiness, nausea and vomiting, food accumulation and Qi stagnation, abdominal distension constipation, cough and asthma due to accumulation of phlegm in the lung.

【药理作用 / Pharmacological effects】

1. 调节胃肠运动　厚朴具有增强胃底平滑肌运动的作用，能够促进胃蠕动，有利胃排空。其增强胃底平滑肌张力作用可被阿托品阻断，说明此作用可能是由 M 受体所介导。厚朴也能够拮抗乙酰胆碱引起的十二指肠平滑肌运动。此外，厚朴碱静脉注射使麻醉猫在体小肠张力下降；厚朴酚和厚朴碱对组胺所致十二指肠痉挛有一定的抑制作用。

(1) Regulate gastrointestinal movement *Hòu pò* can enhance gastric fundus smooth muscle movement, which can promote gastric peristalsis, and lead to gastric empty. The effect of enhancing gastric fundus smooth muscle tension can be blocked by atropine, which means the effect on gastrointestinal smooth muscle movement may be partially mediated by M receptor. *Hòu pò* also has significant antagonistic effects on duodenal smooth muscle strengthening caused by acetylcholine. In addition, magnolia alkaloids with intravenous injection decrease the tension of the small intestine in anesthetized cats; magnolol and magnolia alkaloids have a certain inhibitory effect on duodenal spasm caused by histamine.

2. 抗胃溃疡　生品厚朴、姜炙厚朴煎剂对大鼠幽门结扎型溃疡及应激型溃疡均有明显抑制作用。厚朴乙醇提取物对大鼠盐酸-乙醇所致溃疡有显著抑制作用。厚朴酚对应激和静脉注射胃泌素或卡巴胆碱所致胃酸分泌增多有明显抑制作用。抗溃疡主要有效成分为厚朴酚与和厚朴酚，作用机制与其抑制胃酸分泌有关。

(2) Anti-gastric ulcer Decoction from raw or ginger processed *Hòu pò* have obvious therapeutic effects on gastric ulcer induced by pyloric ligation or stress induced in rat model. It has been proved that ethanol extracts has a significant therapeutic effect on gastric ulcers caused by hydrochloric acid-ethanol in rats. What is more, magnolol can also significantly inhibit gastric acid secretion caused by stress, gastrin or carbamylcholine stimulation. The main active ingredients are magnolol and honokiol. The mechanism is related to the inhibition on excessive secretion of gastric acid.

3. 保肝、利胆　厚朴具有保肝作用，能够减轻四氯化碳（CCl_4）诱导肝损伤小鼠的肝纤维化，降低血液中谷丙转氨酶（ALT）、谷草转氨酶（AST）、碱性磷酸酶（ALP）含量和血糖浓度；减少损伤肝组织中肿瘤坏死因子 –α（TNF-α），白细胞介素 –6（IL-6），干扰素 – γ（IFN- γ）mRNA 的表达，降低 MDA 含量，增加 SOD 活性；保肝作用机制与抗炎、抗氧化相关；主要药效物质基础为厚朴酚、和厚朴酚。厚朴具有利胆作用，能够增加低温麻醉大鼠的胆汁分泌量，对胆固醇、胆汁酸及总胆红素含量无明显影响。

(3) Liver protection and bile secretion promotion *Hòu pò* has a protective effect on the liver. It can lower alanine aminotransferase (ALT), aspartate aminotransferase (AST), alkaline phosphatase (ALP) content and glucose concentration of blood in the mice induced by carbon tetrachloride (CCl_4). *Hòu pò* can also decrease tumor necrosis factor (TNF-α), interleukin-6 (IL-6), interferon- γ (IFN- γ) mRNA expression and MDA content, and increase the activity of SOD injured liver tissue. The mechanisms of its protective effect on the damaged liver may be related to its anti-inflammatory and antioxidant effect. Magnolol and honokiol are the main active substances. *Hòu pò* can promote bile secretion. It can significantly increase the total bile secretion of anesthetized rats under low temperature conditions, but there is no significant change in cholesterol, bile acid and total bilirubin.

4. 抗病原微生物　厚朴煎剂对金黄色葡萄球菌、α– 溶血性链球菌、白喉棒状杆菌、枯草杆菌、痢疾杆菌、伤寒杆菌、副伤寒杆菌、霍乱弧菌、大肠埃希菌、铜绿假单胞菌、须毛癣菌、肺炎链球菌、百日咳鲍特菌均有抑制作用。和厚朴酚对于持续病毒应答（SVR）细胞及人类免疫缺陷病毒（HIV）活性具有较好的抑制作用，对 SVR 细胞的抑制率达 60% 以上；对人淋巴细胞中 HIV 的半数有效浓度（EC_{50}）为 3.3 μmol/L。

(4) Anti-microbial effects The bacteria that can be inhibited by *Hòu pò* decoction include *Staphylococcus aureus*, *α-streptococcus hemolylicus*, *Corynebacterium diphtheriae*, *Bacillus subtilis*, *Shigella dysenteriae*, *Salmonella typhi*, *Salmonella paratyphi*, *Vibrio cholerae*, *Escherichia coli*,

Pseudomonas aeruginosa, *Trichophyton mentagrophytes*, *Streptococcus pneumoniae* and *Bordetella pertussis*. Honokiol has a good inhibitory effect on the sustained virus response (SVR) cells and human immunodeficiency virus (HIV). The inhibition rate of honokiol reaches on SVR cell 60%. The median effective concentration (EC_{50}) of honokiol on HIV in human lymphocytes 3.3μmol/L.

5. 抗炎　厚朴可以抑制 5– 脂氧合酶（5-LO）、白三烯 A_4 水解酶（LTA_4H）和环氧合酶（COX）活性；对二甲苯引起的耳肿胀、角叉菜胶引起的足趾肿胀和乙酸引起的小鼠腹腔毛细血管通透性升高均有明显抑制作用；能影响白细胞功能，抑制炎症介质的生物合成，抑制环氧合酶 –2（COX-2）、诱导型一氧化氮合酶（iNOS）和核转录因子 –κB（NF-κB）调控的前炎症因子表达，发挥改善大鼠炎症和氧化应激的作用。主要物质基础是厚朴乙醇提取物、厚朴酚、和厚朴酚。作用机制与抑制花生四烯酸代谢相关。

(5) Anti-inflammation　*Hòu Pò* has an inhibitory effect on the activity of 5-lipoxygenase (5-LO), leukotriene A_4 hydrolase (LTA_4H) and cyclooxygenase (COX). *Hòu pò* has inhibitory effects on the ear edema of mouse caused by xylene, foot swelling caused by carrageenan, and capillary permeability caused by acetic acid. It also can inhibit inflammation and oxidation by affecting the function of white blood cells, suppressing the biosynthesis of inflammatory mediators, and down-regulating the expression of cyclooxygenase-2 (COX-2), inducible nitric oxide synthase (iNOS) and pro-inflammatory factors regulated by nuclear transcription factor-κB (NF-κB). The main material bases are ethanol extract, magnolol and honokiol. The mechanism may be related to its inhibitory effect on the arachidonic acid metabolic pathway.

6. 抗氧化　多种厚朴提取物及厚朴酚、和厚朴酚对 1, 1– 二苯基 –2– 苦味肼基自由基（DPPH）有清除作用，以乙醇提取物清除能力最强。厚朴乙醇提取物对亚油酸、猪油的脂质过氧化有良好的阻断作用，其抗氧化作用随提取物用量的增加而逐渐增强。

(6) Anti-oxidation　A variety extracts from *Hòu pò*, magnolol and honokiol can scavenge 1,1-diphenyl-2-bitter hydrazine (DPPH) free radicals. Among them, ethanol extract has the strongest ability. The *Hòu Pò* extract has a good blocking effect on lipid peroxidation of linoleic acid or lard, and its antioxidant effect gradually increases with the amount of extract.

7. 肌肉松弛和中枢抑制　厚朴具有肌肉松弛作用，对士的宁、印防己毒素、戊四氮等药物诱发的痉挛有强烈的抑制作用，主要有效成分为木兰箭毒碱、厚朴酚、和厚朴酚。木兰箭毒碱属非去极化型骨骼肌松弛剂，厚朴酚、和厚朴酚具有中枢性肌肉松弛作用。此外，厚朴乙醚提取物、厚朴酚、和厚朴酚具有明显的中枢抑制作用。

(7) Muscle relaxation and central depression　*Hòu Pò* has a muscle relaxation effect, which can inhibit spasm induced by strychnine, tetrodotoxin or pentaerythrazole. Magnocurarine, magnolol and honokiol are the major active ingredients. Magnocurarine is a non-depolarizing relaxant for skeletal muscle. Magnolol and honokiol have a central muscle relaxant effect. What is more, ether extract, magnolol and honokiol have an obvious central depressant effect.

8. 其他作用　厚朴还具有一定的抗肿瘤、神经保护、抗白内障、抗血管新生、降血糖、降血脂、抗惊厥、抗癫痫作用。

(8) Other effects　*Hòu pò* also has anti-tumor, neuroprotective, anti-cataract, anti-angiogenic, hypoglycemic, hypolipidemic, anti-convulsant and anti-epileptic effects.

【不良反应 / Adverse effects 】
　　厚朴具有潜在的呼吸系统和肌肉毒性，主要毒性成分是木兰箭毒碱。木兰箭毒碱在厚朴药材中含量较低，口服后经肠道吸收缓慢，吸收后即经肾脏排泄，血中浓度较低，故口服毒性较小。

厚朴具有较强的眼和皮肤刺激作用，炮制后刺激作用显著减低。腹腔注射厚朴水提液小鼠无异常反应和死亡，最大耐受量为临床的 150 倍。

Hòu pò has potential risk of poisoning respiratory and muscular systems. Magnocurarine is the main toxic ingredients. But owning to the low content in *Hòu pò*, it is slowly absorbed by the intestine after oral administration and quickly excreted by the kidneys after absorption, which leads to a very low level of magnocurarine in the blood. Therefore the toxicity of *Hòu pò* with oral administration is low. *Hòu pò* has strong eye and skin irritation, but the irritative effect of processed *Hòu pò* is significantly reduced. Toxicity study of raw and processed *Hòu pò* showed that *Hòu pò* extract causes no abnormal response and death in mice, and its maximum tolerated amount is 150 times of clinical amount.

苍术 ¦ *Cāng zhú (Atractylodis Rhizoma)*

【来源 / Origin】

本品为菊科植物茅苍术［*Atractylodes lancea* (Thunb.) DC.］或北苍术［*Atractylodes chinensis* (DC.) Koidz.］的干燥根茎。茅苍术主产于江苏、湖北、河南等地，北苍术主产于华北及西北地区。春、秋二季采挖，除去泥沙，晒干，撞去须根。

Cāng zhú is the dried rhizome of *Atractylodes lancea* (Thunb.) DC. or *Atractylodes chinensis* (DC.) Koidz, one of compositae plant. *Máo cāng zhú* is wildly cultivated in Jiangsu province, Hubei province and Henan province in China; *Běi cāng zhú* is widely cultivated in north China and northwest China. *Cāng zhú* is harvested in the spring and autumn, then processed with slit removed, dry and fibrous roots removed by hitting.

【化学成分 / Chemical ingredients】

挥发油含量较高。茅苍术根茎挥发油含量一般为 5%~9%，北苍术根茎挥发油含量一般为 3%~5%。挥发油主要成分包括苍术醇（atractylol）、茅术醇（hinesol）、β-桉叶醇（β-eucalyptol）、苍术酮（atractylone）等。另含十六烷酸甲酯（methyl hexadecanoate）、十八碳二烯酸甲酯（methyl octadecadienoate）、亚油酸乙酯（ethyl linoleate）等。茅苍术尚含鼠李糖（rhamnose）、阿拉伯糖（arabinose）、半乳糖（galactose）、汉黄芩素（baicalein）、香草酸（vanillic acid）等。

Volatile oil is the main ingredient of *Cāng zhú*. The content of volatile oil *Máo cāng zhú* is about 5% to 9%. The content of volatile oil *Běi cāng zhú* is about 3%-5%. Volatile oil includes atractylol, β-eucalyptol, atractylone, etc. It also contains methyl hexadecanoate, methyl octadecadienoate, ethyl linoleate, etc. In addition, rhamnose, arabinose, galactose, baicalein and vanillic acid are found in *Máo cāng zhú*.

【药性与功效 / Chinese medicine properties】

味辛、苦，性温，归脾、胃、肝经。具有燥湿健脾、祛风散寒、明目的功效。用于湿阻中焦、脘腹胀满、泄泻、水肿、脚气痿躄、风湿痹痛、风寒感冒、夜盲、眼目昏涩证。

In Chinese medicine theory, *Cāng zhú* is warm in nature, and acrid and bitter in flavor. It can enter the meridians of the spleen, stomach, liver; *Cāng zhú* can dry dampness and invigorate spleen, disperse wind and dissipate cold, improve eyesight. Clinically it is used for dampness retention in the middle energizer, abdominal distension and fullness, diarrhea, edema, atrophy-flaccidity, rheumatism agonizing arthralgia, common cold and night blindness.

【药理作用 / Pharmacological effects】

1. 调节胃肠运动　苍术对胃肠运动的调节作用与药材产地、给药剂量及机体状态等因素相关。①促进胃肠运动：苍术煎剂、苍术醇提物对正常大鼠胃平滑肌有轻度兴奋作用。苍术乙醇提取物等在一定剂量范围内具有促进肠推进作用。作用机制与提高脾虚证大鼠血清胃泌素、胃动素和P物质水平以及降低血清血管活性肠肽水平相关。②抑制胃肠运动：在一定剂量范围内，苍术煎剂、苍术醇提物能对抗乙酰胆碱、氯化钡所致胃肠平滑肌痉挛；苍术丙酮提取物、β-桉叶醇及茅术醇能对抗卡巴胆碱、Ca^{2+}及电刺激引起的小肠收缩；β-桉叶醇可以对抗新斯的明造模小鼠胃肠运动加快。

(1) Regulation of gastrointestinal movement *Cāng zhú* has a two-way effect on the gastrointestinal movement. The place of origin, the dosage of administration and body state are the main influencing factors. ①The stimulating effect of gastrointestinal movement. The decoction and ethanol extracts have a mild excitatory effect on gastric smooth muscle of normal rats. The inferior intestinal propulsion rate can be improved by water extract or other extract. The mechanism may be related to increasing gastrin, motilin and substance P and decreasing vasoactive intestinal peptide levels. ②The inhibitory effect on gastrointestinal movement. Within a certain dose range, both the water extract and alcohol extract can resist gastrointestinal smooth muscle spasm caused by acetylcholine or barium chloride. Acetone extract, β-eucalyptol and hinesol can resist the contraction of small intestine caused by carbachol, Ca^{2+} and electrical stimulation. β-eucalyptol can inhibit gastrointestinal movement induced by neostigmine.

2. 抗胃溃疡 茅苍术及北苍术提取物具有抗实验性溃疡作用，对多种原因引起的实验性胃溃疡有抑制作用，能够抑制胃液分泌、降低胃液总酸度和胃蛋白酶活力，主要药效物质基础是β-桉叶醇、苍术醇和茅术醇。

(2) Anti-gastric ulcer The extracts from *Cāng zhú* can inhibit experimental gastric ulcer caused by various reasons through decreasing the secretion of gastric juice, and lower the total acidity of gastric juice or pepsin activity. β-eucalyptol, atractylol and hinesol are the main active ingredients of its anti-gastric ulcer effect.

苍术抗溃疡作用机制主要涉及以下方面。①抑制胃酸分泌：β-桉叶醇能抑制胃组织中H_2受体，从而抗胃酸分泌；苍术醇通过抑制甾体激素释放抑制胃酸分泌。②保护胃黏膜：苍术可以增加胃黏膜组织血流量和黏膜修复成分己糖胺的含量，促进溃疡愈合。③抑制胃组织炎症细胞因子过度表达：茅苍术、北苍术及其活性成分能够抑制大鼠胃组织炎症因子白细胞介素-6（IL-6）、白细胞介素-8（IL-8）和TNF-α的过度表达，抗醋酸致慢性胃溃疡。④升高胃泌素和三叶因子促进胃黏膜修复：苍术能升高醋酸性慢性溃疡大鼠血清胃泌素水平；升高大黄、番泻叶、小承气汤加饥饱失常以及饮食不节、潮湿、强迫游泳等致脾虚证模型大鼠血清胃泌素水平。苍术提取物及苍术素能提高醋酸性慢性溃疡大鼠和脾虚证大鼠血清和胃组织表皮生长因子和三叶因子表达，改善模型大鼠胃黏膜形态和胃黏膜细胞超微结构。

The mechanism mainly involves the following aspects. ①Gastric acid secretion inhibition: β-eucalyptol can inhibit gastric acid secretion by inhibiting the expression of histamine H_2 receptors in gastric tissues; atractylol can inhibit gastric acid secretion by decreasing the release of steroid hormones. ② Gastric mucosal protection: *Cāng zhú* can promote ulcer healing by increasing the blood flow and the content of hexosamine which is important for mucosal repair. ③Inhibition of gastric tissue inflammatory cytokine overexpression: *Cāng zhú* and its active ingredients can inhibit the overexpression of inflammatory factors in gastric tissues, such as interleukin-6 (IL-6), interleukin-8 (IL-8) and TNF-α, thereby *Cāng zhú* can play a therapeutic role in combating chronic gastric ulcer caused by acetic acid. ④ Repair gastric mucosa by elevating gastrin and trefoil factor: *Cāng zhú* can increase the level of gastrin in serum and stomach of rats with chronic ulcer caused by vinegar acid, and rats with spleen deficiency syndrome caused by rhubarb or folium sennae or by improper diet, moist environment and forced swimming, or by hunger and satiety disorder. *Cāng zhú* extract and atractylodin can promote the expression of epidermal growth factor and trefoil factor in serum and gastric tissues. As a result, the morphology of gastric mucosa and the active components of abnormal ultrastructure of gastric mucosa cells are improved.

3. 保肝、利胆　苍术具有抗肝毒性作用。苍术挥发油、苍术多糖及苍术水提物能降低 CCl_4 诱导肝损伤小鼠血清 ALT 和 AST 水平。苍术酮能够对抗 CCl_4 诱导肝损伤、叔丁基过氧化物诱导的 DNA 损伤和大鼠肝细胞毒性。苍术能够促进胆汁分泌。苍术乙醇提取物能够促进麻醉大鼠胆汁分泌；苍术醋酸乙酯提取物在 500mg/kg（相当于 10 g 生药 /kg）时，促进大鼠胆汁分泌作用持续 6 小时以上。

(3) Liver protection and bile secretion enhancement　*Cāng zhú* has the function of antihepatotoxicity. The volatile oil, polysaccharide and water extract can decrease ALT and AST in serum of mice with liver injury induced by CCl_4. Atractylone can not only resist liver damage, but also inhibit deoxyribonucleic acid （DNA） damage and hepatotoxicity induced by tert butyl peroxide. *Cāng zhú* can promote bile secretion. Ethanol extract of *Cāng zhú* can promote bile secretion in anesthetized rats. When the dosage of ethyl acetate extract is set at 500mg/kg (equivalent to 10 g crude drug/kg), the last time of bile secretion may be more than 6 hours for rats.

4. 抗病原微生物　苍术对金黄色葡萄球菌、肺炎链球菌、甲型溶血性链球菌、乙型溶血性链球菌，大肠埃希菌、铜绿假单胞菌、枯草芽孢杆菌和幽门螺杆菌均有抑制作用；并能抑制白念珠菌、红色毛癣菌、许兰毛癣菌、奥杜盎小孢子菌、黑曲霉菌、黄曲霉菌、桔青霉菌和酵母菌等真菌。苍术还具有抗病毒和杀虫作用。苍术水煎剂对乙肝病毒具有抑制作用；苍术酮具有杀灭流感病毒的作用；苍术精油能够杀死黑腹果蝇。

(4) Anti-microbial　A variety of pathogenic microbials can be inhibited by *Cāng zhú*, such as *Staphylococcus aureus*, *Diplococcus pneumoniae*, *Streptococcus A helomyticus*, *Streptococcus B helomyticus*, *Escherichia coli*, *Pseudomonas aeruginosa*, *Bacillus subtilis* and *Helicobacter pylori*. It can also inhibit fungi such as *Candida albicans*, *Trichophyton rubrum*, *Trichophyton brevistrium*, *Microsporum auduense*, *Aspergillus niger*, *Aspergillus flavus*, *Penicillium citrinum* and *Saccharomyces*. In addition, *Cāng zhú* also has antiviral and insecticidal effects. *Cāng zhú* decoction has inhibitory effect on HBV. Atractylone can kill influenza virus and volatile oil can kill drosophila melanogaster.

5. 利尿、改善水代谢　生苍术能够提高湿阻中焦证模型大鼠的尿量，主要药效物质基础是正丁醇提取物和苍术挥发油。挥发油中 β– 桉叶醇可通过抑制 Na^+-K^+-ATP 酶活性，阻止 Na^+ 重吸收，增加尿液排出。苍术能够降低 AQP_2 和 AQP_3 的表达，关闭水通道，减少胃、小肠、大肠等组织器官对水液的吸收，改善体内水液代谢。

(5) Dieresis, water metabolism improvement　*Cāng zhú* can increase the urine output of the model rats of dampness retention in middle energizer. N-butanol extract and volatile oil are the active ingredients for its diuretic effect. β-eucalyptol in volatile oil can inhibit the activity of Na^+-K^+-ATPase and prevent sodium ion reabsorption, thereby urine excretion is increased. *Cāng zhú* can turn off the water channels by reducing the expression of AQP_2 and AQP_3, which decreases the absorption of water in the stomach, small intestine, large intestine and other tissues and organs, and improves water metabolism in the body.

6. 抗炎、镇痛　苍术提取物对二甲苯致小鼠耳肿胀、角叉菜胶致大鼠足肿胀、醋酸致小鼠毛细血管通透性升高以及小鼠棉球肉芽肿、大鼠佐剂关节炎等急慢性及免疫性炎症模型都有明显的抑制作用。苍术乙醇提取物、苍术中芹烷二烯酮、苍术烯内酯Ⅰ、苍术烯内酯Ⅱ、苍术烯内酯Ⅲ均具有抗炎活性。苍术还具有镇痛作用。麸炒北苍术挥发油及醇提物能够减少醋酸引起的小鼠扭体反应次数，延长热刺激引起的小鼠甩尾潜伏期。β-桉叶醇和苍术醇为其镇痛主要成分。

(6) Anti-inflammation and analgesia The extract of *Cāng zhú* has inhibitory effects on ear swelling caused by xylene or croton oil, feet swelling and mouse cotton ball granuloma caused by carrageenan and capillary permeability. The ethanol extract, atractyldionone, atractylenolide Ⅰ, atractylenolide Ⅱ, Ⅲ in *Cāng zhú* also have anti-inflammatory activity. *Cāng zhú* has an analgesic effect too. The volatile oil and alcohol extracts from *Cāng zhú* prepared with bran can reduce the frequency of body-twisting and prolong the tail-flicking latency. β-eucalyptol and atractylol are effective ingredients for their analgesic effects.

7. 其他作用　苍术及其活性成分还有一定的降血糖、降血压、抗肿瘤、抗缺氧、抗癫痫等作用。

(7) Other effects *Cāng zhú* and its active ingredients also have effects on hypoglycemic effect, hypotensive effect, anti-tumor, anti-hypoxia and anti-epilepsy, etc.

【不良反应 / Adverse effects】

生苍术挥发油半数致死量（LD_{50}）为2454.71mg/kg，95%可信限为2123.24~2837.92mg/kg。根据化合物经口急性毒性分级标准，生苍术挥发油分级为低毒。主要毒性表现为行动迟缓、静卧、昏睡、呼吸减弱、心率减慢，甚至死亡。毒性症状的轻重与剂量呈正相关。麸炒苍术挥发油无毒性反应。

The median lethal dose (LD_{50}) of raw *Cāng zhú* was 2454.71mg/kg, and the confidence limit of 95% is 2123.24 to 2837.92mg/kg. According to the oral acute toxicity grading standard, raw *Cāng zhú* should be classified as low toxicity. Toxic symptoms include slow action, lying still, lethargy, weakened breathing, slowed heart rate, and even death. The severity of toxic symptoms is positively correlated with dose. However, there is no toxicity for the volatile oil of *Cāng zhú* processed with bran.

广藿香　*Guǎng huò xiāng*（*PogoStemonis Herba*）

【来源 / Origin】

本品为唇形科植物广藿香［*Pogostemon cablin*（Blanco）Benth.］的干燥地上部分。原产菲律宾，我国广东、广西、海南均有栽培。枝叶茂盛时采割，日晒夜闷，反复至干。

Guǎng huò xiāng is the dry aboveground part of *Pogostemon cablin* (Blanco) Benth. The plant is native to the Philippines and cultivated in Guangdong province, Guangxi province and Hainan province in China. The branches and leaves are harvested when they are lush, then processed in the sun to dry during the day and put under cover at night until they are fully dried.

【化学成分 / Chemical ingredients】

主要有挥发油类、黄酮类成分等。挥发油类成分是广藿香的主要有效成分，含量约为1.5%，主要包括广藿香醇（patchouli alcohol）、广藿香酮（pogostone）、β-广藿香烯（β-patchouliene）。广藿香还含有藿香黄酮等10多种黄酮类成分。此外，广藿香尚含有木醛酮（lignanone）、表木醛醇（epilignol）、齐墩果酸（oleanolic acid）等成分。

Chemical ingredients of *Guǎng huò xiāng* are divided into volatile oils, flavonoids, and others. Volatile oils are the main active ingredients of *Guǎng huò xiāng*, taking up about 1.5% of total content. Patchouli alcohol, pogostone and β-patchouliene are the main components of the volatile oil. Research has also suggested that at least 10 kinds of flavonoids can be found in *Guǎng huò xiāng*. In addition, it also contains lignanone, epilignol and oleanolic acid.

【药性与功效 / Chinese medicine properties】

味辛，性微温，归脾、胃、肺经。具有芳香化浊、和中止呕、发表解暑的功效。用于湿浊中阻、脘痞呕吐、暑湿表证、湿温初起、发热倦怠、胸闷不舒、寒湿闭暑、腹痛吐泻、鼻渊头痛等证。

In Chinese medicine theory, *Guǎng huò xiāng* is slightly warm in nature and acrid in flavor. It can enter the meridians of the spleen, stomach, lung; *Guǎng huò xiāng* can resolve turbidity with aroma, harmonize middle and arrest vomiting, release exterior to relieve summerheat. Clinically it is used for dampness turbid obstructing middle, abdominal mass and vomiting, summerheat exterior syndrome, dampness-warm beginning, fever and tiredness, fullness and discomfort in chest, cold dampness blocking summerheat, abdominal pain and diarrhea, nasosinusitis and headache.

【药理作用 / Pharmacological effects】

1. **调节胃肠运动**　广藿香对胃肠运动呈双向调节作用。广藿香水提物、去油水提物和挥发油可以抑制离体家兔肠管自发性收缩和乙酰胆碱及氯化钡引起的肠痉挛性收缩，以广藿香挥发油作用最强。在整体实验中，水提物和去油水提物均能减慢胃排空，抑制正常小鼠和新斯的明引起的小鼠肠推进；挥发油对胃排空和肠推进均无影响。广藿香水提物和去油水提物能减少番泻叶引起的腹泻；挥发油却起协同作用加重腹泻。

(1) Gastrointestinal movement regulation　*Guǎng huò xiāng* has a two-way regulation on gastrointestinal movement. Water extract, oil removed-water extract and volatile oil can inhibit the spontaneous contraction of rabbit intestine tract and spasmodic contraction caused by acetylcholine or by barium chloride, and the volatile oil has the strongest inhibitory effect. What is more, the animal experiment results show that water extract and oil removed-water extract can slow down the gastric emptying, and inhibit the intestinal propulsion in normal mice and mice induced by neostigmine, while the volatile oil has no effect on gastric emptying and intestinal propulsion. In addition, water extract and oil removed-water extract can reduce the frequency of diarrhea caused by folium sennae, while volatile oil can play a synergistic role in aggravating diarrhea.

2. **肠道屏障保护**　广藿香挥发油和水提液具有肠道屏障保护作用，能够降低大鼠血清中一氧化氮（NO）浓度、抑制 TNF-α 水平，保护和维持肠上皮细胞膜的流动性。广藿香还能够提高杯状细胞的分泌功能，增强肠道自身防御功能。广藿香挥发油能够增强感染后肠易激综合征（PI-IBS）模型大鼠结肠黏膜上皮细胞 ZO-1 和 Occludin 蛋白表达，修复肠黏膜紧密连接结构，保护肠黏膜机械屏障。

(2) Intestinal barrier protection　The volatile oil and water extract from *Guǎng huò xiāng* can protect the intestinal barrier by lowering the concentration of nitric oxide (NO) and TNF-α, so as to protect and maintain the fluidity of intestinal epithelial cell membrane. Furthermore, *Guǎng huò xiāng* can improve the intestinal self-defense system by enhancing the secretion function of goblet cells. In addition, volatile oil can enhance the expression of ZO-1 and Occludin protein in colonic epithelial cells of rats with post-infectious irritable bowel syndrome (PI-IBS) model after infection, and repair the tight junction structure of intestinal mucosa, so as to protect the mechanical barrier of intestinal mucosa.

3. **调节胃液分泌**　广藿香挥发油能减少胃酸分泌；水提物和去油水提物能增加胃酸分泌，以去油水提物作用稍强。广藿香水提物、去油水提物和挥发油均可提高胃蛋白酶活性，以水提物和去油水提物作用较强。去油的广藿香水、乙醇、正丁醇、乙酸乙酯、氯仿不同极性部位均能不同程度地增加胃酸分泌，增强胃蛋白酶活性。

(3) Regulation of gastric secretion　Volatile oil can reduce gastric acid secretion. However, water extract and oil removed-water extract can increase gastric acid secretion, and the oil removed-water extract has a slightly stronger effect. The Water extract, oil removed-water extract and volatile oil can improve pepsin activity, and the effect of water extract and oil-water extract are stronger than that of volatile oil. Extracts of *Guǎng huò xiāng*, such as oil-free water extract, extract by alcohol, by n-butanol, by ethyl acetate or by chloroform, can increase gastric acid secretion and pepsin activity.

4. 抗炎、镇痛　广藿香水提取物对 2,4, 6- 三硝基苯磺酸（TNBS）诱导的结肠炎有保护作用。广藿香醇能抑制二甲苯致小鼠耳郭肿胀、角叉菜胶及蛋清致大鼠足肿胀，减少醋酸致小鼠扭体次数。广藿香甲醇提取物对于醋酸致扭体反应、福尔马林致舔爪行为及角叉菜胶致足跖肿胀均有抑制作用。主要药效物质基础为水提液、甲醇提取物、挥发油、广藿香醇和广藿香酮，作用机制与抗氧化和抑制 TNF-α 等炎症介质释放有关。

(4) Anti-inflammation and analgesia　The water extract from *Guǎng huò xiāng* has a protective effect on colitis induced by three nitrobenzene sulphonic acid (TNBS). Patchouli alcohol can inhibit the ear swelling caused by xylene, the feet swelling induced by carrageenan or egg white, and reduce the number of writhing in mice. The methanol extract of *Guǎng huò xiāng* has inhibitory effects on acetic acid-induced writhing, formalin-induced paw licking, and carrageenan-induced foot swelling in mice. The water extract, methanol extract, patchouli alcohol and pogostone may be the material basis for its anti-inflammatory and analgesic effects. The mechanism may be related to antioxidantion and lowering inflammatory mediators, such as TNF-α.

5. 抗病原微生物　广藿香具有抗真菌、抗病毒、抗细菌、抗钩端螺旋体等作用。广藿香酮能抑制金黄色葡萄球菌、肺炎链球菌、溶血性链球菌、大肠埃希菌、痢疾杆菌、铜绿假单胞菌、白念珠菌、新型隐球菌、申克孢子丝菌等。广藿香甲醇提取物及乙酸乙酯提取物具有较高的抗柯萨奇病毒 B_3（CVB_3）作用。藿香水煎液具有抑制或杀灭钩端螺旋体作用。

(5) Anti-microbial effects　*Guǎng huò xiāng* has effects of antifungal, antiviral, antibacterial, and anti-leptospira. Pogostone can inhibit various of bacteria, including *Staphylococcus aureus*, *Streptococcus pneumoniae*, *Streptococcus hemolyticus*, *Escherichia* coli, *Shigella dysenteriae*, *Pseudomonas aeruginosa*, *Candidaalbicans*, *Cryptocaccus neoformans*, *Sporothris schenckii*, etc. Methanol extract and ethyl acetate extract could against coxsackievirus B_3 (CVB_3). The decoction has effects of inhibiting or killing leptospira

6. 其他作用　广藿香还具有抗氧化、调节免疫、镇咳、化痰、平喘、抗肿瘤、通便等作用。

(6) Other effects　*Guǎng huò xiāng* also has effects of antioxidant, immune regulation, relieving cough, resolving phlegm, relieving asthma, anti-tumor, catharsis, etc.

【不良反应 / Adverse effects】

广藿香醇花生油溶液灌胃给药 LD_{50} 约为 4.693g/kg，95% 可信限为 4.038 ~5.498g/kg。小鼠不良反应主要表现为站立不稳、左右摇晃、抽搐、僵直等现象，严重者可发生死亡。死亡小鼠及时进行尸检，主要脏器未见明显异常。

The LD_{50} of patchouli alcohol with intragastric administration is about 4.693g/kg, the upper limit of 95% confidence interval is about 5.498g/kg, and the lower limit is about 4.038g/kg. The main adverse reactions in mice include unsteady standing, shaking left and right, convulsion, rigidity, and even death. No obvious abnormality is found in the main organs of the dead mice.

广藿香醇腹腔注射 LD_{50} 为 3.145g/kg，95% 可信限为 2.663~3.675g/kg。中毒表现与口服给药相似。

The LD_{50} of patchouli alcohol with intraperitoneal injection is about 3.145g/kg, the upper limit of the 95% confidence interval is 3.675g/kg, and the lower limit is 2.663g/kg. The main adverse reactions are similar to those of intragastric administration.

题库

医药大学堂
WWW.YIYAODXT.COM

（李冰涛　李红艳）

第九章　利水渗湿药
Chapter 9　Damp-draining medicines

学习目标｜Objectives

1. **掌握**　利水渗湿药的基本药理作用；茯苓、茵陈与功效相关的药理作用、作用机制和药效物质基础。

2. **了解**　猪苓、泽泻、车前子的主要药理作用和药效物质基础。

1. **Must know**　The main pharmacological effects of damp-draining medicines; the efficacy related pharmacological effects, mechanism of action, and material basis of *Fú líng* and *Yīn chén*.

2. **Desirable to know**　The main pharmacological effects and material basis of *Zhū líng*, *Zé xiè* and *Chē qián zǐ*.

第一节　概述
Section 1　Overview

PPT

微课

　　凡以通利水道、渗泄水湿，治疗水湿内停证为主要功效的药物称为利水渗湿药。本类药物多味甘、淡，主入膀胱、脾、肾经，作用趋向偏于下行。利水渗湿药一般具有利尿的作用，通过利尿而起到渗利水湿的作用，使停滞于体内的水湿之邪从小便而解。部分利水渗湿药还兼有利湿退黄、利尿通淋等作用，可用于湿热黄疸、淋证等。利水渗湿药根据功效可以分为利水消肿药，包括茯苓、猪苓、泽泻、薏苡仁等；利尿通淋药，包括车前子、海金砂等；利湿退黄药，包括茵陈、金钱草、虎杖等。

All Chinese materia medica that are mainly used to regulate water discharge, increase urine excretion and treat internal retention are classified as damp-draining medicines. These medicines mostly are sweet and bland in flavor, enter the bladder, spleen and kidney meridians. The effect tends to be downward. They possess the efficacies of inducing diuresis, by which the purpose of regulating discharge is achieved. The damage of water stagnation in the body can be resolved by urination. Damp-draining medicines also have the effects of draining dampness, relieving jaundice, and removing stranguria, and are commonly used to treat the syndromes of edema, dribbling urinary block, strangury-turbidity. According to their different characters and actions, damp-draining medicines are mainly classified into three types. ①Herbs that induce diuresis and relieve edema include *Fú líng*, *Zhū líng*, *Zé xiè*, *Yì yǐ rén*, etc. ②Herbs that induce diuresis and relieve strangury comprise *Chē qián zǐ, Hǎi jīn shā*, etc. ③Herbs that drain dampness and abate jaundice consist of *Yīn chén, Jīn qián cǎo, Hǔ zhàng*, etc.

水湿内停证，主要为脾、肺、肾、膀胱及三焦等功能失调所致。临床表现为水肿、淋浊、痰饮、泄泻、癃闭等，既可溢于肌肤而呈水肿，也可同其他外邪（如湿热）相夹杂，侵犯人体某一脏腑、部位，如湿热熏蒸而发黄疸。中医认为肺失通调、脾失转运、肾失开合、膀胱气化无权可致水饮内停。水湿内停证与西医学中泌尿系统疾病（感染或结石、肾脏病变）、消化系统疾病（肝胆疾病、腹水）、呼吸系统疾病（慢性支气管炎引起的痰液积留以及胸腔积液）和各种原因所致的水肿、代谢异常、变态反应性疾病等有关。现代药理研究表明，利水渗湿药治疗水湿内停证与下列药理作用有关。

Retention of water-dampness in the body, is mainly due to the dysfunction of spleen, lung, kidney, bladder and triple energizers. The clinical manifestations are edema, strangury-turbidity, phlegm-rheum, diarrhea, dribbling urinary block and, etc. It can also be mixed with other external evils (such as damp heat) to invade a certain part of the body, and then develop to jaundice. According to TCM theories, the failure of the lung in regulation, the spleen in transportation, the kidney in opening and closing, and the bladder in gasify are all related to the stagnation of water. Syndromes caused by water and damp accumulation commonly appear in diseases such as urinary system diseases (infection or stone, kidney disease), digestive system disorders (hepatobiliary disease, ascites), respiratory disorders (sputum accumulation during chronic bronchitis, and pleural effusion), and edema caused by various reasons, metabolic abnormalities, allergic diseases. The effect of damp-draining medicines on water-damp stagnation is related to the following pharmacological effects.

1. 利尿 利水渗湿药均有不同程度的利尿作用，利水消肿类作用较强，作用机制与以下因素有关。①拮抗醛固酮受体。②抑制肾小管对电解质和水的重吸收。③影响 Na^+-K^+-ATP 酶活性。④增加血浆心房钠尿肽（ANP）含量。⑤抑制抗利尿激素（ADH）的分泌。

(1) Diuresis All damp-draining medicines show diuretic effect in varying degrees, and the effect of inducing diuresis and relieving edema medicines is stronger than that of others. The mechanism is generally related to the following factors. ①Antagonizing aldosterone receptor. ② Inhibiting renal tubular reabsorption of electrolyte and water. ③Affecting Na^+-K^+-ATPase activity. ④Increasing plasma ANP content. ⑤Inhibiting the secretion of antidiuretic hormone (ADH).

2. 保肝 利水渗湿药均具有一定的保肝作用，其中利湿退黄类作用较强，可以通过多环节发挥保肝作用。①抗肝炎病毒和抑制病毒复制（茵陈）。②抑制脂质过氧化损伤，促进肝细胞修复（茵陈、泽泻）。③防治肝纤维化（茵陈）。④调节脂质代谢，减轻脂肪肝形成（泽泻）。⑤促进肝细胞再生、恢复肝功能（猪苓多糖）。

(2) Hepatoprotection All damp-draining herbs have certain hepatoprotective effects, and drain dampness and abate jaundice herbs have the stronger effect. They exert hepatoprotective effects in various ways. ①Anti-hepatitis virus and inhibitory virus reproduction (*Yīn chén, Chuí pén cǎo*). ②Inhibiting lipid peroxidation damage and promote liver cell repair (*Yīn chén, Zé xiè*). ③Preventing liver fibrosis (*Yīn chén*). ④Regulating lipid metabolism and reducing fatty liver formation (*zé xiè*). ⑤Promoting liver cell regeneration and restoring liver function (polyporus umbellatus polysaccharide).

3. 利胆 多数利水渗湿药具有利胆作用，其机制可能是促进胆囊动力功能恢复、收缩胆囊、扩张奥迪括约肌、增加胆汁流量、降低胆汁内胆固醇浓度、预防胆固醇结石形成，以及促进胆汁中固体物、胆酸及胆红素排除等。

(3) Promoting function of gallbladder Most of damp-draining herbs have the effect of promoting gallbladder function, and the mechanism may be related to promoting the restoration of gallbladder's dynamic function, contracting the gallbladder, expanding the Oedipal sphincter, increasing bile flow, reducing cholesterol concentration in the bile, preventing the formation of cholesterol stones, and enhancing the excretion of solids, cholic acid and bilirubin in the bile.

4. 排石　部分利水渗湿药具有排石作用，如金钱草、海金沙、车前子、石韦、茯苓、泽泻等。金钱草黄酮类成分、海金沙黄酮苷、茯苓多糖、泽泻的乙酸乙酯四环三萜类化合物等，均具有显著的防石、溶石、排石作用，可治疗肾脏结石、输尿管结石、膀胱结石。

(4) Clearing calculi　Some damp-draining herbs have the effect of clearing calculi, such as *Jīn qián cǎo*, *Chē qián zǐ*, *Hǎi jīn shā*, *Shí wěi*, *Fú líng* and *Zé xiè*. Flavonoids of *Jīn qián cǎo* and *Hǎi jīn shā*, polysaccharides of *Fú líng* and and ethyl acetate tetracyclic triterpenoids of *Zé xiè*, have significant effects of preventing the formation of calculi, helping dissolve the calculi and discharge the calculi from the kidney and bladder.

5. 抗炎　大部分利水渗湿药有抗炎作用，对急慢性前列腺炎，前列腺增生，泌尿系统感染性疾病等急慢性炎症及痛风性关节炎均有一定作用。

(5) Anti-inflammation　Most of damp-draining herbs exhibit anti-inflammation effects, and have certain effects on acute and chronic prostatitis, prostatic hyperplasia, urinary system infectious diseases, other acute and chronic inflammation, and gouty arthritis.

6. 保护前列腺　多与清除尿路致病菌、缓解炎性水肿和尿道梗阻以及增加尿量有关。利水渗湿药还可降低血清睾丸素水平，抑制前列腺增生和前列腺炎。

(6) Prostate protection　The prostatic protective effect of damp-draining herbs is mainly related to removing urinary tract pathogens, alleviating inflammatory edema, alleviating inflammatory urethral obstruction, and increasing urine output. The damp-draining medicines can reduce the level of serum testosterone and have the effects of inhibiting prostatic hyperplasia and prostatitis.

7. 增强免疫与抗肿瘤　茯苓、猪苓、薏苡仁、茵陈、虎杖均具有抗肿瘤作用，作用途径包括以下几种。①直接抑杀肿瘤细胞：诱导肿瘤细胞凋亡、抑制肿瘤细胞增殖、延缓肿瘤生长、改善癌症恶病质、抑制恶性肿瘤转移。②增强机体免疫功能：增强单核巨噬细胞的吞噬功能及细胞免疫和体液免疫的应答反应，促进机体低下的免疫功能恢复正常，提高机体免疫功能而抗肿瘤。③升高白细胞：减弱化疗或放疗药物的毒性反应。

(7) Enhancing immune and anti-tumor　*Fú líng*, *Zhū líng*, *Yì yǐ rén*, *Yīn chén* and *Hǔ zhàng* have antitumor effects. The underlying mechanisms involve the following aspects. ①Inhibiting and killing tumor cells directly, directly inducing apoptosis of tumor cells, inhibiting tumor cell proliferation, arresting cell cycle and preventing malignant tumor cell migration and invasion. ②Enhancing the body's immunity, increasing the phagocytosis of mononuclear macrophage, elevating cellular and humoral immune response, and promoting immune function recovery. ③Increasing the number of white blood cells, and reducing the adverse reaction of chemotherapy or radiotherapy.

8. 降血脂　泽泻、车前子、茵陈、虎杖等均有降血脂作用，作用机制包括以下几方面。①抑制外源性脂质吸收（虎杖及其蒽醌）。②减少内源性脂质的合成（虎杖、泽泻三萜类）。③促进脂质转运和排泄（茵陈）。④抑制3-羟基-3-甲基戊二酰辅酶A还原酶（HMGR）活力，调节脂质代谢。⑤清除自由基、抗氧化（车前子）。⑥改善血液流变性（泽泻）。

(8) Lowering blood lipids　*Zé xiè*, *Chē qián zǐ*, *Yīn chén* and *Hǔ zhàng* all have hypolipidemic effects. Main mechanism may be related to the following aspects. ①Inhibition of exogenous lipid absorption (*Hǔ zhàng* and its anthraquinone). ②Reduction of endogenous lipid synthesis (*Hǔ zhàng*

and triterpenoids of *Zé xiè*). ③Promotion of lipid transport and excretion (*Yīn chén*). ④Inhibition of 3-Hydroxy-3-methylglutaryl-coenzyme A reductase (HMGR) activity and regulation of lipid metabolism. ⑤Elimination of free radicals, antioxidation (*Chē qián zǐ*). ⑥Improvement of hemorheology (*Zé xiè*).

此外，利水渗湿药还具有解酒作用，用于治疗酒精性肝病。常用利水渗湿药的主要药理作用见表 9-1。

Damp-draining herbs also have an anti-alcoholic effect and are used to treat alcoholic liver disease. The main pharmacological effects of commonly used damp-draining medicines are summarized in Table 9-1.

表 9-1　常用利水渗湿药的主要药理作用

类别	药物	利尿	利胆	保肝	抗病原微生物	其他药理作用
利水消肿药	茯苓	+	–	–	–	增强免疫功能、抗肿瘤、降血糖
	猪苓	+	–	–	+	增强免疫功能、抗肿瘤、抗辐射
	泽泻	+	+	+	+	降血脂、降血糖、抗炎
	薏苡仁	+	–	–	–	—
利尿通淋药	海金砂	+	+	–	–	—
	车前子	+	+	–	+	降血脂、降血压、抗炎、抗溃疡
	石韦	–	–	+	–	镇咳、祛痰、平喘
利湿退黄药	茵陈	+	+	+	+	降血脂、降血压、降血糖、解热、抗炎
	金钱草	+	+	–	+	抗心肌缺血、抑制泌尿道结石、抗炎
	虎杖	+	+	+	+	抗炎

注："+"表示有明确作用；"–"表示无作用，或未查阅到相关研究文献

第二节　常用药物

Section 2　Commonly used medicines

PPT

茯苓 ┊ *Fú líng (Poria)*

【来源 / Origin】

本品为多孔菌科真菌茯苓 [*Poria cocos* (Schw.) Wolf] 的干燥菌核。主要分布于安徽、湖北、云南、河南等地。

Fú líng is the dried sclerotia of *Poria cocos* (Schw.) Wolf., family of Polyporaceae. The plant is widely cultivated in Anhui province, Hubei province, Yunnan province, and Hainan province in China.

【化学成分 / Chemical ingredients】

菌核中主要含有茯苓多糖（pachyman），三萜类成分茯苓素（poriatin）、茯苓酸（pachymic acid）、猪苓酸（pachymic acid）等。尚含有蛋白质、麦角甾醇（ergosterol）及无机盐成分钾、钠、镁、磷等。

It mainly contains pachyman, triterpenoids including poriatin, pachymic acid and pachymic acid.

Other minor compounds include protein, ergosterol and inorganic salt components potassium, sodium, magnesium, phosphorus.

【药性与功效 / Chinese medicine properties】

味甘、淡，性平，归心、脾、肾经。具有利水渗湿、健脾宁心的功效。用于水肿尿少、痰饮眩晕、脾虚少食、便溏泄泻、心神不安、惊悸失眠等证。

In Chinese medicine theory, *Fú líng* is sweet or bland in flavor and neutral in nature. It can enter the heart, spleen and kidney meridians. *Fú líng* has the effects of eliminating water and draining dampness, fortifying the spleen and quieting the heart. Clinically it can be used in treatment for edema and little urine, phlegm-fluid retention and vertigo, spleen deficiency and deficiency of food, loose stool and diarrhea, disquieted heart spirit, palpitation and insomnia.

【药理作用 / Pharmacological effects】

1. 利尿　茯苓的利尿作用与动物种属、清醒或麻醉、急性或慢性试验、生理状态以及提取方法有密切关系。慢性试验能明显利尿而急性试验无作用；甲醇或乙醇提取物有明显的利尿作用，茯苓煎剂、水提物均不出现利尿作用；对健康动物和人不具有利尿作用，但可增加水肿患者尿液排出量，尤其对于水肿严重的肾炎或心脏疾病患者，茯苓利尿作用均显著。茯苓素可能为潜在性醛固酮受体拮抗剂，是茯苓利尿的有效成分；茯苓的利水渗湿作用还与对机体水盐调节机制的影响有关。茯苓利尿作用与茯苓所含无机盐无关。

(1) Diuresis　The diuretic effect of *Fú líng* is closely related to different animal species, waking or anesthesia, acute or chronic test, physiological state and extraction method. *Fú líng* has obvious diuretic effects in chronic tests but it shows no effects in acute tests. Methanol or ethanol extracts have obvious diuretic effects, while decoctions and water extracts have no effect. In addition, it does not have diuretic effect on healthy animal and person, but can increase oedema patient urine eduction quantity, especially on dropsy serious nephritis or heart disease patient, its diuretic effect is remarkable. Poriatin, a potential aldosterone receptor antagonist, is an effective diuretic component of *Fú líng*. The effect of *Fú líng* on eliminating water and draining dampness is also related to the effect of water and salt regulation on the body. The diuretic effect has nothing to do with the inorganic salts.

2. 调节免疫　茯苓多糖、羧甲基茯苓多糖、茯苓素具有增强机体免疫功能的作用。①增强巨噬细胞吞噬功能，进而增强机体的免疫应答和非特异性免疫反应。②激活补体。③增强细胞免疫反应，使玫瑰花结形成率及植物血凝素诱发的淋巴细胞转化率明显上升。④增加小鼠抗体分泌细胞数以及抗原结合细胞数，并抑制小鼠迟发型超敏反应。⑤促进淋巴细胞分泌白细胞介素 –2（IL-2），γ– 干扰素（IFN-γ），肿瘤坏死因子 –α（TNF-α），白介素细胞 –6（IL-6）。⑥增强刀豆蛋白（Con A）或脂多糖（LPS）活化的小鼠脾淋巴细胞的增殖反应。⑦增强 T 淋巴细胞、B 淋巴细胞的增殖活性。⑧对抗钴 –60（^{60}Co）照射所致小鼠外周血白细胞减少。茯苓同时具有免疫抑制作用：茯苓提取物能使异位心脏模型大鼠移植心脏存活时间明显延长、减轻病理损伤程度；茯苓能明显抑制小鼠接触性皮炎，呈现一定的量–效关系。茯苓调节免疫作用可认为是其健脾的药理学基础。

(2) Enhancing immunity　*Fú líng* polysaccharides, carboxymethylpachymaran and poriatin are capable of enhancing immunity. ①Strengthening phagocytosis of peritoneal macrophages and enhance the immune response and non-specific immune response. ②Activating complement. ③Enhancing cellular immune response, so that rosette formation rate and plant hemagglutinin induced lymphocyte conversion rate are significantly increased. ④Increasing the number of cells secreted by antibodies and the number of antigen-binding cells, and inhibit the delayed hypersensitivity of mice. ⑤Promoting the secretion of interleukin-2 (IL-2), interferon-γ (IFN-γ), tumor necrosis factor-α (TNF-α) and interleukin-2

(IL-6) by lymphocytes. ⑥Enhancing the proliferation response of spleen lymphocytes activated by concanavalin A (Con A) or lipopolysaccharides (LPS) in mice. ⑦ Enhancing the proliferative activity of T and B lymphocytes. ⑧ Fighting against leukopenia in peripheral blood of mice induced by cobalt-60 (^{60}Co) irradiation. *Fú líng* also has immunosuppressive effect: *Fú líng* extract can significantly prolong the survival time of transplanted heart in heterotopic heart model rats and reduce the degree of pathological damage. *Fú líng* can obviously inhibit contact dermatitis in mice, showing a certain dose-effect relationship. The effect of *Fú líng* in regulating immunity can be considered as the pharmacological basis of fortify the spleen.

3. 镇静　茯苓提取物羧甲基茯苓多糖可增强中枢抑制剂的中枢抑制作用。

(3) Sedation　*Fú líng* has a certain sedative effect, and *Fú líng* extract carboxymethylpachymaran can enhance the central inhibitory effect of the central inhibitor.

4. 保肝　茯苓对实验性肝损伤具有保护作用。

(4) Hepatoprotection　Tuckahoe can protect liver and protect experimental liver injury.

5. 抗肿瘤　茯苓素抑制肿瘤细胞 DNA 合成的多个环节，在体内外均有明显增强巨噬细胞 TNF 的能力；在体内对小鼠移植性肿瘤细胞有明显的抑制生长作用，与 TNF 的水平呈正相关。羧甲基茯苓多糖能显著改善荷瘤小鼠自然杀伤细胞（NK）的杀伤活性，增强荷瘤小鼠 NK 细胞含量，提高小鼠单核巨噬细胞吞噬功能，诱导产生 IL-2、IFN-γ、TNF-α 和 IL-6，从而增强免疫、抗肿瘤。茯苓多糖对生长迟缓的移植性肿瘤抗瘤作用尤为显著，对肝癌细胞 S$_{180}$ 膜磷脂酰肌醇（PI）转换具有明显抑制作用；茯苓多糖、羧甲基茯苓多糖、茯苓素对抗肿瘤药有增效作用。

(5) Antitumor　Poriatin inhibits multiple stages of tumor cell deoxyribonucleic acid (DNA) synthesis. It significantly enhances the capacity of macrophages to produce TNF *in vivo* and *in vitro*. *In vivo*, it has a significant inhibitory effect on mouse transplanted tumor cells, which is positively correlated with the level of TNF. Carboxymethylpachymaran can improve the cytotoxic activity of natural killer cell (NK) in tumor-bearing mice, enhance phagocytosis of mouse mononuclear macrophages and induce cells to produce IL-2，IFN-γ，TNF-α and IL-6, so as to increase immune activity and anti-tumor effects. *Fú líng* pachyman has a particularly significant antitumor effect on transplanted tumors with stunted growth, and it has a significant inhibitory effect on hepatoma cell S$_{180}$ membrane phosphatidylinositol (PI) conversion. Pachyman, carboxymethylpachymaran and poriatin have synergistic effect on anticancer drugs.

6. 其他作用　茯苓可防治某些神经退行性疾病（如阿尔茨海默病、血管性痴呆及帕金森病等）。茯苓多糖具有减少补体 C3 免疫复合物沉积于肾脏的活性，减轻腺嘌呤在肾小管中的沉积，保护残存肾单位，从而改善肾功能，延缓肾功能不全（CRF）进程。茯苓多糖能有效抑制肾内草酸钙结晶的形成和沉积，具有较好的预防结石作用；茯苓提取物和三萜类物质可降低血糖，作用机制与提高胰岛素的敏感性，增强胰岛素的分化诱导活性，降低胰岛素抵抗有关。

(6) Other effects　*Fú líng* can prevent and cure some neurodegenerative diseases (such as Alzheimer's disease, vascular dementia, and Parkinson's disease). Pachyman has the activity of preventing the complement 3 (C3) immune complex from being deposited in the kidney, reducing the deposition of adenine in renal tubules, protecting the remaining nephrons, thus improving renal function and delaying the process of chronic renal failure. *Fú líng* pachyman can effectively inhibit the formation and deposition of calcium oxalate crystals in the kidney and has a good effect on preventing calculi. *Fú líng* extract and triterpenoids can reduce blood sugar, the mechanism is related to the increase in insulin sensitivity, enhance insulin differentiation-inducing activity, and reduction in insulin resistance.

【不良反应 / Adverse effects】

小鼠皮下注射羧甲基茯苓多糖半数致死量（LD_{50}）为 3.13g/kg。

Experimental results in mice show that median lethal dose (LD_{50}) of carboxymethylpachymaran is 3.13g/kg.

猪苓 ┊ *Zhū líng (Polyporus)*

【来源 / Origin】

本品为多孔菌科真菌猪苓 *Polyporus umbellatus* (Pers.) Fries 的干燥菌核。主要分布于河北、山西、内蒙古等地区。

Zhū líng is the dried sclerotia of *Polyporus umbellatus* (Pers.) Fries., family of Polyporaceae. The plant is widely cultivated in Hebei province, Shanxi province, Neimenggu area in China.

【化学成分 / Chemical ingredients】

主要含猪苓多糖（polyporus umbellatus polysaccharides）、麦角甾醇（ergosterol）、蛋白质、无机盐（inorganic salts）等。

Zhū líng mainly contains polyporus umbellatus polysaccharides (PUPs), ergosterol, protein and inorganic salts.

【药性与功效 / Chinese medicine properties】

味甘、淡，性平，归肾、膀胱经。具有利水渗湿的功效。用于治疗小便不利、水肿、泄泻、淋浊、带下等证。

In Chinese medicine theory, *Zhū líng* is sweet or bland in flavor and neutral in nature; it enters the kidney and bladder meridians. *Zhū líng* has the effects of eliminating water and draining dampness. Clinically it can be used for dysuria, edema, diarrhea, strangury-turbidity, and leukorrhea.

【药理作用 / Pharmacological effects】

1. 利尿　猪苓具有显著的利尿作用，其利尿作用在水滞留状态下明显；慢性肾功能不全大鼠灌服猪苓汤后，可促进 Na^+ 和 K^+ 及 Cl^- 的排泄，延长存活时间，表明猪苓利尿作用机制主要是抑制肾小管对电解质和水的重吸收。

(1) **Diuresis**　*Zhū líng* has a significant diuretic effect, and its diuretic effect is obvious in the state of water retention. After ingestion of *zhū líng* decoction in rats with chronic renal insufficiency, the excretion of Na^+, K^+ and Cl^- is promoted, and the survival time is prolonged. This indicates that the diuretic mechanism of *Zhū líng* is mainly to inhibit the reabsorption of electrolyte and water by renal tubules.

2. 抗肿瘤与提高免疫功能　猪苓多糖具有广谱抗肿瘤活性，抑制肿瘤生长和增强肿瘤患者免疫功能，与化学药物配伍使用可增强疗效、减轻副作用。猪苓多糖与 IFN-γ、TNF、IL-2 共同激活细胞的抗肿瘤活性，促进 IFN-γ、TNF-α 水平升高，可使肿瘤细胞癌基因表达下降，抑制肿瘤细胞分裂增殖而发挥抗肿瘤作用。猪苓多糖的免疫调节作用和抗肿瘤作用的机制可能与其促进单核巨噬细胞生成一氧化氮（NO）有关。

(2) **Anti-tumor and enhancing immune function**　PUPs have broad spectrum antitumor activity, which can inhibit tumor growth and enhance immune function of patients with tumors. When PUPs are used in combination with chemical drugs, it can enhance the efficacy and reduce the side effects. PUPs, together with IFN-γ, TNF, and IL-2, activate the anti-tumor activity of cells, promote the increase of IFN-γ, TNF-α level, reduce the expression of oncogenes in tumor cells, and inhibit the proliferation of tumor cells to exert antitumor effect. The mechanism of these effects of PUPs may be related to the

promotion of nitric oxide (NO) production by monocyte macrophages.

3. **保肝降酶** 猪苓多糖能减轻四氯化碳（CCl_4）和 D–氨基半乳糖所致的动物肝损伤，降低谷丙转氨酶（ALT）活性，增加腹腔巨噬细胞数量，促进病变肝脏的再生和修复；猪苓多糖注射液对乙型肝炎 e 抗原（HBeAg）及乙肝病毒的脱氧核糖核酸（HBV-DNA）具有转阴作用。

(3) Hepatoprotection PUPs alleviate carbon tetrachloride (CCl_4) or D-galactosamine-induced liver injury, reduce alanine aminotransferase (ALT) activity, and increase the number of peritoneal macrophages. It also promotes the regeneration and repairs of the diseased liver. PUPs injection facilitates clearance of serum HBeAg and hepatitis B virus DNA.

4. **抗辐射** 猪苓多糖具有防治小鼠急性放射病的作用。初步认为猪苓多糖的抗辐射作用可能是通过调节垂体–肾上腺系统的功能，使机体处于应激状态，从而增强抗辐射损伤的能力。

(4) Anti-radiation PUPs can prevent and treat acute radiation sickness in mice. It is preliminarily believed that the anti-radiation effect of PUPs may be through regulating the function of the pituitary-adrenal system, putting the body in a stress state, thereby enhancing the ability to resist radiation damage.

【不良反应 / Adverse effects】

猪苓多糖注射液可引起皮疹、瘙痒、过敏样反应。

PUPs injection can cause rash, itching and allergic reactions.

泽泻 ┊ *Zé xiè* (*Alismatis Rhizoma*)

【来源 / Origin】

本品为泽泻科植物 [*Alisma orientale* (Sam.) Juzep.] 的干燥块茎。主要分布于福建、广东、广西、四川等地区。

Zé xiè is the dried rhizome of the perennial herb *Alisma orientalis* (Sarm.) Juzep., family of Alismataceae. The plant is widely cultivated in Fujian province, Guangdong province, Guangxi area, and Sichuan province in China.

【化学成分 / Chemical ingredients】

主要含泽泻醇（alismol）、泽泻醇 A–24–醋酸酯（alisol A-24-acetate）、泽泻醇 B–23–乙酸酯（alisol B-23-acetate)、泽泻醇 C (alismol C)、16–23–环氧泽泻醇 B(16-23-epoxysalaris B）等。

Zé xiè contains alismol, alisol A-24-acetate, alisol B-23-acetate, alismol C, 16-23-epoxysalaris B, etc.

【药性与功效 / Chinese medicine properties】

味甘、性寒，归肾、膀胱经。具有利小便、清湿热的功效。用于治疗水肿、小便不利、泄泻、淋浊、痰饮等证。

In Chinese medicine theory, *Zé xiè* has the nature of sweet and cold. It can enter the kidney and bladder meridians. *Zé xiè* possess the efficacies in inducing diuresis, discharging heat. It can be used for the treatment of edema, unfavorable urination, diarrhea, turbidity, phlegm drinking and other symptoms.

【药理作用 / Pharmacological effects】

1. **利尿** 泽泻煎剂和浸膏对人和动物均有明显的利尿作用，使尿中钠、钾、氯、尿素的排泄量增加。泽泻的利尿作用可因药材的采收时间、药用部位和炮制方法的不同而异。冬季采收的正品泽泻利尿效力最强，春季泽泻利尿效力稍差。泽泻须稍有利尿作用，泽泻草根无利尿作用。生品、酒炙、麸炒者有利尿作用，盐炙者无利尿作用。泽泻利尿作用的机制：通过直接作用于肾小管的收集管，抑制肾脏 Na^+-K^+-ATP 酶活性，抑制钠离子的重吸收、钾离子及酸的排泄；显著升高小鼠血浆心钠素（ANF）含量。

(1) Diuresis　The decoction and extracts of *Zé xiè* have significant diuretic effect in human and animals. It can also increase the excretion of sodium, potassium, chloride and urea in urine. The diuretic effect of *Zé xiè* varies depending on the harvest time, medicinal site and processing method of the medicinal material. The diuretic effect of *Zé xiè* collected in winter is the strongest, and the diuretic effect of *Zé xiè* is slightly worse in spring. *Zé xiè* fibril has a little diuretic effect. *Zé xiè* root has no diuretic effect. Raw products, and wine or bran fried products have diuretic effect, while salt-burned ones have no diuretic effect. The mechanisms of diuretic effect include directly acting on the collecting tube of the renal, reducing the activity of Na^+-K^+-ATPase in the kidney and Na^+ reabsorption, K^+ and acid excretion, and increasing concentration of atrial natriuretic peptide (ANF) in plasma in mice significantly.

2. **抗肾结石形成**　泽泻醇提取物、乙酸乙酯浸膏或四环三萜类化合物均能显著抑制大鼠肾草酸钙结石的形成，泽泻较强的利尿作用也有助于大鼠肾结石的排出。可能通过减少结石大鼠肾组织骨桥蛋白（OPN）mRNA 的表达抑制大鼠肾结石的形成。

(2) Inhibiting formation of renal calculi　*Zé xiè* has the activity of inhibiting formation of renal calculi. The alcohol extracts, ethyl acetate extract or tetracyclic triterpenoids of *Zé xiè* can significantly inhibit the formation and growth of crystals of calcium oxalate in artificial urine in rats. The diuretic effect of *Zé xiè* can also help the kidney stones to be excreted in rats. It is possible to inhibit the formation of rat kidney stones by reducing the expression of osteopontin (OPN) mRNA in the kidney tissue of rats with stones.

3. **降血脂**　泽泻醇提取物、泽泻醇浸膏及乙酸乙酯提取物有降低高脂血症动物的血清胆固醇（TC）、甘油三酯（TG）、低密度脂蛋白（LDL），升高高密度脂蛋白（HDL）的作用，对家兔高脂血症有预防和治疗作用。降脂的物质基础及强弱：泽泻醇 A–24– 醋酸酯 > 泽泻醇 B–23– 乙酸酯 > 泽泻醇，作用机制与其干扰外源性胆固醇的吸收和内源性胆固醇的代谢有关。

(3) Lowering blood lipid　*Zé xiè* has the activity of lowering blood lipid. *Zé xiè* alcohol extracts and its ethyl acetate extract parts from alcohol extracts can decrease serum total cholesterol (TC), triglyceride (TG) and low-density lipoprotein (LDL) in high-fat dieting-induced dyslipidemia, and increase high-density lipoprotein (HDL) in hyperlipidemic animals. *Zé xiè* can prevent and treat hyperlipidemia in rabbits. The material basis of lipid-lowering is: alisinol A-24-acetate> alisinol B-23-acetate> alismol. The mechanism may be related to interference of exogenous cholesterol absorption and endogenous cholesterol metabolism.

4. **抗动脉粥样硬化**　泽泻醇溶性部位可抑制实验性动脉粥样硬化，抗动脉粥样硬化的机制与降低血脂，调整动脉壁内微量元素含量，调节前列环素与血栓素 A_2 比值（PGI_2/TXA_2）的动态平衡，降低脂质过氧化物的含量，降低动脉壁内钙异常升高，改善红细胞的变形性及其他血液流变性异常有关。

(4) Anti-atherosclerosis　*Zé xiè* has anti-atherosclerosis activity. *Zé xiè* alcohol soluble parts can suppress atherosclerosis in experimental model. The mechanism may be relate to lowering blood lipids, adjusting the content of trace elements in the arterial wall and the dynamic balance of prostacyclin/thromboxane A_2 (PGI_2/TXA_2), reducing the content of lipid peroxide, reducing the abnormal increase of calcium in the arterial wall, improving the deformability of red blood cells and other abnormal blood rheology.

5. **保肝**　泽泻提取物对各种原因引起的动物脂肪肝均有保护作用。泽泻盐制后能增强保肝降酶的作用，活性成分为泽泻醇类。泽泻缓解 D– 氨基半乳糖及 $CC1_4$ 引起的急性肝损伤，促进肝细胞对脂肪的代谢，增加脂蛋白的合成，抑制肝内脂肪堆积，改善肝功能；增加超氧化物歧化酶

(SOD)、过氧化氢酶（CAT）活性和谷胱甘肽（GSH）含量，减少自由基对肝细胞的损伤。

(5) Hepatoprotective activity *Zé xiè* has hepatoprotective activity. *Zé xiè* extracts has protective effects on animal fatty liver caused by various reasons. *Zé xiè* processed with salt is able to produce stronger hepatoprotective effect. The active ingredient is alismol. *Zé xiè* can relieve acute liver damage caused by D-galactosamine or CCl_4, promote lipid metabolism in the hepatocytes, increase the synthesis of lipoproteins, suppress fat accumulation in the liver, improve the liver function, increase the activity of superoxide dismutase (SOD) and catalase (CAT) and the content of glutathione (GSH), and reduce free radical-induced hepatocyte damage.

6. 其他作用 泽泻还具有抑制血小板聚集、抗血栓形成、降血糖、抗炎等作用。

(6) Other effects *Zé xiè* also has the effects of inhibiting platelet aggregation, anti-thrombosis, hypoglycemia, and anti-inflammatory.

【不良反应 / Adverse effects】

泽泻煎剂小鼠腹腔注射 LD_{50} 为 36.6g/kg；泽泻醇提物 LD_{50} 为 1.27g/kg。泽泻醇提物大鼠长期喂饲未见发育异常，但病理切片显示肝细胞及肾近曲小管有不同程度的肿胀及变性，其中泽泻醇 C，16-23– 环氧泽泻醇 B 可能会引起肾毒性。

The LD_{50} of *Zé xiè* decoction mice injected intraperitoneally is 36.6g/kg. The LD_{50} of *Zé xiè* alcohol extracts intravenously is 1.27g/kg. There is no developmental abnormality after long-term feeding of *Zé xiè* extracts in rats, but pathological sections show varying degrees of edema and degeneration of hepatocytes and renal proximal tubules. Alismol C, 16-23-epoxysalaris B may cause nephrotoxicity.

车前子 ¦ *Chē qián zǐ* (Plantaginis Semen)

【来源 / Origin】

本品为车前科植物车前（*Plantago asiatica* L.）或平车前（*Plantago deprdssa* Willd.）的干燥成熟种子。全国分布，以北方为多。

Chē qián zǐ is the dried mature seed of *Plantago asiatica* L. or *Plantago deprdssa* Willd., family of Plantaginaceae, which is distributed nationwide, but mostly in the north.

【化学成分 / Chemical ingredients】

主要含车前子酸、黄酮、6– 羟基木犀草素、熊果酸及环烯醚萜苷（车前苷、车前烯醇酸、梓醇）等，此外还含有黏液质，属多糖类成分，即车前多糖（又称车前胶）。

Chē qián zǐ contains plantenolic acid, flavone, 6-hydroxylluteolin, ursolic acid and iridoid glycoside (plantaginin, plantenolic acid, catalpol), etc. In addition, it contains phlegm, which is a polysaccharide component, also known as plantago-mulilage (or called psyllium gum).

【药性与功效 / Chinese medicine properties】

味甘，性寒，归肝、肾、肺、小肠经。具有清热利尿通淋、渗湿止泻、明目、祛痰等功效。用于治疗热淋涩痛、水肿胀满、目赤肿痛、痰热咳嗽等证。

In Chinese medicine theory, *Chē qián zǐ* are sweet and bland in flavor, cold in property, enter the liver, kidney, lung, and small intestine. They have the effects of inducing diuresis and relieving stranguary, draining dampness and checking diarrhea, improving eyesight and dispelling phlegm. Plantago seed are commonly used to treat heat stranguary and difficult and painful urination, edema and distention and fullness, swelling and pain of the eye, endogenous cough with phlegm-heat syndrome.

【药理作用 / Pharmacological effects】

1. 利尿 车前子提取物能增加水负荷后的排尿量和尿中 Na^+ 和 K^+ 及 Cl^- 含量，降低尿酸含量。

(1) Diuresis *Chē qián zǐ* has diuresis effects. The extracts of Plantago seed can increase urine output and the excretion of Na^+, K^+ and Cl^- in urine after water loading, and reduce uric acid levels.

2. 预防肾结石　车前子提取液可增强尿中草酸钙结晶排泄，抑制肾脏草酸钙结晶沉淀，预防肾结石形成。

(2) Preventing formation of renal calculi *Chē qián zǐ* has the effects of preventing the formation of renal calculi. Plantago seed can enhance the excretion of crystals of calcium oxalate in the urine, suppress the formation of calcium oxalate crystals in the renal tubules, thereby preventing the formation of renal calculus.

3. 降血脂　车前子可以降低高脂血症大鼠血清 TC 和 TG 水平，升高血清高密度脂蛋白胆固醇（HDL-C）水平和 HDL-C/TC，增强机体抗氧化能力，减轻脂质代谢紊乱引起的脂质过氧化。

(3) Lowering blood lipid *Chē qián zǐ* has the effects of lowering blood lipid. Plantago seed can decrease serum TC and TG levels in hyperlipidemia rats, increase serum high density lipoprotein-cholesterol (HDL-C) levels and HDL-C/TC ratios, enhance the antioxidant capacity in organism and reduce lipid peroxidation caused by disorders of lipid metabolism.

4. 镇咳、平喘　车前子煎剂能使气管分泌物增加，有明显的祛痰作用。车前苷有兴奋分泌神经的作用，能促进气管及支气管黏液的分泌。车前草水煎剂有镇咳作用，尤其是对电刺激和氨水引起的咳嗽；有松弛气管作用，尤其是对组胺或氯乙酰胆碱引起的气管兴奋。

(4) Antitussive and antiasthmatic *Chē qián zǐ* has antitussive and antiasthmatic effects. Plantago seed decoction can increase tracheal secretion and have obvious expectorant effect. Plantaginin can excite the secretory nerves, promote the secretion of tracheal and bronchial mucus. Plantain decoction has antitussive effects, especially on coughs caused by electrical stimulation and ammonia. Plantain decoction can relax the trachea, especially on those caused by histamine or acetylcholine chloride.

5. 抗病原微生物　车前子中的熊果酸可以杀灭多种葡萄球菌、革兰阳性菌、革兰阴性菌等；6-羟基木犀草素可以杀灭金黄色葡萄球菌、铜绿假单胞菌、表皮葡萄球菌等。

(5) Anti-pathogenic microorganisms Ursolic acid in Psyllium can kill a variety of bacteria such as staphylococcus, Gram-positive bacteria, and Gram-negative bacteria. 6-hydroxylluteolin can kill *Staphylococcus aureus*, *Pseudomonas aeruginosa*, *Epidermis staphylococcus speidermidis*, etc.

茵陈 ┆ *Yīn Chén (Artemisiae Scopariae Herba)*

【来源 / Origin】

本品为菊科植物滨蒿（*Artemisia scoparia* Waldst. et Kit.）或茵陈蒿（*Artemisia capillaris* Thunb.）的干燥地上部分。主要分布于陕西、山西、安徽等地区。

Yīn Chén is the dried aboveground part of *Artemisia scoparia* Waldst. et Kit. or *Artemisia Capillaris* Thunb. It is mainly distributed in Shaanxi, Shanxi, Anhui and other regions.

【化学成分 / Chemical ingredients】

主要有效成分有茵陈色原酮（capillarisin）、6,7-二甲氧基香豆素（6,7-dimethylesculetin）、绿原酸（chlorogenic acid）、水溶性多糖（water-soluble polysaccharide）、水溶性多肽（water-soluble polypeptide）、滨蒿内酯（scoparone）、对羟基苯乙酮（p-hydroxy acetophenone）、咖啡酸（caffeic acid）、7-甲氧基香豆素（7-methoxycoumarine）、蓟黄素（cirsimaritin）、6,7-二甲氧基七叶苷元（6,7-dimethoxyescin）、挥发油（volatile oil）、微量元素（trace elements）等。

Yīn chén contains capillarisin, 6,7-dimethylesculetin, chlorogenic acid, water-soluble polysaccharide, water-soluble polypeptide, scoparone, p-hydroxy acetophenone, caffeic acid, 7-methoxycoumarine, cirsimaritin, 6,7-dimethoxyescin, volatile oil, trace elements, etc.

【药性与功效 / Chinese medicine properties 】

味苦、辛，性微寒，归脾、胃、肝、胆经。具有清湿热、退黄疸的功效。主治湿热黄疸、湿疮瘙痒等证。

Yīn chén is bitter, pungent in flavor, slightly cold in nature. It can enter the spleen, stomach, liver and gallbladder meridians. Clinically it can be used for clearing heat and removing dampness, discharging bile and relieving jaundice.

【药理作用 / Pharmacological effects 】

1. 利胆退黄　在茵陈的诸多有效成分中，茵陈色原酮利胆作用最强。茵陈的利胆退黄作用与其诱导肝微粒体尿苷二磷酸葡萄糖醛酸基转移酶（UDPGT）活性密切相关，可促进胆红素的葡萄糖醛酸化，使结合胆红素生成增加，从而促进胆红素代谢。茵陈可减轻糖尿病对胆囊微血管的损害，其机制可能与提高抗氧化酶活性、降低脂质过氧化和降血脂有关。

(1) **Promoting function of gallbladder**　*Yīn chén* obviously promotes the discharge of bile to relieve jaundice. Among the active ingredients of *Yīn chén*, capillarisin has the strongest cholecystic effect. This effect is closely related to inducing the activity of uridine diphospho glucuronyl transferase (UDPGT) in hepatic microsomal. This enzyme promotes the bilirubin glucuronidation, and increases the conjugated bilirubin production, thereby promoting bilirubin metabolism. *Yīn Chén* can reduce the damage of gallbladder microvessels by diabetes, and its mechanism may be related to increasing antioxidant enzyme activity, reducing lipid peroxidation, and lowering blood lipids.

2. 保肝　茵陈的保肝作用表现为抑制肝炎模型肝脏系数上升；明显降低 ALT、谷草转氨酶（AST）；显著提高人血白蛋白（ALB），降低血清球蛋白（GLB），升高 A/G；6,7- 二甲氧基香豆素能抑制 D- 氨基半乳糖损伤过程中 TC 及 TG 的升高，具有防止肝细胞坏死及肝脂肪变性的作用；6,7- 二甲氧基香豆素具有抗脂质过氧化作用，阻止丙二醛（MDA）的形成，该活性可能是其肝保护作用的主要原因。

(2) **Hepatoprotection**　*Yīn chén* has a strong liver protective effect. It is manifested in inhibiting the increase of liver coefficient caused by the hepatitis model; significantly reducing ALT and aspartate aminotransferase (AST); significantly increasing human serum albumin (ALB), reducing serum globulin (GLB), increasing A/G ratio; 6,7-dimethoxycoumarin can inhibit the level of TC and TG in serum damaged by D-aminogalactose to prevent hepatocyte necrosis and hepatic steatosis; 6,7-dimethoxycoumarin has anti-lipid peroxidation effect and prevents the formation of malondialdehyde (MDA). This activity may be the main reason for its hepatoprotective effect.

3. 提高免疫力　茵陈有显著提高机体免疫功能和诱生干扰素作用，能清除乙肝病毒，提高机体免疫能力，用于调整机体功能，治疗乙型肝炎。

(3) **Improving immunity**　*Yīn chén* can significantly improve the body's immune function and induce interferon, clear the hepatitis B virus and improve the body's immune ability. It is used to adjust the body's function and treat hepatitis B.

4. 利尿　6,7- 二甲氧基香豆素为利尿的有效成分，在不同程度上有效地增加尿液的排泄，减轻水肿。

(4) **Diuresis**　6,7-dimethoxycoumarin is an effective component of diuresis, which can effectively increase urine excretion and reduce edema to varying degrees.

5. 降血脂　茵陈能够降低高血脂动物血脂水平，降低主动脉壁中 TC 含量，防止血管壁和内脏的脂肪沉着，具有抗动脉粥样硬化作用。

(5) Reducing blood lipid and anti-atherosclerosis　*Yīn chén* can reduce the blood lipid level of hyperlipidemic animals, reduce the TC content in the aortic wall, prevent the fat deposits in the vascular wall and viscera, exerting anti-atherosclerotic effect.

6. 抗菌　茵陈对金黄色葡萄球菌、甲型和乙型溶血链球菌、流感嗜血杆菌、肺炎链球菌、炭疽杆菌、白喉棒状杆菌、大肠埃希菌、奈瑟菌等均有不同程度的体外抑制作用。

(6) Antibacterial　*Yīn Chén* inhibits has different degrees of *in vitro* inhibitory effect on *Staphylococcus aureus*, *A, B Streptococcus hemolyticus*, *Haemophilus influenzae*, *Diplococcus pneumoniae*, *Bacillus anthracis*, *Corynebacterium diphtheriae*, *Escherichia. coli*, *Neisseria*, etc.

7. 抗肿瘤　茵陈对肿瘤细胞有明显的细胞毒作用，使肿瘤细胞被阻滞于 G_0/G_1 期；对致癌物黄曲霉毒素 B_1 或亚硝酸钠或 N– 亚硝基甲基苄胺致癌致突变作用有明显的抑制作用；显著抑制人肝癌细胞 BEL_{7402}、恶性黑色素瘤、肾癌、前列腺癌、移植性 MethA 肿瘤生长。

(7) Anti-tumor　*Yīn chén* has obvious cytotoxic effects on tumor cells, so that tumor cells are blocked at G_0/G_1 phase; *Yīn chén* has obvious carcinogenic mutation effects on carcinogens aflatoxin B_1 or sodium nitrite or N-nitrosylmethylbenzylamine; *Yīn chén* can significantly inhibit the growth of human liver cancer cell BEL_{7402}, malignant melanoma, kidney cancer, prostate cancer, and transplanted MethA tumors.

【**不良反应 / Adverse effects**】

茵陈二炔酮小鼠灌胃 LD_{50} 为 6.98mg/kg；6,7– 二甲氧基香豆素小鼠灌胃 LD_{50} 为 497mg/kg，死亡前有阵发性惊厥。

The LD_{50} of glaucoma diacetylone in mice is 6.98mg/kg; the LD_{50} of 6,7-dimethoxycoumarin in mice is 497mg/kg, and previous paroxysmal convulsions occurs when mice die.

题库

（华永庆　李红艳）

第十章　温里药
Chapter 10　Interior-warming medicines

学习目标┊ Objectives

　　1. **掌握** 温里药主要的药理学作用以及与功效的相关性；附子与功效相关的药理作用、作用机制、药效物质基础和不良反应。

　　2. **了解** 干姜、肉桂、吴茱萸、花椒的主要药理作用和药效物质基础。

　　1. **Must know** The main pharmacological effects and connection with efficacy of interior-warming medicines; The efficacy related pharmacological effects, mechanism of actions, material basis, and adverse effects of *Fù zǐ*.

　　2. **Desirable to know** The efficacy related pharmacological effects and material basis of *Gān jiāng, Ròu guì, Wú zhū yú*, and *Huā jiāo*.

第一节　概述
Section 1　Overview

PPT

　　凡以温里祛寒，治疗里寒证为主要功效的药物，称为温里药。本类药物多味辛，药性温热，主入脾、胃、肝、肾经。具有辛散温通、散寒止痛、补火助阳等功效，主要用于寒邪内盛、心肾阳衰所呈现的各种里寒证候。

　　All Chinese materia medica that are mainly used to warm interior and dispel cold are classified as interior-warming medicines. The medicines in the category are traditionally used to treat interior cold syndrome. They generally have acrid flavor and warm medicinal nature. They majorly enter the meridians of spleen, stomach, liver and kidney. The medicines in the category can disperse stasis by acrid flavor, warm and dredge the channels and vessels, dispel cold to relieve pain, and tonify fire to help Yang. They are mainly used for all kinds of interior cold syndrome caused by pathogenic cold in interior and Yang failure of heart and kidney.

　　里寒证常见两方面病证：一是寒邪入里，脾胃阳气受抑所表现的脾胃受寒或脾胃虚寒证；二是心肾阳虚，寒从内生，或心肾阳衰。还与某些神经、肌肉、关节等炎症有关。温里药多依据中医"寒者热之"的治疗原则而立法，属于"八法"中的"温法"，即用具有温热作用的温里药温扶人体的阳气。所谓温热作用，一般指兴奋或激动的作用；所谓阳气，一般指人体各种生理调节

医药大学堂
WWW.YIYAODXT.COM

的代偿功能。温扶人体的阳气就是指兴奋或激动人体生理调节的代偿功能。

There are usually two aspects of disease and syndrome in interior cold syndrome. One is pathogenic cold in interior, and Yang failure of spleen and stomach which causes the syndrome of invading or deficiency cold in spleen and stomach. The other is Yang deficiency of heart and kidney which causes pathogenic interior cold, or Yang failure of heart and kidney. In addition, they are related to the inflammation in some nerves, muscles, joints etc. Interior-warming medicines are based on the therapeutic principle of cold syndrome treated by warming property, which is the warming principle of eight principles. It means interior-warming medicines with heating therapy can warm and recuperate Yang Qi. Heating therapy is approximately considered as the effect of excitation or activation. Yang Qi is approximately considered as compensation functions of various physiological regulations. Thus, warming and recuperating Yang Qi mean stimulating or activating compensation functions of various physiological regulations.

里寒证是人体各种生理调节的代偿功能下降所致，临床可见胀满冷痛、呕吐泄泻，或腰膝冷痛、畏寒肢冷、夜尿频多，或呼吸微弱、四肢厥冷、脉微欲绝等病理反应。与西医学中消化系统疾病、慢性心功能不全、休克、缓慢性心律失常及肾衰竭等疾病的症状表现相似。现代药理研究表明，温里药治疗里寒证与下列药理作用有关。

In western medicine, interior cold syndrome is caused by decline compensation function of various physiological regulations. In clinic, there are pathological reactions, such as distention and cold pain, vomiting and diarrhea, or knee cold pain, chilliness and cold hands and feet, nocturia, or weak breathing, peripheral coldness, and faint pulse. Therefore, interior cold syndrome has the similar symptoms to those diseases in western medicine, including digestive system diseases, chronic cardiac insufficiency, shock, slow arrhythmia, and renal failure. The efficacy of interior-warming medicines function is related to the following pharmacological effects.

1. 强心 温里药一般具有不同程度的正性肌力、正性频率和正性传导作用。例如，附子、干姜、肉桂及吴茱萸等均有强心作用，可使心肌收缩力增强，心率加快，心输出量增加；消旋去甲乌药碱是附子强心的主要成分，是β受体部分激动剂；肉桂的强心作用与其促进交感神经末梢释放儿茶酚胺有关；干姜的醇提液有直接兴奋心肌作用。

(1) Cardiotonic actions Interior-warming medicines exhibit positive inotropic, chronotropic and conductive effects. For instance, *Fù zǐ*, *Gān jiāng*, *Ròu guì*, possess the cardiotonic actions through enhancing cardiac contractility, heart rate and cardiac output. Higenamine is the active constituent of *Fù zǐ* in terms of cardiotonic actions, which is the partial agonist of β receptor. Cardiotonic actions of *Ròu guì* is correlated with catecholamine released from sympathetic nerve endings. Alcohol extracts of *Gān jiāng* result in myocardium excitation directly.

2. 影响心率 附子能改善维拉帕米（异搏定）所致小鼠缓慢性心律失常的房室传导功能，恢复正常窦性心律；对甲醛所致家兔窦房结功能低下也有改善作用。干姜、肉桂、荜澄茄、荜茇也有加快心率作用，但吴茱萸提取物能减慢心率。

(2) Heart rate effects *Fù zǐ* improves rat slow-type arrhythmia induced by verapamil, through developing the electric conduction speed between atrium and ventricular, and converses to normal sinus rhythm. Moreover, *Fù zǐ* ameliorates rabbit sinus node dysfunction by formaldehyde. *Gān jiāng*, *Ròu guì*, *Bì chéng qié* and *Bì bá* accelerate heart rate. On the contrary, extracts from *Wú zhū yú* reduce heart rate.

3. 扩张血管，改善血液循环 附子、肉桂、吴茱萸、荜澄茄、荜茇等能扩张冠脉，增加冠脉血流量，改善心肌供血；附子、肉桂、干姜等可扩张脑血管，增加脑血流量，改善脑循环；胡椒、干姜、肉桂等所含的挥发油或辛辣成分可使体表血管、内脏血管扩张，改善循环，使全身产生温热感。温里药能"助阳""散寒"，治疗四肢厥逆（冷）主要与其改善循环作用有关。

(3) Dilate vessels and improve blood circulation The medicines, including *Fù zǐ*, *Ròu guì*, *Wú zhū yú*, *Bì chéng qié*, and *Bì bá*, dilate coronary artery, increase coronary blood flow and enhance myocardial blood supply. *Fù zǐ*, *Ròu guì* and *Gān jiāng* dilate cerebral vessels, increase cerebral blood flood and improve cerebral circulation. Volatile oils or pungency components of *Hú jiāo*, *Gān jiāng* and *Ròu guì* can improve circulation and warm the body. Effects of interior-warming medicines on "reinforcing Yang" "dispelling cold", and peripheral coldness may be related to improvement of circulation.

4. 抗休克 附子、肉桂及干姜等对失血性、内毒素性、心源性及肠系膜上动脉夹闭性休克等均能提高动脉压，延长实验动物存活时间和提高存活百分率，对单纯缺氧性、血管栓塞性休克等亦有防治作用。其抗休克的作用机制主要与其强心、扩张血管、改善微循环有关。

(4) Antishock effects In various shock models caused by hemorrhage, endotoxin, cardiogenic factors and superior mesenteric artery occlusion, *Fù zǐ*, *Ròu guì* and *Gān jiāng* can raise arterial pressure, prolong rat living time, and increase survival percentage. At the same time, these medicines prevent simple hypoxic and thrombosis shock. The mechanism of antishock effects are related to strengthening heart, dilating vessels and improving microcirculation.

5. 影响胃肠运动 温里药大多具有增强胃肠运动、健胃祛风的作用。干姜、肉桂、吴茱萸、丁香、胡椒、荜澄茄等性味辛热，含有挥发油，对胃肠道有温和的刺激作用，能使肠管兴奋，增强胃肠张力，促进蠕动，排出胃肠积气。另外，附子、丁香、小茴香等能抑制小鼠胃排空，吴茱萸、干姜、肉桂能缓解胃肠痉挛性收缩。

(5) Influence gastrointestinal motility Several interior-warming medicines have the effects of enhancing gastrointestinal motility, invigorating stomach and dispelling wind. The medicines, including *Gān jiāng*, *Ròu guì*, *Wú zhū yú*, *Dīng xiāng*, *Hú jiāo* and *Bì chéng qié*, are acrid in taste and hot in nature and contain volatile oils. They embody mild stimulations of gastrointestinal tract, intestine activation, gastrointestinal tension enhancement, peristalsis promotion, and gastrointestinal pneumatosis excretion. In addition, *Fù zǐ*, *Dīng xiāng* and *Xiǎo huí xiāng* delay mice gastric empty. *Wú zhū yú*, *Gān jiāng* and *Ròu guì* can relieve gastric enterospasm contraction in mice.

6. 促进消化 干姜的芳香和辛辣成分能直接刺激口腔和胃黏膜，改善局部血液循环，增加胃液分泌，增加胃蛋白酶和唾液淀粉酶活性，有助于提高食欲，促进消化吸收。丁香、高良姜、草豆蔻可增加胃酸排出量，提高胃蛋白酶活力。

(6) Promote digestion Aromatic and piquancy components of *Gān jiāng* can promote appetite, digestion and absorption through stimulating oral and stomach local circulation, increasing gastric secretion, and improving pepsin and salivary amylase activation. *Dīng xiāng*, *Gāo liáng jiāng* and *Cǎo dòu kòu* can increase gastric acid output and pepsin amylase activation.

7. 利胆、镇吐、抗溃疡 干姜、肉桂、高良姜等能促进胆汁分泌。干姜、吴茱萸、丁香有镇吐作用。附子、干姜、肉桂、吴茱萸、花椒、小茴香、丁香等还有抗胃溃疡的作用。

(7) Cholagogic, antiemetic and antiulcer effects *Gān jiāng*, *Ròu guì* and *Gāo liáng jiāng* promote bile secretion. Antiemetic effects are found in *Gān jiāng*, *Wú zhū yú* and *Dīng xiāng*. Antiulcer actions are found in *Fù zǐ*, *Gān jiāng*, *Ròu guì*, *Wú zhū yú*, *Huā jiāo*, *Xiǎo huí xiāng* and *Dīng xiāng*.

8. 影响肾上腺皮质系统功能 附子、肉桂、干姜对垂体–肾上腺皮质系统有兴奋作用，可使肾上腺中维生素 C、胆固醇含量降低，促进肾上腺皮质激素合成，发挥抗炎作用。附子、肉桂均可使阴虚动物模型的阴虚证进一步恶化，而使阳虚动物模型的阳虚证得到改善。

(8) Influence adrenal system function *Fù zǐ*, *Ròu guì*, and *Gān jiāng* stimulate hypophyseal-adrenocortical system for anti-inflammation through decreasing vitamin C and cholesterol in adrenal gland and increasing adrenal cortical hormone secretion. Yin deficiency syndrome are deteriorated in Yin deficiency model, while Yang deficiency syndrome are improved in Yang deficiency model after using *Fù zǐ* and *Ròu guì*.

9. 影响神经系统功能 附子、肉桂、吴茱萸、小茴香等有镇静作用。附子、干姜、肉桂、吴茱萸、花椒、小茴香、丁香、高良姜等有不同程度的镇痛作用。附子、乌头、花椒有局部及黏膜麻醉作用。附子、干姜、肉桂、四逆汤能兴奋交感神经，使产热增加，有祛寒作用。

(9) Affect nervous system function *Fù zǐ*, *Ròu guì*, *Wú zhū yú*, and *Xiǎo huí xiāng* induce sedation. *Fù zǐ*, *Gān jiāng*, *Ròu guì*, *Wú zhū yú*, *Huā jiāo*, *Xiǎo huí xiāng*, *Dīng xiāng* and *Gāo liáng jiāng* process different degrees of analgesic effects. *Fù zǐ*, *Wū tóu* and *Huā jiāo* have local and mucosa anesthetic actions. *Fù zǐ*, *Gān jiāng*, *Ròu guì* and *Sini decoction* excite sympathetic nerves, increase thermogenesis, and dispel cold.

常用温里药的主要药理作用见表 10-1。

The main pharmacological effects of commonly used interior-warming medicines are summarized in Table 10-1.

表 10-1 常用温里药的主要药理作用

药物	强心	扩张血管	抗休克	健胃	镇吐	抗炎	镇静	镇痛	兴奋交感神经	其他药理作用
附子	+	+	+	+	–	+	+	+	+	增强免疫、局部麻醉、抗血栓
干姜	+	+	–	+	+	+	+	+	+	抗菌、增强免疫、抗血栓
肉桂	–	+	–	+	+	+	+	+	+	抗菌、抗缺氧、抗血栓
吴茱萸	–	+	–	+	–	+	+	+	–	抗菌、止泻、抗血栓
花椒	–	–	–	–	–	+	–	+	–	影响消化系统、抗菌杀虫、抗肿瘤、抗氧化
丁香	–	–	–	+	+	–	–	–	–	抗菌、驱虫、兴奋子宫
胡椒	–	+	–	+	–	–	–	–	–	升压、产生全身温热感
小茴香	–	–	–	+	–	–	–	–	–	增强胃肠运动、抗溃疡
荜澄茄	–	–	–	+	–	–	+	+	–	抗过敏、抗菌

注："+"表示有明确作用；"–"表示无作用，或未查阅到相关研究文献

微课

第二节 常用药物

Section 2 Commonly used medicines

附子 ┆ *Fù zǐ (Aconiti Lateralis Radix Preparata)*

【来源 / Origin】

本品为毛茛科植物乌头（*Aconitum carmichaelii* Debx.）子根的加工品。主要分布于四川、湖北、陕西等地区。

Fù zǐ is the processed daughter roots of *Aconitum carmichaelii* Debx., a plant of Ranunculaceae. The plant is widely cultivated in Sichuan province, Hubei province, and Shaanxi province in China.

【化学成分 / Chemical ingredients】

主要含多种生物碱，主要有乌头碱（aconitine）、新乌头碱（mesaconitine）、次乌头碱（hypaconitine）等。此外，主要有效成分为消旋去甲乌药碱（higenamine），氯化甲基多巴胺（methyl chloride dopamine）、去甲猪毛菜碱（salsolinol）等。

There are several alkaloids in *Fù zǐ*, including aconitine, mesaconitine, and hypaconitine. Additionally, the main effective components are higenamine, methyl chloride dopamine, and salsolinol.

【药性与功效 / Chinese medicine properties】

味辛、甘，性大热，有毒，归心、肾、脾经。具有回阳救逆、补火助阳、散寒止痛的功效。用于治疗亡阳虚脱、肢冷脉微、阳痿、宫冷、心腹冷痛、虚寒吐泻、阴寒水肿、寒湿痹痛等证。

In Chinese medicine theory, *Fù zǐ* is acrid and sweet in flavor, extremely hot and toxic in nature. It enters the meridians of heart, kidney, and spleen. *Fù zǐ* can revive Yang for resuscitation, tonify fire to help Yang, and dispel cold to relieve pain. Clinically it can be used for Yang-exhaustion, faint pulse and cold limbs, impotence, cold uterine, precordial and abdominal pain with cold sensation, vomiting and diarrhea with cold deficiency, Yin-cold edema, and cold-dampness arthralgia pain.

【药理作用 / Pharmacological effects】

1. 强心 附子对离体和在体心脏、正常及衰竭心脏均具有强心作用，能增强心肌收缩力、加快心率、增加心输出量、增加心肌耗氧量。消旋去甲乌药碱、氯化甲基多巴胺和去甲猪毛菜碱是附子强心的主要物质基础。目前研究认为，消旋去甲乌药碱是β受体部分激动剂，其强心作用与兴奋β受体有关。去甲猪毛菜碱也能兴奋心脏，加快心率，对α受体和β受体都有激动作用，但对α受体的激动作用较弱。氯化甲基多巴胺亦有强心作用，为α受体激动剂。

(1) **Cardiotonic actions** *Fù zǐ* has cardiotonic actions in isolating hearts, hearts *in vivo*, normal hearts, and failing hearts. It enhances cardiac contractility, heart rate, cardiac output, and myocardial oxygen consumption. The main effective components of cardiotonic actions are higenamine, methyl chloride dapamine, and salsolinol in *Fù zǐ*. Higenamine, as the partial agonist of β receptor, has cardiotonic actions related to activating β receptor. Salsolinol excites heart and accelerates heart rate because of α receptor and β receptor activation, but it shows weak interaction of α receptor. Methyl chloride dopamine is the agonist of α receptor with cardiotonic actions.

2. 影响血管和血压 静脉注射附子注射液或消旋去甲乌药碱有扩张血管作用，均可使麻醉犬心输出量、冠状动脉血流量、脑血流量及股动脉血流量增加，血管阻力降低。附子既有升压又有降压作用，与其所含成分有关。研究证明，消旋去甲乌药碱是其降压的物质基础，具有兴奋β受体及阻断α₁受体的双重作用。氯化甲基多巴胺为α受体激动剂，去甲猪毛菜碱对β受体和α受体均有兴奋作用，二者是其升压作用的主要物质基础。

(2) Effects on vessels and pressure *Fù zǐ* or higenamine injections dilate vessels, which can increase anesthesia dog heart output, coronary, cerebral, and femoral artery blood flow, and reduce vascular resistance. *Fù zǐ* has not only pressor but also hypotensive effects, which is related to the components. Higenamine is the important material basis of hypotensive effects, with the double functions of activating β receptor and blocking $α_1$ receptor. Methyl chloride dopamine is the agonist of α receptor. Salsolinol stimulates both α receptor and β receptor. Methyl chloride dopamine and salsolinol are main material basis of pressor effects.

3. 抗休克 针对失血性休克、内毒素性休克、心源性休克及肠系膜上动脉夹闭性休克，附子能改善心输出量、提高平均动脉压，延长休克动物存活时间及存活百分率。消旋去甲乌药碱、氯化甲基多巴胺和去甲猪毛菜碱是附子抗休克的主要物质基础。附子的抗休克作用与其强心、扩张血管、改善循环等作用有关。

(3) Antishock effects In various shock models caused by hemorrhage, endotoxin, cardiogenic factors and superior mesenteric artery occlusion, *Fù zǐ* can increase heart output and arterial pressure, prolong rat living time and increase survival percentage. The main effective components of antishock effects are higenamine, methyl chloride dopamine, and salsolinol in *Fù zǐ*. The antishock effects of *Fù zǐ* are related to strengthening heart, dilating vessels and improving microcirculation.

4. 抗心律失常 附子有抗缓慢性心律失常作用。消旋去甲乌药碱是其抗缓慢性心律失常的主要物质基础。该成分对维拉帕米所致小鼠缓慢性心律失常，能改善房室传导，加快心率和恢复窦性心律。对甲醛所致的家兔窦房结功能低下，能使窦房结和房室结功能趋于正常，提高心率，恢复窦性心律，使ST段及T波恢复正常。附子抗缓慢性心律失常作用与消旋去甲乌药碱兴奋β受体有关。此外，附子也具有抗快速性心律失常的作用。附子水溶性部分、附子注射液可分别对抗乌头碱、垂体后叶素所致大鼠的心律失常，附子正丁醇、乙醇及水提物均对三氯甲烷所致小鼠室颤有预防作用。说明附子对心肌电生理的不同作用与其物质基础有关。

(4) Anti-arrhythmia effects *Fù zǐ* improves slow-type arrhythmia. As main material basis, higenamine improves mice slow-type arrhythmia induced by verapamil through developing the electric conduction speed between atrium and ventricular, fastening heart rate, and conversing to normal sinus rhythm. In rabbit sinus dysfunction induced by formaldehyde, it also recovers sinus and atrioventricular nodes function, rises heart rate, regains sinus rhythm, normalizes ST segment and T wave. The effects of *Fù zǐ* on slow-type arrhythmia are related to the activation of β receptor by higenamine. Moreover, *Fù zǐ* inhibits fast-type arrhythmia. Water-soluble components in *Fù zǐ* and *Fù zǐ* injection refine rat arrhythmia inducing by aconitine or pituitrin. Butanol, ethanol, and water-soluble extracts of *Fù zǐ* recover mice ventricular fibrillation induced by chloroform. It shows that different effects of *Fù zǐ* on myocardial electrophysiology are related to material basis.

5. 抗心肌缺血 静脉注射附子注射液能对抗垂体后叶素所引起的大鼠急性实验性心肌缺血，对心电图ST段升高有抑制作用。消旋去甲乌药碱具有扩张冠状动脉和增加心肌营养性血流量的作用，附子抗心肌缺血作用可能与增加心肌血氧供应有关。

(5) Anti-myocardial ischemia effects After injecting *Fù zǐ*, rat acute experimental myocardial ischemia induced by pituitrin is improved with the inhibition of rising ST segment. Higenamine dilates coronary artery, and enhances myocardial blood supply. Anti-myocardial ischemia effects of *Fù zǐ* are correlated with strengthening myocardial blood and oxygen supply.

6. 提高耐缺氧能力　腹腔注射附子注射液能提高小鼠对常压缺氧的耐受能力，延长小鼠在缺氧条件下的存活时间。

(6) Increasing hypoxia tolerance capability　After peritoneal injection of *Fù zǐ*, anoxia tolerance capability is improved, and the survival time of rats are prolonged.

7. 抗寒冷　附子冷浸液和水煎液均能抑制寒冷环境引起的鸡和大鼠体温下降，延长生存时间，减少死亡数。附子抗寒冷作用与其强心、扩张血管、增加血流量等作用有关，也与增强 β 受体、环磷酸腺苷（cAMP）系统的反应性有关。

(7) Cold tolerance effects　Liquid and water decoctions of *Fù zǐ* can inhibit the decrease in temperature of chickens and rats in cold situation. At the same time, they also prolong the survival time and reduce death count. The cold tolerance of *Fù zǐ* are related to strengthening heart, dilating vessels, increasing blood flow, enhancing β receptor and cyclic adenosine monophosphate (cAMP) system reaction.

8. 影响消化系统　附子煎剂能兴奋离体兔空肠平滑肌的收缩运动，此作用可被阿托品、肾上腺素或苯海拉明阻断，推测附子具有胆碱样、组胺样和抗肾上腺素样作用。黑附片水煎剂对阿托品抑制的胃肠推进运动和酚妥拉明促进的胃肠推进运动有对抗作用，说明附子对整体动物的胃肠运动有一定的调节作用。附子水煎剂还能抑制小鼠水浸应激性和大鼠盐酸（HCl）损伤性胃溃疡的形成。

(8) Digestive system effects　*Fù zǐ* decoction promotes the contraction of isolated rabbit jejunal smooth muscles, which is abolished by atropine, epinephrine, or diphenhydramine. It is suggested that *Fù zǐ* possesses cholinergic, histamine, or antiadrenoid effects. Prepared *Fù zǐ* decoction not only enhances the gastrointestinal propulsive motility inhibited by atropine, but also resists the gastrointestinal propulsive motility promoted by phentolamine. The results show that *Fù zǐ* has the certain regulation on gastrointestinal propulsive motility in vivo. *Fù zǐ* decoction also inhibits gastric ulcer formation by water immersion stress in mice, and hydrochloride (HCl) damage in rat.

9. 抗炎　附子对多种实验性炎症有抑制作用。附子能抑制巴豆油所致的小鼠耳郭肿胀和甲醛、蛋清、组胺、角叉菜胶等所致的大鼠足跖肿胀，对抗醋酸所致的小鼠毛细血管通透性增加。附子也能抑制佐剂诱导的关节炎，并对佐剂诱发的关节炎大鼠的骨变性、纤溶功能下降具有抑制作用。乌头碱、新乌头碱、次乌头碱是其抗炎的主要物质基础。附子抗炎作用与兴奋下丘脑-垂体-肾上腺皮质系统有关。但是动物切除双侧肾上腺后，附子仍有抗炎作用。因此，附子的抗炎作用可能是通过多途径实现的。

(9) Anti-inflammation effects　*Fù zǐ* exhibits the inhibitory effect in various experimental inflammation models, including mice ear edema by croton oil, rat metatarsal swelling by formaldehyde, albumen, histamine, or carrageenan. *Fù zǐ* inhibits the increase of mice capillary permeability by acetic acid. Meanwhile, *Fù zǐ* inhibits adjuvant arthritis through decrease of bone degeneration and fibrinolytic function. Anti-inflammation effects are mainly based on aconitine, mesaconitine, and hypaconitine. In spite of relationship between *Fù zǐ* anti-inflammation effects and hypothalamus-pituitary-adrenal system activation, *Fù zǐ* remains anti-inflammation effects in bilaterally adrenalectomized animal. Thus, there are multi-ways for anti-inflammation activities in *Fù zǐ*.

10. 镇痛　生附子及乌头碱能抑制醋酸所致的小鼠扭体反应。生附子能提高小鼠尾根部加压致痛法的痛阈。附子水煎醇沉液对热刺激所致小鼠疼痛有镇痛作用。乌头碱是其镇痛的主要物质基础。

(10) Analgesic effects　Aconite roots and aconitine decrease the mice writhes caused by acetic acid. Aconite roots ameliorates pain threshold in tail-pressure mice. Water extracts precipitated with alcohol of *Fù zǐ* has analgesic effect in heat induced pain mice. The main effective component of analgesic effects is aconitine.

11. 其他作用

(11) Other effects

（1）增强免疫功能　附子对非特异性及特异性免疫功能有促进作用。附子水煎液能促进小鼠脾淋巴细胞分泌白细胞介素 –2（IL-2），附子注射液可增加小鼠补体含量。附子水煎液还能增加豚鼠 T 淋巴细胞玫瑰花环形成率（RFC）和家兔 T 淋巴细胞转化率（LTT）。附子水溶性提取物能提高阳虚模型小鼠脾细胞产生抗体的能力。

1) Immunity enhancement　*Fù zǐ* strengthens the non-specific and specific immunologic functions. *Fù zǐ* decoction stimulates the secretion of interleukin-2 (IL-2) in mice spleen lymphocytes. *Fù zǐ* injection increases mice complement levels. *Fù zǐ* decoction augments rosette forming percentage (RFC) of T lymphocytes in guinea pig, rabbit T lymphocyte transformation percentage (LTT). In Yang deficiency model, water-soluble extracts in *Fù zǐ* improve antibody production ability of spleen cells in mice.

（2）镇静　生附子能抑制小鼠自发活动，延长环己巴比妥所致的小鼠睡眠时间。

2) Inducing sedation　Aconite roots decrease mice spontaneous activities, and prolongs sleeping time caused by cyclobarbital.

（3）局部麻醉　附子能刺激局部皮肤，使皮肤黏膜的感觉神经末梢兴奋，产生瘙痒与灼热感，继之麻醉，丧失知觉。

3) Local anesthetic action　*Fù zǐ* stimulates local skins to activate sensory nerve ending in mucocutaneous, with pruritus and burning heat sensation. Then anesthesia happens and perception is lost.

【不良反应 / Adverse effects 】

附子为毒性较大的中药，其毒性主要为双酯型乌头碱类生物碱引起。附子经过炮制、水解、合理配伍，双酯型生物碱含量大大降低，毒性也降低。乌头碱经水解后生成毒性较小的苯甲酰乌头原碱，毒性仅为乌头碱的 1/1000 左右，其继续水解生成乌头原碱，其毒性为乌头碱的 1/2000。生附子给小鼠灌服、腹腔注射、静脉注射的半数致死量（LD$_{50}$）分别是 5.49g/kg、0.71g/kg、0.49g/kg，炮制后 LD$_{50}$ 分别是 161g/kg、11.5g/kg、2.8g/kg，毒性降低。新乌头碱小鼠口服的 LD$_{50}$ 为 5.64mg/kg。乌头碱的不良反应主要涉及神经系统、循环系统和消化系统，其中对心脏毒性最大。

Fù zǐ is the Chinese herb with great toxicity which is mainly caused by di-ester type aconitum alkaloids. After processing, hydrolysis, and rational compatibility, di-ester type alkaloids are reduced greatly to low toxicity. Aconitine is hydrolyzed to benzoylaconine with less toxity, which is about 1/1000 toxicity of aconitine. Benzoylaconine is continually hydrolyzed to aconine, which is 1/2000 toxicity of aconitine. 50% lethal doses (LD$_{50}$) of aconite roots are 5.49g/kg, 0.71g/kg, 0.49g/kg by gavage, intraperitoneal and intravenous injection in mice. Processed aconite has less toxicity, whose LD$_{50}$ are 161g/kg, 11.5g/kg, 2.8g/kg. LD$_{50}$ of mesaconitine is 5.64mg/kg in mice oral administration. Adverse effects of aconitine are involved in nervous, circulation and digestive systems, especially cardiac toxicity.

干姜 ┆ *Gān jiāng* (*Zingiberis Rhizoma*)

【来源 / Origin】

本品为姜科植物姜（*Zingiber officinale* Rosc.）的干燥根茎。主要分布于四川、湖北、广东、广西、福建、贵州等地。

Gān jiāng is the dry rhizome of *Zingiber officinale* Rosc., one of Zingiberanceous plants. The plant is widely cultivated in Sichuan province, Hubei province, Guangdong province, Guangxi province, Fujian province and Guizhou province in China.

【化学成分 / Chemical ingredients】

含挥发油和姜辣素（gingerols）。挥发油中主要有效成分为姜烯（zingiberene），占 33.9%，其次为姜醇（zingiberol）、姜烯酮（ginger ketene）等。姜辣素中含姜酚（gingerol）和姜酮（zingerone）等。

There are volatile oils and gingerols in *Gān jiāng*. 33.9% of volatile oils is zingiberene, then zingiberol and ginger ketene. Gingerols include gingerol and zingerone.

【药性与功效 / Chinese medicine properties】

味辛，性热，归脾、胃、心、肺经。具有温中散寒、回阳通脉、燥湿消痰的功效。用于治疗脘腹冷痛、呕吐泄泻、肢冷脉微、痰饮喘咳等证。

In Chinese medicine theory, *Gān jiāng* has the nature of acrid and hot. It can enter the meridians of spleen, stomach, heart, and lung. *Gān jiāng* can warm middle-jiao to dispel cold, promote coronary circulation by restoring Yang, eliminate dampness and phlegm. Clinically it can be used for cold pain of gastric cavity and abdomen, vomiting and diarrhea, cold limbs and weak pulse, cough and asthma due to phlegm in lung.

【药理作用 / Pharmacological effects】

1. **调节胃肠平滑肌运动**　干姜对胃肠平滑肌运动的影响与成分及平滑肌功能状态有关。干姜挥发油对消化道有轻度刺激作用，可使肠张力、节律及蠕动增强。姜辣素的主要成分姜酚可通过激动 M 受体、H_1 受体而发挥收缩肠管效应。干姜醇提物对阿托品、多巴胺引起的胃排空减慢有促进作用，而挥发油能竞争性拮抗乙酰胆碱（ACh）、组胺所致离体回肠收缩。干姜石油醚提物、水提物能分别对抗蓖麻油、番泻叶引起的腹泻，但不影响小鼠胃肠蠕动。

(1) **Gastrointestinal motility regulations**　The effects of *Gān jiāng* on gastrointestinal muscle motility are correlated with smooth muscles function. Volatile oils of *Gān jiāng* can slightly stimulate digestive tracts to enhance intestinal tension, rhythm, and peristalsis. As the major ingredient of gingerols, gingerol acts on systolic intestine through activating M receptor and H_1 receptor. Alcohol extractions of *Gān jiāng* enhance the gastrointestinal propulsive motility inhibited by atropine and dopamine. Volatile oils of *Gān jiāng* perform competitive antagonism of acetylcholine (ACh) and histamine to resist systolic ileum actions in vitro. Petroleum ether and water-soluble extracts in *Gān jiāng* inhibit diarrhea by castor oil and senn, without influencing gastrointestinal peristalsis.

2. **抗溃疡**　干姜有保护胃黏膜和抗溃疡的作用。干姜水煎液给大鼠灌服，对应激性溃疡、醋酸诱发胃溃疡、幽门结扎性胃溃疡均有抑制作用。干姜石油醚提物能对抗水浸应激性、吲哚美辛加乙醇性、HCl 性和结扎幽门性胃溃疡的形成。干姜抗溃疡作用与抑制血栓素 A_2（TXA_2）的合成和促进前列腺素 I_2（PGI_2）合成有关，TXA_2 及 PGI_2 分别对胃黏膜起损伤和保护作用。

(2) **Antiulcer effects**　*Gān jiāng* can protect gastric mucosa and inhibit ulcer. *Gān jiāng* decoction by gavage restrains rat stomach ulcer induced by stress, acetic acid, and pyloric ligated. Petroleum ether extracts in *Gān jiāng* inhibit stomach ulcer formation induced by water immersion stress, indomethacin

plus ethanol, HCl, and pyloric ligated. Antiulcer effects of *Gān jiāng* are associated with decrease of thromboxane A_2 (TXA_2) and increase of prostacyclin I_2 (PGI_2). TXA_2 has a damaging effect on gastric mucosa while PGI_2 has a protective effect on gastric mucosa.

3. **镇吐**　干姜对硫酸铜致犬呕吐有抑制作用，但对家鸽由洋地黄、犬由阿扑吗啡诱发的呕吐无抑制作用，提示干姜镇吐作用是末梢性的。姜酮及姜烯酮是其镇吐的主要物质基础。

(3) Antiemetic effects　*Gān jiāng* prohibits canine vomiting caused by copper sulfate. There are no obvious effects in pigeon vomiting induced by digitalis, and canine vomiting induced by apomorphine. It suggests that antiemetic effects of *Gān jiāng* are peripheral produce. Ginger ketene and zingerone are suggested to be the main material basis for antiemetic effects.

4. **抗炎**　干姜水提物、醚提物、挥发油、姜烯酮等具有抗炎作用。干姜水提物和醚提物能抑制二甲苯引起的小鼠耳郭肿胀，可拮抗角叉菜胶引起的大鼠足跖肿胀。姜烯酮能抑制组胺和醋酸所致小鼠毛细血管通透性增加，抑制肉芽增生，减轻幼年大鼠胸腺重量，并使肾上腺重量增加。干姜水提物、干姜挥发油或干姜酚酸性部位给大鼠灌服能降低肾上腺中维生素 C 的含量。说明干姜的抗炎作用与促进肾上腺皮质功能有关。

(4) Anti-inflammation effects　Water-soluble, petroleum ether extracts, volatile oils of *Gān jiāng* and ginger ketene have anti-inflammation effects. Water-soluble and petroleum ether extracts of *Gān jiāng* exhibits the inhibition effect in mice ear edema by xylene, and rat metatarsal swelling by carrageenan. Ginger ketene inhibits the increase of mice capillary permeability by histamine and acetic acid, prevents granulation hyperplasia, decreases thymus weight, and augments adrenal gland weight in juvenile rats. Water-soluble, volatile oils, and phenol acid sites of *Gān jiāng* lessen vitamin C in adrenal gland. Anti-inflammation effects of *Gān jiāng* are correlated to active adrenal cortex functions.

5. **镇痛**　干姜醚提物和水提物都有镇痛作用。给小鼠灌服醚提物或水提物，均能使乙酸引起的小鼠扭体反应次数减少，且呈量–效关系，还能延长小鼠热刺激反应潜伏期。干姜挥发油也有镇痛作用。

(5) Analgesic effects　Petroleum ether and water-soluble extracts of *Gān jiāng* have analgesic effects. Using petroleum ether and water-soluble extracts of *Gān jiāng* by gavage, mice writhes caused by acetic acid decrease and it shows dose-effect relationship. Meantime they also extend thermal stimulation latency in mice. Volatile oils of *Gān jiāng* also have analgesic effects.

6. **强心**　干姜醇提物对麻醉猫有直接兴奋心脏作用，能增强心肌收缩力。姜酚给犬静脉注射，可使心肌收缩力增强、心率加快。干姜甲醇提取物可使离体豚鼠心房自主运动增强。姜烯酮和姜酚是其强心的主要物质基础。

(6) Cardiotonic actions　Alcohol extractions of *Gān jiāng* directly promote cat heart to enhance cardiac contractility. After injection of gingerol, cardiac contractility is strengthened, and heart rate become faster. Methanol extracts of *Gān jiāng* can improve atria independent movements in guinea pig. Ginger ketene and gingerol are suggested to be the main material basis for cardiotonic action.

7. **影响血管和血压**　干姜挥发油和姜辣素有扩张血管作用。姜烯酮能抑制去甲肾上腺素（NA）对肠系膜静脉的收缩作用。姜酚能使血管扩张，促进血液循环。姜酚静脉注射可使大鼠血压出现一过性降低后上升，以后又持续下降的三相性变化。

(7) Effects on vessels and pressure　Volatile oils of *Gān jiāng* and gingerols dilate vessels. Ginger ketene inhibits systolic mesenteric veins by noradrenaline (NA). Gingerol dilates vessels and improves microcirculation. Using gingerol injection, blood pressure in rat shows triphasic changes, downregulation after transient upregulation, and continuous downregulation.

8. **抑制血小板聚集和抗血栓形成** 干姜水提物对二磷酸腺苷（ADP）、胶原诱导的血小板聚集有抑制作用，能延迟实验性血栓形成，姜烯酮还对家兔血小板环氧化酶活性和人 TXA_2 的生成有抑制作用。干姜挥发油也具有抗血栓形成的作用，并能延长白陶土部分凝血活酶时间。

(8) Anti-platelet aggregation and antithrombotic effects Water-soluble extracts of *Gān jiāng* prevent platelet aggregation induced by adenosine diphosphate (ADP) and collagen, and delay experimental thrombus formation. Ginger ketene interferes rabbit platelet cyclooxygenase activity and human TXA_2 formation. Volatile oils of *Gān jiāng* prolong kaolin thromboplastin time for anti-thrombosis.

9. **抗病原微生物** 姜酮、姜烯酮等对伤寒杆菌、霍乱弧菌、葡萄球菌、肺炎链球菌等有抑制作用。

(9) Antipathogenic microorganism effects Ginger ketene and zingerone can inhibit *Salmonella typhi*, *Vibrio cholerae*, *Staphylococcus*, and *Streptococcus pneumoniae*.

10. **其他作用**

(10) Other effects

（1）抗缺氧 干姜醚提物能延长常压密闭缺氧和氰化钾中毒模型小鼠的存活时间，延长断头小鼠的张口动作持续过程。

1) Anti-hypoxia effects Petroleum ether extracts of *Gān jiāng* extend the survival time of closed normobaric hypoxia and potassium cyanide poisoned mice. They also lengthen decapitation-induced gasping duration in mice.

（2）抗氧化 干姜能提高脑组织中超氧化物歧化酶（SOD）活性和 Na^+-K^+-ATP 酶的活性，抑制家兔脑组织丙二醛（MDA）的生成，减轻体内自由基造成的神经细胞膜损伤，减轻脑水肿。

2) Antioxidation *Gān jiāng* activates superoxide dismutase (SOD) and Na^+-K^+-ATPase in cerebral tissue, inhibits malondialdehyde (MDA) formation in rabbit cerebral tissue, and decreases of neuron membrane damage and cerebral edema caused by free radicals *in vivo*.

（3）镇静 干姜醇提物及挥发油可抑制实验动物的自主活动，延长环己巴比妥诱发的睡眠时间，对抗戊四氮引起的兴奋。干姜醇提物还可使兔皮质脑电图（EEG）由低幅快波（LVFW）变为高幅慢波（HVSW）。说明干姜镇静作用与加强皮质抑制过程有关。

3) Inducing sedation Alcohol extracts and volatile oils of *Gān jiāng* decrease mice spontaneous activities, prolong sleeping time caused by cyclobarbital, and inhibit pentylenetetrazol-induced convulsions. Alcohol extracts of *Gān jiāng* change from low voltage fast waves (LVFW) to high voltage slow waves (HVSW) in rabbit electroencephalogram (EEG). It is suggested that *Gān jiāng* sedation effects are related to enhancement of cortical inhibition.

此外，干姜还具有解热、利胆、保肝、抗过敏、镇咳和增强免疫功能等作用。

Gān jiāng also has antipyretic, cholagogic, liver protection, antiallergic, antitussive, and enhancing immune effects.

【**不良反应 / Adverse effects**】

干姜水提物 120g 生药 /kg 小鼠灌胃，观察 7 天，无死亡。干姜醇提物小鼠灌胃 LD_{50} 为 108.9g/kg；干姜醚提物小鼠灌胃 LD_{50} 为 16.3 ± 2.0ml/kg。干姜醇提物 18g/kg、10g/kg，大鼠灌胃 2 个月，大鼠体重、血液学和血液生化学指标、脏器病理学检查均无异常。

After being given water-soluble extracts of *Gān jiāng* (120g crude drug/kg) by gavage, no death among mice are observed in 7 days. LD_{50} of alcohol and petroleum ether extracts of *Gān jiāng* are 108.9g/kg, and 16.3 ± 2.0ml/kg by gavage respectively in mice. 18g/kg and 10g/kg of alcohol extracts in *Gān jiāng*

have no obvious influence on rat weight, hematologic and biochemical indices, organs pathological examination for two months by gavage.

肉桂 ┊ *Ròu guì (Cinnamomi Coriex)*

【来源 / Origin】

本品为樟科植物肉桂（*Cinnamomum cassia* Presl）的干燥树皮。主要分布于广东、广西、云南等地。

Ròu guì is the dried cortex of *Cinnamomum cassia* Presl, one of lauraceous plants. The plant is widely cultivated in Guangdong province, Guangxi area, and Yunnan province in China.

【化学成分 / Chemical ingredients】

主要含挥发油［桂皮油（cinnamon oils）］，含量为 1%~2%。挥发油中的主要有效成分为桂皮醛（cinnamaldehyde），约占挥发油总量的 85%，其次为桂皮酸（cinnamic acid）、醋酸桂皮酯（acetate cinnamon ester）、桂二萜醇（diterpenoid alcohol）、乙酰桂二萜醇（ethyl-diterpenoid alcohol）等。此外，尚含多糖（polysaccharides）、肉桂苷（cinnamon glycosides）和香豆素（coumarin）等。

Volatile oils (cinnamon oils) of *Ròu guì* are the main components with 1%-2%. Cinnamaldehyde is the important effective constituents in 85% percentage of total volatile oils. As following, there are cinnamic acid, acetate cinnamon ester, diterpenoid alcohol, and ethyl-diterpenoid alcohol. In addition, polysaccharides, cinnamon glycosides, and coumarin are found in volatile oils.

【药性与功效 / Chinese medicine properties】

味辛、甘，性大热，归脾、肾、心、肝经。具有补火助阳、引火归元、散寒止痛、温通经脉的功效。用于治疗阳痿宫冷、腰膝冷痛、肾虚作喘、虚阳上浮、眩晕目赤、心腹冷痛、虚寒吐泻、寒疝腹痛、痛经经闭等证。

In Chinese medicine theory, *Ròu guì* has the nature of acrid, sweet, and extremely hot. It can enter the meridians of spleen, kidney, heart, and liver. *Ròu guì* can tonify fire to help Yang, conduct fire into its origin, dispel cold to relieve pain, warm and dredge collaterals. Clinically it can be used for impotence and uterine cold, knee cold pain, asthma by kidney deficiency, floating Yang-deficiency, vertigo and bulbar conjunctiva congestion, precordial and abdominal cold pain, vomiting and diarrhea by deficiency and cold, abdominal pain by cold hernia, dysmenorrhea and amenorrhea.

【药理作用 / Pharmacological effects】

1. 强心 肉桂中桂皮醛能增强豚鼠离体心脏的收缩力，增加心率。肉桂强心作用与促进交感神经末梢释放儿茶酚胺有关。

(1) Cardiotonic actions Cinnamaldehyde in *Ròu guì* can improve atria independent movements and heart rate in guinea pig. Cardiotonic effects of *Ròu guì* are associated with inducing catecholamine release from sympathetic nerve endings.

2. 影响血管和血压 肉桂、桂皮醛、桂皮酸钠等有扩张冠脉、脑血管和外周血管作用。可使冠脉和脑血流量增加，外周血管阻力下降，血压降低。肉桂可降低肾上腺再生高血压大鼠的血压和尿醛固酮24小时总排出量，而给犬肾上腺动脉注射桂皮醛可引起血压升高。

(2) Effects on vessels and pressure *Ròu guì*, cinnamaldehyde, cinnamic acid sodium can dilate coronary artery, cerebral and peripheral vessels, which increases coronary and cerebral blood flow, reduces peripheral vascular resistance and pressure. *Ròu guì* decreases blood pressure and urinary aldosterone levels within 24 hours in rat adrenal-inducing hypertension. When injected cinnamaldehyde to dog abdominal artery, blood pressure raises.

3. **影响内分泌系统** 肉桂使幼鼠肾上腺中维生素 C 含量下降，可使阳虚模型小鼠肾上腺中胆固醇含量降低，提示肉桂可提高肾上腺皮质功能。肉桂水煎液能提高性功能，提高血浆睾酮水平，还能降低血浆三碘甲状腺原氨酸（ T_3 ）水平。

(3) Endocrine system effects *Ròu guì* lessens vitamin C of adrenal gland in juvenile mice, and cholesterol of adrenal gland in Yang-deficiency mice. It can be surmised that *Ròu guì* actives adrenal cortex functions. *Ròu guì* decoction improves sexual function, increases testosterone and decreases triiodothyronine (T_3) in serum.

4. **调节胃肠运动** 肉桂对胃肠平滑肌有不同的作用。肉桂水煎液可抑制大鼠和小鼠的小肠蠕动。肉桂水提物和醚提物能减少蓖麻油引起的小鼠腹泻次数。桂皮油可促进兔肠蠕动，也能解除内脏平滑肌痉挛、缓解痉挛性疼痛。

(4) Gastrointestinal motility regulations *Ròu guì* has the different effects on gastrointestinal muscles. *Ròu guì* decoction can inhibit intestinal peristalsis in rats and mice. Water-soluble, petroleum ether extracts of *Ròu guì* reduce diarrhea caused by castor oil. Cinnamon oils stimulate rabbit intestinal peristalsis. Besides, cinnamon oils relieve visceral smooth muscle spasm and spastic pain.

5. **抗溃疡** 肉桂对多种实验性溃疡模型有抑制作用。肉桂水提物、乙醚提取物和肉桂苷对大鼠应激性溃疡以及吲哚美辛、氢氧化钠、醋酸、5–羟色胺（5-HT）等所致的胃溃疡均有抑制作用。肉桂水提物腹腔注射能抑制大鼠胃液分泌和胃蛋白酶活性，增加胃黏膜氨基己糖的含量，促进胃黏膜血流量，改善微循环，抑制溃疡的形成。

(5) Antiulcer effects *Ròu guì* shows inhibition effects in plenty of experimental ulcer models. Water-soluble, petroleum ether extracts of *Ròu guì* and cinnamon glycosides inhibit rat stomach ulcer induced by stress, indomethacin, sodium hydroxide, acetic acid, and 5-hydroxytryptamine (5-HT). Water-soluble extracts of *Ròu guì* exhibit antiulcer effects by intraperitoneal injection through inhibiting gastric secretion and pepsin amylase activation, enlarging hexosamine levels in gastric mucosa, promoting gastric mucosa blood flow and microcirculation.

6. **利胆** 肉桂水提物和醚提物大鼠十二指肠给药、桂皮醛大鼠灌胃均能增加胆汁分泌。

(6) Cholagogic effects Rat bile secretions increase after duodenal administration of water-soluble and petroleum ether extracts of *Ròu guì*, or intragastric administration of cinnamaldehyde.

7. **抗炎** 肉桂提取物对角叉菜胶致大鼠足跖肿胀、二甲苯致小鼠耳郭肿胀和棉球致大鼠肉芽组织增生均有抑制作用。

(7) Anti-inflammation effects Extractions of *Ròu guì* show anti-inflammation effects on rat metatarsal swelling caused by carrageenan, mice ear edema caused by xylene, rat granuloma proliferation after being implanted cotton pellets.

8. **镇痛** 肉桂水煎液能减少醋酸引起的小鼠扭体次数，同时能延长小鼠热刺激反应潜伏期，对热刺激、化学刺激及压尾刺激引起的疼痛均有抑制作用。

(8) Analgesic effects *Ròu guì* decoction decreases the mice writhes caused by acetic acid, and at the same time, extends the withdrawal latency to heat stimulation. *Ròu guì* decoction has analgesic effects in heat, chemistry induced, tail-pressure mice.

9. **抑制血小板聚集和抗凝血** 肉桂提取物、桂皮醛对 ADP 诱导的体外大鼠血小板聚集有抑制作用。肉桂水煎剂及水溶性甲醇部分体外还能延长大鼠血浆复钙时间，具有抗凝血作用。

(9) Anti-platelet aggregation and antithrombotic effects Extractions of *Ròu guì* and cinnamaldehyde prevent rat platelet aggregation *in vitro* induced by ADP. *Ròu guì* decoction and water-soluble methanol fractions show antithrombotic effects through prolonging serum recalcification time of rats *in vitro*.

10. 其他作用

(10) Other effects

（1）镇静、抗惊厥　肉桂油、桂皮酸钠、桂皮醛等具有镇静、抗惊厥作用。桂皮醛使动物自发活动减少，延长环己巴比妥钠的麻醉时间，可对抗苯丙胺引起的动物活动过多。桂皮醛还可延缓士的宁引起的强直性惊厥，延长存活时间。

1) Inducing sedation and anticonvulsant actions　Cinnamon oils, cinnamic acid sodium, and cinnamaldehyde exhibit sedation and anticonvulsant actions. Cinnamaldehyde decreases animal spontaneous activities, prolongs anesthetized time caused by cyclobarbital, and antagonizes excessive activities by amphetamine. It also delays tetanic convulsion leaded by strychnine, and extends survival time.

（2）延缓衰老　肉桂水煎液能提高老龄大鼠血清总抗氧化能力（T-AOC），增强红细胞 SOD 活性，降低脑脂褐素（LPF）和肝脏 MDA 含量，起到延缓衰老作用。

2) Anti-aging effects　*Ròu guì* decoction possesses anti-aging effects, such as developing total antioxidant capacity (T-AOC) and SOD, reducing cerebral lipofuscin (LPF) and liver MDA.

（3）抗菌　桂皮油对革兰阳性菌有抑制作用。桂皮煎剂及桂皮的醇、醚浸液对红色毛癣菌、白念珠菌等多种致病性皮肤真菌均有抑制和杀灭作用。肉桂醛对 22 种 31 株条件致病性真菌具有抗菌作用，具有抗菌谱广、毒性低的特点。

3) Antibacterial effects　Cinnamon oils inhibit Gram-positive bacteria. Decoction, alcohol and ether immersion liquids of cinnamon have inhibitory and killing effects on various pathogenic dermatophytes, such as *Trichophyton rubrum* and *Candida albicans*. Cinnamaldehyde has the characteristics of broad antibacterial spectrum and low toxicity, with antibacterial actions on 22 species 31 strains of opportunistic fungi.

此外，肉桂还有调节免疫功能、松弛支气管平滑肌、抗缺氧、抗心律失常等作用。

Ròu guì also has effects of regulating immune, relaxing bronchial smooth muscle, antioxidation, anti-arrhythmia.

【不良反应 / Adverse effects】

肉桂挥发油的 LD_{50} 为 5.04g/kg（相当于 236.53g 生药 /kg）。肉桂醚提取物的 LD_{50} 为 8.24 ± 0.50ml/kg。

LD_{50} of *Ròu guì* volatile oils is 5.04g/kg (equal to 236.53g crude drug/kg). LD_{50} of petroleum ether extracts of *Ròu guì* is 8.24 ± 0.50ml/kg.

吴茱萸 ｜ *Wú zhū yú (Evodiae Fructus)*

【来源 / Origin】

本品为芸香科植物吴茱萸［*Euodia rutaecarpa* (Juss.) Benth.］、石虎［*Euodia rutaecarpa* (Juss.) Benth. Var. *officinalis* (Dode) Huang］或疏毛吴茱萸［*Euodia rutaecarpa* (Juss.) Benth. Var. *bodinieri* (Dode) Huang］的近成熟果实。主要分布于贵州、广西、湖南、云南、陕西、浙江、四川等地。

Wú zhū yú is the fruit of *Euodia rutaecarpa* (Juss.) Benth., *Euodia rutaecarpa* (Juss.) Benth. Var. *officinalis* (Dode) Huang, *Euodia rutaecarpa* (Juss.) Benth. Var. *bodinieri* (Dode) Huang, one of Rutaceae plants. The plant is widely cultivated in Guizhou province, Guangxi area, Hunan province, Yunnan province, Shaanxi province, Zhejiang province, and Sichuan province in China.

【化学成分 / Chemical ingredients】

主要含有挥发油和生物碱，挥发油主要为吴茱萸烯（evodene）、罗勒烯（ocimene）、月桂烯（myrcene）、吴茱萸内酯（limonin）等。生物碱主要为吴茱萸碱（evodiamine）、吴茱萸次碱（rutaecarpine）、吴茱萸素（evoxine）等。此外，还含吴茱萸酸（fructus evodiae acid）、吴茱萸苦素（evodine）、芳香胺（aromatic amines）。

Wú zhū yú contains volatile oils and alkaloids. Volatile oils mainly include evodene, ocimene, myrcene, and limonin. Alkaloids of *Wú zhū yú* contain evodiamine, rutaecarpine, and evoxine. There are fructus evodiae acid, evodine, and aromatic amines.

【药性与功效 / Chinese medicine properties】

味辛、苦，性热，有小毒，归肝、肾、脾、胃经。具有散寒止痛、降逆止呕、助阳止泻的功效。用于治疗寒凝疼痛、胃寒呕吐、虚寒泄泻。

In Chinese medicine theory, *Wú zhū yú* has the nature of acrid, bitter, hot, and slightly toxic. It enters the meridians of liver, kidney, spleen, and stomach. *Wú zhū yú* can dispel cold to relieve pain, lower Qi adverse flow for antiemetic actions, tonify fire for anti-diarrhea. Clinically it can be used for cold coagulation pain, gastric cold vomiting, deficiency cold diarrhea.

【药理作用 / Pharmacological effects】

1. 强心　吴茱萸碱能明显增加在体兔心肌收缩幅度及心肌收缩能力，使心输出量、心脏指数增大，血压升高。吴茱萸碱可缩短心室肌细胞动作电位持续时间，其强心作用不通过 β 受体，而是直接活化膜电位依赖 Ca^{2+} 电流。

(1) Cardiotonic actions　Evodiamine improves the degree of myocardial contraction, myocardial contractility, stroke volume, cardiac index, and elevates blood pressure. Evodiamine shortens action potential duration of ventricular myocyte. Cardiotonic actions of *Wú zhū yú* are directly activate Ca^{2+} current of membrane potential dependence, not β receptor.

2. 促进血液循环、升高体温　吴茱萸具有增加组织器官血流量的作用。吴茱萸甲醇提取物灌胃可增加大鼠背部皮肤血流量，使其直肠温度上升，对水浸应激造成的血流量减少和温度下降有恢复作用。正常家兔静脉注射吴茱萸乙醇提取物，有上升体温和增加四氢萘胺上升体温的作用。吴茱萸乙醇提取物、吴茱萸碱、吴茱萸次碱是其升高体温的主要物质基础。

(2) Improving circulation and increasing temperature　*Wú zhū yú* increases circulation in tissues and organs. Methanol extracts of *Wú zhū yú* enhance the skin blood flow in rat back, raise rectal temperature, recover the blood flow and temperature decreased by water stress. After injection in normal rabbits, ethanol extracts of *Wú zhū yú* increase the temperature and have the synergistic effect with tetrahydro-naphthalenamine on rising temperature. Ethanol extracts of *Wú zhū yú*, evodiamine, and rutaecarpine are suggested to be the active ingredients for rising temperature.

3. 抗心肌缺血　猫发生心肌缺血后，吴茱萸能部分改善缺血心电图（ECG），减少血中肌酸激酶（CK）及乳酸脱氢酶（LDH）的释放，缩小心肌梗死面积。

(3) Anti-myocardial ischemia effects　After cat myocardial ischemia, *Wú zhū yú* partly refines ischemia electrocardiogram (ECG), decreases serum creatine kinase (CK) and lactate dehydrogenase (LDH) release, and lessens infarct area of myocardium.

4. 调节血压　吴茱萸注射液对大鼠和麻醉犬均有一过性升压然后降压的作用，并与剂量呈依赖关系。其作用与兴奋 α 受体有关。但脱氢吴茱萸次碱对麻醉大鼠则具有降血压作用。

(4) Blood pressure regulations　*Wú zhū yú* injection shows hypotensive effects after transient pressor effects with dose-dependent manner in rats and anesthetized dogs, which is related to the activation of α receptor. However, dehydrogenation rutaecarpine shows the hypotensive effects in anesthetized rats.

5. **抗血栓**　吴茱萸水煎剂可对抗大鼠在冰水应激状态下内源性儿茶酚胺分泌增加所致的血小板聚集。吴茱萸水提物有抗血栓作用，能延长白陶土部分凝血活酶时间和Ⅴ因子时间，可使大鼠血栓形成时间明显延长。

(5) Antithrombotic effects　*Wú zhū yú* decoction antagonizes platelet aggregation induced by endogenous CA secretion in cold water stress rats. Water-soluble extracts of *Wú zhū yú* show antithrombotic effects through delaying kaolin thromboplastin, Ⅴ factor, and thrombus formation time.

6. **镇痛、镇静**　吴茱萸水煎液小鼠灌胃能减少醋酸引起的扭体反应次数，延长热刺激致痛的反应潜伏期。吴茱萸水煎液延长戊巴比妥钠引起的小鼠睡眠时间。吴茱萸水煎液和乙醇提取物、吴茱萸碱、吴茱萸次碱、吴茱萸内酯等均具有镇痛作用。

(6) Analgesic and inducing sedation effects　*Wú zhū yú* decoction by gavage decreases mice writhes caused by acetic acid, at the same time, extends the withdrawal latency to heat stimulation. *Wú zhū yú* decoction prolongs sleeping time caused by pentobarbital. *Wú zhū yú* decoction, ethanol extracts of *Wú zhū yú*, evodiamine, rutaecarpine, and limonin express the analgesic effects.

7. **止泻、镇吐**　吴茱萸水煎液对蓖麻油和番泻叶引起的小鼠腹泻具有止泻作用，且随剂量增大，作用持续时间延长。吴茱萸还能抑制正常小鼠的胃肠推进，抑制大鼠胃自发活动，抑制ACh引起的胃痉挛性收缩，具有镇吐的效果。

(7) Anti-diarrhea and antiemetic effects　*Wú zhū yú* decoction inhibits mice diarrhea by castor oil and senna. The anti-diarrhea durations are extended with dose increase. *Wú zhū yú* processes antiemetic effects through restraining gastrointestinal propulsive motility in mice, gastric self-motility in rats, and gastric enterospasm contraction by ACh.

8. **抗溃疡**　吴茱萸水煎液具有抗溃疡作用，能显著抑制吲哚美辛加乙醇引起的小鼠胃溃疡形成和大鼠HCl性、水浸应激性及结扎幽门性胃溃疡形成。吴茱萸中的喹诺酮生物碱还具有抗幽门螺杆菌的作用。

(8) Antiulcer effects　*Wú zhū yú* decoction can inhibit stomach ulcer induced by indomethacin plus ethanol in mice, HCl, water immersion stress, and pyloric ligated in rats. Furthermore, quinolone alkaloids of *Wú zhū yú* inhibit *helicobacter pylori*.

9. 其他作用

(9) Other effects

（1）抗炎　吴茱萸水煎液能抑制二甲苯引起的小鼠耳郭肿胀，降低乙酸所致的小鼠腹腔毛细血管通透性增加，抑制角叉菜胶引起的大鼠足趾肿胀。

1) Anti-inflammation effects　*Wú zhū yú* decoction prevents mice ear edema caused by xylene, mice capillary permeability increased by acetic acid, and rat metatarsal swelling by carrageenan.

（2）调节子宫功能　吴茱萸次碱、芳香胺有兴奋子宫作用，能使子宫收缩，这种作用与兴奋5-HT受体和刺激前列腺素合成有关。

2) Uterus regulations　Rutaecarpine and aromatic amines upregulate and contract uterus. It is due to the activation of 5-HT receptor and prostaglandin formation.

此外，吴茱萸还有利胆、局部麻醉、驱除蛔虫、利尿、抗肿瘤、抗缺氧等作用。

Wú zhū yú also has cholagogic, local anesthesia, treating ascaris, diuretic, anti-tumor, and anti-hypoxia effects.

【不良反应 / Adverse effects】

灌胃给予吴茱萸挥发油14天，测得 LD_{50} 为1.708ml/ (kg·d)。吴茱萸水煎液或水提物分别连续给药21天或7天，导致小鼠肝损伤。

LD_{50} of *Wú zhū yú* volatile oils is 1.708ml/(kg·d) for 14 days by gavage. After administration of *Wú zhū yú* decoction or water-soluble extracts of *Wú zhū yú* for 21 or 7 days separately, there are liver damages in mice.

花椒 ┊ *Huā jiāo (Zanthoxyli Pericarpium)*

【来源 / Origin】

本品为芸香科植物青椒（*Zanthoxylum schinifolium* Sieb. et Zucc.）或花椒（*Zanthoxylum bungeanum* Maxim.）的干燥成熟果皮。我国大部分地区有分布，但以四川产者为佳。

Huā jiāo is the dried mature peel of *Zanthoxylum schinifolium* Sieb. et Zucc. or *Zanthoxylum bungeanum* Maxim., one of rutaceae plants. The plant is widely cultivated in most areas in China, especially best in Sichuan province.

【化学成分 / Chemical ingredients】

主要含有挥发油、生物碱、酰胺（amides）、香豆素（coumarins）、木质素（lignans）、黄酮（flavonoids）等。

There are volatile oils, alkaloids, amides, coumarins, lignans, and flavonoids in *Huā jiāo*.

【药性与功效 / Chinese medicine properties】

味辛，性温，归脾、胃、肾经。具有温中止痛、杀虫止痒的功效。用于治疗中寒腹痛、寒湿吐泻、虫积腹痛、湿疹、阴痒。

In Chinese medicine theory, *Huā jiāo* has the nature of acrid and warm. It can enter the meridians of spleen, stomach, and kidney. *Huā jiāo* can warm middle-jiao to dispel cold, killing parasites to relieve itching. Clinically it can be used for abdominal pain by middle-jiao cold, vomiting and diarrhea by cold-dampness, abdominal pain due to parasitic infestation, eczema, and pruritus vulvae.

【药理作用 / Pharmacological effects】

1. 镇痛 花椒和青椒水提液均有镇痛作用。花椒水提物和醚提物能减少乙酸引起的小鼠扭体反应次数，但对于热刺激致痛并无作用。

(1) Analgesic effects Decoctions of *Huā jiāo* and *Qīng jiāo* have analgesic effects. Water-soluble, petroleum ether extracts of *Huā jiāo* decrease the mice writhes caused by acetic acid, but they show no effect on heat stimulation.

2. 影响消化系统 花椒具有止泻、保肝的作用。花椒对蓖麻油和番泻叶引起的腹泻均有对抗作用，抑制四氯化碳（CCl_4）诱发的肝损伤。花椒对胃肠平滑肌具有高浓度抑制、低浓度兴奋的双向作用。

(2) Digestive system regulations *Huā jiāo* has anti-diarrhea and liver protective effects. *Huā jiāo* can inhibit mice diarrhea caused by castor oil and senna. It can also reduce liver damage caused by carbon tetrachloride (CCl_4). *Huā jiāo* has remarkable biphasic effects on gastrointestinal muscle motility, which are mean to prevent in high concentration and promote in low concentration.

3. 抗菌杀虫 花椒对 10 种革兰阳性菌和多种肠内致病菌有抑制作用，对 11 种皮肤癣菌和 4 种深部真菌都有抑制和杀灭作用。

(3) Antibacterial and insecticidal effects *Huā jiāo* can inhibit 10 species of Gram-positive bacteria and lots of enteral pathogenic bacteria. It also expresses bacteriostatic and bactericidal effects on 11 species dermatophyte fungi and 4 species of deep fungi.

4. 其他作用 花椒还能抗炎、抗肿瘤、抗氧化等作用。

(4) Other effects *Huā jiāo* also has anti-inflammation, anti-tumor, and antioxidation effects.

【不良反应 / Adverse effects】

予小鼠花椒挥发油灌胃、腹腔注射、肌内注射和皮下注射 1 次，测得 LD_{50} 分别为 2.27g/kg、2.03g/kg、4.64g/kg、5.32g/kg。予花椒和青椒口服，测得 LD_{50} 分别为 51.14 ± 4.47g/kg 和 78.02 ± 6.86g/kg。

LD_{50} of volatile oils of *Huā jiāo* are 2.27g/kg, 2.03g/kg, 4.64g/kg, 5.32g/kg by gavage, intraperitoneal, intravenous and subcutaneous injection once in mice. LD_{50} of *Huā jiāo* and *Qīng jiāo* are 51.14 ± 4.47g/kg and 78.02 ± 6.86g/kg by oral administration in mice.

（陈 怡 李红艳）

第十一章　理气药
Chapter 11　Qi-regulating medicines

第一节　概述
Section 1　Overview

微课

PPT

　　凡以疏畅气机、调整脏腑功能为主要功效，用于治疗气滞证、气逆证的药物，称为理气药。本类药物性味多辛、苦、温而芳香，主要归脾、胃、肝、胆、肺经。辛香行散，苦能降泄，温能通行，故本类药物具有理气健脾、疏肝解郁、理气宽胸、行气止痛、破气散结等功效。

　　All Chinese materia medica that can regulate Qi system and movement, treat Qi stagnation syndrome and Qi counterflow syndrome are known as Qi-regulating medicines. Most of them are pungent, fragrant, bitter, warm and mainly enter the meridians of spleen, stomach, liver, gallbladder and lung. They can disperse with pungent and fragrant property, descend and purge with bitter property and promote smooth flow with warm property. Therefore, they have the efficiency of regulating Qi to invigorate the spleen, soothing the liver and relieving depression, rectifying Qi and loosening the chest, moving Qi and relieving pain, breaking Qi and dissipating knots.

　　气升降出入运行全身，是人体生命活动的根本。若人体某一脏腑或经络发生病变，则影响气的疏通，导致气机不畅。气机不畅有气滞证和气逆证之分。气滞的临床特点是胀、闷、痛。由于气机阻滞的脏腑部位不一，临床证候也有不同表现。脾胃为气机升降之枢纽，脾胃气滞者，症见脘腹胀满、嗳气、呕恶、便秘或腹泻等，与西医学中溃疡、肠炎、胃炎、消化不良等消化系统疾

医药大学堂
WWW.YIYAODXT.COM

病或症状相似；肝主疏泄，调畅气机，肝气郁滞者，症见胸胁胀闷、乳房胀痛或结块、疝气疼痛、月经不调等，与西医学中急慢性肝炎、胆囊炎、焦虑症、抑郁症、疝气疼痛、月经不调、乳房胀痛等疾病或症状相似；肺主一身之气，肺失宣降，肺气壅滞者常见胸闷咳喘，与西医学中咳嗽、支气管哮喘等疾病或症状相似。气逆证则有呕吐、呃逆或喘息等主要临床症状，其中，胃气上逆常见呕吐、反胃、呃逆等，与西医学中各种胃炎、胆囊炎等相似；肺气上逆常见咳嗽、喘息等，与西医学中各种呼吸道感染、支气管哮喘等疾病或症状相似。理气药治疗气滞证和气逆证与下列药理作用有关。

The ascending and descending of Qi movement throughout the body is the basis of human life activities. Dysfunction of Zangfu organs may cause the disorder of the movement of Qi. Disorder of Qi movement refers to syndromes caused by various pathogenic factors such as emotional depression, drinking and eating irregularly, invasion of exogenous pathogen, resulting in dysfunction of Zangfu, meridian and collateral. Disorder of Qi movement principally can be divided into two types: Qi stagnation syndrome and Qi counterflow syndrome. Qi stagnation syndrome usually manifests as distension, oppression and pain. Due to the different parts of Qi stagnation syndrome, the clinical syndromes also have different manifestations. Spleen and stomach control the ascending and descending of Qi movement, symptoms of spleen and stomach Qi stagnation include fullness and distention of epigastrium and abdomen, vomiting, nausea, belching, constipation or diarrhea. Therefore, Qi stagnation of spleen and stomach is related to digestive system diseases including various kinds of gastritis, indigestion, ulcer disease, etc. Liver governs free coursing and regulates Qi movements. Symptoms of liver Qi stagnation shows rib-side pain, choking sensation in chest. Qi stagnation of liver is usually observed in acute and chronic hepatitis, cholecystitis, cholelithiasis, distending pain of the breast, irregular menstruation, colic pain, melancholia, anxiety neurosis, etc. Lung governs Qi of whole body. Symptoms of lung Qi stagnation involve oppression in the chest, cough and dyspnea, so congestion of lung Qi usually appears in the disease of respiratory system such as bronchial asthma. As for syndrome of Qi counterflow, it manifests itself chiefly as nausea and vomiting or dyspnea. Symptoms of lung Qi ascending counterflow include cough and pant, etc. Lung Qi ascending counterflow is related to respiratory system diseases such as bronchial asthma, respiratory infection. Symptoms of stomach Qi ascending counterflow involve emesia, nausea, hiccup. Therefore, stomach Qi ascending counterflow is related to digestive system diseases such as various kinds of gastritis and cholecystitis. The main pharmacological effects of Qi-regulating medicines are as follows.

1. **调节胃肠运动**　理气药对胃肠运动一般具有双向调节作用，通过兴奋或抑制作用，可使紊乱的胃肠功能恢复正常。①兴奋胃肠运动：部分理气药能兴奋胃肠平滑肌，增强胃肠运动。如枳实、枳壳、木香、大腹皮对大鼠胃排空具有促进作用；木香、大腹皮、陈皮有促进小鼠小肠蠕动作用。②抑制胃肠运动：多数理气药对离体胃肠平滑肌或痉挛状态的胃肠平滑肌具有解痉作用。如青皮、枳实与枳壳、香附等可降低家兔离体肠管的紧张性，减小其收缩幅度，减慢节律；对乙酰胆碱、毛果芸香碱、氯化钡等引起的肠肌痉挛抑制作用更明显。理气药抑制胃肠运动作用主要与阻断 M 胆碱受体有关，也有部分药物与兴奋 α 受体和直接抑制胃肠平滑肌有关。

(1) Regulating gastrointestinal motility　Qi-regulating medicines usually have dual-directional regulation effects on gastrointestinal movement. They can adjust the gastrointestinal function to normal state by stimulating or inhibiting action. ①Exciting gastrointestinal movement: most Qi-regulating herbs can stimulate gastrointestinal smooth muscle and enhance its movement. *Zhǐ shí*, *Zhǐ qiào*, *Mù xiāng*, *Dà fù pí* can promote gastric emptying in rats, and *Mù xiāng*, *Dà fù pí*, *Chen pí* can promote small intestine peristalsis of mice. ②Restraining gastrointestinal hypermobility: most Qi-regulating medicines can reduce the gastrointestinal muscle tensile *in vivo* or relieve spasm of gastrointestinal muscle when the smooth muscle is in the spasmodic state. *Qīng pí*, *Zhǐ shí*, *Zhǐ qiào*, *Xiāng fù*, etc., reduce the tension of isolated ileum in rabbits, decrease the contractile amplitude and the rhythm of ileum muscle. They relax the spastic intestinal smooth muscle stimulated by acetylcholine, pilocarpine, and barium chloride. The effects on restraining gastrointestinal hypermobility are mainly related to blocking choline M receptor, directly inhibiting on gastrointestinal peristalsis, and partly related to stimulating α receptor.

2. 调节消化液分泌　理气药大多对消化液的分泌起双向调节作用，这与药物所含不同成分和机体功能状态有关。多数理气药性味芳香，含挥发油，对胃肠黏膜具有轻度刺激作用，促进消化液分泌，提高消化酶活性，呈现健胃和助消化作用，如陈皮、木香等所含挥发油能促进消化液的分泌。部分理气药又可对抗病理性胃酸分泌增多，如理气药中所含的甲基橙皮苷对病理性胃酸分泌增多有降低作用，可减少幽门结扎性胃溃疡大鼠胃液分泌，降低溃疡发病率。

(2) Regulating secretion of digestive juice　Qi-regulating medicines can either inhibit or enhance the secretion of digestive juice depending on the different ingredients contained in the specific herb and functional state of the body. Most of Qi-regulating medicines are fragrant and contain volatile oil, which can slightly stimulate gastrointestinal mucosa, promote the secretion of digestive juice, improve the activity of digestive enzyme, and present the functions of invigorating stomach and helping digestion. *Chen pí*, *Mù xiāng* can stimulate the secretion of digestive juices including gastric juice, intestinal juice, pancreatic juice, etc., and enhance the activities of digestive enzyme. Moreover, partial Qi-regulating medicines antagonize the increase of pathologic gastric acid secretion. The hesperidin contained in the Qi-regulating medicines has a decreasing effect on the increase of pathological gastric acid secretion. It can reduce the secretion of gastric juice of the pyloric ligation gastric ulcer in rats and reduce the incidence rate of ulcers.

3. 利胆　肝的疏泄功能与胆汁的排泄有关。大多数理气药具有促进胆汁分泌的作用，如香附、木香、陈皮、青皮、枳壳，能促进实验动物和人的胆汁分泌，使胆汁流量增加，其作用与收缩胆囊平滑肌和松弛胆道平滑肌有关。青皮和陈皮能显著增加胆汁中胆酸盐含量。

(3) Cholagogic effect　The free coursing function of liver is related to biliary excretion. Most Qi-regulating medicines can promote bile secretion. For example, *Xiāng fù*, *Mù xiāng*, *Chén pí*, *Qīng pí* and *Zhì qiào*, improve bile secretion and increase bile flow in experimental animals and human beings, this effect is related to contraction of gallbladder smooth muscle and relaxation of bile duct smooth muscle. *Qīng pí* and *Chen pí* significantly increase the content of cholate in bile.

4. 松弛支气管平滑肌　多数理气药有松弛支气管平滑肌作用。枳实、陈皮、香橼、沉香等均可松弛支气管平滑肌；青皮、陈皮、香附、木香能缓解组胺所致的支气管痉挛，扩张支气管，降低气道阻力。作用机制与直接松弛支气管平滑肌、抑制亢进的迷走神经功能、拮抗抗过敏介质释放、兴奋支气管平滑肌 β 受体有关。

(4) Relaxing bronchial smooth muscle　Most Qi-regulating medicines, such as *Zhǐ shí*, *Chen pí*, *Xiāng yuán* and *Chén xiāng* can relax the smooth muscle of bronchus. *Qīng pí*, *Chen pí*, *Xiāng fù* and *Mù xiāng* can alleviate bronchospasm caused by histamine, dilate the bronchi and reduce airway resistance. Its mechanism of action may be related to the direct relaxation of bronchial smooth muscle, inhibition of hypervagus function, antagonizing the release of anti-allergic mediators, and stimulation of β receptor of bronchial smooth muscle.

5. 调节子宫平滑肌张力　枳实、枳壳、陈皮、木香等能兴奋子宫平滑肌；香附、青皮等则抑制子宫平滑肌，使痉挛的子宫平滑肌松弛，张力减小，并有微弱的雌激素样作用。

(5) Regulating the tension of uterine smooth muscle *Zhǐ shí*, *Zhǐ qiào*, *Chen pí*, *Mù xiāng* can activate uterine smooth muscle, while *Xiāng fù* and *Qīng pí* can inhibit the contraction of uterine smooth muscle, relax the spasmodic uterine smooth muscle, reduce the tension, and have a weak estrogen like effect.

6. 影响心血管系统 含有昔奈福林和 N– 甲基酪胺的理气药，如枳实、枳壳、青皮等，静脉注射给药时能表现出心血管药理活性，具有强心、升压、抗休克的作用。中医古代文献未见理气药有类似升压或抗休克的记载，该作用在静脉注射给药时才显示出来，是理气药研究的新进展。

(6) Effects on the cardiovascular system The Qi-regulating medicines containing synephrine and N-methyl-tyramine, such as *Zhǐ shí*, *Zhǐ qiào*, *Qīng pí*, show cardiovascular pharmacological activity when administered intravenously. They have the effects of heart strengthening, pressure boosting and anti shock. The modern researches reveal that some Qi-regulating medicines exhibit the effects of raising blood pressure or anti-shock, which were not documented in the ancient literature of TCM during oral administration.

常用理气药的主要药理作用见表 11-1。

The main pharmacological effects of commonly used Qi-regulating medicines are summarized in Table 11-1.

表 11-1　常用理气药的主要药理作用

药物	调节胃肠运动		促进消化液分泌	利胆	松弛支气管平滑肌	调节子宫功能		升压	强心	其他药理作用
	兴奋	抑制				兴奋	抑制			
枳实（枳壳）	+	+	–		+	–	–	+	+	利尿、抗炎、抗溃疡、镇静、镇痛等
陈皮	+	+	+	+	+	–	+	+	+	抗溃疡、保肝、祛痰、抗炎等
青皮	–	+						+	+	祛痰、抗休克等
木香	+	+	+	+		–	–			抗溃疡、镇痛、抗菌、降压、抑制血小板聚集
香附	–	+		+	+	–	+	–	+	镇痛、抗炎、雌激素样作用等

注："+"表示有明确作用；"–"表示无作用，或未查阅到相关研究文献

第二节　常用药物

Section 2　Commonly used medicines

PPT

枳实（枳壳）┊ *Zhǐ shí* (*Aurantii Fructus Immaturus*) [*Zhǐ qiào* (*Aurantii Fructus*)]

【来源 / Origin】

枳实为芸香科植物酸橙（*Citrus aurantium* L.）及其栽培变种或甜橙（*Citrus sinensis* Osbeck）的干燥幼果；枳壳为酸橙（*Citrus aurantium* L.）及其栽培变种的干燥近成熟果实。主要分布于四川、江西、福建、江苏等省。枳实于 5~6 月间采收，收集自落的幼果，除去杂质，切片，晒干或

低温干燥，生用或麸炒用；枳壳于 7 月果皮尚绿时采收，自中部横切为两半，去瓤，晒干或低温干燥。生用或麸炒用。

Zhǐ shí is the dried immature fruits of *Citrus aurantium* L. or *Citrus sinensis* Osbeck., *Zhǐ qiào* is the dried near mature fruits of *Citrus aurantium* L., family of Rutaceae. They are mainly distributed in Sichuan province, Jiangxi province, Fujian province, Jiangsu province and other places in China. *Zhǐ shí* is harvested between May and June, and obtained through collecting fallen immature fruits, removing impurities, slicing, drying in the sun or at low temperature. It is used in raw form or after stir-fried with wheat bran. *Zhǐ qiào* is harvested when the peel is still green in July cut into two parts from the middle, with the pulp removed, dried in the sunshine or at low temperature. It is used in raw form or after stir-fried with wheat bran.

【化学成分 / Chemical ingredients】

二者主要含有挥发油、黄酮苷及生物碱等成分，其中柠檬烯（limonene）是挥发油的主要成分；黄酮苷有新橙皮苷（neohesperidin）、橙皮苷（hesperidin）和柚皮苷（naringin）等；生物碱类成分有 N– 甲基酪胺（N-methyl-tyramine）和昔奈福林（synephrine）。

Zhǐ shí and Zhǐ qiào mainly contain volatile oil, flavonoid glycosides and alkaloids. Limonene is the main component of volatile oil. Flavonoid glycosides contains neohesperidin, hesperidin and naringin, N-methyl-tyramine and synephrine are the two most important active ingredients of alkaloids.

【药性与功效 / Chinese medicine properties】

味苦、辛、酸，性微寒，归脾、胃经。枳实具有破气消积、化痰散痞之功效，主治积滞内停、痞满胀痛、泻痢后重、大便不通、痰滞气阻、胸痹、结胸、脏器下垂；枳壳具有理气宽中、行滞消胀之功效，主治胸胁气滞、胀满疼痛、食积不化、痰饮内停、脏器下垂。

In Chinese medicine theory, *Zhǐ shí* (*Zhǐ qiào*) has the nature of bitter, pungent, sour, and slightly cold. It can enter the meridians of spleen and stomach. *Zhǐ shí* has the efficacies of breaking Qi and removing food retention, resolving phlegm and dissipating nodule. Clinically, it can be used for accumulation and stagnation internally, stuffiness and fullness and distending pain, diarrhea with rectal heaviness, constipation, phlegm stagnation due to Qi obstruction, chest impediment, chest bind, visceral ptosis, etc. *Zhǐ qiào* has the efficacies of regulating Qi to soothe the middle and moving stagnation to relieve distension. Clinically, it can be used for Qi stagnation in the chest and rob-side, distention and fullness and pain, food accumulation syndrome, phlegm-rheum collecting internally, visceral ptosis, etc.

【药理作用 / Pharmacological effects】

1. 调节胃肠平滑肌　枳实、枳壳对胃肠平滑肌和胃肠运动呈双向调节作用，既可兴奋胃肠平滑肌，使其收缩加强、蠕动加快；又可降低胃肠平滑肌张力，减缓蠕动。枳实、枳壳煎液灌胃可促进胃瘘、肠瘘犬胃肠运动，使胃肠收缩节律增加；枳实水煎液灌胃可兴奋家兔胃平滑肌。枳实、枳壳对在体肠平滑肌的兴奋作用与兴奋 M 受体有关。枳实、枳壳对小鼠、豚鼠和家兔离体肠平滑肌皆呈抑制效应，且能对抗乙酰胆碱、氯化钡、磷酸组胺的肠肌兴奋作用。枳实、枳壳对胃肠平滑肌呈双向调节作用与胃肠功能状态、药物浓度、实验手段、动物种属、体内外环境之间的差别等有关。

(1) Regulating gastrointestinal smooth muscle　*Zhǐ shí* and *Zhǐ qiào* have dual-directional regulation effects on gastrointestinal movement. They can not only excite gastrointestinal smooth muscle, strengthen its contraction and accelerate peristalsis, but also reduce the tension of gastrointestinal smooth muscle and slow down peristalsis. Gastrointestinal administration of water decoction of *Zhǐ shí* and *Zhǐ qiào* to gastric fistula and intestinal fistula dogs can promote gastrointestinal movement and increase gastrointestinal contraction rhythm. *Zhǐ shí* decoction can excite the smooth muscle of rabbit stomach. The excitatory effect of *Zhǐ shí* and *Zhǐ qiào* on intestinal smooth muscle *in vivo* is related to activating M receptor. *Zhǐ shí* and *Zhǐ qiào* have inhibitory effects on isolated intestinal smooth muscle of mice, guinea pigs and rabbits, and can counteract the intestinal muscle excitatory effects of acetylcholine, barium chloride, and histamine phosphate. The dual-directional regulation effects of *Zhǐ shí* and *Zhǐ qiào* on gastrointestinal movement may be related to the functional state of the gastrointestinal tract, drug concentration, experimental means, species of animals, differences between the environment *in vivo* and *in vitro*.

2. **抗溃疡**　枳实、枳壳挥发油能减少大鼠胃液分泌量、降低胃蛋白酶活性，预防溃疡形成。枳实还对幽门螺杆菌有杀灭作用。

(2) Anti-ulcer　The volatile oil of *Zhǐ shí* and *Zhǐ qiào* can reduce the secretion of gastric juice and the activity of pepsin which prevent the formation of ulcer. *Zhǐ shí* can also kill *Helicobacter pylori*.

3. **调节子宫平滑肌运动**　枳实与枳壳的水煎液、酊剂、流浸膏对家兔子宫（离体或在体、未孕及已孕）呈兴奋作用，表现为收缩力增强，张力增加，收缩频率加快，甚至出现强直性收缩；但对小鼠离体子宫，不论未孕或已孕，皆呈抑制效应，提示枳实（枳壳）对子宫的影响与动物种属有关。枳实提高子宫紧张性的作用为其临床治疗子宫脱垂提供了药理学基础，也为揭示《本草备要》"枳实孕妇忌用"的合理性提供了药理学依据。

(3) Regulating the tension of uterine smooth muscle　The decoction, tincture and liquid extract of *Zhǐ shí* and *Zhǐ qiào* have excitatory effect on rabbit uterus (*in vitro* or *in vivo*, unpregnant and pregnant), It shows that the contractile force is increased, the tension is increased, the contractive frequency is accelerated, and even the rigidity contraction appeared. However, it has inhibitory effect on mouse uterus *in vitro*, whether it is unpregnant or pregnant, suggesting that it has different effects on uterus of different species of animals. *Zhǐ shí* are generally utilized to treat descensus uteri in clinic. The effect of *Zhǐ shí* on increasing uterine tonicity may be the pharmacological basis for the treatment to descensus uteri. In addition, an ancient Chinese medicine literature, *Essentials of Materia Medica* recorded that "*Zhǐ shí* is contraindicated in pregnancy". The most existing research results demonstrate that it is reasonable.

4. **对心血管系统的作用**

(4) Effects on the cardiovascular system

(1) **升压**　枳实、枳壳注射液静脉注射可使麻醉犬血压升高，其升压特点为作用迅速、持续时间较长。昔奈福林和 N- 甲基酪胺是其升压的主要物质基础。N- 甲基酪胺对 α 受体、β 受体皆有兴奋作用，昔奈福林主要兴奋 α 受体。枳实与枳壳升压作用主要与兴奋 α 受体，使血管收缩、总外周阻力提高有关；兴奋心脏 β 受体，增强心肌收缩力，增加心输出量，也是其升压的作用机制之一。

1) Increase blood pressure　*Zhǐ shí* and *Zhǐ qiào* injection can increase the blood pressure of anesthetized dogs, which is characterized by rapid action and long duration. N-methyl-tyramine and synephrine are the main substance bases of increasing blood pressure. N-methyl-tyramine can excite both α and β receptors, and mainly excites α receptor of hydroxyfordrine. Synephrine can excite β-adrenergic receptor. The effect of *Zhǐ shí* and *Zhǐ qiào* on raising blood pressure are mainly related to activate α adrenergic receptor, contract blood vessel, improve the total peripheral resistance of blood vessels. This effects on raising blood pressure are also related to stimulate the β adrenergic receptor of the heart, enhance myocardial contractility, increase the output of the heart.

（2）**强心**　枳实与枳壳注射液、N- 甲基酪胺、昔奈福林对动物离体和在体心脏均有兴奋作用，能增强心肌收缩力，增加心输出量，呈现强心作用，该作用与兴奋心脏 β 受体有关。N- 甲基酪胺、昔奈福林是其强心的主要物质基础。N–甲基酪胺、昔奈福林易被碱性肠液破坏，故枳实与枳壳心血管作用需要静脉给药才能体现出来。

2) Cardiotonic effect   *Zhǐ shí* and *Zhǐ qiào* injection, N-methyl-tyramine and synephrine can stimulate the isolated and *in vivo* hearts of animals, enhance the myocardial contractility, increase the cardiac output, and show a strong cardiotonic action which is related to the activation of β-adrenergic receptor. N-methyl-tyramine and synephrine are the main material bases of heart strengthening. N-methyl-tyramine and synephrine are easily destroyed by alkaline intestinal fluid. The cardiovascular effects of *Zhǐ shí* and *Zhǐ qiào* can be observed only by intravenous administration.

陈皮（青皮） ┊ *Chen pí (Pericarpium Citri Reticulata)* [*Qīng pí (Pericarpium Citri Reticulata Viride)*]

【来源 / Origin】

陈皮为芸香科植物橘（*Citrus reticulata* Blanco）及其栽培变种的干燥成熟果皮；青皮为芸香科植物橘（*Citrus reticulata* Blanco）及其栽培变种的干燥幼果或尚未成熟果实的果皮。主要分布于广东、四川、浙江、江西等省。陈皮在秋末冬初采摘，剥取成熟果实的果皮，切丝，晒干或低温干燥，生用。青皮于5~6月间采收，收集自落的幼果，晒干，称为"个青皮"；7~8月间采收未成熟的果实，在果皮上纵制成四瓣至基部，除尽瓤瓣，切厚片或丝，晒干，习称"四花青皮"，生用或醋拌炒用。

Chen pí is the dried of fruit of *Citrus reticulata* Blanco and its cultivated varieties, family of Rutaceae. *Qīng pí* is the dried of immature fruit of *Citrus reticulata* Blanco and its cultivated varieties, family of Rutaceae. They are mainly distributed in Guangdong province, Sichuan province, Jiangxi province, Zhenjiang province, etc. *Chen pí* are picked at late autumn and early winter, The mature fruits of *Citrus reticulata* Blanco are picked, peeled, sliced, dried in the sun or at low temperature, and are used in raw form. *Qīng pí* are harvested between May and June, the fallen immature fruits are collected and dried in the sunshine, which are called *Gè Qīng pí*. *Qīng pí* are collected from July to August, these immature fruits are cut vertically into four parts. After removing the pulp, they are cut into thick pieces or slices and dried in the sunshine, which are called *Sì huā Qīng pí*. It is used in raw form or after stir-fried with vinegar.

【化学成分 / Chemical ingredients】

二者主要含挥发油、黄酮苷、生物碱等。挥发油中的主要有效成分为柠檬烯（limonene）。黄酮苷中含新橙皮苷（neohesperidin）、橙皮苷（hesperidin）、甲基橙皮苷（methyl hesperidin）等。生物碱中含昔奈福林（synephrine）等。

Chen pí and *Qīng pí* mainly contain volatile oil, flavonoid glycosides and alkaloids, etc. Limonene is the main component of volatile oil. Flavonoid glycosides contains neohesperidin, hesperidin, methyl hesperidin, alkaloids contains synephrine.

【药性与功效 / Chinese medicine properties】

陈皮味苦、辛，性温，归肺、脾经。具有理气健脾、燥湿化痰之功效，主治脘腹胀满、食少吐泻、咳嗽痰多等证。青皮味苦、辛，性温，归肝、胆、胃经。具有疏肝破气、消积化滞之功效，主治胸胁胀痛、疝气疼痛、乳癖、乳痈、食积气滞、脘腹胀痛等证。

In Chinese medicine theory, *Chen pí* has the nature of bitter, pungent and warm. It can enter the meridians of lung, spleen. *Chen pí* has the efficacies to rectify Qi and fortify the spleen, dry dampness and transform phlegm. It can be used for distention in stomach duct and abdomen; less-eating, vomiting and diarrhea; cough and phlegm. *Qīng pí* has the nature of bitter, pungent and warm. It can enter the meridians of liver, gallbladder and stomach. *Qīng pí* has the efficacies to soothe liver and break Qi, resolve food retention and relieve stagnation. It can be used for distending pain in the chest and rob-side, hernia pain, mammary hyperplasia, acute mastitis, food accumulation and Qi stagnation, distending pain in stomach duct and abdomen.

【药理作用 / Pharmacological effects】

1. 对消化系统的作用

(1) Effects on digestive system

（1）调节胃肠平滑肌运动　对在体胃肠平滑肌，陈皮具有兴奋作用，而青皮具有抑制作用。对离体胃肠平滑肌，陈皮与青皮均表现为抑制作用，且青皮的作用强于陈皮。

1) Regulating gastrointestinal smooth muscle movement　*Chen pí* can excite the smooth muscle of gastrointestinal tract *in vivo*, while *Qīng pí* shows inhibition effect. Both *Chen pí* and *Qīng pí* shows inhibitory effect on gastrointestinal smooth muscle *in vitro*, and the effect of *Qīng pí* was stronger than that of *Chen pí*.

（2）促进消化液分泌　陈皮与青皮的挥发油对胃肠道有温和的刺激作用，能促进消化液分泌，排除胃肠积气。

2) Promoting secretion of digestive fluid　The volatile oil of *Chen pí* and *Qīng pí* has a mild stimulating effect on gastrointestinal tract, which can promote the secretion of digestive fluid and eliminate gastrointestinal gas accumulation.

（3）利胆　陈皮与青皮均具有利胆、促进胆汁分泌作用。青皮能松弛奥迪括约肌，收缩胆囊，促进胆汁排泄。

3) Cholagogic effect and liver protection　Both *Chen pí* and *Qīng pí* have the functions of cholagogue and promoting bile secretion. *Qīng pí* can strengthen the contraction of gallbladder or relax the sphincter of choledochus and increase bile flow.

2. 对呼吸系统的作用　陈皮与青皮的挥发油均有刺激性祛痰作用，柠檬烯是其祛痰的主要物质基础。陈皮与青皮均具有松弛支气管平滑肌的作用，发挥平喘作用。

(2) Effects on respiratory system　The volatile oil of *Chen pí* and *Qīng pí* can stimulate expectoration. Limonene in *Chen pí* and *Qīng pí* is the main effect component of expectoration. Both *Chen pí* and *Qīng pí* have the function of relaxing the smooth muscle of bronchus, which shows antiasthmatic effect.

3. 松弛子宫平滑肌　陈皮与青皮均能松弛子宫平滑肌。陈皮煎剂、甲基橙皮苷对离体子宫平滑肌有抑制作用，对 ACh 所致子宫平滑肌痉挛有拮抗作用。青皮煎剂能松弛子宫平滑肌，降低收缩幅度，减慢收缩频率，且呈浓度依赖性增强。

(3) Relaxing uterine smooth muscle　*Chen pí* and *Qīng pí* relax uterine smooth muscle. Decoction of *Chen pí* and methyl hesperidin have the inhibitory effect on isolated uterine smooth muscle, and can antagonize the effect on uterine smooth muscle spasm induced by ACh. Decoction of *Qīng pí* can relax the smooth muscle of uterus, reduce the contractile amplitude, slow down the contractile frequency, which increases in a concentration dependent manner.

4. 对心血管系统的作用

(4) Effects on cardiovascular system

（1）升血压　青皮与陈皮注射液静脉注射均具有升血压作用。昔奈福林是其升血压的主要物质基础。

1) Increasing blood pressure　The injection of *Qīng pí* and *Chen pí* have the effects of increasing

blood pressure. Synephrine is the main active ingredient of increasing blood pressure.

（2）兴奋心脏　青皮与陈皮均有兴奋心脏的作用。陈皮水提物、橙皮苷、甲基橙皮苷注射液和青皮注射液均能增强实验动物的心肌收缩力，增加心输出量。

2) Exciting heart　Both *Chen pí* and *Qīng pí* can excite heart. Decoction of *Chen pí*, hesperidin, methyl hesperidin, *Qīng pí* injection can increase the force of myocardial contraction and increase the cardiac output.

木香 ┊ *Mù xiāng (Aucklandiae Radix)*

【来源 / Origin】

本品为菊科植物木香（*Aucklandia lappa* Decne.）的干燥根。产于我国云南、广西者，称为"云木香"；产于印度、缅甸者，称为"广木香"。秋、冬二季采挖，除去须根，切段。干燥后去粗皮，生用或煨用。

Mù xiāng is the dried root of *Aucklandia lappa* Decne., family of Composite. Those in Yunnan and Guangxi area in china are called *Yún Mù xiāng*, and those in India and Myanmar are called *Guǎng Mù xiāng*. The roots are dug and collected in autumn and winter. After fibrous roots are removed, they are cut into sections, and the rough bark are bumped away after being dried. The raw or roasted are used for Chinese medicinal preparation.

【化学成分 / Chemical ingredients】

主要含有挥发油、木香碱、菊糖等。挥发油中的主要有效成分为木香内酯（costuslactone）、去氢木香内酯（dehydrocostus lactone）、二氢木香内酯（dihydrocostulactone）、木香烃内酯（costunolide）、木香酸（costic acid）、α–木香烯（α-costene）等。

Mù xiāng contains volatile oil, sausurine, synanthrin. The components of volatile oil include costuslactone, dehydrocostus lactone, dihydrocostulactone, costunolide, costic acid, α-costene, etc.

【药性与功效 / Chinese medicine properties】

味辛、苦，性温，归脾、胃、大肠、三焦、胆经。具有行气止痛、健脾消食之功效。主治胸胁和脘腹胀痛、泻痢后重、食积不消、不思饮食等证。

In Chinese medicine theory, *Mù xiāng* has the nature of bitter, pungent and warm. It can enter the meridians of spleen, stomach, large intestine, triple energizer and gallbladder. *Mù xiāng* has the efficacies to move Qi to stop pain, reinforce spleen to promote digestion. It can be used for distending pain in the chest and rob-side, stomach duct and abdomen, diarrhea with rectal heaviness, food retention, no appetite, etc.

【药理作用 / Pharmacological effects】

1. 对消化系统的影响

(1) Effects on digestive system

（1）调节胃肠运动　不同剂量的木香水煎剂对胃肠排空及肠推进均有促进作用。木香总生物碱、挥发油能对抗 ACh、组胺或 BaCl₂ 所致的肠痉挛，木香烃内酯、去氢木香内酯能对抗阿托品引起的胃排空减慢，二氢木香内酯可使离体肠运动节奏变慢，呈较强的抑制作用。

1) Regulating gastrointestinal motility　Different doses of *Mù xiāng* decoction can promote gastrointestinal emptying and intestinal propulsion. The total alkaloid and volatile oil of *Mù xiāng* can antagonize the intestinal spasm caused by ACh, histamine or BaCl₂. Costun olide and dehydrocostus lactone can antagonize the slow gastric emptying caused by atropine. Dihydrocostulactone can slow down the rhythm of intestinal motility *in vitro*.

（2）保护胃肠黏膜　木香的丙酮与乙醇提取物对盐酸–乙醇、氢氧化钠、氨水诱发的大鼠急性胃肠黏膜损伤均有保护作用。

2) Protection gastrointestinal mucosa　Acetone extract and ethanol extract of *Mù xiāng* have protective effects on acute gastrointestinal mucosal injury in rats induced by hydrochloric-acid ethanol, sodium hydroxide, and ammonia.

（3）止泻　木香乙醇提取物能减少蓖麻油引起的小鼠小肠性腹泻和番泻叶引起的小鼠大肠性腹泻次数，对小鼠墨汁胃肠推进运动也有一定的抑制作用。

3) Antidiarrheal effects　The ethanol extract of *Mù xiāng* can reduce the diarrhea of small intestine in mice caused by castor oil and the diarrhea of large intestine in mice caused by senna leaf, and can also inhibit the gastrointestinal propulsion of ink.

（4）利胆　木香水煎剂能增强空腹时胆囊的收缩，促进胆汁分泌。木香烃内酯和去氢木香内酯是其利胆的主要物质基础。其促进胆囊收缩的作用机制是使血中的胆囊收缩素或胃动素水平增高。

4) Cholagogic effects　Decoction of *Mù xiāng* shrinks the gallbladder volume on an empty stomach, promotes the biliary secretion. The active ingredients in *Mù xiāng* are dehydrocostus lactone, costunolide. The effects of *Mù xiāng* on promoting gallbladder contraction are related to an increase in the level of cholecystokinin and motilin in blood.

2. 松弛支气管平滑肌　木香对支气管平滑肌有解痉作用。木香水提液、醇提液、挥发油、生物碱对豚鼠的气管、支气管收缩均有对抗作用。

(2) Relaxing bronchial smooth muscle　*Mù xiāng* has the spasmolysis effect on bronchial smooth muscle. Decoction, alcohol extract, volatile oil, total alkaloids of *Mù xiāng* can antagonize spastic contraction of trachea and bronchia in guinea pig induced by histamine or acetylcholine.

3. 抗炎、镇痛　木香醇提取物能抑制二甲苯引起的小鼠耳郭肿胀、角叉菜胶引起的小鼠足跖肿胀和乙酸引起的小鼠腹腔毛细血管通透性增加，具有抗炎作用。75% 木香乙醇提取物有一定的镇痛作用。

(3) Anti inflammatory and analgesic　The extract of *Mù xiāng* inhibit auricle swelling caused by xylene and paw swelling caused by carrageenan in mice. It can also inhibit the increase of permeability of capillaries in abdominal cavity of mice induced by acetic acid. 75% ethanol extract of *Mù xiāng* has analgesic effect.

4. 抗病原微生物　木香挥发油对链球菌、金黄色与白色葡萄球菌均有抑制作用。木香煎剂对多种真菌有抑制作用。

(4) Anti-pathogenic microorganisms　Volatile oil of *Mù xiāng* can inhibit the growth of bacteria such as *Streptococcus*, *Staphylococcus aureus*, *Staphylococcus albus*, and also inhibit the growth of pathogenic dermatophyte.

【不良反应 / Adverse effects】
部分使用木香者皮肤可出现粟粒样红色丘疹、瘙痒。

Some people who use *Mù xiāng* have miliary red papule and itch.

香附　┊　*Xiāng fù* (Cyperi Rhizoma)

【来源 / Origin】
本品为莎草科植物莎草（*Cyperus rotundus* L.）的干燥根茎。主要分布于广东、四川、浙江、山东等地。秋季采挖，燎去毛须，碾碎或切薄片，晒干。生用或醋炒用。

Xiāng fù is the dried rhizome of *Cyperus rotundus* L., family of Cyperaceae. It is mainly distributed in Guangdong province, Sichuan province, Zhejiang province, Shandong province in China. The rhizomes are dug and collected in autumn. After the fibrous roots are burned away, they are pulverized or sliced and then dried in the sunshine. The raw or those stir-fried with vinegar are used for Chinese medicinal preparation.

【化学成分 / Chemical ingredients 】

主要含有挥发油，含量约为1%。其中α–香附酮（α-cyperone)、香附烯 (cyperene) Ⅰ和Ⅱ是香附挥发油中的主要成分，占香附挥发油的28.85%，此外还有香附子醇 (cyperol)、异香附醇（isocyperol)、柠檬烯（limonene）等。尚含有黄酮类、三萜类化合物及生物碱等。

Xiāng fù mainly contains volatile oil, the content of volatile oil is about 1%, among which, α-cyperone, cyperene Ⅰ and Ⅱ are the main components, accounting for 28.85% of the total volatile oil. In addition, cyperol, isocyperol, limonene, etc., are the components in the volatile oil. Besides the volatile oil, it also contains flavonoids, triterpenoids and alkaloids.

【药性与功效 / Chinese medicine properties 】

味辛、微苦、微甘，性平，归肝、脾、三焦经。具有疏肝解郁、理气宽中、调经止痛之功效。主治肝郁气滞、胸胁胀痛、疝气疼痛、乳房胀痛、脾胃气滞、胸脘痞闷、胀满疼痛、月经不调、经闭痛经等证。

In Chinese medicine theory, *Xiāng fù* is pungent, slightly bitter, slightly sweet, and neutral in nature. It can enter the meridians of liver, spleen, triple energizer. *Mù xiāng* has the efficacies to soothe liver to relieve depressed Qi, regulate Qi to comfort the middle energizer, regulate menstruation to relieve pain, etc. It can be used for liver depression and Qi stagnation, distending pain in the chest and rob-side, hernia pain, distending pain in the breasts, Qi stagnation of spleen and stomach, chest and epigastric fullness and distress, distention and fullness and pain, menstrual irregularities, amenorrhea and dysmenorrhea.

【药理作用 / Pharmacological effects 】

1. 松弛子宫平滑肌　香附浸膏对豚鼠、兔、猫、犬等动物的离体子宫平滑肌活动，无论已孕还是未孕，都呈抑制作用，使其收缩力减弱，肌张力降低。α–香附酮是其抑制子宫平滑肌的主要物质基础。香附抑制子宫平滑肌作用与抑制前列腺素的合成和释放有关。

(1) **Relaxing uterine smooth muscle**　Extractum of *Xiāng fù* can inhibit the smooth muscle activity of isolated uterus of guinea pigs, rabbits, cats, dogs and other animals, whether pregnant or not, and reduce its contractility and muscle tension. α-cyperone is main active component of its inhibition of uterine smooth muscle. The inhibition of α-cyperene on uterine smooth muscle is related to the inhibition of prostaglandin synthesis and release.

2. 雌激素样作用　香附挥发油对去卵巢大鼠有轻度雌激素样作用，皮下注射或阴道给药可促进阴道上皮细胞角质化。香附烯Ⅰ是其雌激素样作用的主要物质基础。

(2) **Estrogen-like effect**　The volatile oil of *Xiāng fù* has mild estrogen-like activity in ovariectomized rats. Volatile oil of *Xiāng fù* can promote the keratinization of vaginal epithelial cells by subcutaneous injection or vaginal delivery. Cyperene Ⅰ is the main active component of estrogen-like effect.

3. 抑制肠道平滑肌　香附醇提物对离体兔回肠平滑肌有直接抑制作用，丙酮提取物、挥发油可对抗乙酰胆碱、K⁺所致肠平滑肌收缩，能使肠平滑肌张力下降，收缩幅度降低。

(3) **Relaxing gastrointestinal**　Ethanol extract of *Xiāng fù* has direct inhibitory effect on ileal smooth muscle of rabbits *in vitro*. Acetone extract and volatile oil can resist the contraction of intestinal smooth muscle caused by acetylcholine and K^+, and reduce the tension and contraction range of intestinal smooth muscle.

4. 利胆、保肝　香附水煎液十二指肠给药对正常大鼠有较强利胆作用，可促进胆汁分泌，增加胆汁流量，对四氯化碳所致肝损伤大鼠的胆汁分泌也有明显促进作用，并可降低其 ALT，对肝细胞有保护作用。

(4) Cholagogic effect and liver protection　The decoction of *Xiāng fù* by duodenal administration can promote bile secretion and increase bile flow in normal rats. It also improves bile secretion of liver injury rats caused by carbon tetrachloride, decreases the activity of serum transaminase, protects the function of liver cells.

5. **镇痛、抗炎**　香附石油醚、乙酸乙酯、醇提物均具有镇痛作用。香附醇提物对角叉菜胶和甲醛引起的大鼠足跖肿胀有抑制作用。α- 香附酮是香附抗炎、镇痛的主要活性成分，该作用与抑制前列腺素的合成和释放有关。

(5) Easing pain and anti-inflammation　The petroleum ether, ethyl acetate and alcohol extract of *Xiāng fù* have analgesic effect. The alcohol extract of *Xiāng fù* can alleviate foot swelling in rats induced by carrageenan and formaldehyde. α-cyperone is the main active component of anti-inflammatory and analgesic effects of *Xiāng fù*, which is related to the inhibition of prostaglandin synthesis and release.

6. **解热**　香附醇提物可降低内毒素、酵母菌引起的大鼠体温升高，解热见效快、持续时间较长。

(6) Relieving fever　The alcohol extract of *Xiāng fù* can reduce the temperature rise of rats caused by endotoxin and yeast, and has rapid antipyretic effect and a longer duration.

7. **抗病原微生物**　香附挥发油对金黄色葡萄球菌和痢疾杆菌有抑制作用，其抗菌作用的主要成分是香附烯Ⅰ和香附烯Ⅱ。

(7) Anti-pathogenic microorganisms　The volatile oil of *Xiāng fù* has inhibitory effect on *Staphylococcus aureus* and *Shigella dysenteriae in vitro*. Cyperene Ⅰ and Ⅱ are the main antibacterial active components.

题库

（汪　宁　李红艳）

第十二章 消食药

Chapter 12 Digestant medicines

学习目标 | Objectives

1. **掌握** 消食药的基本药理作用；山楂与功效相关的药理作用及其调节心血管系统的药效物质基础与机制。

2. **了解** 神曲、莱菔子的主要药理作用。

1. **Must know** The main pharmacological effects of digestant medicines; the efficacy-related pharmacological effects of *Shān zhā*, the material basis and main mechanism of its effect on cardiovascular system.

2. **Desirable to know** The main pharmacological effects of *Shén qū* and *Lái fú zǐ*.

微课

第一节 概述

Section 1 Overview

PPT

　　凡以消食化积为主要功效，主治饮食积滞的药物，称为消食药。本类药物多味甘，性平，主入脾、胃经，具有消食导滞、健脾益胃、促进消化的功效。部分药物尚兼有行气散瘀、回乳消胀、降气化痰等功效。消食药主要用于饮食积滞或脾胃虚弱所致的脘腹胀满、嗳腐吞酸、恶心呕吐、不思饮食、大便失常等。

All Chinese materia medica that are mainly used to disperse food and eliminate stagnation are classified as digestant medicines. The medicines in the category are traditionally used to treat food stagnation. They are mainly sweet in flavor and neutral in nature. They majorly enter the meridians of spleen and stomach. These medicines can disperse food and abduct stagnation, fortify the spleen and boost the stomach, promote digestive function. Some medicines also have the effects of moving Qi and dissipating stasis, terminating lactation and dispersing distention, downbearing Qi and transforming phlegm, and so on. Digestant medicines are mainly used for those symptoms caused by food accumulation or weakness of spleen and stomach, such as distention in stomach and abdomen, belching and acid regurgitation, nausea and vomiting, no appetite, abnormal stool and so on.

　　中医学认为饮食积滞通常是饮食不节、贪食过饱或恣食生冷，损伤脾胃，纳运不及所致，治宜消食导滞。从食滞胃肠的临床表现来看，主要与西医学中消化系统疾病如胃肠神经官能症、消化不良、急慢性胃肠炎、胃下垂、消化性溃疡等有关。常用的消食药有山楂、神曲、鸡内金、莱菔子、麦芽、谷芽等。现代药理学研究表明，消食药治疗宿食不化、脘腹胀满、纳差等证与下列药理作用有关。

According to TCM theories, food stagnation is usually caused by dietary irregularities, rapacious appetite and overeating, or indulgence in raw and cold foods. The spleen and stomach are damaged and poor to transport, so it is appropriate for them to disperse food and abduct stagnation. From the clinical manifestations of gastrointestinal stagnation, it is mainly related to digestive system diseases in western medicine, such as gastrointestinal neurosis, dyspepsia, acute and chronic gastroenteritis, gastroptosis, peptic ulcer and so on. The commonly used digestant medicines include *Shān zhā*, *Shén qū*, *Jī nèi jīn*, *Lái fú zǐ*, *Mài yá*, *Gǔ yá*, etc. Modern pharmacological studies have shown that the therapeutic effects of digestant medicines on food stagnation, distention in stomach and abdomen, poor appetite are related to the following pharmacological effects.

1. **助消化**　食物在胃肠道的消化分解主要依靠消化道腺体分泌的消化酶、肝脏分泌的胆汁以及肠道细菌合成的有关酶，通过上述化学性消化，食物成为可被吸收的小分子物质。消食药多含有消化酶、维生素等，能增强消化系统的消化功能。如山楂、神曲含有脂肪酶，有利于脂肪消化，中医称之擅长消"肉积"；麦芽、谷芽、神曲含有淀粉酶，能促进碳水化合物消化，擅长消"米面食积"；神曲为酵母制剂，还含有胃蛋白酶、胰酶、蔗糖酶等，能分解多种营养成分，促进消化吸收。

(1) Aiding digestion　The digestion and decomposition of food in the gastrointestinal tract mainly depends on digestive enzymes secreted by digestive glands, bile secreted by liver and related enzymes synthesized by intestinal bacteria. Through the above-mentioned chemical digestion, food transforms to small molecular substances that can be absorbed by the body. Digestant medicines mostly contains digestive enzymes and vitamins, which can enhance the digestive function of digestive system. For example, *Shān zhā* and *Shén qū* contain lipase are beneficial to the digestion of fat in food, which are thought to be good at eliminating "meat accumulation" by TCM practioner; *Mài yá*, *Gǔ yá*, and *Shén qū* contain amylase, which can promote the digestion of carbohydrates are thought to be good at eliminating "rice and noodles accumulation"; *Shén qū* is a yeast preparation, which contains pepsin, pancreatin, sucrase and so on can decompose a variety of nutrients and promote the digestion and absorption of these ingredients.

有机酸也有助于食物的消化和吸收。山楂含山楂酸、柠檬酸等有机酸，能提高胃蛋白酶活性，促进蛋白质消化。鸡内金能增强胃蛋白酶、胰脂肪酶活性。有些药物能促进消化液分泌，如鸡内金促进胃液分泌，使胃中游离酸和胃蛋白酶含量升高，胆汁分泌增加。

Organic acids also contribute to the digestion and absorption of food. *Shān zhā* contains organic acids such as maslinic acid, citric acid, which can improve the activity of pepsin and promote the digestion of protein. *Jī nèi jīn* can promote pepsin and pancreatic lipase activity. Some medicines can promote secretion of digestive juice, such as *Jī nèi jīn* promotes gastric juice secretion, which increases the contents of free acid and pepsin in the stomach, and also increases bile secretion.

有些药物自身含有多种维生素，如麦芽、谷芽含有 B 族维生素；山楂含有大量维生素 C；神曲含有丰富的复合维生素 B；鸡内金含有维生素 B_1、维生素 B_2、烟碱及维生素 C 等。补充 B 族维生素可增进食欲，对维持正常消化功能有一定作用。另外，神曲、麦芽、谷芽中含有酵母菌，也有一定助消化作用。

Some medicines contain a variety of vitamin components, such as *Mài yá* and *Gǔ yá* contain vitamin B; *Shān zhā* contains a lot of vitamin C; *Shén qū* is rich in vitamin B complex; *Jī nèi jīn* contains vitamin B_1, B_2, nicotinic acid and vitamin C, etc. Supplement of vitamin B can increase appetite and play a certain role in maintaining normal digestive function. In addition, *Shén qū*, *Mài yá* , and *Gǔ yá* contain yeast have certain effects on aiding digestion.

2．调节胃肠道运动 食物中营养成分的消化吸收、食物残渣的排出有赖于正常的胃肠黏膜功能和胃肠道平滑肌的规律蠕动。消食药大多有不同程度的调节胃肠活动功能，有的能增强胃蠕动，提高胃排空速率，如鸡内金、山楂；有的可增强回肠节律性收缩，如莱菔子；有的对胃肠平滑肌功能呈双向调节作用，如山楂。

(2) Regulating gastrointestinal motility   The digestion and absorption of nutrients in food and the excretion of food residues also depend on the normal function of gastrointestinal mucosa and the regular peristalsis of gastrointestinal smooth muscle. Most of the digestant medicines have different degrees of regulating gastrointestinal activity. Some can enhance gastric peristalsis, increase the rate of gastric emptying, such as *Jī nèi jīn* and *Shān zhā;* some can enhance the rhythmic contraction of ileum, such as *Lái fú zǐ;* and some have a two-way regulatory effect on the function of gastrointestinal smooth muscle, such as *Shān zhā*.

3．调节肠道菌群状态 有些消食药能调节肠道内菌群，抑制腐败菌繁殖，防止肠道内异常发酵，减少肠道内毒素产生，发挥调节肠道功能的作用。

(3) Regulating the state of intestinal flora   Some digestant medicines can regulate intestinal flora, inhibit the reproduction of spoilage bacteria, prevent abnormal fermentation in the intestinal tract, reduce the production of intestinal endotoxin, and play a role in regulating intestinal function.

常用消食药的主要药理作用见表 12-1。

The main pharmacological effects of commonly used digestant medicines are summarized in Table 12-1.

表 12-1 常用消食药的主要药理作用

药物	助消化	调节胃肠运动	调节肠道菌群状态	其他药理作用
山楂	+	+	+	调血脂、抗动脉粥样硬化、抗心肌缺血、抗脑缺血、改善心脏功能、降压、抗氧化
神曲	+	+	+	—
鸡内金	+	+	-	改善血液流变学、调血脂、降血糖、促进锶排泄、抗乳腺增生
麦芽	+	-	-	回乳、降压
谷芽	+	-	-	—
莱菔子	-	+	-	镇咳祛痰平喘、调血脂、抗肿瘤、降压、抗菌

注："+"表示有明确作用；"–"表示无作用，或未查阅到相关研究文献

第二节　常用药物

Section 2　Commonly used medicines

PPT

山楂 ｜ *Shān zhā (Crataegi Fructus)*

【来源 / Origin】

本品为蔷薇科植物山里红（*Crataegus pinnatifida* Bge. var. major N. E. Br.）或山楂（*Crataegus pinnatifida* Bge.）的干燥成熟果实。主要分布于山东、河南、河北、辽宁。

Shān zhā is derived from the dry ripe fruit of *Crataegus pinnatifida* Bge. var. major N. E. Br. or *Crataegus pinnatifida* Bge., family Rosaceae. The plant is widely cultivated in Shangdong province, Henan province, Hebei province, and Liaoning province in China.

【化学成分 / Chemical ingredients】

主要成分为黄酮类、有机酸类和萜类。黄酮类有槲皮素（quercetin）、牡荆素（vitex）、金丝桃苷（hyperoside）、芦丁（rutin）等；有机酸类主要有枸橼酸（organic acid），含量占 5% 以上，还有琥珀酸（succinic acid）、苹果酸（malic acid）、绿原酸（chlorogenic acid）等；三萜类主要有山楂酸（maslinic acid）、熊果酸（ursolic acid）、齐墩果酸（oleanolic acid）。还含有少量的维生素（维生素 C、烟酸、维生素 B_1、维生素 B_2）及多种氨基酸等。

Shān zhā mainly contains flavonoids, organic acid and terpenoids compounds. The main flavonoids are quercetin, vitex, hyperoside, rutin, etc. Citric acid is the main organic acids, accounting for more than 5%. It also contains succinic acid, malic acid, chlorogenic acid and so on. Terpenoids contains maslinic acid, ursolic acid, oleanolic acid. Moreover, there is also a small amount of vitamins C, nicotinic acid, B_1, B_2, and a variety of amino acids can be found in *Shān zhā*.

【药性与功效 / Chinese medicine properties】

味酸、甘，性微温，归脾、胃、肝经。具有消食健胃、行气散瘀、化浊的功效。用于治疗肉食积滞、胃脘胀满、泻痢腹痛、瘀血经闭、产后瘀阻、心腹刺痛、胸痹心痛、疝气疼痛等证。

In Chinese medicine theory, *Shān zhā* has the nature of sour, sweet and warm. It can enter the meridians of spleen, stomach and liver. *Shān zhā* can disperse food and fortify the stomach, move Qi and dissipate stasis, and transform turbidity. It can be used for the treatment of meat and food accumulation, distention of stomach, diarrhea and abdominal pain, blood stasis and amenorrhea, postpartum blood stasis, stabbing pain in heart and abdomen, chest stuffiness and heartache, hernia pain and other syndromes.

【药理作用 / Pharmacological effects】

1. 促进消化　山楂能增加胃液分泌量、胃液总酸度和总酸排出量，还能增加胃蛋白酶的分泌。山楂含有的有机酸和维生素 C 可以提高胃蛋白酶活性，这些作用可促进蛋白质的消化与吸收。山楂含有少量脂肪酶，可直接将脂肪分解成小分子的脂肪酸，更易于肠道吸收，故山楂能减轻"肉食积滞"。

(1) Promoting digestion　*Shān zhā* can significantly promote the secretion of gastric juice in stomach, increase total acidity of gastric juice and total acid output, also promote the secretion of pepsin. The organic acids and vitamin C contained in *Shān zhā* can increase the activity of pepsin, which promote the digestion and absorption of protein. *Shān zhā* contains a small amount of lipase, it can directly decompose fat into small molecules of fatty acids, which are easier to be absorbed by the intestine, so *Shān zhā is* thought to be good at eliminating "meat accumulation".

2. 调节胃肠运动 山楂对胃肠功能紊乱有调整作用，促进食糜消化和胃肠道内积食积气排出，达到健胃消食功效。山楂的不同炮制品均能促进小鼠胃排空，增强肠推进，其中以生品作用最强。山楂能促进松弛的大鼠胃平滑肌收缩，还能拮抗 ACh 或钡离子对家兔肠平滑肌的兴奋，对胃肠活动有双向调节作用。

(2) Regulating gastrointestinal motility *Shān zhā* can adjust gastrointestinal dysfunction. It can promote digestion of chyme and discharging of accumulated food and Qi in gastrointestinal tract, so as to achieve the effect of strengthening stomach and digesting food. Experiments have showed that different processed products of *Shān zhā* could promote gastric emptying and intestinal motility in mice, while raw *Shān zhā* has the strongest effect. Furthermore, *Shān zhā* can promote contraction of the relaxed gastric smooth muscle, and also inhibit the excitatory effect of ACh or Ba^{2+} on the intestinal smooth muscle of rabbits, so it has a two-ways adjustment effect on gastrointestinal activity.

3. 调节血脂，抗动脉粥样硬化 山楂能明显降低高血脂患者血清总胆固醇（TC）、甘油三酯（TG）和低密度脂蛋白胆固醇（LDL-C）水平，升高高密度脂蛋白胆固醇（HDL-C）水平。山楂可通过抑制胆固醇的合成来调节血脂，山楂及其成分如槲皮素、金丝桃苷等能抑制胆固醇合成限速酶 3- 羟基 -3- 甲基戊二酸单酰辅酶 A（HMG-CoA）还原酶的活性。金丝桃苷和熊果酸为山楂调节血脂的主要物质基础。

(3) Regulating blood lipid and anti-atherosclerosis *Shān zhā* can significantly reduce the serum levels of cholesterol (TC), triacylglycerol (TG) and low-density lipoprotein cholesterol (LDL-C) and increase high-density lipoprotein cholesterol (HDL-C) level in patients with hyperlipidemia. Experiments has proved *Shān zhā* can regulate blood lipid by inhibiting the synthesis of cholesterol. *Shān zhā* and its components such as quercetin and hypericin can inhibit the activity of cholesterol synthesis rate-limiting enzyme 3-hydroxy-3-methylglutaryl-coenzyme A (HMG-CoA) reductase. Hypericin and ursolic acid are the main material basis of *Shān zhā* for regulating blood lipid.

山楂具有抗实验性动脉粥样硬化（AS）病变的作用，能减小主动脉斑块面积，减轻主动脉及冠状动脉病变。山楂能增强内皮细胞对有害因素的抵抗力和耐受性，有效地保护内皮细胞免受氧化型低密度脂蛋白的损伤，从而预防 AS 发生发展。山楂对氧自由基和羟自由基均有较强的清除效果，对抗超氧自由基的损害，可以保护心脑血管。抗氧化的主要活性物质为黄酮类。山楂还可通过调节肠道菌群治疗脂质代谢异常。

Shān zhā also has the effect of anti-atherosclerosis (AS), reducing the area of aortic plaque, reducing the pathological changes of aorta and coronary artery. It can enhance the resistance and tolerance of endothelial cells to harmful factors, effectively protect endothelial cells from oxidative LDL damage, so as to prevent the development of AS. Moreover, *Shān zhā* has a strong scavenging effect on scavenging oxygen free radicals and hydroxyl free radicals, which can against the damage of superoxide free radicals and protect the heart and brain vessels. The main active substances of antioxidation are flavonoids. Furthermore, *Shān zhā* can treat the abnormal lipid metabolism through regulating intestinal flora.

4. 调节心脑血管系统功能

(4) Regulating function of cardiovascular system

（1）抗心肌缺血 山楂能预防和减轻实验性心肌缺血，机制与其扩张冠状动脉、增加冠脉血流量、降低心肌耗氧量、扩张外周血管、降压、减轻心脏负荷等作用有关。

1) Anti-myocardial ischemia *Shān zhā* can prevent and alleviate experimental myocardial

ischemia. The mechanism is related to dilation of coronary artery and increasement of coronary blood flow, reduction of myocardial oxygen consumption, dilation of peripheral vessels, lowering blood pressure, reduction heart load and so on.

（2）抗脑缺血 山楂对缺血性脑损伤有保护作用，能改善脑代谢，减少缺血时神经元损伤。

2) Anti-cerebral ischemia *Shān zhā* has protective effect on ischemic brain injury, it can improve brain metabolism and reduce neuron injury during ischemia.

（3）改善心脏功能 山楂提取物、山楂黄酮能增强在体及离体蟾蜍心脏的收缩力。山楂增强心肌收缩力时减慢心率，但仍能增加心输出量，改善全身血液循环。山楂提取物能对抗静脉注射乌头碱、垂体后叶素等引起的实验性心律失常。山楂黄酮和萜类是其发挥心血管效应的主要物质基础。

3) Improving cardiac function *Shān zhā* extract and its flavonoids can enhance the contractility of bufonid heart *in vivo* and *in vitro*. It can reduce the heart rate when it increases myocardial contractility, but still increases cardiac output, improves systemic blood circulation. *Shān zhā* extracts can resist experimental arrhythmia caused by intravenous injection of aconitine and pituitrin. *Shān zhā* flavonoids and terpenes are the main material basis for exerting cardiovascular effect.

（4）降血压 山楂具有缓慢持久的降压作用，机制与扩张外周血管、降低外周阻力有关。山楂能缓解家兔血管平滑肌痉挛，对氯化钾引起的离体主动脉条收缩痉挛有明显的松弛作用。

4) Lowering blood pressure *Shān zhā* has a slow and lasting antihypertensive effect. The antihypertensive mechanism is related to the dilation of peripheral blood vessels and the reduction of peripheral resistance. *Shān zhā* can relieve the vasospasm of rabbit, it has obvious relaxation effect on contraction and spasm of isolated aortic strips caused by potassium chloride.

【不良反应 / Adverse effects】

山楂有轻微促子宫收缩作用，孕妇慎用。进食高蛋白及高脂肪食物后再进食山楂易引起胃石症。

Pregnant women should use *Shān zhā* with caution for it has a slight contractile effect on uterus. In addition, eating *Shān zhā* after food with high-protein and high fat may cause gastrolith.

神曲 ┆ *Shén qū (Medicata Fermentata Massa)*

【来源 / Origin】

本品为面粉或麸皮与杏仁泥、赤小豆粉以及新鲜青蒿、苍耳、辣蓼汁，按一定比例混匀后经自然发酵的干燥品。全国各地均有生产。生用或炒用。

Shén qū is obtained by mixing flour or bran with almond mud, red bean powder, and fresh artemisia annua, xanthium sibiricum and polygonum hydropiper juice in a certain proportion, and being dried by natural fermentation. It is produced all over the country. Raw or fried.

【化学成分 / Chemical ingredients】

主要含有酵母菌（yeast）、乳酸杆菌（*lactobacillus*）、淀粉酶（amylase）、蔗糖酶（sucrase）、脂肪酶（lipase）、胰酶（trypsin）、B 族维生素（vitamin B）、挥发油（volatile oil）等。

Shén qū mainly contains yeast, *lactobacillus*, amylase, sucrase, lipase, trypsin, vitamin B, volatile oil and so on.

【药性与功效 / Chinese medicine properties】

味甘、辛，性温，归脾、胃经。具有消食和胃的功效。用于治疗食积不化、脘腹胀满、恶心呕吐、肠鸣腹泻等证。

Shén qū has the nature of sweet, pungent, and warm. It can enter the meridians of spleen and stomach. It has the effect of eliminating food and harmonizing stomach, and is used to treat syndrome such as food stagnation, distention in stomach and abdomen, nausea and vomiting, intestinal ringing and diarrhea.

【药理作用 / Pharmacological effects】

1. 促进消化、改善食欲　神曲含有脂肪酶、淀粉酶、蔗糖酶、胰酶等多种消化酶，可以将脂肪、蛋白质、多糖分解为小分子物质，B族维生素促进这些小分子物质在肠道吸收。

(1) **Promoting digestion and improving appetite**　*Shén qū* contains lipase, amylase, sucrase, trypsin and other digestive enzymes, which can decompose fat, protein and polysaccharides into small molecular substances. vitamin B promote the absorption of these small molecular substances in the intestinal tract.

2. 调节肠道菌群　神曲中含有的酵母菌和乳酸杆菌具有调节肠道微生态作用。乳酸杆菌在肠道内可分解糖类产生乳酸，抑制腐败菌繁殖，防止肠道内异常发酵，减少肠道内毒素吸收而发挥作用。

(2) **Regulating the state of intestinal flora**　*Saccharomyces* and *Lactobacillus* contained in *Shén qū* can regulate intestinal microecology. Lactobacilli can decompose sugars in the intestine to produce lactic acid, inhibit the reproduction of spoilage bacteria, prevent abnormal fermentation in the intestine, and reduce the absorption of intestinal endotoxin.

莱菔子 ┆ *Lái fú zǐ* (Raphani Semen)

【来源 / Origin】

本品为十字花科植物萝卜（*Raphanus sativus* L.）的干燥成熟种子。

Lái fú zǐ is derived from the dry mature seed of *Raphanus sativus* L. of crucifer plant.

【化学成分 / Chemical ingredients】

含有芥子碱及其硫酸氢盐和脂肪油（约含30%），另含有莱菔子素（SNF）、植物甾醇、维生素类等。

Lái fú zǐ mainly contains sinapine, hydrogen sulfate and fat oil (about 30%), and also contains sulforaphane, phytosterol, vitamins, etc.

【药性与功效 / Chinese medicine properties】

味辛、甘，性平，归脾、胃、肺经。具有消食除胀、降气化痰之功效。用治饮食停滞、脘腹胀痛、大便秘结、积滞泻痢、痰壅喘咳等。

Lái fú zǐ has the nature of acridity, sweet and neutral. It can enter the meridians of spleen, stomach and lung. *Lái fú zǐ* can disperse food and eliminate distention, downbear Qi and resolve phlegm. It can be used to treat food accumulation, abdominal distention and pain, constipation, food stagnation and diarrhea, asthma and cough caused by phlegm stagnation, etc.

【药理作用 / Pharmacological effects】

1. 促进胃肠动力　生或炒莱菔子均有增强胃、十二指肠节律性收缩作用，有利于食物的机械性消化，缓解腹胀。脂肪油部分能显著增加大鼠血浆胃动素（MTL）的含量，明显促进肠推进。

(1) **Promoting gastrointestinal motility**　Raw or fried *Lái fú zǐ* can enhance the rhythmic contraction of stomach and duodenum, which is beneficial to the mechanical digestion of food and relieving abdominal distension. Fatty oil can significantly increase the content of plasma motilin (MTL) and promote intestinal propulsion in rats.

2. 镇咳、祛痰、平喘　炒莱菔子水提液可减少刺激性咳嗽，能延长乙酰胆碱（ACh）对豚鼠的引喘潜伏期，体外能对抗组胺引起的离体气管收缩。生莱菔子可促进呼吸道分泌液排泌而祛痰。

(2) Antitussive, expectorant and antiasthetic The aqueous extract of fried *Lái fú zǐ* can reduce irritant cough, prolong the incubation period of asthma induced by acetylcholine (ACh) in guinea pigs, and resist the contraction of isolated trachea caused by histamine *in vitro*. Raw *Lái fú zǐ* can promote the secretion of respiratory tract and eliminate phlegm.

3. 调节血脂 莱菔子水溶性生物碱对载脂蛋白 E（ApoE）基因敲除小鼠有降血脂作用，能提高 HDL-C 的含量，降低 TC 和 TG 及 LDL-C 含量。芥子碱对高脂血症模型大鼠有降血脂作用。

(3) Regulating blood lipid Water soluble alkaloids of *Lái fú zǐ* can reduce blood lipid of apolipoprotein E (ApoE) knockout mice. It can increase HDL-C serum levels and reduce TC, TG and LDL-C levels. In addition, sinapine can reduce blood lipid in hyperlipemia rats model.

4. 降血压 莱菔子注射液、莱菔子正丁醇提取部位、莱菔子水溶性生物碱、莱菔子素等均具有降压作用，与血管紧张素转化酶（ACE）抑制作用和抗氧化有一定关系。莱菔子水溶性生物碱还能改善自发性高血压大鼠的心室重构。

(4) Antihypertensive *Lái fú zǐ* injection, n-butanol extract of *Lái fú zǐ*, water soluble alkaloids of *Lái fú zǐ* and sulforaphane (SFN) all have antihypertensive effect, which are related to the inhibition of angiotensin converting enzyme (ACE) and antioxidation activity. Water soluble alkaloids also can improve ventricular remodeling in spontaneously hypertensive rats.

5. 抗肿瘤 莱菔子素为异硫代氰酸盐衍生物，可诱导机体产生Ⅱ型解毒酶，增加对致癌物的代谢解毒作用，可预防化学致癌物诱导的 DNA 损伤和多种肿瘤的发生。

(5) Anti-tumor SFN is a derivative of isothiocyanate, which can induce the body to produce type Ⅱ detoxification enzyme, increase the metabolic detoxification effect on carcinogens, and prevent DNA damage and the occurrence of multiple tumors induced by chemical carcinogens.

6. 抗菌 SFN 是抑菌有效成分，1 mg/ml 浓度能抑制多种革兰阳性菌和革兰阴性菌生长。

(6) Antibacterial SFN is an effective bacteriostatic component, it can inhibit the growth of various Gram-positive bacteria and Gram-negative bacteria at a concentration of 1mg/ml.

题库

（陈艳芬 李红艳）

第十三章 止血药
Chapter 13 Hemostatic medicines

学习目标 ┊ **Objectives**

1. **掌握** 止血药的基本药理作用；三七的药理作用、作用机制及药效物质基础。
2. **了解** 蒲黄、白及的药理作用及药效物质基础。

1. **Must Know** The basic pharmacological effects of hemostatic medicines; the pharmacological effects, mechanism of action and material basis of efficacy of *Sān qī*.

2. **Desirable to know** The pharmacological effects and material basis of *Pú huáng* and *Bái jí*.

第一节 概述
Section 1 Overview

凡能促进血液凝固，制止体内外出血的药物称为止血药。本类药物多味苦、涩，入肝、肺、心、脾经。止血药都有止血作用，部分药物尚有清热解毒、消肿、止痛、利尿等作用，可用于各种出血证，如咯血、衄血、吐血、尿血、便血、崩漏、紫癜及创伤出血等。

All Chinese materia medica that can promote blood coagulation and stop various bleeding internally or externally are classified as hemostatic medicines. The medicines is bitter and astringent, enters the liver, lung, heart, spleen meridians. Usually they have effects of hemostasis, some medicines still have clearing heat and detoxification, detumescence, analgesic, diuretic and other effects. They are applied to a variety of bleeding patterns, such as hemoptysis and epistaxis, hematemesis, hematuria, blood in the stool, flooding and spotting, purpura and trauma hemorrhage.

出血证多为寒热失调、情志内伤、气血功能紊乱或外伤，导致血不循常道溢于脉外。出血证与西医学中出血、紫癜、凝血障碍等的症状相似。

Hemorrhagic diseases are due to cold and heat disorders, internal damage caused by mental disorders, dysfunction of Qi and blood , which leads to the abnormal blood benefiting the outside of the pulse. Bleeding syndrome is similar to the symptoms of bleeding, purpura and coagulation disorders in western medicine.

西医学揭示机体的血液系统存在凝血和纤维蛋白溶解两种对立又统一的生理过程，二者相辅相成并保持动态平衡，既能使血液在血管内不停地流动，也能在血管损伤的局部迅速启动凝血机制而止血。在病理状态下，打破上述平衡就会发生出血性或血栓栓塞性疾病。造成出血的主要病因有：血管损伤、血管通透性和脆性增加；凝血过程障碍，如血小板减少或功能障碍、凝血因子缺乏或功能障碍；纤维蛋白溶解系统功能亢进等。

Western medicine reveals that there is a unity of opposite in the blood coagulation and anti-coagulation system. They complement each other, maintaining dynamic balance, and keeping blood flowing in the blood vessels constantly, as well as rapidly coagulating and stopping bleeding in the injured local blood vessels. In pathological condition, the balance is broken, leading to thromboembolic disease or hemorrhagic disease. The hemorrhage may be due to vessel wall damage, increasing vascular permeability and fragility, or dysfunction of the coagulation process, the hyperthyroidism of the fibrinolytic system, and so on.

根据主要功效，止血药可分为化瘀止血、收敛止血、凉血止血、温经止血 4 类。常用止血药有三七、蒲黄、白及、大蓟、小蓟、仙鹤草、侧柏叶、地榆、槐花、紫珠及茜草等。现代药理研究表明，止血药治疗出血与下列药理作用有关。

According to the main efficacies, hemostatic medicines can be classified into four types: stasis-resolving hemostatic medicines, astringent hemostatic medicines, blood-cooling hemostatic medicines and meridian-warming hemostatic medicines. The frequently used herbs are *Sān qī*, *Bái jí*, *Pú huáng*, *Dà jì*, *Xiǎo jì*, *Xiān hè cǎo*, *Cè bǎi yè*, *Dì yú*, *Huái huā*, *Zǐ zhū*, *Qiàn cǎo*. The main pharmacological effects are as followings.

1. **影响局部血管** 止血药可收缩局部血管，减慢血流，促进血栓形成而止血。如三七、小蓟、紫珠、槐花等可收缩局部小血管；槐花、白茅根还能降低毛细血管通透性。

(1) Affect local blood vessel Contract local blood vessels, slow down blood flow, promote thrombosis and stop bleeding. *Sān qī*, *Xiǎo jì*, *Zǐ zhū* and *Huáo huā* can contract local small blood vessels; *Huái huā* and *Bái máo gēn* can reduce capillary permeability.

2. **促进凝血因子生成** 三七增加凝血酶含量，大蓟促进凝血酶原激活物生成，白茅根促进凝血酶原生成，小蓟含有凝血酶样活性物质，这些都有利于使血液凝固的关键凝血酶增加。

(2) Promote coagulation factors *Sān qī* can increase the content of thrombin; *Dà jì* can promote the production of prothrombin activator; *Bái máo gēn* can promote the production of prothrombin; *Xiǎo jì* has thrombin like activity substance all of which are conducive to the increase of thrombin.

3. **提高血小板数量和功能** 三七可增加血小板数量，提高血小板的黏附性，促进血小板聚集；白及可增强血小板因子Ⅲ的活性；地榆可增加血小板功能；仙鹤草、小蓟、紫珠、蒲黄可增加血小板数量，提高其功能，促进生理性止血。

(3) Improve platelet activity *Sān qī* can increase the number of platelet, improve the adhesion of platelet, and promote the release and aggregation of platelet; *Bái jí* can enhance the activity of platelet factor Ⅲ; *Dì yú* can improve the function of platelet; *Xiān hè cǎo*, *Xiǎo jì*, *Zǐ zhū* and *Pú huáng* can raise platelet count and improve their function and promote physiological hemostasis.

4. **抗纤维蛋白溶解** 白及、紫珠、小蓟、艾叶通过抗纤维蛋白溶解而促进凝血。

(4) Antifibrinolysis *Bái jí*, *Zǐ zhū*, *Xiǎo jì* and *Ài yè* can inhibit fibrinolysis and hemostasis.

常用止血药的主要药理作用见表 13-1。

The main pharmacological effects of common hemostatic medicines are summarized in Table 13-1.

表 13-1　常用止血药的主要药理作用

类别	药物	收缩局部血管	促凝血	抗纤溶	其他药理作用
化瘀止血	三七	+	+	-	抗血栓、促进造血、调节心血管功能、抗炎、保肝、镇痛、镇静
	蒲黄	-	+	-	抑制血小板聚集、调节心血管功能、兴奋子宫、抗肾损伤
收敛止血	茜草	-	-	-	抗凝血、升高白细胞、抗肿瘤
	白及	-	+	-	保护胃黏膜、抗菌
	仙鹤草	-	+	-	抗凝血、杀虫、抗菌、抗肿瘤
	紫珠	+	+	-	抗菌
凉血止血	小蓟	+	+	+	降血脂、强心、升压、利尿、利胆
	大蓟	-	+	-	降压、抗菌
	地榆	-	+	-	抗菌、抗炎、抗溃疡、保肝
	槐花	+	-	-	抗炎、解痉、抗溃疡、降血脂
温经止血	艾叶	-	+	+	平喘、镇咳、祛痰、利胆

注："+"表示有明确作用；"-"表示无作用，或未查阅到相关研究文献

第二节　常用药物
Section 2　Commonly used medicines

PPT

三七 ┊ *Sān qī*（*Notoginseng Radix et Rhizoma*）

【来源 / Origin】

本品为五加科植物三七 [*Panax notoginseng*（Burk.）F. H. Chen] 的干燥根和根茎。主产于广西、云南两地。秋季花开前采挖，洗净，分开主根、支根及根茎，干燥。

Sān qī derives from the dried root and root lotus of *Panax notoginseng* (Burk.) F. H. Chen. *Sān qī* is mainly cultivated in Guangxi area and Yunnan province. It is excavated and washed in autumn,then removed the main root,branch root and rhizome,and dried them.

【化学成分 / Chemical ingredients】

主要含有多种皂苷，总皂苷含量可达 8%~12%，分别是人参皂苷 Rb、人参皂苷 Rd、人参皂苷 Re、人参皂苷 Rg_1、人参皂苷 Rg_2、人参皂苷 Rh、人参皂苷 R_1、人参皂苷 R_2、人参皂苷 R_3、人参皂苷 R_4、人参皂苷 R_6，还含有三七多糖 A、三七氨酸、挥发性成分等。

Sān qī mainly contains a variety of notoginsenoside, the total content of which can reach 8%-12%, which is similar to ginsenoside. They are ginsenoside Rb, Rd, Re, Rg_1, Rg_2, Rh, R_1, R_2, R_3, R_4, R_6, and also contain notoginseng polysaccharide A, notoginseng amino acid, volatile components, etc.

【药性与功效 / Chinese medicine properties】

味甘、微苦，性温，归肝、胃经。具有散瘀止血、消肿定痛的功效。用于治疗咯血、吐血、衄血、便血、崩漏、外伤出血、胸腹刺痛、跌打肿痛等证。

In Chinese medicine theory, *Sān qī* has the nature of sweet, slightly bitter, warm. It can enter the meridians of liver and stomach. It has the effect of dissipate stasis to stop bleeding, alleviate edema to relieve pain. It is used to treat hemoptysis, hematemesis, hematemesis, hematochezia, metrorrhagia, traumatic bleeding, chest and abdomen stabbing pain, bruise and swelling pain.

【药理作用 / Pharmacological effects】

1. 止血　三七不同制剂和给药途径均有明显的止血作用。给麻醉犬灌服三七粉后，犬颈动脉血体外凝血时间和凝血酶原时间都缩短。静脉注射三七注射液后的家兔凝血时间、凝血酶原时间和凝血酶时间也缩短。无论是三七溶液灌胃，还是三七注射液腹腔注射，小鼠的凝血时间和出血时间都缩短。三七氨酸对正常动物及其出血模型均有良好的止血作用。三七氨酸是三七发挥止血作用的主要物质基础，但其受热易被破坏，故生用三七止血效果好。三七止血的作用机制与增加血小板数量、增强血小板黏附性、增加血液中凝血酶含量、收缩局部血管有关。

(1) Hemostasis *Sān qī* has obvious hemostatic effect in different preparations and administration ways. The clotting time and prothrombin time of carotid blood in anesthetized dogs were shortened. The clotting time, prothrombin time and thrombin time of rabbits were also shortened after intravenous injection of *Sān qī* injection. The clotting time and bleeding time of mice were shortened no matter whether it was intragastric injection or intraperitoneal injection of *Sān qī* injection. It has a good hemostatic effect on normal animals and their bleeding models. Notoginsenic acid is the main material basis for its hemostasis, but it is easy to be damaged by heat, it should be used raw to stop bleeding. The hemostatic mechanism of *Sān qī* is related to the increase of platelet number, platelet adhesiveness, thrombin content in blood and the contraction of local blood vessels.

2. 促进造血　三七有"补血"作用。三七及其皂苷能明显改善各种血液损伤动物模型的病理状态。三七注射液能促进急性失血大鼠红细胞、网织红细胞浓度的恢复，提高血红蛋白的含量。三七总皂苷（PNS）还对环磷酰胺所致的小鼠白细胞减少有促进恢复作用。三七能促进造血干细胞增殖、分化，提高血液中粒细胞、红细胞、白细胞的数量和功能，产生"补血"作用，正常的血细胞数量和功能有利于发挥生理性止血作用。

(2) Promoting hematopoiesis *Sān qī* has the function of "tonifying blood". *Sān qī* and its saponins can obviously improve the pathological state of various animal models of blood injury. *Sān qī* injection can promote the recovery of red blood cell and reticulocyte concentration and increase the content of hemoglobin in rats with acute hemorrhage. PNS can also promote the recovery of leucopenia induced by cyclophosphamide. *Sān qī* can promote the proliferation and differentiation of hematopoietic stem cells, improve the number and function of granulocytes, erythrocytes and leukocytes in the blood, and produce "tonifying blood" effect. Normal blood cell number and function are conducive to play a physiological hemostatic role.

3. 抗血栓　三七活血散瘀与抗血栓形成有密切关系。血液高黏和（或）高血脂患者口服生三七粉后可显著降低体内血浆纤维蛋白原的含量，抑制血栓形成。静脉注射三七总皂苷后能抑制大鼠实验性血栓形成。在大鼠弥散性血管内凝血模型实验中，静脉注射三七皂苷能显著抑制血小板的减少和纤维蛋白降解物的增加。三七总皂苷在大鼠体外或家兔体内均能显著抑制胶原、ADP诱导的血小板聚集。三七可抑制凝血酶诱导的纤维蛋白原降解及血栓形成过程，并能激活尿激酶，促进纤维蛋白溶解。

(3) Anti-thrombosis *Sān qī* promoting blood circulation and dissipating blood stasis is closely related to anti-thrombosis. The content of plasma fibrinogen can be significantly reduced and the formation of thrombus can be inhibited in patients with high viscosity or hyperlipidemia. PNS can inhibit experimental thrombosis in rats. Intravenous injection of PNS can significantly inhibit the decrease of platelets and the increase of fibrin degradation in the model experiment of disseminated intravascular coagulation in rats. PNS can significantly inhibit platelet aggregation induced by collagen and ADP *in vitro* and *in vivo*. *Sān qī* can inhibit fibrinogen degradation and thrombosis induced by thrombin, activate urokinase and promote fibrinolysis.

4. 调节心血管功能　血瘀证产生和发展与循环系统的功能障碍密不可分。三七及其有效成分调节心血管系统功能是其产生活血散瘀功效的药理学基础。

(4) Regulating the cardiovascular system　The origin and development of blood stasis syndrome are closely related to the dysfunction of circulatory system. *Sān qī* and its active ingredients regulate the function of cardiovascular system is the pharmacological basis of its effect of promoting blood circulation and removing blood stasis.

（1）调节心功能　三七总皂苷具有降低心肌收缩力、减慢心率的作用。给麻醉猫、犬静脉注射三七总皂苷，其左心室内压与左心室内压最大上升速率均显著降低，达到峰值所用时间显著延长，心率减慢，但心输出量、心脏指数不下降或有增加。三七总皂苷能拮抗 $CaCl_2$ 引起的豚鼠离体心肌收缩力和收缩频率的增加，缩短心肌细胞动作电位平台期。

1) Regulating heart function　PNS can reduce myocardial contractility and heart rate. After intravenous injection of PNS into anesthetized cats and dogs, the maximum rate of rise of left ventricular internal pressure and left ventricular internal pressure decreased significantly, the time to reach the peak value prolonged significantly, the heart rate slowed down, but the cardiac output and cardiac index did not decrease or increase. PNS can antagonize the increase of contractile force and contractile frequency caused by $CaCl_2$, and shorten the action potential platform period of cardiomyocytes.

（2）扩张血管、降血压　三七及 PNS 对犬、猫、自发性高血压大鼠等多种动物具有降压作用，以降低舒张压更为明显。PNS 主要扩张肾动脉、肠系膜动脉和门静脉、下腔静脉及软脑膜微血管，作用较强，对大动脉扩张作用不明显。三七总皂苷作用比单体强，Rb_1 的作用强于 Rg_1。三七扩血管、降血压作用可能与阻止 Ca^{2+} 内流有关。PNS 能特异性地阻断血管平滑肌上受体依赖性钙通道，减少 Ca^{2+} 内流，也能明显减少去甲肾上腺素引起的 Ca^{2+} 内流。

2) Dilating blood vessels and reducing blood pressure　*Sān qī* and PNS have hypotensive effects on dogs, cats, spontaneously hypertensive rats and other animals, especially in reducing diastolic blood pressure. PNS mainly dilates renal artery, mesenteric artery, portal vein, inferior vena cava and pia mater microvasculature, and has strong effect, but has no obvious effect on large artery dilation. The effect of PNS is stronger than that of monomer, Rb_1 is stronger than Rg_1. The vasodilator and hypotensive effects of *Sān qī* may be related to the inhibition of Ca^{2+} influx. PNS can specifically block receptor-dependent calcium channels on vascular smooth muscle, reduce Ca^{2+} influx, and also significantly reduce Ca^{2+} influx caused by noradrenaline.

（3）抗心肌缺血　三七对多种实验性心肌缺血模型有保护作用。三七、三七总黄酮及三七根提取物能对抗垂体后叶素所致家兔急性心肌缺血性 T 波升高。三七注射液可显著减轻实验性急性心肌梗死犬心电图 ST 段的偏移和病理性 Q 波的出现。PNS 能显著扩张冠脉，降低冠脉阻力，增加冠脉血流量。三七抗心肌缺血的作用机制如下。①扩张冠脉，增加冠脉血流量，促进心肌梗死区侧支循环，改善缺血心肌血氧供应。②降低心肌收缩力，减慢心率，降低外周血管阻力，降低心肌耗氧量。③抗过氧化，提高 SOD 活性，减少 MDA 生成。④提高耐缺氧能力，明显延长小鼠在常压缺氧条件下的存活时间。

3) Anti-myocardial ischemia　*Sān qī* has protective effects on a variety of experimental myocardial

ischemia models. *Sān qī*, *Sān qī* total flavonoids and *Sān qī* root extract can resist the T wave elevation of acute myocardial ischemia induced by pituitrin in rabbits. *Sān qī* injection can significantly reduce ST segment shift and pathological Q wave in dogs with experimental acute myocardial infarction. PNS can significantly expand coronary artery, reduce coronary resistance and increase coronary blood flow. The mechanism of *Sān qī* against myocardial ischemia includes: dilating coronary artery, increasing coronary blood flow, promoting collateral circulation in myocardial infarction area, improving blood oxygen supply of ischemic myocardium; inhibiting myocardial contractility, slowing heart rate and reducing peripheral blood vessels resistance, reduce myocardial oxygen consumption; anti-peroxidation, improving SOD activity, reducing MDA production; improving hypoxia tolerance, significantly prolong the survival time of mice under atmospheric hypoxia.

（4）抗心律失常　三七、三七总皂苷及其二醇苷（PDS）、三醇苷（PTS）对多种实验性心律失常模型有明显保护作用。对多种药物诱导的实验性心律失常均有明显改善作用。三七及其有效成分抗心律失常机制涉及阻滞钙通道，阻滞钙内流；PTS与胺碘酮对心脏细胞的电生理作用相似，主要是延长动作电位时程（APD）及有效不应期 (ERP)，阻断期前收缩的冲动传导而发挥抗心律失常作用。

4) Anti-arrhythmia　*Sān qī*, PNS and diol glycosides (PDS) and triol glycosides (PTS) have obvious protective effects on a variety of experimental arrhythmia models. It can obviously improve the experimental arrhythmia induced by various drugs. The antiarrhythmic mechanism of *Sān qī* and its active ingredients involves slow calcium channel, which blocks calcium influx; PTS and amiodarone have similar electrophysiological characteristics to heart cells, mainly including prolonging action potential duration (APD) and effective refractory period (ERP), blocking impulse conduction of premature beat and playing an antiarrhythmic role.

（5）抗动脉粥样硬化　给家兔腹腔注射三七总皂苷，其能显著抑制实验性动脉粥样硬化家兔动脉内膜斑块的形成，稳定血管内环境。

5) Anti-atherosclerosis　*Sān qī* can significantly inhibit the formation of atherosclerotic plaque and stabilize the vascular environment.

5. 调节代谢　三七对糖代谢有双向调节作用。三七皂苷 C_1 能降低血糖并拮抗胰高血糖素的升血糖作用，而 PNS 则与胰高血糖素有协同升血糖作用。三七甲醇提取物可拮抗高胆固醇饮食大鼠脂蛋白、磷脂及游离脂肪酸的升高。三七根乙醇提取物能促进小鼠肝、肾和睾丸等脏器的蛋白质合成，三七皂苷能促进小鼠脑中蛋白质含量的增加。Rb_1 能提高 RNA 聚合酶的活性，促进大鼠肝细胞 RNA 合成。

(5) Regulating metabolize　*Sān qī* has two-way regulation on glucose metabolism. Notoginsenoside C_1 can reduce blood glucose and antagonize the hypoglycemic effect of glucagon, while PNS and glucagon have synergistic effect. The methanol extract of *Sān qī* can inhibit the increase of lipoproteins, phospholipids and free fatty acids in rats fed with high cholesterol diet. The ethanol extract of *Sān qī* root can promote the protein synthesis of liver, kidney, testis and other organs of mice, and PNS can promote the protein content in the brain of mice. Rb_1 can enhance the activity of RNA polymerase and promote RNA synthesis of rat hepatocytes.

6. 抗炎　三七有抗炎作用。三七总皂苷对多种物质引起的毛细血管通透性增高有明显的抑制作用，能明显抑制实验性大鼠足跖肿胀、棉球肉芽肿形成和小鼠耳郭肿胀。皂苷是其抗炎的主要物质基础，以人参二醇皂苷为主。

(6) anti-inflammation　*Sān qī* has anti-inflammatory effect. PNS can significantly inhibit the

increase of capillary permeability caused by various substances, and can significantly inhibit the experimental rat paw swelling, cotton ball granuloma formation and mouse auricle swelling. Ginsenoside is the main material basis of anti-inflammatory, mainly panaxadiol saponin.

7. 抗肿瘤　人参皂苷 Rh_1 对离体肝癌细胞有抑制作用。Rh_2 可抑制小鼠黑色素瘤 B_{16} 的生长，并呈浓度依赖关系。

(7) anti-tumor　Ginsenoside Rh_1 has an inhibitory effect on hepatoma cells in vitro. Rh_2 inhibited the growth of B_{16} in a concentration dependent manner.

8. 镇痛　三七为治疗跌打损伤的常用药，有确切的镇痛作用。三七能提高多种疼痛模型动物的痛阈，显示明显的镇痛效应。PNS 与电针有相似的抗炎镇痛效应，并可被纳洛酮阻断。人参二醇皂苷是其镇痛的主要物质基础。

(8) Analgesic　*Sān qī* is a commonly used medicine for the treatment of traumatic injury, which has a definite analgesic effect. *Sān qī* can improve the pain threshold of various pain model animals and show obvious analgesic effect. PNS has similar anti-inflammatory and analgesic effects as electroacupuncture, and can be blocked by naloxone. Panaxadiol saponin is the main material basis of analgesia.

9. 其他作用　三七还具有抑制中枢、调节免疫功能、延缓衰老、保肝、利胆等作用。

(9) Other effects　*Sān qī* also has the functions of inhibiting central nervous system, regulating immune function, delaying aging, protecting liver and benefiting gall.

【不良反应 / Adverse effects 】

有使用三七出现过敏反应、胃肠道不适及出血倾向的个案病例报告，表现为痰中带血、牙龈出血、月经增多等；有超剂量服用（口服生三七粉 10g 以上）引起房室传导阻滞的个案病例报告。

Cases of allergic reaction, gastrointestinal discomfort and bleeding tendency were reported, including blood in the sputum, gingival bleeding, increased menstruation, etc.; cases of atrioventricular block caused by over dose administration (more than 10g of oral *Sān qī* powder) were reported.

蒲黄　*Pú huáng*(*Typhae Angustifoliae*)

【来源 / Origin 】

本品为香蒲科植物水烛香蒲（*Typha angustifolia* L.）、东方香蒲（*Typha orientalis* Presl）或同属植物的干燥花粉。全国大部分地区多有生产。夏季采收蒲棒上部的黄色雄花序，晒干后碾轧，筛取花粉。

Pú huáng is the dried pollen of *Typha angustifolia* L., *Typha Orientalis* Presl or the same plant. The plant is widely cultivated in most provinces of china. The yellow male infloresceneces on the upper part of the dandelion are collected in summer, then dried,milled and screened for pollen.The male flowers are cut and dried after sun exposure.

【化学成分 / Chemical ingredients 】

主要成分为黄酮类，如槲皮素（quercetin）、山奈酚（kaempferol）、异鼠李素（isorhamnetin）、柚皮素（naringenin）、泡桐素（paulownin）、香蒲新苷、异鼠李素 –3–O– 芸香糖苷、异鼠李素 –3–O– 新橙皮糖苷（isorhamnetin-3-O-neohesperidoside）、槲皮素 –3–O–(2G–α–L– 鼠李糖基)– 芸香糖苷及山奈酚 –3–O– 新橙皮糖苷等。还含有甾醇类，如 β– 谷甾醇（β-sitosterol）、β– 谷甾醇葡萄糖苷（β-sitosterol glucoside）等，另外还含有多种多糖和氨基酸。

The main components of *Pú huáng* are flavonoids, such as quercetin, kaempferol, isorhamnetin, naringenin, paulownin, typhoside, isorhamnetin-3-O-rutoside, isorhamnetin-3-O-neohesperidoside, quercetin-3-O-(2G-α-L-rhamnosyl)-rutoside and kaempferol-3-O-neohesperidin. It also contains sterols, such as β-sitosterol, β-sitosterol glucoside, and many kinds of polysaccharides and amino acids.

【药性与功效 / Chinese medicine properties】

味甘，性平，归肝、心包经。具有止血、化瘀、通淋之功效。用于吐血、衄血、咯血、崩漏、外伤出血、经闭痛经、脘腹刺痛、跌扑肿痛、血淋涩痛。

In Chinese medicine theory, *Pú huáng* has the nature of sweet and flat. It can enter the meridians of liver and pericardium. It has the effect of hemostasis, removing blood stasis and dredging drench. It is used for emesis, bleeding, hemoptysis, metrorrhagia, traumatic bleeding, dysmenorrhea, abdominal pain, tumefacient pain and astringent pain.

【药理作用 / Pharmacological effects】

1. 止血　蒲黄可缩短凝血时间和出血时间，又能改善血液流变学。有研究认为，蒲黄中的黄酮类物质在一定温度下可转化为具有止血作用的鞣质，增强止血作用。炮制的蒲黄炭品可以通过影响实验动物凝血系统的多个环节发挥止血作用。生蒲黄也具有止血作用，能缩短活化部分凝血酶原时间（APTT），但对血瘀大鼠凝血酶原时间（PT）无明显影响。

(1) **Hemostasis**　*Pú huáng* can shorten coagulation time and bleeding time, and can improve hemorheology at the same time. Some studies have shown that the flavonoids in *Pú huáng* can be converted into tannins with hemostatic effect at a certain temperature and enhance the hemostatic effect. The processed *Pú huáng* charcoal can play a role in hemostasis by influencing the coagulation system of experimental animals. Raw *Pú huáng* has hemostatic effect and can shorten APTT, but has no significant effect on PT in blood stasis rats.

2. 抗血小板聚集　生蒲黄可延长小鼠凝血时间，较大剂量时可促进纤维蛋白溶解。蒲黄煎剂能抑制磷酸二酯酶活性，升高血小板内 cAMP，减少 TXA_2 的合成，使细胞内 Ca^{2+} 浓度降低，减少 5-HT 释放，抑制 ADP、花生四烯酸和胶原诱导的家兔体内外血小板聚集。蒲黄水浸液可增加家兔实验性颈静脉血栓的溶解率，抑制血小板黏附和聚集，轻度增加抗凝血酶Ⅲ的活性。蒲黄水提取液可分解纤维蛋白，促进纤维蛋白溶解，且不依赖纤溶酶系统存在。蒲黄黄酮类物质能刺激主动脉内皮细胞产生前列环素，促进纤溶酶原激活物（t-PA）活性，从而抑制血小板聚集，抗血栓形成。蒲黄有机酸能抑制花生四烯酸诱导的家兔体外血小板聚集。蒲黄异鼠李素Ⅱ在体内外均能抑制 ADP 诱导的大鼠血小板聚集，并明显延长复钙时间。

(2) **Antiplatelet aggregation**　*Pú huáng* can prolong the clotting time of mice and promote the fibrinolysis in large dose. *Pú huáng* decoction can inhibit phosphodiesterase activity, increase camp in platelets, reduce TXA_2 synthesis, reduce Ca^{2+} concentration in cells, reduce 5-HT release, and inhibit platelet aggregation induced by ADP, arachidonic acid and collagen in rabbits. The aqueous extract of *Pú huáng* can increase the dissolution rate of experimental jugular vein thrombosis, inhibit platelet adhesion and aggregation, and slightly increase the activity of antithrombin Ⅲ. The aqueous extract of *Pú huáng* can decompose fibrin, promote the dissolution of fibrin, and does not depend on the existence of plasmin system. Typhae flavonoids can stimulate the production of prostacyclin and promote the activity of plasminogen activator (t-PA), thus inhibiting platelet aggregation and antithrombotic. *Pú huáng* organic acid can inhibit the platelet aggregation induced by arachidonic acid in vitro. *Pú huáng* isorhamnetin Ⅱ can inhibit the platelet aggregation induced by ADP *in vivo* and *in vitro*, and prolong the time of calcium recovery.

3. 对心血管系统的作用

(3) **Effect on cardiovascular system**

（1）抗心肌缺血　蒲黄可增加离体心脏、冠状动脉血流量，增加整体动物耐低气压、低氧的能力，改善心肌营养性血流量。蒲黄提取物可对抗垂体后叶素引起的心肌缺血。

1) Anti-myocardial ischemia　*Pú huáng* can increase the blood flow of isolated heart and coronary artery, increase the ability of the whole animal to bear low pressure and hypoxia, and improve the myocardial nutritional blood flow. The extract of Typhae can resist the myocardial ischemia caused by pituitrin.

（2）调节血脂、抗动脉粥样硬化　蒲黄能抑制脂质在主动脉壁的沉积，抑制肠道对外源性胆固醇的吸收，并促进胆固醇的排泄，升高高密度脂蛋白胆固醇（HDL-C），降低血小板黏附和聚集，同时保护血管内皮细胞，减轻高脂血症对血管内皮的损伤，改善血液流变性与红细胞流变性，进而改善血液循环和微循环，有利于内皮细胞的正常代谢，抑制动脉粥样硬化斑块形成。

2) regulating blood lipid and anti-atherosclerosis　*Pú huáng* can inhibit the deposition of lipid in the aortic wall, inhibit the absorption of intestinal exogenous cholesterol, promote the excretion of cholesterol, increase HDL-C, reduce platelet adhesion and aggregation, protect vascular endothelial cells, reduce the damage of hyperlipidemia on vascular endothelial, improve hemorheology and RBC rheology, and improve blood circulation and microcirculation. Circulation is conducive to the normal metabolism of endothelial cells and the inhibition of atherosclerotic plaque formation.

4. 兴奋子宫　蒲黄对多种动物在体、离体子宫均有兴奋作用，剂量较大时甚至引起子宫痉挛性收缩。蒲黄具有良好的引产作用，对早期、中期妊娠均有明显效果。

(4) Excite the uterus　*Pú huáng* can excite the uterus *in vivo* and *in vitro*, and even cause the spasmodic contraction of uterus when the dosage is large. *Pú huáng* has good induction effect, and has obvious effect on early and middle pregnancy.

5. 对抗肾损伤　蒲黄对多种肾脏损伤动物模型具有保护作用，可降低血肌酐和尿 N– 乙酰 –β–D– 氨基葡糖苷酶，减少近曲小管上皮细胞坏死及囊腔内有红细胞的肾小球数目。

(5) Against renal injury　*Pú huáng* has protective effect on many kinds of renal injury animal models. It can reduce serum creatinine and urinary N-acetyl-β-D-glucosaminidase (Nag enzyme), reduce the necrosis of proximal tubule epithelial cells and the number of glomeruli with red cells in the capsule.

6. 其他作用　蒲黄尚具有加速血肿吸收，促进骨折愈合、骨母细胞及软骨细胞增生、骨痂形成及抗疲劳作用。此外，蒲黄还具有糖皮质激素样作用，可抑制体液及细胞免疫。

(6) Other effects　*Pú huáng* can accelerate the absorption of hematoma, promote fracture healing, proliferation of osteoblasts and chondrocytes, callus formation and anti fatigue effect. In addition, *Pú huáng* has glucocorticoid like effect, which can inhibit humoral and cellular immunity.

白及 ｜ *Bái jí*（Bletillae Rhizoma）

【来源 / Origin】

本品为兰科植物白及 [*Bletilla striata* (Thunb.) Reichb. f.] 的干燥块茎。夏秋二季采挖，除去须根，洗净，置沸水中煮或蒸至无白心，晒至半干，除去外皮，晒干。

Bái jí is the dried root and rhizome of [*Bletilla striata* (Thunb.) Reichb. f.], family of Orchidaceae. It is excavated in summer and autumn, then removed fibrous, washed, boiled or steamed in boiling water until there is no white heart, dried to half dry, removed skin, and dried them.

【化学成分 / Chemical ingredients】

主要化学成分有白及胶（含联苄类化合物）、菲类衍生物（二氢菲类化合物、联菲类化合物、双菲醚类化合物、二氢菲并吡喃类化合物、菲类糖苷化合物等）、苄类化合物等。此外，尚含有大黄素甲醚、对羟基苯甲酸、对羟基苯甲醛等。

The main chemical components of *Bái jí* are gum bletilla (including bibenzyls), phenanthrene derivatives (dihydro-phenanthrene-based compounds, biphenyl phenanthrene compound, bis philippines ethers, dihydro-phenanthrene benzopyran compounds, phenanthrene glycoside compounds, etc.), benzyl compounds and so on. In addition, it contains physcion, hydroxybenzoic acid, p-hydroxybenzaldehyde.

【药性与功效 / Chinese medicine properties】

味苦、甘、涩，性微寒，归肺、肝、胃经。具有收敛止血、消肿生肌之功效。用于咯血、吐血、外伤出血、疮疡肿毒、皮肤皲裂。

In Chinese medicine theory, *Bái jí* has the nature of bitter, sweet, astringent in flavor, and slightly cold. It can enter the meridians of lung, liver and stomach. It has the effect of astringent hemostasis, detumescence and muscle growth. It is used for hemoptysis, hematemesis, traumatic bleeding, sore, swelling and toxic, chapped skin.

【药理作用 / Pharmacological effects】

1. **止血**　白及可通过缩短凝血时间、凝血酶生成时间，抑制纤维蛋白溶解系统，轻度增强血小板因子Ⅲ的活性，并加速红细胞沉降率而发挥较好的止血效果。白及的止血作用通常认为与其所含胶状成分有关。

(1) Stopping bleeding　*Bái jí* can shorten the clotting time, thrombin generation time, inhibit fibrinolysis system, mildly enhance the activity of platelet factor Ⅲ, accelerate erythrocyte sedimentation rate and achieve better hemostatic effect. The *Bái jí* hemostatic effects are generally considered to be related to a gel composition.

2. **保护黏膜**　白及煎剂对多种因素导致的胃黏膜损伤具有较好的保护作用，可促进溃疡愈合。其作用机制与增加胃壁黏液分泌量和胃黏膜血流量，刺激胃黏膜合成和释放内源性前列腺素有关。

(2) Protecting mucosa　*Bái jí* decoction have better protection of the gastric mucosal against injury caused by a variety of factors, promotes ulcer healing. The mechanism is associated with increasing mucus secretion and gastric mucosal blood flow, stimulating the synthesis and release of endogenous gastric prostaglandin.

3. **促进伤口愈合**　白及能明显加快伤口的愈合速度，促进创伤的愈合，其作用机制与其能提高创面组织中羟脯氨酸和蛋白质含量有关。另外，白及所含胶状成分可作为外源性重组人表皮生长因子载体，显著促进创面细胞 DNA 的合成，提高细胞的增殖能力，缩短伤口愈合时间，加速伤口愈合。白及多糖可通过增加羟脯氨酸含量、促进成纤维细胞增殖而显著促进糖尿病溃疡创面愈合。

(3) Promoting wound healing　*Bái jí* can significantly accelerate wound healing, promote healing, and its mechanism is associated with improving the content of hydroxyproline and protein in wound. In addition, the composition of *Bái jí* gum as exogenous recombinant human epidermal growth factor support, significantly promote the synthesis of cellular DNA in wound, and improve the ability of proliferation, shorten healing time, accelerate wound healing. *Bái jí* polysaccharide can promote wound healing in diabetic ulcers by increasing hydroxyproline content, significant promoting the proliferation of fibroblasts.

4. **抗菌**　白及联菲类化合物在体外对金黄色葡萄球菌、枯草杆菌、蜡样芽孢杆菌和加得那诺卡菌有一定抑制作用；对真菌如白念珠菌和须毛癣菌的抑制作用较弱。白及联菲 A、白及联菲 B、白及联菲 C 对金黄色葡萄球菌以及与龋齿形成有关的突变链球菌也有抑制作用，其中白及联菲 B 的作用较强。

(4) Anti-bacteria *Bái jí* phenanthrene compounds have a certain inhibition of *Staphylococcus aureus*, *Bacillus subtilis*, *Bacillus cereus* and Gardrernocandia *in vitro*; the inhibition of fungus such as *Candida albicans* and *Trichophyton mentagrophytes* are weak. *Bái jí* philippines A, B, C has inhibitory effects on *Staphylococcus aureus* and dental caries related *Staphylococcus*. *Bái jí* philippines B is suggested to be more stronger.

（屈 飞）

第十四章 活血化瘀药
Chapter 14 Blood invigorating and stasis dissolving medicines

 学习目标 | Objectives

1. **掌握** 活血化瘀药的主要药理作用；丹参、川芎、延胡索、银杏叶、红花的主要药理作用和药效物质基础。

2. **了解** 益母草、莪术、水蛭、桃仁、姜黄的主要药理作用和药效物质基础。

1. **Must Know** The main pharmacological effects of blood invigorating and stasis dissolving medicines; the main pharmacological effects and material basis of *Dān shēn*, *Chuān xiōng*, *Yán hú suŏ*, *Yín xìng yè*, and *Hóng huā*.

2. **Desirable to know** The main pharmacological effects and material basis of of *Yì mǔ cǎo*, *É zhú*, *Shuǐ zhì*, *Táo rén*, and *Jiāng huáng*.

第一节 概述
Section 1 Overview

PPT

　　凡以疏通血脉、祛除瘀血为主要功效，临床用于治疗血瘀证的药物，称为活血化瘀药。本类药物主要归肝、心经，入血分，药性较温和，味多辛、苦。辛能散瘀化滞，温可通行经脉、促进血行，故本类药物除了能通利血脉、祛瘀通滞、破瘀消癥之外，尚有活血调经、通经下乳、通痹解结、疗伤止痛、活血消痈、化瘀止血及去瘀生新等功效。

All Chinese materia medica that have the functions of dredging the blood vessels and dissipating static blood and are clinically used to treat blood stasis, are classified as blood invigorating and stasis dissolving medicines. They majorly enter the meridians of liver and heart and invade the blood level. They mainly have mild medicinal nature and usually bitter and acrid flavor. Because acrid flavor helps to dissipate stasis and dissolve stagnation, and warm nature helps to unblock channels and promote blood flow, hence in addition to the functions of dredging the blood vessels to promote circulation, dissipating stasis to remove stagnation, breaking up stasis to disperse concretions, the medicines in the category can invigorate blood to regulate menstruation, unblock the channels to promote lactation, diffuse Bi to remove knot, promote healing to relieve pain, invigorate blood to disperse abscess, dissolve stasis to stanch bleeding, and dissipate stasis to promote regeneration.

凡离经之血不能及时排除或消散，停留于体内，包括因血行不畅而壅遏于经脉之内以及瘀积于脏腑、组织、器官，均称为瘀血。导致血瘀的原因有很多，脏腑之气血功能障碍、七情所伤等都可致血瘀，常见成因主要有以下几种。①寒凝致瘀：血液遇冷会发生凝滞，导致血液瘀滞或原有瘀血加重。②热邪致瘀：血受热邪熬煎凝聚成瘀。③气滞血瘀：气为血之帅，气行则血行，气滞则血瘀。④气虚血瘀：血液循脉流动主要依赖于气的推动，心气不足、推动无力可导致血瘀。⑤外伤血瘀：各类外伤致恶血在内不去则凝结成瘀。

If the extravagated blood cannot be eliminated or dissipated in time, it would stay in the body, i. e., being confined in the blood vessels due to poor blood flow or being confined in Zangfu organs, tissues and organs, resulting in static blood. In general, static blood is caused by the dysfunction of Qi and blood of viscera and bowels, or the damages caused by the seven emotions. The common causes are as follows. ①Congealing cold: when blood is cold, it will clot into static blood or the original static blood will deteriorate. ②Pathogenic heat: when the blood is suffering from the pathogenic heat, it would be coagulated into stasis. ③Qi stagnation: Qi is the commander of blood and blood is the mother of Qi, hence the blood moves when Qi moves, while blood stasis occurs when qi is stagnated. ④Qi deficiency: the blood flow mainly depends on the promotion of Qi; when the heart Qi is insufficient, the blood circulation is not adequately promoted and thereby blood stasis occurs. ⑤Traumatic injury: extravagated blood caused by various traumas will be condensed into blood stasis if it cannot be eliminated or dissipated in time.

瘀血内阻引起的病变即为血瘀证。血瘀证的主证有面色晦暗，口唇青紫，爪甲色青，舌紫暗、有瘀斑，脉涩或结代等。中医认为"瘀"为"积血"，"瘀证"为"积血之病"，可见瘀与血液停滞不能流通有关。研究表明，血瘀证至少存在以下病理生理改变。①血液处于高黏状态。②血液循环、微循环障碍。③血小板活化、黏附、聚集。④血液凝固与纤溶系统改变。⑤血栓形成。⑥组织和细胞代谢异常、免疫功能障碍等。总体来说，血瘀证与西医学中心脑血管疾病症状相似，因此活血化瘀药可用于治疗冠心病、心绞痛、高血压、脑动脉硬化、缺血性中风、头痛等。

Blood stasis is the pathological changes caused by static blood induced internal obstruction. The main clinical manifestations of blood stasis include dark complexion, blue lips, blue claws, dark tongue, ecchymosis, choppy pulse, and knotted and (or) intermittent pulse. According to TCM theories, "stasis" is "accumulation"; hence "blood stasis" is diseases caused by blood accumulation. It can be concluded that blood stasis is related to the stoppage of blood flow. Researches showed that at least the following pathophysiological changes exist in blood stasis. ①Increase of blood viscosity. ②Disorders of systemic circulation and microcirculation. ③Activation, adhesion, and aggregation of platelets. ④Changes of blood coagulation and fibrinolytic systems. ⑤Formation of thrombus. ⑥Abnormalities of tissue and cell metabolism, dysfunction of immune system, etc. In general, the symptoms of blood stasis are similar to those of cardiovascular and cerebrovascular diseases. Hence, the medicines in the category can be used for the treatment of coronary heart diseases, angina pectoris, hypertension, cerebral arteriosclerosis, ischemic stroke, and headache.

常用的活血化瘀药有丹参、川芎、延胡索、银杏叶、红花、益母草、莪术、水蛭、桃仁、姜黄等。药理研究表明，活血化瘀药治疗血瘀证与下列药理作用有关。

Commonly used blood invigorating and stasis dissolving medicines include *Dān shēn*, *Chuān xiōng*, *Yán hú suǒ*, *Yín xìng yè*, *Hóng huā*, *Yì mǔ cǎo*, *É zhú*, *Shuǐ zhì*, *Táo rén*, and *Jiāng huáng*. Their blood invigorating and stasis dissolving functions are related to the following pharmacological effects.

1. **抗血栓** 活血化瘀药具有抗血栓形成作用，此作用与抑制血小板活化聚集和黏附、抗凝血、提高纤溶系统活性等作用有关。例如，丹参中的多种成分具有抗血栓作用，其中，丹酚酸B可抑制凝血系统的激活、抑制血小板与暴露的内皮下胶原黏附；隐丹参酮可抑制血小板黏附内皮细胞；丹参总酚酸盐可提高血浆组织型纤溶酶原激活物（t-PA）水平，同时降低纤溶酶原激活物抑制剂–1（PAI-1）水平，使纤溶能力增强。川芎嗪在体外对诱导剂二磷酸腺苷（ADP）、胶原、凝血酶所致的血小板聚集有强烈的抑制作用。

(1) Anti-thrombotic effects The anti-thrombotic effects of blood invigorating and stasis dissolving medicines are related to their effects of inhibiting the activation, aggregation, and adhesion of platelets, prolonging clotting time, and improving the activity of fibrinolytic system. Salvianolic acid B inhibits the activation of the coagulation system, inhibits platelet adhesion to exposed subendothelial collagen; cryptotanshinone can inhibit the adhesion of platelets to endothelial cells; total phenolic salts of *Dān shēn* can increase the plasma level of tissue type plasminogen activator (t-PA) and reduce the levels of plasminogen activator inhibitor-1 (PAI-1), and thus enhance the fibrinolytic capacity; ligustrazine has strong *in vitro* inhibitory effects on platelets aggregation induced by adenosine diphosphate (ADP), collagen, and thrombin.

2. **改善血液流变学** 活血化瘀药可以降低血液黏度、降低血细胞比容、减慢红细胞沉降率、加快红细胞或血小板电泳速度、增加红细胞变形能力等。其中以丹参、川芎、益母草等作用较为明显。

(2) Improve hemorheology Blood invigorating and stasis dissolving medicines can reduce blood viscosity, reduce hematocrit, slow down the sedimentation rate of erythrocytes, accelerate the electrophoresis speed of erythrocytes or platelets, and increase the deformability of erythrocytes. Among them, the effects of *Dān shēn*, *Chuān xiōng*, and *Yì mǔ cǎo* are significant.

3. **改善微循环** 活血化瘀药可改善微循环，表现为改善微血流，使原本流动缓慢的血流加速；缓解微血管痉挛；减轻微循环内红细胞淤滞和聚集；减少或消除微血管襻顶淤血，使微血管轮廓清楚、形态趋于正常；降低毛细血管通透性，减少微血管周围渗血；促进建立侧支循环等。

(3) Improve microcirculation Blood invigorating and stasis dissolving medicines can speed up the blood flow of microcirculation, alleviate the spasm of micro-vessels, reduce the stasis and aggregation of red blood cells in the microcirculation, reduce or eliminate the stasis of micro-vessel crest, restore the clear outline and normal morphology of the micro-vessels, reduce capillary permeability and blood leakage around micro-vessels, and promote the establishment of collateral circulation.

4. **改善血流动力学** 多种活血化瘀药具有扩张外周血管、增加冠脉血流量、降低外周阻力、增加组织器官血流量的作用。丹参、川芎、益母草、桃仁、水蛭、莪术、延胡索等均有不同程度的降低血管阻力和增加器官血流量的作用。丹参酮 II_A 是丹参扩张冠状动脉的活性成分。此外，川芎的主要活性成分川芎嗪也有明显的舒张血管作用，可对抗多种诱发因素引起的血管收缩。

(4) Improve hemodynamics Several blood invigorating and stasis dissolving medicines have the effects of dilating peripheral blood vessels, increasing coronary blood flow, reducing peripheral resistance, and increasing blood flow to tissues and organs. The medicines including *Dān shēn*, *Chuān xiōng*, *Yì mǔ cǎo*, *Táo rén*, *Shuǐ zhì*, *É zhú*, and *Yán hú suǒ* have varying degrees of effects on reducing vascular resistance and increasing organ blood flow. Tanshinone II_A is the active constituent of *Dān shēn* in terms of dilating coronary arteries. In addition, ligustrazine has a significant vasodilating effect, which can counteract the contraction of vascular segments caused by different inducing factors.

5. 其他作用 活血化瘀药通常还有抗炎、抗氧化、抑制组织异常增生等作用，某些活血化瘀药还具有镇痛、调节子宫等作用。

(5) Others effects Blood invigorating and stasis dissolving medicines have other effects like anti-inflammation, anti-oxidation, and inhibiting abnormal tissue proliferation. In addition, some blood invigorating and stasis dissolving medicines have the effects of analgesia and regulating uterus.

常用活血化瘀药的主要药理作用见表14-1。

The main pharmacological effects of commonly used blood invigorating and stasis dissolving medicines are summarized in Table 14-1.

表 14-1　常用活血化瘀药的主要药理作用

类别	药物	改善血液流变学、抗血栓	抗炎、抗氧化	镇痛	调节子宫	其他药理作用
活血止痛药	丹参	+	+	+	–	抗肿瘤、保肝、抗菌
	川芎	+	+	+	+	保护心肌细胞、舒张血管
	延胡索	+	+	+	–	镇静催眠、抗溃疡、抗肿瘤
	银杏叶	+	+	–	–	抗动脉粥样硬化、平喘、改善记忆力
	姜黄	+	+	–	–	抗肿瘤、抗菌、神经保护
活血调经药	益母草	+	+	–	+	利尿、保护肾脏
	红花	+	+	+	+	保护血管内皮细胞、抗糖尿病肾病
	桃仁	+	+	+	+	抗组织纤维化、镇咳、润肠通便
破血消癥药	莪术	+	+	+	–	抗肿瘤、抗溃疡、保肝
	水蛭	+	+	–	–	抗动脉粥样硬化、抗纤维化、抗肿瘤

注："+"表示有明确作用；"–"表示无作用，或未查阅到相关研究文献

第二节　常用药物

Section 2　Commonly used medicines

PPT

丹参 ┆ *Dān shēn (Salvia miltiorrhiza Bge.)*

【来源 / Origin】

本品为唇形科植物丹参（*Salvia miltiorrhiza* Bge.）的干燥根和根茎。主产于安徽、江苏、山东、四川等省。秋季采挖，除去茎叶、泥沙、须根，晒干。

Dān shēn is the dried roots and rhizomes of *Salvia miltiorrhiza* Bge.. It is mainly produced in Anhui, Jiangsu, Shandong, Sichuan and other provinces. It is excavated in autumn, then removed stems, leaves, silt and fibrous roots, and dried after sun exposure.

【化学成分 / Chemical ingredients】

有效成分有水溶性及脂溶性两大类。水溶性主要是酚酸类化合物，如丹参酸 A(又称丹参素)、丹参酸 B、丹参酸 C，丹酚酸 A、丹酚酸 B、丹酚酸 C、丹酚酸 D、丹酚酸 E、丹酚酸 F、

丹酚酸 G、丹酚酸 H、丹酚酸 I、丹酚酸 J 等。丹参的脂溶性成分主要是二萜醌类化合物，现已细分到 40 余种，包括丹参酮类（邻醌型）和罗列酮类（邻羟基对醌型），根据其不同的化学结构分为丹参酮 I、丹参酮 II_A、丹参酮 II_B、隐丹参酮、异隐丹参酮、15,16- 二氢丹参酮，羟基丹参酮、丹参酸甲酯等化合物。

The active ingredients of *Dān shēn* are water-soluble and fat-soluble. Among them, the water-solubility is mainly phenolic compounds, such as salvianic acid A (Danshensu), salvianic acid B, salvianic acid C, salvianolic acid A, salvianolic acid B, salvianolic acid C, salvianolic acid D, salvianolic acid E, salvianolic acid F, salvianolic acid G, salvianolic acid H, salvianolic acid I, salvianolic acid J, etc. The fat-soluble components of salvia miltiorrhiza are mainly diterpene quinones, which have been classified into more than forty types, including tanshinones (o-quinone type) and rositone (o-hydroxy-p-quinone type). According to their different chemical structures, they are divided into tanshinone I, tanshinone II_A, tanshinone II_B, cryptotanshinone, iso cryptotanshinone, 15,16-dihydrotanshinone, hydroxytanshinone, methyl tanshinate and other compounds.

【药性与功效 / Chinese medicine properties】

味苦，性微寒，归心、肝经。具有活血祛瘀、通经止痛、清心除烦、凉血消痈的功效。主治胸痹心痛、脘腹胁痛、热痹疼痛、心烦不眠、月经不调、痛经经闭、疮疡肿痛。

In Chinese medicine theory, *Dān shēn* has a bitter taste and a slightly cold nature. It can enter the meridians of the heart and liver. *Dān shēn* can promote blood circulation and remove blood stasis, pass through menstruation and relieve pain, clear the heart and remove annoyance, and cool blood to eliminate diarrhea; Clinically it can be used to treat chest pain, heartache, abdominal pain, heat pain, upset and insomnia, irregular menstruation, dysmenorrhea, aches and swellings.

【药理作用 / Pharmacological effects】

1. 改善微循环　丹参提取物能有效抑制高胆固醇膳食家兔血清总胆固醇水平，减轻动脉粥样硬化所致髂动脉狭窄、降低血浆纤溶酶原水平、提高纤溶蛋白原水平，可在一定程度上抑制纤溶系统活性进而改善微循环，发挥抗动脉粥样硬化等作用。另外，丹参提取物喷鼻剂可有效缩小脑缺血大鼠脑梗死面积、抑制脑缺血大鼠全身微动脉收缩，进而改善脑缺血大鼠局部组织微循环、促进局部组织血流灌注恢复等；丹参酮 II_A 磺酸钠注射液（STS）可有效降低动脉粥样硬化所致脑梗死恢复期患者血清 D- 二聚体水平并调节凝血-纤溶系统平衡，进而改善缺血病灶微循环及患者预后。

(1) Improve microcirculation　The extract of *Dān shēn* can effectively inhibit the serum total cholesterol levels of rabbits with a high cholesterol diet, alleviate iliac artery stenosis caused by atherosclerosis, reduce plasma plasminogen levels, and increase fibrinoprotein levels, which can inhibit fibrinolytic system activity to improve the microcirculation to a certain extent, and exert anti-atherosclerotic effects. In addition, the extract of *Dān shēn* nasal spray can effectively reduce the cerebral infarction area of cerebral ischemia rats, inhibit the contraction of systemic arterioles in rats with cerebral ischemia, thereby improving the local tissue microcirculation in cerebral ischemia rats, and promoting local tissue blood perfusion, recovery, etc; tanshinone II_A sodium sulfonate injection (STS) can effectively reduce the serum D-dimer level and adjust the coagulation-fibrinolytic system balance of patients with cerebral infarction caused by atherosclerosis, thereby improving the microcirculation of ischemic lesions and patient prognosis.

2. 改善缺血再灌注损伤　丹参酮 II_A 磺酸钠注射液在临床主要用于冠心病的治疗，具有一定的改善心律失常和心绞痛症状、抑制炎症因子的作用。另外，STS 可降低局灶性脑缺血再灌注模型大鼠的脑梗死体积百分比、脑含水量、血清中肿瘤坏死因子 – α（TNF-α）的量，改善神经功能缺损。实验表明丹参酮 II_A 是丹参心肌保护作用的主要有效成分。

(2) Improving ischemia-reperfusion injury Tanshinone II_A sodium sulfonate injection is clinically used for the treatment of coronary heart disease, and has certain effects on improving the symptoms of arrhythmia and angina pectoris and inhibiting inflammatory factors. STS can reduce cerebral infarction volume percentage, brain water content, and tumor necrosis factor-α (TNF-α) in serum in focal cerebral ischemia-reperfusion model rats, and improve neurological deficits. Experiments show that tanshinone II_A is the main active ingredient of myocardial protection of salvia miltiorrhiza.

3. 抗肿瘤 丹参酮类化合物可抑制多种肿瘤细胞的生长、增殖，包括大肠癌、肺癌、肝癌、胰腺癌和胃癌细胞等。TanI 能阻断内皮细胞介导的血管生成起始阶段及全过程。隐丹参酮可显著抑制 4T1 肿瘤细胞的增殖。在划痕、Transwell 和斑马鱼肿瘤转移模型实验中，隐丹参酮在体内外均能显著抑制人乳腺癌 MDA-MB-231 细胞的转移作用，且在体外对抑制肿瘤细胞增殖也表现出一定作用。

(3) Antitumor Tanshinones can inhibit the growth and proliferation of a variety of tumor cells, including colorectal cancer, lung cancer, liver cancer, pancreatic cancer, and gastric cancer cells. TanI can block the initial stage and the whole process of endothelial cell-mediated angiogenesis. Cryptotanshinone can significantly inhibit the proliferation of 4T1 tumor cells. In scratch, Transwell, and zebrafish tumor metastasis model experiments, cryptotanshinone can significantly inhibit the metastasis of human breast cancer MDA-MB-231 cells *in vitro* and *in vivo*, and it can also inhibit tumor cell proliferation in vitro.

4. 保肝 给小鼠腹腔注射脂多糖（LPS），建立小鼠免疫性肝损伤模型，其血清 ALT 和 AST 较正常对照组显著升高，而提前灌胃一定剂量的丹参多糖，连续 7 天，每天 1 次，则可显著缓解 LPS 引起的血清 ALT 和 AST 升高。表明丹参多糖对免疫性肝损伤具有良好的保护作用。

(4) Hepatoprotective The mice were injected intraperitoneally with LPS to establish the mouse immune liver injury models. The serum ALT and AST were significantly higher than those in the normal control group, and a certain dose of salvia polysaccharide was administered to the stomach for 7 days in a row, once a day, significantly relieving the increase of serum ALT and AST caused by LPS. It shows that the salvia miltiorrhiza polysaccharide has a good protective effect on immune liver injury.

5. 抗菌 丹参酮类化合物对革兰阳性球菌，特别是金黄色葡萄球菌具有较强的抗菌作用。隐丹参酮对金黄色葡萄球菌、耐甲氧西林金黄色葡萄球菌和 β– 内酰胺酶阳性的金黄色葡萄球菌具有明显的抑制作用，表明丹参具有抗菌作用，其抗菌作用主要有效成分是隐丹参酮。

(5) Antibacterial Tanshinones have a strong antibacterial effect on Gram-positive cocci, especially on *Staphylococcus aureus* (SA). Cryptanthinone has a significant inhibitory effect on *Staphylococcus aureus*, methicillin-resistant *Staphylococcus aureus*, and β-lactamase-positive *Staphylococcus aureus*, indicating that *Dān shēn* has an antibacterial effect, and its main active ingredient is cryptotanshinone.

6. 抗炎 丹参提取物对感染性炎症和非感染性炎症都具有抗炎作用。动物实验表明，丹参煎煮后经灌胃方式给药，可有效降低关节炎小鼠关节液炎症因子水平；临床研究发现，丹参多酚酸盐（salvia polyphenolate）能有效提高急性冠脉综合征患者脂联素水平并抑制炎症反应，从而改善患者近、远期预后。

(6) Anti-inflammatory The extract of *Dān shēn* has a strong anti-inflammatory effect on infectious inflammation and a certain anti-inflammatory effect on non-infective inflammation. Animal experiments show that oral administration of Chinese medicine *Dān shēn* after decoction can effectively reduce the levels of inflammatory factors in the joint fluid of arthritic mice; clinical studies have found that *Dān shēn*

polyphenolate can effectively increase adiponectin levels and inhibit inflammation in patients with acute coronary syndrome response, thereby improving the short-term and long-term prognosis of patients.

7. 抗血栓　在丹参注射液干预的下肢深静脉血栓模型犬实验中，将预防组于造模前一周进行干预，治疗组造模成功后给药，并于第 2 天、第 9 天、第 20 天采空腹静脉血，并进行血液黏度、凝血酶原时间、纤维蛋白原等血液流变学指标检测。结果显示，丹参注射液能明显改善血液流变学各项指标，减轻血液高凝状态，但预防组效果明显优于治疗组，提示丹参注射液预防用药可有效预防下肢深静脉血栓形成。

(7) Antithrombotic　In the experiment of Danshen injection on lower extremity deep venous thrombosis model dogs, the prevention group was intervened early one week before the modeling, and the treatment group was administered after the successful modeling, and the fasting vein was collected on the 2nd, 9th, and 20th days. Hematology blood viscosity, prothrombin time, fibrinogen and other blood rheology indicators were tested. The results showed that Danshen injection can significantly improve the values of various hemorheology parameters and reduce the hypercoagulable state of the blood in the treatment group. It was suggested that Danshen injection can effectively prevent deep vein thrombosis of lower limbs.

8. 其他作用　丹参还具有抗凝血、扩血管、降血脂、降血压，抗氧化、雌激素样作用等；在治疗心血管系统疾病、消化系统疾病及神经系统疾病方面也有显著疗效。

(8) Other effects　*Dān shēn* also has anticoagulant, vasodilator, hypolipidemic, hypotensive, antioxidant, estrogen-like effects, protection of the digestive system and nervous system, etc., in the treatment of cardiovascular system diseases, digestive system diseases and nervous system diseases, it shows significant effects.

【不良反应 / Adverse effects 】

丹参注射液不良反应有头晕、头痛、心悸、红肿、疼痛、全身乏力、嗜睡、畏冷、寒战等；还可能出现变态反应，表现为过敏性休克、咽喉水肿等。临床有患者出现药源性肝炎、肌肉震颤等不良反应，严重时可诱发死亡。丹参口服类制剂不良反应为胃肠道不适，包括胃黏膜充血、水肿，胃肠道出血、糜烂性胃炎。此外，患者还有休克、高血压、心绞痛定时发作、晕厥、阴道出血、牙龈增生等症状。

The adverse reactions of *Dān shēn* injection include dizziness, headache, palpitations, redness and swelling, pain, general weakness, drowsiness, chills, chills, etc.; allergic reactions may also occur, including anaphylactic shock, sore throat. Clinically, patients also have adverse reactions such as drug-induced hepatitis and muscle tremor, which can induce death in severe cases. *Dān shēn* adverse reactions of oral preparations are occasional gastrointestinal discomfort, including gastric mucosal hyperemia, edema, occasional gastrointestinal bleeding and erosive gastritis. In addition, the patient also developed symptoms of shock, hypertension, timing of angina pectoris, syncope, vaginal bleeding, and gingival hyperplasia.

川芎 ｜ *Chuān xiōng (Ligusticum chuan xiong Hort.)*

【来源 / Origin 】

本品为伞形科植物川芎（*Ligusticum chuanxiong* Hort.）的干燥根茎。主产于我国四川、云南、贵州及广西等地。夏季当茎上的节盘显著突出并略带紫色时采挖，除去泥沙，晒后烘干，再去须根。

*Chuān xiōng i*s the dried rhizome of *Ligusticum chuanxiong* Hort.. The plant is mainly cultivated in Sichuan province, Yunnan province, Guizhou province, and Guangxi area in China. In summer, when the

微课

nodal disc on the stem is prominent and slightly purple, the plant is dug to remove the sediment, dried after sun exposure, and then removed the fibrous root.

【化学成分 / Chemical ingredients】

种类较多，主要为挥发油、有机酸、生物碱和多糖类成分。挥发油类约占1%，主要有苯酞类（藁本内酯、丁基酞内酯、丁烯基酞内酯、蛇床内酯、新蛇床内酯）和萜烯类（松油烯、香桧烯、月桂烯）；有机酸类有阿魏酸、咖啡酸、芥子酸、琥珀酸、油酸等；生物碱类有川芎嗪、三甲胺、黑麦碱、胆碱、腺苷、腺嘌呤、尿嘧啶等。

There are many chemical components in *Chuān xiōng*, such as essential oil, organic acid, alkaloid, polysaccharide, etc. Among them, the essential oil is about 1%, mainly including phthalides (Z-ligustilide, 3-n-butylphthalide, Z-3-butylidenephthalide, cnidilide, neocnidilide) and terpenes (terpinene, sabinene, 7-methyl-3-methyleneocta-1, 6-diene). Organic acids have ferulic acid, caffeic acid, sinapic acid, succinic acid, oleic acid, etc., In addition, the common alkaloids of *Chuān xiōng* have tetramethylpyrazine, trimethylamine, pelolyrine, choline, adenosine, adenine, uracil, etc.

【药性与功效 / Chinese medicine properties】

味辛，性温，归肝、胆、心包经。具有活血行气、祛风止痛的功效。临床主要用于胸痹心痛、胸胁刺痛、跌扑肿痛、月经不调、经闭痛经、癥瘕腹痛、头痛、风湿痹痛等。

In the theory of traditional Chinese medicine, *Chuān xiōng* is pungent in flavor and warm in nature. It can enter the meridians of liver, gallbladder and pericardium. It has the effect of promoting blood circulation and promoting Qi, dispelling wind and relieving pain. It is mainly used for chest pain, chest and flank tingling, tumbling pain, irregular menstruation, amenorrhea, abdominal pain, headache, rheumatic arthralgia, etc.

【药理作用 / Pharmacological effects】

1. **保护心肌细胞** 川芎水煎液能显著提高心肌细胞清除氧自由基的能力，提高线粒体抗氧化能力，拮抗心肌中琥珀酸脱氢酶及细胞色素氧化酶活性的降低，减少线粒体功能的损伤程度，从而发挥心脏功能的预保护作用。川芎中的川芎嗪、香兰素、大黄酚及阿魏酸等成分可直接作用于心肌细胞膜上的 α 受体或 β₁ 受体，川芎嗪可通过阻断脂多糖信号传导，拮抗脂多糖所引起的心肌细胞凋亡来发挥心肌细胞保护作用，洋川芎内酯 A 可保护新生大鼠心肌细胞免受缺氧–复氧损伤，同时可保护心肌微血管内皮细胞不受缺氧–复氧的影响。

(1) **Protect cardiomyocytes** The decoction of *Chuān xiōng* can significantly improve the ability of myocardial cells to scavenge oxygen free radicals, improve the antioxidant capacity of mitochondria, antagonize the decline of succinate dehydrogenase and cytochrome oxidase activity in myocardium, reduce the damage degree of mitochondrial function, so as to play the pre-protective role in heart function. Ligustrazine, vanillin, chrysophanol and ferulic acid in *Ligusticum Chuān xiōng* can directly act on α receptor or β₁ receptor on the myocardial cell membrane. Ligustrazine can protect myocardial cells by blocking lipopolysaccharide signaling and antagonizing the apoptosis of myocardial cells caused by lipopolysaccharides. Senkyunolide A can protect myocardial cells in neonatal rats from hypoxia-reoxygenation injury, and protect myocardial microvascular endothelial cells from hypoxia-reoxygenation.

2. **改善心肌缺血** 川芎煎剂能明显提高小鼠心肌营养血流量，降低小鼠心肌耗氧量。川芎生物碱能对抗垂体后叶素引起的心肌缺血性心电图变化。藁本内酯能够显著抑制血清游离脂肪酸的升高，阿魏酸能显著降低急性心肌缺血犬血清的乳酸水平。川芎嗪可减少结扎静脉造成的犬实验性心肌梗死的梗死范围，减轻病变程度，减少心肌坏死量。

(2) Improve myocardial ischemia *Chuān xiōng* decoction can significantly increase myocardial nutritional blood flow and reduce myocardial oxygen consumption in mice. The alkaloids of *Chuān xiōng* can resist myocardial ischemic ECG changes induced by the posterior pituitary. Ligustilide can significantly inhibit the increase of serum free fatty acids, and ferulic acid can significantly reduce the serum lactic acid level in dogs with acute myocardial ischemia. Ligustrazine can reduce the infarct range of experimental myocardial infarction in dogs caused by ligation of veins, reduce the degree of lesions, and decrease the amount of myocardial necrosis.

3. **改善脑缺血**　川芎嗪具有改善微循环作用，可通过增加脑皮质血流量，促进神经功能恢复。川芎嗪还能通过调节凋亡基因及促凋亡基因表达，减少缺血缺氧性脑组织损伤。川芎苯酞和川芎素也能改善局部缺血性脑损伤，后者主要通过增强大脑皮质细胞外信号调节激酶，以起到减少脑梗死面积作用，有利于改善神经功能缺损。

(3) Improve microcirculation Ligustrazine has the effect of improving microcirculation and can promote the recovery of nerve function by increasing the blood flow in the cerebral cortex. Ligustrazine can also reduce ischemic and hypoxic brain tissue damage by regulating the expression of apoptotic genes and pro-apoptotic genes. The phthalide of *Chuān xiōng* and chuanxiusin can also improve ischemic brain damage, the latter mainly enhances extracellular signal-regulated kinases in the cerebral cortex to reduce the area of cerebral infarction, which is beneficial to improve neurological deficits.

4. **舒张血管**　川芎嗪有利于舒张血管平滑肌，预防微血栓的形成，减轻血管内皮细胞的损伤程度，延缓早期动脉粥样硬化病变。丁烯基酞内酯对血管有较强的舒张作用。洋川芎内酯 A 和藁本内酯均具有血管舒张作用，并表现出对血管收缩剂的拮抗作用，藁本内酯血管舒张作用强于洋川芎内酯 A。藁本内酯和正丁基苯酞与大鼠主动脉平滑肌细胞具有亲和性，并能显著抑制由碱性成纤维细胞生长因子介导的大鼠血管平滑肌细胞的异常增殖。

(4) Effect on blood vessels Ligustrazine can relax vascular smooth muscle, prevent the formation of microthrombosis, reduce the damage degree of vascular endothelial cells, and delay the progress of early atherosclerosis. Butylphthalide has a strong vasodilative effect on blood vessels. Both senkyunolide A and ligustilide have vasodilation effect, and show the antagonistic effect on vasoconstrictor. Ligustilide had a stronger vasodilatory effect than senkyunolide A did. Ligustilide and n-butylphthalide have an affinity with rat aortic smooth muscle cells and can significantly inhibit the abnormal proliferation of rat vascular smooth muscle cells mediated by basic fibroblast growth factor.

5. **抗血栓**　川芎可通过降低血小板聚集率和改善血液流变学来抑制血栓的形成。川芎嗪对 ADP、胶原、凝血酶所引起的血小板聚集具有一定的抑制作用，其机制可能与减少血小板 TXA_2 生成，增加血小板 cAMP 含量，抑制血小板内容物有关。阿魏酸、洋川芎内酯 H、洋川芎内酯 I 可通过抑制 Con A 诱导的红细胞变形能力指数和定向指数的下降、降低红细胞聚集率来发挥抗血栓作用。

(5) Antithrombotic *Chuān xiōng* can inhibit the formation of thrombus by reducing platelet aggregation rate and improving hemorheology. Ligustrazine has a certain inhibitory effect on platelet aggregation caused by ADP, collagen and thrombin, and its mechanism may be related to the reduction of TXA_2 generation of platelets, the increase of platelet cAMP content, and the inhibition of platelet contents. Ferulic acid, senkyunolide H and senkyunolide I can play an antithrombotic role by inhibiting the Con A-induced decrease of erythrocyte deformability index and orientation index and reducing the erythrocyte aggregation rate.

6. **抗凝血**　采用注射盐酸肾上腺素和冰水浴共同复制急性血瘀大鼠模型，测定不同浓度川芎提取物给药前后大鼠的血浆纤维蛋白原（FIB）、凝血酶原时间（PT）和活化部分凝血酶原时间（APTT）的含量，比较不同浓度川芎提取物对急性血瘀大鼠凝血功能的影响。结果显示，应用川芎后大鼠的 FIB 含量明显升高，PT 和 APTT 明显减少，表明川芎对血瘀大鼠的凝血功能异常具有明显的改善作用，且具有剂量依赖性。

(6) Anticoagulant The model of acute blood stasis rats was established by injecting adrenaline hydrochloride and ice water bath. The contents of FIB, PT and APTT were measured before and after administration of different concentrations of *Chuān xiōng* extract. The effects of different concentrations of *Chuān xiōng* extract on the coagulation function of acute blood stasis rats were compared. The results showed that the FIB content of rats significantly increased, and the PT and APTT decreased significantly after the application of *Chuān xiōng*, which showed that *Chuān xiōng* had a significant improvement on blood coagulation dysfunction in rats with blood stasis, and had a dose-dependent effect.

7. 镇痛 通过改良椎管插线方法建立神经根型颈椎病大鼠神经根性疼痛模型，将大鼠随机分为 5 组：川芎高、中、低剂量组，模型组，颈复康组，每组 8 只。干预前及干预后 10 天分别进行疼痛行为及步态评估、左正中神经体感诱发电位（SEP）测量。干预结束后取受损颈髓及神经根组织，进行病理切片，观察形态学变化。结果显示，川芎高、中、低剂量灌胃给药后，可以明显改善模型大鼠根性疼痛的相关行为，恢复受损神经 SEP 的潜伏期、波幅及传导速度等，与模型组相比有显著性差异（*P*<0.05），并可发挥神经保护作用，减轻受损神经根的水肿变性、髓鞘脱失等损伤。说明川芎提取物可以明显减轻模型大鼠的颈神经根性疼痛，其作用可能与神经保护作用有关。

(7) Analgesic A modified spinal cannula method was used to establish a nerve root pain model in rats with cervical spondylotic radiculopathy. The rats were randomly divided into 5 groups: high-dose, medium-dose, and low-dose groups of *Chuān xiōng*, model group, and neck rehabilitation group, 8 rats in each group. Pain behavior, gait assessment and left median somatosensory evoked potential (SEP) measurements were performed before and 10 days after the intervention. The injured cervical spinal cord and nerve root tissue were taken after the intervention, and pathological sections were performed to observe the morphological changes. The results showed that high-dose, medium-dose, and low-dose intragastric administration of *Chuān xiōng* could significantly improve the related behaviors of root pain in model rats, restore the latency amplitude and conduction velocity of SEP in the damaged nerves (*P*<0.05), and exert a neuroprotective effect to reduce edema degeneration of injured nerve root, demyelination and other injuries. This shows that *Chuān xiōng* extract can significantly relieve cervical nerve root pain in model rats, and its effect may be related to neuroprotective effect.

8. 其他作用 川芎还具有降血压、降血脂、兴奋子宫平滑肌、镇静、抗痉挛、提高免疫及造血功能、保护神经、解热、消炎、抗肿瘤、抗氧化、治疗哮喘、孕激素样作用等。

(8) Other effects *Chuān xiōng* has the hypotensive, hypolipidemic, antispasmodic, antipyretic, anti-inflammatory, anti-tumor and anti-oxidation activities. Meanwhile, it can exert the effects of sedation, nerve protection, exciting uterine smooth muscle, improving immunity and hematopoietic function, treating asthma and curing progesterone like, etc.

【不良反应 / Adverse effects】

川芎的毒性和副作用不明显。小鼠连续 7 天以 125g/kg 剂量灌胃给予川芎水提物，未发现死亡。川芎水煎液小鼠腹腔注射与肌内注射的半数致死量分别为 65.86g/kg 和 66.42g/kg。川芎嗪小鼠静脉注射的半数致死量为 239mg/kg。亚急性毒性试验连续给药 4 周（每天 5~10mg/kg），在实验中犬未见中毒表现及明显病理变化。

The toxicity of *Chuān xiōng* is not obvious, The mice were administered orally with water extract of ligusticum chuanxiong at a dose of 125g/kg for 7 consecutive days, and no death was found. The half lethal doses of Chuanxiong decoction for intraperitoneal and intramuscular injection in mice were 65.86g/kg and 66.42g/kg, respectively. Half of the lethal dose of ligustrazine in mice was 239mg/kg. The subacute toxicity test was continuously administered for 4 weeks (5-10mg/kg per day). No poisoning and obvious pathological changes were observed in the experiment.

延胡索 ┊ *Yán hú suǒ*（*Rhizoma Corydalis*）

【来源 / Origin 】

本品为罂粟科植物延胡索（*Corydalis yanhusuo* W. T. Wang）的干燥块茎。主产于浙江、江苏、湖北等地。夏初茎叶枯萎时采挖，除去须根，洗净，置沸水中煮至恰无白心时，取出，晒干，生用或炙用。

Yán hú suǒ is a dried tuber of the poppy family *Corydalis yanhusuo* W. T. Wang. It is mainly produced in Zhejiang province, Jiangsu province, Hubei province in China. When its stems and leaves are withered in early summer, the plant is dug, removed the fibrous roots, washed , boiled in boiling water until there is almost no white heart, and then dried. It is usually used after drying in the sun or cooking.

【化学成分 / Chemical ingredients 】

有效成分为叔胺碱类和季胺碱类生物碱，含量分别约为 0.65% 和 0.30%。生物碱中主要成分是异喹啉类生物碱，包括延胡索甲素、四氢帕马丁（THP）、脱氢紫堇碱、巴马汀等；另有延胡索丙素、小檗碱、d– 海罂粟碱、α– 别隐品碱等。此外，尚含有挥发油、萜类、有机酸等。

Yán hú suǒ contains tertiary amine bases and quaternary amine base alkaloids, and the content is about 0.65% and 0.30%, respectively. The main components of alkaloids are isoquinoline alkaloids, including d-corydaline, tetrahydropalmatine (THP), dehydrocordaline, palmatine, etc. Additionally, it contains protopine, berberine, d-glaucine, α-allocryptopine , etc. *Yán hú suǒ* also contains volatile oils, terpenes, organic acids

【药性与功效 / Chinese medicine properties 】

味辛、苦，性温，归肝、脾经。具有活血、行气、止痛的功效。主治气血瘀滞引起的痛症。

In Chinese medicine theory, *Yán hú suǒ* hasthe pungent, bitter, and warm nature. It can enter the meridians of liver and spleen. *Yán hú suǒ* has the functions of activating blood and moving Qi to relieve pain. Clinically, it can be used for pain due to Qi stagnation and blood stasis.

【药理作用 / Pharmacological effects 】

1. 镇痛　用二甲基亚砜将四氢帕马丁配制成不同浓度（3mg/ml、6mg/ml、12mg/ml），制备模型前一小时按 1ml/kg 标准给大鼠灌胃，发现四氢帕马丁（3mg/ml、6mg/ml、12mg/ml）能明显减少福尔马林致痛模型大鼠的缩腿、舔爪时间。此外，与吗啡等麻醉性镇痛药相比，延胡索副作用少且安全，没有成瘾性。如给猴每天剂量从 60mg/kg 开始，逐渐增加至 200mg/kg，连续给药 3 个多月，停药后没有出现戒断症状。

(1) **Analgesic**　Use dimethyl sulfoxide to configure tetrahydropalmatine to different concentrations (3mg/ml, 6mg/ml, 12mg/ml). One hour before the model was prepared, rats were intragastrically administered at the standard of 1ml/kg, It was found that THP (3mg/ml, 6mg/ml, 12mg/ml) can significantly reduce the leg shrinking and paw licking time in formalin-induced pain rats. In addition, compared with narcotic analgesics such as morphine, *Yán hú suǒ* has fewer side effects, is safe, and is not addictive. For example, the daily dose of monkeys was started from 60mg/kg, gradually increased to

200mg/kg, and continuously administered for more than 3 months. No withdrawal symptoms occurred after stopping the drug.

2. **镇静、催眠** 小白鼠腹腔注射四氢帕马丁或丑素（corydalis L）40~200mg/kg，或癸素（corydalis J）10~50ml/kg。5~10分钟相继出现安静反应，匍匐笼角或互相依偎，以乙素最为明显，丑素次之，癸素最差。

(2) Sedative and hypnotic The mice were injected intraperitoneally with tetrahydropalmatine or corydalis L (40-200mg/kg), or corydalis J (10-50ml/kg). After about 5-10 minutes, the mice appeared to have a quiet effect one after the other, crept in the cage or snuggled each other. The order of strong and weak effects is tetrahydropalmatine, the most obvious, followed by corydalis L, the worst corydalis J.

3. **减轻脑缺血再灌注损伤** 利用大鼠脑缺血再灌注模型，设置对照组和四氢帕马丁组，观察到 THP 组的脑缺血再灌注海马组织中超氧化物歧化酶（SOD）、谷胱甘肽过氧化物酶（GSH-P_X）活性升高，同时脂质过氧化物丙二醛（MDA）明显降低，表明 THP 能抑制氧自由基及脂质过氧化物形成，从而减轻大鼠脑缺血再灌注损伤。此外，THP 能显著提高 Na^+-K^+-ATP 酶、Ga^{2+}-THP 酶的活性和阻滞钙通道，促进细胞内外离子的平衡恢复，避免细胞因钙超载而引起损害，防止线粒体结构和功能遭破坏所致的能量代谢失衡，从而减轻大鼠脑缺血再灌注损伤。

(3) Reduce cerebral ischemia-reperfusion injury Using a rat cerebral ischemia-reperfusion model, a control group and a THP group were set up, It was observed that the activities of superoxide dismutase (SOD) and glutathione peroxidase (GSH-P_X) in hippocampus of cerebral ischemia-reperfusion rat model of THP group were enhanced, while lipid peroxidation malondialdehyde aldehyde (MDA) was significantly reduced; this indicates that THP can inhibit the formation of oxygen free radicals and lipid peroxides, thereby reducing cerebral ischemia-reperfusion injury in rats. In addition, THP can significantly enhance the activity of Na^+-K^+-ATPase and Ga^{2+}-THP enzyme, and can also block calcium channels, promote the restoration of the balance of ions inside and outside the cell, avoid damage caused by calcium overload, and prevent energy metabolism imbalance caused by the disruption of mitochondrial structure and function, thereby alleviating cerebral ischemia-reperfusion injury in rats.

4. **减轻心肌缺血再灌注损伤** 四氢帕马丁是抗心肌缺血再灌注损伤的主要有效成分。在用自由基发生系统 $FeSO_4$/抗坏血酸（0.1μmol/L）致离体大鼠心肌缺血再灌注损伤时，在体系中加入 THP（1μmol/L、10μmol/L）、谷胱甘肽（10μmol/L）后，心肌中 MDA 含量减少，LDH 释放减少，SOD 和 GSH-P_X 活力明显增加，再灌注室颤的发生率明显降低，窦性节律时间显著延长。说明 THP 对外源性自由基发生系统 $FeSO_4$/抗坏血酸加重离体大鼠心肌缺血再灌注损伤具有保护作用。

(4) Reduce myocardial ischemia-reperfusion injury Tetrahydropalmatine is the main effective component against myocardial ischemia and reperfusion injury. When the free radical generating system $FeSO_4$/ascorbic acid (0.1 μmol/L) was used to treat ischemia-reperfusion injury in isolated rat hearts, THP (1 μmol/L, 10 μmol/L) and glutathione were added to the system. after that, the content of MDA and the release of LDH in myocardium decreased, SOD and GSH-P_X activities improved significantly, obviously reduced the incidence of reperfusion ventricular fibrillation, and significantly prolonged the time of sinus rhythm. This shows that THP has a protective effect on the ischemia-reperfusion injury of isolated rat hearts exacerbated by the exogenous free radical generation system $FeSO_4$ / ascorbic acid.

5. **抗溃疡** 用 dl-THP 15mg/kg、30mg/kg、45mg/kg 给胃黏膜损伤大鼠灌胃，1日2次，共5次。dl-THP（15mg/kg、30mg/kg、45mg/kg）能抑制大鼠胃黏膜损伤，且呈剂量依赖关系，dl-THP

30mg/kg 对大鼠慢性胃溃疡的抑制率为 75.8%，与雷尼替丁 30mg/kg 的抑制率 67.7% 相仿。说明了 dl-THP 有明显的抗实验性胃溃疡作用。

(5) Anti-ulcer The rats with gastric mucosal injury were administrated with dl-THP (15mg/kg, 30mg/kg, 45mg/kg) twice a day for 5 times. It was observed that dl-THP (15mg/kg, 30mg/kg, 45mg/kg) can inhibit gastric mucosal injury in rats in a dose-dependent manner. The inhibition rate of dl-THP 30mg/kg on chronic gastric ulcer in rats was 75.8%, which was similar to that of raney（67.7%）at a dose of 30mg/kg. It shows that dl-THP has the obvious anti-experimental gastric ulcer effect.

6. 抗肿瘤 用四甲基偶氮唑盐（MTT）法研究得出，延胡索脂溶性非酚性生物碱组分对肝肿瘤细胞杀伤活性最强，可有效抑制 SMMC-7721 细胞的生长，半数抑制浓度（IC_{50}）约为 35μg/ml。延胡索碱对人鼻咽喉细胞株 KB 的增殖也有抑制作用，其 IC_{50} 约为 10μmol/L。此外，当延胡索碱的浓度为 4.7μmol/L 和 10μmol/L 时，均能较好地抑制人胃癌细胞株 BGC 细胞和人鼻咽喉细胞株 KB 的增殖。

(6) Antitumor It was found by MTT method that the fat-soluble non-phenolic alkaloid component of *Yán hú suǒ* had the strongest killing activity on liver tumor cells. It could effectively inhibit the growth of SMMC-7721 cells with IC_{50} of about 35μg/ml. Corydaline also inhibited the increase of KB in human nasopharyngeal cell lines, with IC_{50} of about 10 μmol/L. In addition, when the concentration of corydaline is 4.7μmol/L and 10μmol/L, it had a high activity in inhibiting the increase of the human gastric cancer cell line BGC cells and the human nasopharyngeal cell line KB.

7. 抗血栓 采用电刺激法刺激实验性大鼠颈总动脉，可激活外源性凝血系统导致血栓形成，成功复制大鼠体内血栓模型，进一步实验得出延胡索提取物高、中剂量组和阳性对照药组动物体内血栓形成所需时间明显大于正常对照组；低剂量组动物体内血栓形成所需时间与正常对照组比较虽无显著性差异，但有一定的增加趋势。上述实验结果表明，延胡索提取物能显著抑制活体状态下动脉血栓的形成，提示其具有抗血栓的作用，从而有效避免了血栓形成的潜在风险，充分体现了延胡索提取物具有活血化瘀的功能。

(7) Antithrombotic By stimulating the common carotid artery of experimental rats with electrical stimulation, the external coagulation system can be activated to cause thrombosis. successfully making the thrombus model in rats. Further experiments showed that the thrombus formation time in the high dose group, the middle dose group and the positive control group was significantly longer than that in the normal control group. Although the time required for thrombus formation in the low-dose group was not significantly different from that in the normal control group, there was a certain increasing trend. The above experimental results show that yanhusuo extract can significantly inhibit the formation of arterial thrombosis *in vivo*, showing its antithrombotic effect, thus effectively avoiding the potential risk of thrombosis, fully reflecting the function of yanhusuo extract in promoting blood circulation and removing blood stasis.

8. 其他作用 延胡索还具有抗凝血、抗心律失常、保护心肌、降血压、增强抗氧化能力并延缓衰老、抑制胃酸分泌、提高抗应激能力、增强记忆以及用于成瘾药物的戒断等作用。

(8) Other effects *Yán hú suǒ* also has the functions of anticoagulation, antiarrhythmia, myocardial protection, lowering blood pressure, enhancing antioxidant capacity and delaying aging, inhibiting gastric acid secretion, antiulcer, improving antistress ability, enhancing memory and memory, treating the drug withdrawal and other effects.

【不良反应 / Adverse effects】
　　延胡索及其生物碱的不同剂型在临床应用时，未发现一般剂量下的显著毒性或副反应；当给药剂量达到 40g/kg 时，小鼠活动减少、呼吸缓慢、行动姿势改变。

In the clinical application of different formulations of *Yán hú suǒ* and its alkaloids, no significant side effects were found at the general dose; when the dose reached 40g/kg, the mice became quiet , and had the symptoms of breathing slowly, changing posture, tachycardia.

银杏叶 ⋮ *Yín xìng yè*（*Ginkgo biloba*）

【来源 / Origin】

本品为银杏科植物银杏（*Ginkgo biloba* L.）的干燥叶。主产于江苏、浙江、山东、湖北等地。秋季叶尚绿时采收，及时干燥。内服煎汤、外用煎水洗或捣敷。

Yín xìng yè is the dried leaf of *Ginkgo biloba* L.. The plant is mainly produced in Jiangsu province, Zhejiang province, Shandong province, Hubei province and other places. In autumn, when they are still green, the leaves of *Ginkgo biloba* are picked and dried in time, decoctions is used orally, and if used externally, it is washed or applied.

【化学成分 / Chemical ingredients】

药效成分主要是黄酮类物质，有 40 多种，含量占 24%。主要包括单黄酮类、双黄酮类以及儿茶素类，其中单黄酮类中的山奈素、槲皮素和异鼠李素含量最高，被认为是银杏总黄酮中真正有活性的物质。此外，银杏叶中还含有银杏酸和银杏二萜内酯类化合物，二萜内酯主要有倍半萜内酯（即白果内酯）及银杏内酯 A、银杏内酯 B、银杏内酯 C、银杏内酯 M、银杏内酯 J 等。

The main medicinal ingredient in *Yín xìng yè* is flavonoids. It has about 40 kinds of flavonoids, and their content can reach 24% in the total extract. It mainly includes monoflavones, diflavones, and catechins. Among them, kaempferin, quercetin, and isorhamnetin are the the most abundant in monoflavones, and they are considered to be truly active substances in total flavones of ginkgo. In addition, ginkgo biloba leaves also contain ginkgo acid and ginkgo diterpene lactones. Diterpene lactones mainly include sesquiterpene lactones, namely ginkgolide and ginkgolide A、ginkgolide B、ginkgolide C、ginkgolide M、ginkgolide J, etc.

【药性与功效 / Chinese medicine properties】

味甘、苦、涩，性平，归心、肺经。具有活血化瘀、通络止痛、敛肺平喘、化浊降脂的功效。主治瘀血阻络、胸痹心痛、中风偏瘫、肺虚咳喘、高脂血症。

In Chinese medicine theory, *Yín xìng yè* has the nature of sweet and flat, bitter, and astringent. It can enter the meridians of the heart and lungs. *Yín xìng yè* can promote blood circulation and remove blood stasis, Tongluo analgesic, convergence of lungs, asthma, Huazhuo and lipid-lowering effects. Clinically, it is used to treat blood stasis and obstruction, chest pain, heartache, stroke, hemiplegia, lung deficiency, asthma and hyperlipidemia.

【药理作用 / Pharmacological effects】

1. 扩张血管、调节血脂　豚鼠或大鼠注射银杏叶提取物后，可使其后肢血管扩张，双黄酮类对大鼠后肢血管也有扩张作用。另外，银杏叶提取物（GBE）可调节血脂，对大鼠血脂调节作用的研究实验表明，银杏叶提取物可有效降低高脂饲料饲喂大鼠的血清 TC 和 TG 水平。在临床试验中，对比口服辛伐他汀片组发现口服银杏叶胶囊也具有明显的降血脂和血液黏度作用，研究还发现其在降脂的同时，也能有效地降低血清中甘油三酯和脂蛋白胆固醇的含量，能够较好地改善或减轻高脂血症患者临床症状。

(1) Dilate blood vessels and regulate blood lipids　After the injection of *Yín xìng yè* extract into guinea pigs or rats, the blood vessels of their hind limbs can be dilated, and the biflavones in the leaves can also dilate the blood vessels of the hind limbs of rats. In addition, the extract of *Yín xìng yè* can regulate blood lipids, and studies on blood lipid regulation effects in rats have shown that the extract of *Yín xìng yè* can effectively reduce serum TC and TG levels in high-fat feed rats. In clinical experiments, compared with the oral simvastatin tablet group, it was found that oral *Yín xìng yè* capsule also had a significant effect on lowering blood lipids and lowering blood viscosity. Studies have also found that while reducing blood lipids, it can also effectively reduce the content of triglycerides and lipoprotein cholesterol in serum, which can better improve or reduce clinical symptoms of hyperlipidemia.

2. **抗脑血管缺血再灌注损伤**　在沙鼠结扎一侧颈动脉造成的脑缺血模型与三乙基锡（triethyltin）细胞毒损伤的大鼠脑水肿模型都观察到银杏叶有保护脑组织、对抗脑缺血与脑水肿的作用，能防止缺血缺氧引起的氧化磷酸化脱偶联反应，保持细胞内线粒体的正常呼吸，阻止脑缺血造成的细胞膜离子转运紊乱，从而防止细胞内 Ca^{2+} 超负荷及脑细胞损伤。另一作用机制是清除自由基，防止细胞膜脂质过氧化。

(2) Anti-cerebrovascular ischemia-reperfusion injury　Both cerebral ischemia model caused by ligating one carotid artery and cerebral edema rat model induced by triethyltin cytotoxic had observed that *Yín xìng yè* can protect brain tissue against cerebral ischemia and cerebral edema. It could prevent the oxidative phosphorylation uncoupling reaction caused by ischemia and hypoxia, keep the normal respiration of mitochondria in cells, prevent the disorder of ion transport in cell membrane caused by cerebral ischemia, so as to prevent the overload of Ca^{2+} in cells and the damage of brain cells. Another mechanism of action is the action of scavenging free radicals to prevent lipid peroxidation of the cell membrane.

3. **抑制血小板聚集、抗血栓**　以血小板活化因子（PAF）作为血小板聚集诱导剂，将银杏二萜内酯分别加入采集的兔血中，经检验，各银杏二萜内酯化合物对 PAF 诱导家兔血小板聚集均有一定抑制作用，且呈量–效关系。实验表明银杏二萜内酯类化合物对 PAF 受体具有拮抗作用，抑制血小板聚集能力依次为 GK>GB>GA>GC>GM>GJ>GL。其不仅可以抑制血栓形成，还可以抑制 PAF 过度释放导致的神经炎症、细胞凋亡、氧化损伤等。

(3) Inhibition of platelet aggregation and antithrombotic　PAF was used as an inducer of platelet aggregation, and ginkgo diterpene lactones were added to the collected rabbit blood. After examination, each of the gingko diterpene lactone compounds had a certain effect on PAF-induced rabbit platelet aggregation, and there was a dose-effect relationship. Experiments showed that gingko diterpenoid lactones had antagonistic effect on PAF receptor, and the ability of inhibiting platelet aggregation was in the order of GK>GB>GA>GC>GM>GJ>GL, which could not only inhibit thrombosis, but also inhibit neuroinflammation, apoptosis, oxidative damage and the increase of vascular permeability caused by excessive release of PAF.

4. **抗动脉粥样硬化**　临床试验和动物实验均表明银杏叶能有效降低血脂浓度，改善血管内皮功能。通过观察 GBE 对高胆固醇饲料喂养大鼠 NF-κB 表达的影响，发现 GBE 组 TC、TG、LDL-C 水平和 NF-κB 表达阳性率均低于高脂组，高脂组的血管内皮细胞存在明显的崩解现象，可见斑块形成，而 GBE 组损伤轻微。因此 GBE 可以通过调节血脂、抑制 NF-κB 表达，起到减轻动脉粥样斑块局部的炎症反应、保护血管内皮细胞而发挥防治动脉粥样硬化的作用。

(4) Anti-atherosclerotic　Clinical tests and animal experiments have shown that *Yín xìng yè* can effectively reduce the blood lipid concentration of atherosclerosis, and can significantly improve vascular endothelial function. by observing the effect of *Yín xìng yè* extract on the expression of NF-κB in high cholesterol-fed rats, it was found that the levels of cholesterol (TC), triacylglycerol (TG), low-density lipoprotein cholesterol (LDL-C) and the positive rate of NF-κB expression were lower than those in the high-fat group. The vascular endothelial cells in the high-fat group had obvious disintegration, and plaque formation was visible, while the GBE group had minor damage. Therefore, GBE can play a role in preventing and treating atherosclerosis by regulating blood lipids and inhibiting NF-κB expression, reducing the local inflammatory response of atherosclerotic plaques, protecting vascular endothelial cells.

5. 平喘　采用卵蛋白等致敏物构建大鼠哮喘模型，以 2mg/d 的银杏黄酮提取物为治疗组，经与模型组对比，治疗组支气管壁和平滑肌增厚程度显著小于模型组。结果表明，高剂量的银杏黄酮能通过有效抑制哮喘大鼠肺组织的 HIF-1α 和 VEGF 的表达，抑制气道壁和平滑肌增生，改善肺组织的缺氧环境，抑制哮喘模型大鼠的气道重塑，从而起到平喘的作用。

(5) Antiasthmatic　Before the stimulation to rat asthma model constructed with allergens such as egg protein, 2 mg/d ginkgo flavonoid extract was injected intraperitoneally as a treatment group. Comparing with the model group, the thickness of the bronchial wall and smooth muscle in the treatment group was significantly smaller than that in the model group. It is concluded that high-dose ginkgo flavonoids can inhibit the expression of HIF-1α and VEGF in the lung tissue of asthmatic rats, inhibit the airway wall and smooth muscle proliferation, improve the hypoxic environment of lung tissue, and further inhibit airway remodeling in asthmatic rats. Thus, it can relieve asthma.

6. 改善学习记忆力　银杏黄酮能提高抗氧化酶活性，调节氧化与抗氧化系统平衡，增强清除氧自由基的能力，抑制氧化应激，改善学习记忆能力。在对东莨菪碱（scopolamine）建立大鼠获得性记忆障碍模型观察中发现，银杏黄酮能明显缩短大鼠寻找平台的潜伏期，并显著增加其穿越目标象限平台位置次数，提示银杏黄酮能有效改善东莨菪碱诱导的记忆障碍大鼠模型所致的学习记忆能力下降。

(6) Improve learning and memory　Ginkgo flavonoids can increase the activity of antioxidant enzymes, regulate the balance between oxidation and antioxidant systems, enhance the ability to scavenge oxygen free radicals, inhibit oxidative stress, and improve learning and memory functions. In the rat scopolamine model of acquired memory impairment, ginkgo flavonoids could significantly shorten the latency period for rats to find a platform and significantly increase the number of times they cross the target quadrant platform position, indicating that ginkgo flavone could effectively improve the learning and memory ability of scopolamine-induced memory impairment rats.

7. 其他作用　银杏叶还有提高免疫力、抗炎、抗病毒、抗过敏、抗肿瘤、抗骨质疏松、抗流感病毒等多种作用。

(7) Other effects　*Yín xìng yè* also has improving immunity, anti-inflammatory, anti-viral, anti-allergic, anti-tumor and anti-osteoporosis effects.

【不良反应 / Adverse effects】

给犬静脉注射大剂量银杏叶乙醇提取物"舒血宁"一周，每天 1 次，每次用量相当于成人用量的 10~40 倍，可出现流涎、恶心、呕吐、腹泻、食欲减退等症状。临床应用副作用较少，少数患者有食欲减退、恶心、腹胀、大便稀、口干、鼻塞、头晕、头痛和耳鸣等症状，个别患者会出现过敏性皮疹。

Dogs were given a large dose of *Yín xìng yè* ethanol extract "Shuxuening" once a day for a week, and the dosage is equivalent to 10 to 40 times of the adult dosage, which has caused drooling, nausea, vomiting, diarrhea, and loss of appetite. There are few side effects in clinical application, a few patients have anorexia, nausea, abdominal distention, loose stool, dry mouth, nasal obstruction, dizziness, headache and tinnitus, and some patients have allergic rash.

红花 ︱ *Hóng huā (Carthami Flos)*

【来源 / Origin】

本品为菊科植物红花（*Carthamus tinctorius* L.）的干燥花。中国大部分地区均有栽培，主产于河南、四川、浙江、新疆等地。夏季花由黄变红时采摘。阴干或晒干。

Hóng huā is the dried flower of *Carthamus tinctorius* L. The plant is widely cultivated in China, mainly in Henan province, Sichuan province, Zhejiang province, and Xinjiang Uygur Autonomous region. It is harvested in summer when the flower changes from yellow to red. After being dried in the shade or in the sun, the flower is used for Chinese medicinal preparation.

【化学成分 / Chemical ingredients】

主要含黄酮类、脂肪酸、多糖等成分。黄酮类主要为红花黄色素（SY），是一种含有多种成分的水溶性混合物，以羟基红花黄色素 A（HSYA）含量最高。

Hóng huā contains flavonoids, fatty acids, polysaccharides and other constituents. The main flavonoid is safflower yellow (SY), a water-soluble mixture of various constituents. The content of hydroxysafflor yellow A (HSYA) is the highest in SY.

【药性与功效 / Chinese medicine properties】

味辛，性温，归心、肝经。具有活血通经、散瘀止痛之功。主治经闭痛经、恶露不行、癥瘕痞块、胸痹心痛、瘀滞腹痛、胸胁刺痛、跌扑损伤、疮疡肿痛。

In Chinese medicine theory, *Hóng huā* has the flavor of acrid and the nature of warm. It can enter the meridians of heart and liver. *Hóng huā* can invigorate blood to promote menstruation and dissipate stasis to relieve pain. Clinically it can be used for menstrual block, painful menstruation, inhibited lochia, concretions (fixed lower abdominal masses of definite shape) and conglomerations (movable lower abdominal masses of indefinite shape), chest Bi caused heart pain, abdominal pain due to blood stasis and Qi stagnation, stabbing pain in the chest and rib-side, injuries (from falls, fractures, contusions and strains), sores and ulcers induced swelling and pain.

【药理作用 / Pharmacological effects】

1. 抗凝血、抗血栓 红花对内源性和外源性凝血均有显著抑制作用，可延长大鼠血浆凝血酶原时间、凝血酶时间、活化部分凝血酶原时间并降低血浆中纤维蛋白原含量。红花黄色素能缩短血栓长度、减轻血栓重量，具有抗血栓作用。红花抗血栓作用与抗凝血有关，也与抗血小板聚集有关。红花可抑制二磷酸腺苷、胶原、血小板活化因子等诱导的血小板聚集，对已聚集的血小板也有解聚作用。羟基红花黄色素 A 已被证实为 PAF 受体拮抗剂。此外，红花抗血栓也与提高血浆中组织型纤溶酶原激活物活性、促进纤溶酶原转变为纤溶酶有关。

(1) Anti-coagulation and anti-thrombosis *Hóng huā* has strong inhibitory effects on endogenous and exogenous coagulation. *Hóng huā* can prolong the prothrombin time (PT), thrombin time (TT), activated partial thromboplastin time (APTT) and reduce the plasma content of fibrinogen in rats. SY can shorten the length and reduce the weight of thrombus, showing anti-thrombotic effects. The anti-thrombotic effect of *Hóng huā* is related to its inhibitory effects on coagulation and platelet aggregation. *Hóng huā* can inhibit platelet aggregation induced by adenosine diphosphate (ADP), collagen, and platelet activating factor (PAF). Furthermore, it can disperse the aggregated platelets. HSYA has been identified as a PAF receptor antagonist. In addition, the anti-thrombotic effect of *Hóng huā* is also related to its role in improving the activity of tissue-type plasminogen activator (t-PA) in plasma and promoting the transformation of plasminogen into plasmin.

2. 保护血管内皮细胞 红花水提物、红花黄色素、羟基红花黄色素 A 对氧化低密度脂蛋白（ox-LDL）、溶血卵磷脂（LPC）、过氧化氢（H_2O_2）所致血管内皮细胞损伤均有保护作用。羟基红花黄色素 A 保护血管内皮作用与提高线粒体活性、提高缺氧耐受性、抑制氧化应激损伤及凋亡、促进增殖、促进组织黏附、抗炎等机制有关。

(2) Vascular endothelial cells (VECs) protection *Hóng huā* water extract, SY, and HSYA have protective effects on VECs treated with oxidized low density lipoprotein (ox-LDL), lysophosphatidylcholine (LPC), and hydrogen peroxide (H_2O_2). The protective effect of HSYA on VECs is related to the mechanisms of improving mitochondrial activity, improving hypoxia tolerance, inhibiting damage and apoptosis caused by oxidative stress, promoting proliferation, promoting tissue adhesion, and anti-inflammation.

3. 抗心肌缺血 红花黄色素对多种心肌梗死动物模型具有显著保护作用，可缩小心肌梗死范围，缓解微结构损伤，减少乳酸脱氢酶（LDH）和磷酸激酶（CPK）漏出，并改善缺血引起的心功能减退和心电图改变。抗心肌缺血机制主要如下。①抗凝血、抗血栓及抗血小板聚集，改善血流动力学，增加冠脉流量，减慢心率，改善心肌缺血缺氧状态。②缓解心肌线粒体肿胀及膜流动性下降，缓解缺血再灌注时三磷酸腺苷（ATP）合成障碍，改善心肌能量代谢。③提高超氧化物歧化酶活性，清除氧自由基，抑制脂质过氧化反应，抑制氧化应激所致心肌细胞凋亡。羟基红花黄色素 A 为查尔酮类结构，其分子中含多个酚羟基，其抗氧化作用与这些酚羟基有关。

(3) Anti-myocardial ischemia SY has significant protective effects on model animals of myocardial infarction. It can reduce the scope of myocardial infarction, alleviate the damage of microstructure, reduce the leakage of lactate dehydrogenase (LDH) and creatine phosphokinase (CPK), and improve the myocardial dysfunction and electrocardiogram (ECG) changes caused by ischemia. The mechanisms are mainly as follows. ①Improves the state of ischemia and hypoxia by inhibiting coagulation, preventing thrombosis, reducing platelet aggregation, improving hemodynamics, increasing coronary blood flow, and slowing down the heart rate. ②Improves myocardial energy metabolism by alleviating myocardial mitochondrial swelling and decreased membrane fluidity, and alleviating ATP synthesis disorders during ischemia-reperfusion. ③Inhibits oxidative stress induced apoptosis of cardiomyocytes by increasing superoxide dismutase (SOD) activity, scavenging oxygen free radicals, and inhibiting lipid peroxidation. The antioxidant effect of HSYA is related to its chalcone structure, which contains multiple phenolic hydroxyl groups.

4. 抗脑缺血 红花黄色素及羟基红花黄色素 A 均能显著增加缺血再灌注后局部脑血流量，降低脑组织含水量，缩小脑梗死面积，减轻缺血所致病理学变化，并改善神经行为学症状。抗脑缺血机制主要如下。①抗凝血、抗血栓及抗血小板聚集，改善脑供血。②提高脑线粒体 ATP 酶活性，保护缺血脑细胞线粒体，改善能量代谢。③清除氧自由基，抑制脂质过氧化，抑制氧化应激所致神经细胞凋亡。④抑制神经元及小胶质细胞炎症反应。⑤抑制 N- 甲基 -D- 天冬氨酸（NMDA）受体表达及介导的细胞内 Ca^{2+} 浓度的增加，从而抑制兴奋性氨基酸毒性作用。⑥激活脑缺血再灌注损伤脑组织自噬信号通路。⑦增强星形胶质细胞活性。

(4) Anti-cerebral ischemia SY and HSYA can significantly increase the local cerebral blood flow after ischemia-reperfusion, reduce the water content of brain tissue, reduce the scope of cerebral infarction, alleviate the pathological changes caused by ischemia, and improve the neurobehavioral symptoms. The anti-cerebral ischemia mechanisms are mainly as follows. ①Improving cerebral blood supply through anti-coagulation, anti-thrombosis and anti-platelet aggregation. ②Improving energy metabolism of ischemic brain cells through increasing the ATPase activity and protecting the integrity of mitochondria. ③Scavenging oxygen free radicals, inhibiting lipid peroxidation, and inhibiting neuron apoptosis caused by oxidative stress. ④Inhibiting inflammatory response of neurons and microglia. ⑤Inhibiting N-methyl-D-aspartic acid (NMDA) receptor expression and the increase of intracellular Ca^{2+} concentration mediated by NMDA receptor, thus inhibiting the toxic effect of excitatory amino acids. ⑥Activating autophagy signaling pathway in brain tissue. ⑦ Increasing the activity of astrocytes.

5. 抗炎、镇痛　红花黄色素对组胺所致大鼠皮肤毛细血管通透性增加、甲醛性大鼠足肿胀（炎性渗出）及大鼠棉球肉芽肿的形成均有显著抑制作用，表明其具有多环节抗炎作用。例如，红花黄色素可抑制 PAF 诱发的血小板聚集，并缓解其作为炎症介质介导的炎症反应过程。此外，红花黄色素对热板及醋酸所致小鼠疼痛反应均有强且持久的抑制作用，表明其对锐痛（热刺痛）及钝痛（化学性刺痛）均有效。

(5) Anti-inflammation and analgesia　SY has significant inhibitory effects in rats on histamine-induced capillary permeability increase of skin, formaldehyde caused foot swelling, and cotton balls caused granuloma, indicating that SY has multiple anti-inflammatory effects. For example, SY can inhibit platelet aggregation induced by PAF, thus inhibiting PAF mediated inflammatory response. In addition, SY has strong and long-lasting inhibitory effects on the pain response of mice induced by hot plate and acetic acid, indicating that it is effective for acute pain (hot tingling) and dull pain (chemical tingling).

6. 调节子宫　红花对子宫的调节作用与子宫状态有关。红花煎剂对小鼠、兔、犬等多种动物离体及在体子宫有兴奋作用，表现为子宫收缩张力和频率均显著增加，大剂量甚至可以使子宫痉挛。对妊娠子宫的作用更加显著。红花对子宫的兴奋作用与激动组胺 H_1 受体及肾上腺素 α 受体有关。但对处于缩宫素引起痉挛状态的子宫，羟基红花黄色素 A 则可显著抑制其收缩频率和张力。

(6) Uterus regulation　The regulative effects of *Hóng huā* on uterus are related to the state of uterus. *Hóng huā* decoction has both *in vitro* and *in vivo* excitatory effects on the uterus of mice, rabbit, and dog. This excitatory effect is manifested by a significant increase in uterine contraction tension and frequency. Large doses of *Hóng huā* decoction can even cause uterine spasm. *Hóng huā* decoction has a stronger excitatory effect on the pregnant uterus. The effect is related to the activation of histamine H_1 receptor and adrenaline α receptor. However, HYSA can significantly inhibit the contractile frequency and tension of uterus in the spasm state caused by oxytocin.

7. 其他作用　红花尚有抗糖尿病肾病、抗肿瘤、降血脂等作用。

(7) Other effects　*Hóng huā* has anti-diabetic nephropathy, anti-tumor, and hypolipidemic effects.

【不良反应 / Adverse effects】

红花口服可引起口干、鼻出血、女性月经一过性延长或提前、共济失调。偶见过敏反应。剂量过大（超过 15 g）则可产生镇静作用，表现为嗜睡、萎靡不振、活动减少。红花黄色素注射给药还可引起患者发热、瘙痒、皮疹、头晕、头昏、头胀痛、牙龈出血等不良反应。

Oral *Hóng huā* can cause dry mouth, epistaxis, prolonged or advanced menstruation, and ataxia. Anaphylaxis is occasionally observed. Overdose of *Hóng huā* (over 15 g) can induce sedation, manifested by drowsiness, muzzy, and reduced activity. SY injection can cause fever, pruritus, rash, dizziness, headache, and gum bleeding.

益母草┊*Yì mǔ cǎo* (*Leonuri Herba*)

【来源 / Origin】

本品为唇形科植物益母草（*Leonurus japonicus* Houtt.）的新鲜或干燥地上部分。全国各地均有野生或栽培。生用或熬膏用。

Yì mǔ cǎo is the fresh or dry aboveground part of *Leonurus japonicus* Houtt. The plant is wild or cultivated all over China. The raw material or decocted extract is used for Chinese medicinal preparation.

【化学成分 / Chemical ingredients 】

含益母草碱、水苏碱等生物碱类成分，还含有黄酮类、二萜类、脂肪酸类、挥发油等物质。

Yì mǔ cǎo contains alkaloids such as leonurine and stachydrine, as well as flavonoids, diterpenoids, fatty acids, volatile oils, and other constituents.

【药性与功效 / Chinese medicine properties 】

味苦、辛，性微寒，归心、肝、膀胱经。具有活血调经、利尿消肿、清热解毒的功效。主治月经不调、痛经经闭、恶露不尽、水肿尿少、疮疡肿毒。

In Chinese medicine theory, *Yì mǔ cǎo* has the flavor of bitter and acrid, and has the nature of mild cold. It can enter the meridians of heart, liver, and bladder. *Yì mǔ cǎo* can invigorate blood to regulate menstruation, promote urination to remove edema, clear heat and resolve toxins. Clinically it can be used for irregular menstruation, painful menstruation, amenorrhoea, lochiorrhea, edema and lack of urine, toxins inducing sores, ulcers and swelling.

【药理作用 / Pharmacological effects 】

1. 调节子宫　益母草对子宫的调节作用与子宫状态有关，即兴奋正常状态的子宫而松弛痉挛状态的子宫。兴奋作用主要与水溶性生物碱、黄酮类成分有关，而抑制作用主要与脂溶性生物碱有关。兴奋作用表现为使子宫张力增强、收缩幅度增大、频率加快。该作用与兴奋子宫平滑肌 H_1 受体、α 受体及增加子宫平滑肌细胞胞质 Ca^{2+} 浓度有关。兴奋子宫可继而减少药物流产后子宫出血量，缩短出血时间，显著减少宫内滞留物。益母草能显著拮抗缩宫素及前列腺素 E_2（PGE_2）所致类痛经反应，作用机制除与缓解子宫平滑肌痉挛有关外，也与改善子宫炎症状况、降低子宫平滑肌上 $PGF_2α$ 及 PGE_2 的含量、升高体内孕激素水平等有关。

(1) Uterus regulation　The regulatory effects of *Yì mǔ cǎo* on uterus are related to its state, that is, to excite normal uterus but relax spasmodic uterus. The excitatory effect is mainly attributed to water-soluble alkaloids and flavonoids, while the inhibitory effect is mainly attributed to liposoluble alkaloids. The excitatory effects are manifested by the increase of uterine tension, contraction amplitude and frequency. The excitatory effects are related to the activation of H_1 receptor, α receptor and the increase of cytosolic Ca^{2+} concentration in uterine smooth muscle cells. Exciting the uterus can then reduce the amount of uterine bleeding, shorten the bleeding time, and significantly reduce intrauterine retention after medical abortion. On the other hand, *Yì mǔ cǎo* can significantly antagonize dysmenorrhea induced by oxytocin and prostaglandin E_2 (PGE_2). The mechanism of action is not only to alleviate the spasm of uterine smooth muscle, but also to improve the inflammation of uterus, reduce the content of $PGF_2α$ and PGE_2 in uterine smooth muscle, and increase the level of progesterone.

2. 改善血液流变学、抗血栓　益母草能显著降低血细胞比容、血液黏度和红细胞聚集指数，从而改善血液流变学。益母草也可使血栓形成时间延长，血栓长度缩短、质量减轻，产生抗血栓作用。益母草可延长 PT，减少血浆纤维蛋白原，减少血小板计数，降低血小板聚集功能，缩短优球蛋白溶解时间。

(2) Hemorheology improvement and anti-thrombosis　*Yì mǔ cǎo* can significantly reduce hematocrit, blood viscosity and erythrocyte aggregation index, thus improving hemorheology. *Yì mǔ cǎo* can also prolong the time of thrombosis, shorten the length and reduce the weight of thrombus, thus having anti-thrombotic effect. In terms of mechanism, *Yì mǔ cǎo* can prolong PT, educe the plasma content of fibrinogen, reduce platelet count, weaken platelet aggregation, and shorten euglobulin dissolution time.

3. **抗心肌缺血** 益母草抗心肌缺血机制与增强 SOD 活性（提高心肌抗氧化能力）、稳定心肌细胞膜（减少心肌酶释放）、缓解细胞内钙超负荷、抑制心肌细胞凋亡有关。此外，益母草亦能对抗缺血再灌注诱发的心律失常。益母草生物碱和黄酮类成分是抗心肌缺血作用的活性成分。

(3) Anti-myocardial ischemia The anti-myocardial ischemia mechanism of *Yì mǔ cǎo* is related to enhancing SOD activity (improving myocardial antioxidant capacity), stabilizing myocardial cells membrane (reducing the release of myocardial enzymes), alleviating the intracellular calcium overload and inhibiting myocardial cells apoptosis. In addition, *Yì mǔ cǎo* can also resist the arrhythmias induced by ischemia-reperfusion. The alkaloids and flavonoids of *Yì mǔ cǎo* are the active constituents.

4. **利尿、保护肾脏** 水苏碱及益母草碱均能显著增加大鼠尿量，水苏碱作用迅速，而益母草碱作用较为和缓。此外，益母草水提物及益母草碱对急性肾衰竭有保护作用，并可防治急性肾小管坏死。

(4) Diuresis and renal protection Both stachydrine and leonurine can significantly increase the urine output of rats. Stachydrine work quickly, while leonurine works more slowly. In addition, *Yì mǔ cǎo* extract and leonurine have protective effect on acute renal failure and can prevent and treat acute tubular necrosis.

5. **抗炎、镇痛** 益母草水提物抗炎及镇痛作用与阿司匹林强度相近或稍弱。能延长小鼠对热刺激疼痛反应潜伏期，减少醋酸所致扭体次数，并显著减轻二甲苯所致耳郭肿胀、角叉菜胶所致大鼠足跖肿胀。益母草碱可通过部分抑制 NF-κB 信号通路发挥抗炎作用。

(5) Anti-inflammation and analgesia The anti-inflammatory and analgesic effects of the water extract of *Yì mǔ cǎo* are similar to or slightly weaker than those of aspirin. The water extract of *Yì mǔ cǎo* can prolong the latency of pain response to heat stimulation, reduce the number of writhing caused by acetic acid, and significantly reduce the auricle swelling caused by xylene and the plantar swelling caused by carrageenan. Leonurine exerts anti-inflammatory effects by partially inhibiting the NF-κB signaling pathway.

【 不良反应 / Adverse effects 】

益母草可导致呕吐、过敏、多汗、血压过低甚至休克、乏力甚至肢体麻痹等不良反应。子宫兴奋作用可引起阵发性剧烈宫缩痛、孕妇流产等生殖系统不良反应。用药不当可导致腰痛、血尿、蛋白尿、肾间质轻度炎症及纤维组织增生、肾小管轻度脂肪变性等肾脏不良反应。

Yì mǔ cǎo may induce adverse reactions such as vomiting, allergies, sweating, hypotension and even shock, fatigue and limb paralysis. The exciting effect of *Yì mǔ cǎo* on uterus can lead to paroxysmal severe uterine contraction pain, abortion of pregnant women and other adverse reactions of reproductive system. The improper use of *Yì mǔ cǎo* can lead to kidney adverse reactions such as lumbago, hematuria, proteinuria, mild inflammation of renal interstitium, hyperplasia of fibrous tissue, mild fatty degeneration of renal tubules, etc.

莪术 ┆ *É zhú (Rhizoma Curcumae)*

【 来源 / Origin 】

本品为姜科植物蓬莪术（*Curcuma phaeocaulis* Val.）、广西莪术（*Curcuma kwangsiensis* S. G. Lee et C. F. Liang）或温郁金（*Curcuma wenyujin* Y. H. Chen et C. Ling）的干燥根茎。蓬莪术主产于四川、福建、广东等地；广西莪术主产于广西壮族自治区；温郁金（温莪术）主产于浙江、四川等地。生用或醋炙。

É zhú is the dried rhizome of *Curcuma phaeocaulis* Val., *Curcuma kwangsiensis* S. G. Lee et C. F. Liang, or *Curcuma wenyujin* Y. H. Chen et C. Ling. *Curcuma phaeocaulis* Val. is mainly produced in

Sichuan province, Fujian province, Guangdong province. *Curcuma kwangsiensis* S. G. Lee et C. F. Liang is mainly produced in Guangxi Zhuang Autonomous region. *Curcuma wenyujin* Y. H. Chen et C. Ling is mainly produced in Zhejiang province and Sichuan province. After being dried, the raw or vinegar fried rhizome is used for Chinese medicinal preparation.

【化学成分 / Chemical ingredients】

含挥发油和姜黄素类成分，挥发油中活性成分包括莪术醇、β-榄香烯、莪术二酮、呋喃二烯、吉马酮、莪术酮等。

É zhú contains volatile oil and curcuminoids. Active constituents in volatile oil include curcumol, β-elemene, curdione, furandadiene, germacrone and curzerenone.

【药性与功效 / Chinese medicine properties】

味辛、苦，性温，归肝、脾经。具有行气破血、消积止痛的功效。主治癥瘕痞块、瘀血经闭、胸痹心痛、食积胀痛。

In Chinese medicine theory, *É zhú* has the flavor of acrid and bitter, and has nature of warm. It can enter the meridians of the liver and the spleen. *É zhú* can move Qi to break up static blood, disperse accumulation to relieve pain. Clinically it can be used for concretions (fixed lower abdominal masses of definite shape) and conglomerations (movable lower abdominal masses of indefinite shape), menstrual block due to blood stasis, chest Bi caused heart pain, and food accumulation induced distending pain.

【药理作用 / Pharmacological effects】

1. 抗肿瘤　莪术挥发油对妇科肿瘤包括卵巢癌、子宫内膜癌、宫颈癌、乳腺癌等有效，尤其以抗卵巢癌为研究热点。莪术挥发油对肺癌、胃癌、直肠癌、肝癌等也有效。抗肿瘤作用机制主要包括抑制增殖、诱导凋亡、直接破坏、抑制转移与侵袭、抑制血管生成、增强化疗药物敏感性、增强机体免疫功能等。β-榄香烯、莪术醇、莪术二酮、吉马酮、莪术酮等均为抗肿瘤活性成分。莪术挥发油抗肿瘤同时不易引起肿瘤细胞突变，而且具有一定的肿瘤选择性。

(1) Anti-tumor　*É zhú* volatile oil is effective for gynecological tumors, including ovarian cancer, endometrial cancer, cervical cancer, and breast cancer. In particular, the effect on ovarian cancer is a research hotspot. *É zhú* volatile oil is also effective for lung cancer, gastric cancer, rectal cancer, and liver cancer. The anti-tumor mechanisms of *É zhú* volatile oil mainly include inhibition of proliferation, induction of apoptosis, direct destruction, inhibition of metastasis and invasion, inhibition of angiogenesis, enhancement of the sensitivity of chemotherapeutics, and enhancement of the body's immune function. The active constituents include β-elemene, curcumol, curdione, germacrone, and curzerenone. *É zhú* volatile oil seldom induces tumor cell mutation, and it has certain tumor selectivity.

2. 改善血液流变学、抗血栓　莪术挥发油能抑制血小板聚集、抗血栓形成，改善血液流变学，其活性成分为姜黄素、β-榄香烯、莪术二酮等。

(2) Hemorheology improvement and anti-thrombosis　*É zhú* volatile oil has effects of inhibiting platelet aggregation, anti-thrombotic formation and improving hemorheology. The active constituents include curcumin, β-elemene, and curdione.

3. 影响消化系统　莪术挥发油能直接兴奋平滑肌，对大鼠慢性、幽门结扎性、水浸应激性胃溃疡均有显著治疗作用。莪术醇可通过兴奋 M 受体、抑制 α 和 β 受体、促进外钙内流等机制促进大鼠离体十二指肠平滑肌收缩。此外，莪术挥发油对四氯化碳（CCl_4）和硫代乙酰胺（TAA）引起的小鼠实验性肝损伤有保护作用。

(3) Effects on the digestive system　*É zhú* volatile oil can stimulate the smooth muscle directly, and has significant therapeutic effect on chronic gastric ulcer, pyloric ligation induced gastric ulcer and

water immersion stress induced gastric ulcer in rats. Curcumol can promote the contraction of isolated duodenal smooth muscle in rats through mechanisms such as activating M receptors, inhibiting α and β receptors, and promoting external calcium influx. In addition, *É zhú* volatile oil has protective effects on experimental liver injury in mice caused by carbon tetrachloride (CCl_4) and thioacetamide (TAA).

4. **抗炎、镇痛**　莪术挥发油对动物醋酸性腹膜炎有抑制作用，对小鼠局部水肿、炎症及大鼠棉球肉芽肿有显著抑制作用。莪术不同炮制品对化学刺激、热刺激所致疼痛均有较强的镇痛作用，其中醋炙莪术的镇痛作用强而持久。

(4) Anti-inflammation and analgesia　*É zhú* volatile oil has inhibitory effect on vinegar acid induced peritonitis, local edema and inflammation in mice, and granuloma induced by cotton ball in rats. Various processed products of *É zhú* have strong analgesic effects on pain caused by chemical stimulation and thermal stimulation, among which the analgesic effect of vinegar fried *É zhú* is strong and lasting.

【不良反应 / Adverse effects 】

莪术水煎剂较为安全，但莪术油注射液不良反应较多，包括变态反应（严重者可出现过敏性休克甚至死亡）、呼吸系统不良反应（呼吸困难、紫绀等）以及神经系统及血液系统损害等。

É zhú decoction is safe. However, *É zhú* volatile oil injection may induce various adverse reactions, including allergic reactions (anaphylactic shock or death in severe cases), adverse respiratory reactions (dyspnea, cyanosis, etc.), and damage to the nervous system and blood system.

水蛭 ┆ *Shuǐ zhì (Hirudo)*

【来源 / Origin 】

本品为水蛭科动物蚂蟥（*Whitmania pigra* Whitman）、水蛭（*Hirudo nipponica* Whitman）或柳叶蚂蟥（*Whitmania acranulata* Whitman）的干燥全体。全国大部分地区均产。生用或滑石粉烫后用。

Shuǐ zhì is the dried body of *Whitmania pigra* Whitman, *Hirudo nipponica* Whitman, or *Whitmania acranulata* Whitman, which is distributed in most parts of China. After being dried, the raw or scalded body is used for Chinese medicinal preparation.

【化学成分 / Chemical ingredients 】

含水蛭素、吻蛭素、类肝素等蛋白质及多肽类大分子物质，蝶啶类、糖脂类、羧酸酯类和甾体类等小分子物质以及某些微量元素。

Shuǐ zhì contains proteins and polypeptides such as hirudin, hementin and heparan. *Shuǐ zhì* also contains small molecules such as pteridine, glycolipids, carboxylic esters and steroids, as well as some trace elements.

【药性与功效 / Chinese medicine properties 】

味苦、咸，性平，有小毒，归肝经。具有破血通经、逐瘀消癥的功效。主治血瘀经闭、癥瘕痞块、中风偏瘫、跌扑损伤。

In Chinese medicine theory, *Shuǐ zhì* has the flavor of bitter and salty and neutral nature. *Shuǐ zhì* has little poison. It can enter the meridian of liver. *Shuǐ zhì* can break up static blood to promote menstruation, expel stasis to disperse concretions. Clinically it can be used for menstrual block due to blood stasis, concretions (fixed lower abdominal masses of definite shape) and conglomerations (movable lower abdominal masses of indefinite shape), wind-strike caused hemiplegic paralysis, and injuries (from falls, fractures, contusions and strains).

【药理作用 / Pharmacological effects 】

1. **抗凝血、抗血栓**　水蛭具有显著抗凝血活性，但经高温煎煮后显著降低。研究表明，经超细粉碎后直接入药药效优于其水煎液。水蛭素是水蛭抗凝活性物质之一，也是迄今活性最强的天然凝血酶抑制剂。水蛭素对凝血酶的抑制作用不依赖于其他内源性抗凝因子。水蛭素与血浆中游离及与纤维蛋白结合的凝血酶均可特异性地、快速地形成稳定的非共价复合物，使凝血酶的活性丧失，从而抑制凝血过程、凝血酶诱导的血小板聚集以及血液凝固触发的血栓形成，产生显著的抗凝血及抗血栓作用。

(1) Anti-coagulation and anti-thrombosis *Shuǐ zhì* has strong anti-coagulant effects. However, the activity is significantly reduced after decocting with high temperature. Studies have shown that the effect of *Shuǐ zhì* taken directly after superfine crushing is better than its decoction. Hirudin is one of the anti-coagulant substances of *Shuǐ zhì*, and it is by far the most active natural thrombin inhibitor. The inhibitory effect of hirudin on thrombin is independent of other endogenous anti-coagulants. Hirudin can specifically and quickly form a stable non-covalent complex with thrombin which is free in plasma or binding with fibrin. The formation of the complex leads to lose of thrombin activity thus inhibiting the coagulation process, platelet aggregation induced by thrombin and thrombosis triggered by blood coagulation, so as to produce significant anti-coagulant and anti-thrombotic effects.

2. 抗动脉粥样硬化 水蛭可通过调节脂代谢、保护内皮细胞、抑制平滑肌细胞增殖、抑制炎症反应等多环节发挥抗动脉粥样硬化作用。调节脂代谢作用表现为降低血清总胆固醇、甘油三酯、低密度脂蛋白胆固醇及 ox-LDL 的水平，升高高密度脂蛋白胆固醇的水平。凝血酶可引起血管内皮细胞中 Ca^{2+} 浓度增加、通透性增强、形态改变，导致血管内皮损伤。水蛭素可通过抑制凝血酶而保护血管内皮细胞。水蛭素还可通过抗氧化（降低丙二醛、血清过氧化脂质含量，增加 SOD 活性）、升高舒血管活性物质—氧化氮（NO）及前列环素（PGI_2）水平、抑制内皮素（ET）过表达、改善血液流变学等发挥保护血管内皮作用。此外，水蛭可通过抑制平滑肌细胞收缩表型蛋白下调和降低主动脉壁基质金属蛋白酶 -2（MMP-2）和 MMP-9 的表达等机制，抑制平滑肌细胞表型转化、增殖和迁移。

(2) Anti-atherosclerosis *Shuǐ zhì* exerts anti-atherosclerotic effects by regulating lipid metabolism, protecting endothelial cells, inhibiting smooth muscle cell proliferation, and inhibiting inflammatory responses. The regulation of lipid metabolism is manifested in the decrease of serum total cholesterol (TC), triglyceride (TG), low-density lipoprotein cholesterol (LDL-C), oxidized low-density lipoprotein (ox-LDL), and the increase of high-density lipoprotein cholesterol (HDL-C). Thrombin can cause increased intracellular Ca^{2+} concentration, enhanced permeability, and morphological changes in vascular endothelial cells, leading to vascular endothelial damage. Hirudin can protect vascular endothelial cells by inhibiting thrombin. Furthermore, hirudin can protect vascular endothelium by reducing the content of malondialdehyde (MDA) and serum peroxidized lipid (LPO), increasing the activity of SOD, increasing the levels of vasoactive substances nitric oxide (NO) and prostacyclin (PGI_2), inhibiting endothelin (ET) expression, and improving hemorheology. In addition, *Shuǐ zhì* can inhibit the phenotype transformation, proliferation and migration of smooth muscle cells by inhibiting the down regulation of contraction phenotype protein and reducing the expression of matrix metalloproteinase (MMP) including MMP-2 and MMP-9 in the aortic wall.

3. 抗炎、抗纤维化 水蛭对以血浆蛋白渗出、肿胀度为指标的急性炎症模型和以肉芽组织增生为特征的慢性炎症模型均有改善作用，提示水蛭对炎症早期及后期的病理改变均有抑制作用。凝血酶是炎症细胞的化学诱导物，可诱导炎症的发生，而且可激活内皮细胞，刺激成纤维细胞增殖，促进纤维化的形成。水蛭素抑制凝血酶可有效地抑制炎症的发生，并抑制成纤维细胞的增殖和细胞外基质的产生。

(3) Anti-inflammation and anti-fibrosis　*Shuǐ zhì* can improve the plasma protein exudation and swelling degree of acute inflammation model animals, and improve the granulation tissue hyperplasia of chronic inflammation model animals, suggesting that *Shuǐ zhì* can inhibit the pathological changes in both the early and late stage of inflammation. Thrombin is a chemical inducer of inflammatory cells. It can induce inflammation, activate endothelial cells, stimulate fibroblast proliferation and promote the formation of fibrosis. The inhibitory effect of hirudin on thrombin can effectively inhibit the occurrence of inflammation, and thus inhibit the proliferation of fibroblasts and the production of extracellular matrix.

4. 抗肿瘤　水蛭可通过促进肿瘤细胞凋亡、抑制肿瘤细胞增殖、提高机体细胞免疫功能、抑制新生血管生成等发挥抗肿瘤作用。水蛭备受关注的是其抑制肿瘤转移作用，机制与改善血液黏度有关。已知水蛭及其某些活性多肽可抑制肺癌、黑色素瘤、乳腺癌、前列腺癌、膀胱癌、结肠癌、白血病、淋巴癌等多种肿瘤转移。

(4) Anti-tumor　*Shuǐ zhì* exerts anti-tumor effects by promoting tumor cell apoptosis, inhibiting tumor cell proliferation, improving the body's cellular immune function and inhibiting neovascularization. *Shuǐ zhì* has attracted much attention for its inhibitory effects on tumor metastasis. The mechanism is related to improving blood viscosity. *Shuǐ zhì* and some of its active polypeptides are known to inhibit the metastasis of various tumors such as lung cancer, melanoma, breast cancer, prostate cancer, bladder cancer, colon cancer, leukemia, and lymphoma.

【不良反应 / Adverse effects】

治疗量水蛭不良反应少，但可引起过敏。用量过大则可引起恶心、呕吐、子宫出血、胃肠出血、尿血及昏迷等毒性反应。

The therapeutic dose of *Shuǐ zhì* has fewer adverse reactions but can cause allergic reactions. However, overdose of *Shuǐ zhì* can cause toxic reactions such as nausea, vomiting, uterine bleeding, gastrointestinal bleeding, hematuria and coma.

桃仁　┊　*Táo rén (Semen Persicae)*

【来源 / Origin】

本品为蔷薇科植物桃［*Prunus persica* (L.) Batsch］或山桃［*Prunus davidiana* (Carr.) Franch.］的干燥成熟种子。全国各地均产，果实成熟后采收。晒干后生用或炒用。

Táo rén is the dried mature seeds of *Prunus persica* (L.) Batsch or *Prunus davidiana* (Carr.) Franch. The plant is wild or cultivated all over China. The seeds are harvested after the fruit has matured. After being dried, the raw or fried seeds are used for Chinese medicinal preparation.

【化学成分 / Chemical ingredients】

含脂肪酸类、苷类、蛋白质、多糖、氨基酸及其他成分。苷类包括苦杏仁苷、野樱苷等氰苷。

Táo rén contains fatty acids, glycosides, proteins, polysaccharides, amino acids and other constituents. The glycosides include cyanogenic glycosides such as amygdalin and prunasin.

【药性与功效 / Chinese medicine properties】

味苦、甘，性平，有小毒，归心、肝、大肠经。具有活血祛痰、润肠通便、止咳平喘的功效。主治经闭痛经、癥瘕痞块、肺痈肠痈、肠燥便秘、咳嗽气喘、跌扑损伤。

In Chinese medicine theory, *Táo rén* has the flavor of bitter and sweet and neutral nature. *Táo rén* has little poison. It can enter the meridians of heart, liver, and large intestine. *Táo rén* can invigorate blood to dispel phlegm, moisten the intestines to promote defecation, relieve cough and suppress panting. Clinically it can be used for amenorrhea, painful menstruation, concretions (fixed lower abdominal masses of definite shape) and conglomerations (movable lower abdominal masses of indefinite shape), lung abscess and intestine abscess, intestinal dryness induced constipation, cough and panting, and injuries (from falls, fractures, contusions and strains).

【药理作用 / Pharmacological effects】

1. **影响血液和循环系统**　桃仁提取物可显著降低血液黏度、降低血细胞比容、降低纤维蛋白原含量、扩张血管、增加器官血流量，改善血流动力学。桃仁提取物灌胃能使小鼠、家兔出血时间、凝血时间显著延长，显示抗凝血作用。桃仁水提物、桃仁脂肪油、苦杏仁苷均可显著抑制ADP诱导的血小板聚集。桃仁水煎液不影响纤溶酶活性，但桃仁含有纤溶成分，具有直接溶栓作用。桃仁提取物能降低急性心肌梗死大鼠心电图ST段抬高，降低血清中CPK和LDH含量，缩小梗死面积。桃仁提取物还能抑制寒、热两证大鼠血管内皮细胞凋亡。

(1) Effects on blood and circulatory systems　*Táo rén* extract can significantly reduce blood viscosity, reduce hematocrit, reduce fibrinogen content, expand blood vessels, and increase organ blood flow, thereby improving hemodynamics. Oral *Táo rén* extract can significantly prolong the bleeding time and coagulation time of mice and rabbits, showing anti-coagulant effect. The water extract of *Táo rén*, *Táo rén* fat oil and amygdalin can significantly inhibit ADP induced platelet aggregation. The decoction of *Táo rén* does not affect the activity of plasmin, but it contains fibrinolytic constituents and has direct thrombolytic effect. *Táo rén* extract can reduce the ST segment elevation of the electrocardiogram in rats with acute myocardial infarction, reduce the content of CPK and LDH in serum, and reduce the infarct area. *Táo rén* extract can also inhibit the apoptosis of VECs in model rats of cold or heat syndrome.

2. **抗组织纤维化**　桃仁提取物能提高肝组织胶原酶活性，可有效地抑制CCl_4及血吸虫病性肝纤维化胶原的合成，并促进已沉积胶原的降解和吸收。桃仁提取物还能提高机体抗氧化能力，防止乙醇和CCl_4等所致的肝脂质过氧化损伤。此外，桃仁提取物可延缓梗阻性肾病肾间质纤维化及硅沉着病纤维化的发生。

(2) Anti-fibrosis　*Táo rén* extract can improve collagenase activity of liver tissue, effectively inhibit the synthesis of collagen in liver fibrosis caused by carbon tetrachloride (CCl_4) and schistosomiasis, and promote the degradation and absorption of deposited collagen. *Táo rén* extract can also improve the antioxidant capacity and prevent liver lipid peroxidation damage caused by alcohol and CCl_4. In addition, *Táo rén* extract can delay the occurrence of renal interstitial fibrosis and silicosis fibrosis.

3. **镇咳**　苦杏仁苷经苦杏仁苷酶水解后产生苯甲醛和氢氰酸，后者具有中枢性镇咳作用。

(3) Cough suppression　Amygdalin is hydrolyzed by amygdalase to produce benzaldehyde and hydrocyanic acid. Hydrocyanic acid has central antitussive effect.

4. **润肠通便**　桃仁含丰富的脂肪油，可润滑肠道，利于排便。

(4) Defecation promotion　*Táo rén* is rich in fat oil, which can lubricate intestines and facilitate defecation.

5. **其他作用**　桃仁提取物还具有调节子宫、抗肿瘤、调节免疫、保护神经、促进黑色素合成、抗炎、抗氧化、镇痛等作用。

(5) Other effects　*Táo rén* extract has the effects of uterus regulation, anti-tumor, immunity regulation, neuroprotection, melanin synthesis promotion, anti-inflammation, anti-oxidation and analgesia.

【不良反应 / Adverse effects】

剂量过大可引起中枢神经系统损害，出现眩晕、头痛、烦躁不安、瞳孔扩大等反应，严重者神志不清、抽搐，甚至呼吸麻痹而死亡。苦杏仁苷经过桃仁本身或肠道菌群中的苦杏仁苷酶分解后产生氢氰酸。氢氰酸可抑制线粒体呼吸链从而引发毒性反应。

Overdose of *Táo rén* can cause damage to the central nervous system, resulting in dizziness, headache, restlessness, pupil dilation and other reactions. In serious cases, people are delirious, convulsive, and even died of respiratory paralysis. Hydrocyanic acid produced after amygdalin decomposition by *Táo rén* or intestinal flora contained amygdalase causes the toxic reactions via inhibiting mitochondrial respiratory chain.

姜黄 ┊ *Jiāng huáng*（*Turmeric*）

【来源 / Origin】

本品为姜科植物姜黄（*Curcuma Longa* L.）的干燥根茎。主产于广东、广西及云南。冬季茎叶枯萎时采挖，洗净，煮或蒸至透心，晒干，除去须根。

Jiāng Huáng is the dried rhizome of *curcuma longa* L.. It is mainly produced Guangdong provinces, Guangxi area and Yunnan provinces in China. When its stems and leaves wither in winter, it is picked, cleaned, boiled or steamed until it is thoroughly soaked, dried in the sun, and then fibrous roots are removed.

【化学成分 / Chemical ingredients】

有效成分为姜黄素类化合物和挥发油，姜黄素类化合物含量为 3%~8%，主要成分是姜黄素、去甲氧基姜黄素、双去甲氧基姜黄素、四氢姜黄素、环姜黄素等。此外，还含有月桂烯、α-姜黄酮、芳姜黄酮、二氢黄酮醇、芹菜素等。

The effective components of *Jiāng huáng* are curcumin compounds and volatile oil, and the content of curcumin compounds is 3% to 8%. The main components of curcumin compounds are curcumin, demethoxycurcumin, bisdemethoxycurcumin, tetrahydrocurcumin, and cyclocurcumin. In addition, *Jiāng huáng* also contains myrcene, α-turmerone, ar-turmerone, dihydroflavonol and apigenin.

【药性与功效 / Chinese medicine properties】

味辛、苦，性温，归脾、肝经。具有活血行气、通经止痛的功效。主治胸胁刺痛、闭经、癥瘕、风湿肩臂疼痛、跌扑肿痛。

In Chinese medicine theory, *Jiāng huáng* has the nature of pungent, bitter, and warm. It can enter the meridians of liver and spleen. *Jiāng huáng* has the functions of breaking blood stasis and moving Qi, dredging channels and relieving pain. Clinically, it can be used for fullness and discomfort in chest and hypochondrium, chest impediment and heart pain, amenorrhea and dysmenorrheal, shoulder and arm pain induced by wind-dampness, swelling and pain.

【药理作用 / Pharmacological effects】

1. 抗肿瘤　在体内试验中，每天以 50mg/kg 的剂量给肉瘤 S_{180} 小鼠腹腔注射姜黄素，结果显示，药物组抑瘤率高达 76%，表明姜黄素对肿瘤具有较好的抑制作用。将姜黄素（5μmol/L、10μmol/L、20μmol/L、40μmol/L）加入人肝癌细胞系 Huh7 的培养液中，用 CCK-8 检测细胞增殖水平变化。结果显示姜黄素能抑制 Huh7 细胞的增殖，且细胞凋亡率随着姜黄素浓度的升高而上升。

(1) **Antitumor**　*In vivo* experiments, 50mg/(kg·d) curcumin was injected intraperitoneally to the sarcoma S_{180} mice, and the tumor inhibition rate could be as high as 76%, indicating that *Jiāng huáng* has a good inhibitory effect on tumors. In addition, curcumin (5μmol/L, 10μmol/L, 20μmol/L, 40μmol/L) was added to the culture fluid of human liver cancer cell line Huh7, and changes in cell proliferation were

detected with CCK-8. The results showed that *Jiāng huáng* could inhibit the proliferation of Huh7 cells, and the apoptosis rate increased with the increase of curcumin concentration.

2. 抗菌　姜黄素可以抑制链球菌、葡萄球菌、大肠埃希菌、铜绿假单胞菌、肺炎克雷伯菌等细菌的生长。利用尾静脉注射 041184 大肠埃希菌标准菌悬液建立细菌脓毒症小鼠模型，设置对照组、模型组和姜黄素组，观察到姜黄素组血清 AST、ALT、TNF-α 和 NO 含量明显低于模型组，病理检查见脏器损害亦明显减轻；24 小时存活率为 90%，明显高于模型组（50%）。表明姜黄素可减少细菌脓毒症小鼠 TNF-α、NO 和氧自由基的产生，减轻其脏器病理损害。

(2) Antibacterial　*Jiāng huáng* can inhibit the growth of *Streptococcus, Staphylococcus, Escherichia coli, Pseudomonas aeruginosa, Klebsiella* and other bacteria. The mouse model of bacterial sepsis was established by injecting 041184 *Escherichia coli* standard bacterial suspension into the tail vein. The control group, model group and curcumin group were set up. It was observed that the content of AST, ALT, TNF-α and NO in serum of curcumin group was significantly lower than that of model group, and the pathological examination showed that the organ damage was also significantly alleviated. The 24-hour survival rate was 90%, which was significantly higher than that of model group (50%). It suggested that *Jiāng huáng* could reduce the production of TNF-α, NO and oxygen free radicals in mice with bacterial sepsis and alleviate the pathological damage of organs.

3. 抗炎　利用金黄色葡萄球菌感染小鼠造成急性肺损伤模型研究发现，姜黄素能减少中性粒细胞的渗透及Ⅰ型纤溶酶原激活物抑制因子的活性，降低炎症因子、趋化因子的分泌水平，此外，姜黄素治疗组肺组织中性粒细胞的渗出数量减少，水肿程度与肺泡壁厚度较未处理组明显好转。姜黄素衍生物 CMC2.24 可作用于表面活性剂脱辅基蛋白 B（SP-B），减轻金黄色葡萄球菌引起的肺损伤，减少炎症细胞的聚集、NF-κB 的表达及基质金属蛋白酶的活性，改善生存率。

(3) Anti-inflammatory　By the mouse model with acute lung injury induced by *Staphylococcus aureus* infection, it was found that curcumin can attenuate the permeation of neutrophils and neutrophils Ⅰ type plasminogen activator suppressor activity, reduce inflammatory cytokines, chemokines secretion factor. In addition, in the curcumin-treated group, the number of exuded neutrophils decreased, and the degree of edema and the thickness of the alveolar wall were significantly improved compared with the untreated group. Curcumin derivative CMC2.24 can act on surfactant apoprotein B (SP-B), reduce lung damage caused by *Staphylococcus aureus*, reduce the aggregation of inflammatory cells, NF-κB expression and matrix metalloproteinase activity and improve survival rate.

4. 抗氧化　通过高糖（25mmol/L 葡萄糖，7 天）培养新生大鼠心肌细胞（NRVCs）诱导自然衰老的模型研究表明，与衰老组比较，姜黄素组心肌细胞 β-半乳糖苷酶活性减少，ROS 及 MDA 水平降低，抗氧化酶 SOD 及 GSH-Px 活力升高，衰老相关蛋白表达下调，且呈剂量相关性，姜黄素高剂量组改善最为明显。

(4) Antioxidant　A model study of natural aging induced by high glucose (25 mmol/L glucose, 7d) culture of neonatal rat cardiomyocytes (NRVCs) showed that compared with the aging group, β-galactosidase activity in the myocardial cells of the curcumin group was attenuated. The levels of ROS and MDA decreased, the activities of antioxidant enzymes SOD and GSH-Px increased, the expression of senescence-related proteins was down-regulated, and there was a dose correlation, the improvement was highest in the high-dose curcumin group.

5. 保护神经　通过鼠脑微血管内皮细胞制备的体外 BBB 模型发现，姜黄素可增加过氧化氢刺激诱导的跨内皮细胞电阻值，且其值越高，表明 BBB 完整性越好，并且通过 C57BL/6J 雄性小鼠的体内试验发现，姜黄素可改善 CIRI 诱导的 BBB 的破坏，进一步研究发现水通道蛋白 –4(AQP-4）与 BBB 开放密切相关，说明姜黄素可通过下调脑缺血损伤中 AQP-4 的表达，减少 BBB 开放，保护 BBB 的完整性，从而抑制脑水肿，改善神经功能。

(5) Nerve protection *In vitro* BBB model prepared with rat brain microvascular endothelial cells, it was found that *Jiāng huáng* can increase the resistance value of transendothelial cells induced by hydrogen peroxide stimulation. The higher the value was, the better the integrity of the BBBwas, and *in vivo* studies of C57BL/6J male mice, it was found that curcumin improved CIRI-induced destruction of BBB. In addition, aquaporin-4 (AQP-4) is closely related to BBB opening. Curcumin can down-regulate the expression of AQP-4 in cerebral ischemic injury, reduce BBB opening, protect the integrity of BBB, thereby inhibiting brain edema and improving neural functions.

6. 抗凝血及抗血栓 在一项体外试验中，采用家兔血浆复钙时间法、凝血酶时间法及体外血栓法、全血血块法，分别对姜黄素、去甲氧基姜黄素、双去甲氧基姜黄素的体外抗凝血与抗血栓活性进行测定。结果发现姜黄素、去甲氧基姜黄素、双去甲氧基姜黄素均能延长家兔血浆复钙时间及凝血酶时间，且均能加快体外血栓及全血凝块的溶解，其中去甲氧基姜黄素的作用最强。从而表明姜黄素类化合物具有较好的体外抗凝血和抗血栓作用，结合结构分析发现空间不对称结构能加强姜黄素类化合物结构母核的抗凝活性。

(6) Anticoagulant and antithrombotic *In vitro* experiment, the anticoagulant and antithrombotic activities of three natural curcumin compound curcumins, normethoxycurcumin and dideoxycurcumin were measured by the methods of rabbit plasma calcium recovery time, thrombin time, *in vitro* thrombus and whole blood clot. It was observed that curcumin, demethoxycurcumin and didymethoxycurcumin could prolong the time of plasma calcium recovery and thrombin in rabbits, and can accelerate the dissolution of thrombus *in vitro* and whole blood clot, Among them, demethoxycurcumin worked best. The results showed that curcumin compounds had good anticoagulant and antithrombotic effects *in vitro*, and the asymmetric structure could enhance the anticoagulant activity of curcumin compounds.

7. 保护肾脏 将 30 只 C57BL/6J 小鼠随机分成假手术对照组（NC）、5/6 肾结扎模型组（LIG）和姜黄素治疗组（LIG+CUR），每组 10 只，按照改良的 5/6 肾结扎方法制作 CKD 动物模型，检测纤维化指标 α-SMA 及参与慢性肾病纤维化的 Hippo 通路转录激活子 Yap。肾功能检测结果显示，与假手术组相比，结扎组中的尿素氮（BUN）、血肌酐（Scr）显著增高，给予姜黄素可以有效缓解肾功能损伤；另外，HE 和 Masson 及免疫组化实验结果均显示，结扎组小鼠的肾出现明显肾小管病变和一定程度的纤维化改变，给予姜黄素后纤维化程度显著减轻；而 Yap 蛋白在造模后 mRNA 和蛋白水平均升高，姜黄素处理后则显著下降。

(7) Kidney-protecting Thirty C57BL/6J mice were randomly divided into sham operated control group (NC), 5/6 renal ligation model group (LIG) and curcumin treatment group (LIG+ CUR), 10 in each group. CKD animal model was made according to the improved 5/6 renal ligation method. α-SMA and Yap, the transcription activator of the Hippo pathway involved in chronic renal fibrosis, were detected. The results of renal function test showed that compared with the sham operation group, bun and SCR in the ligation group were significantly higher, and curcumin could effectively protect the renal function from damage; HE, Masson and immunohistochemistry results showed that the kidney in the ligation group showed obvious renal tubular lesions and certain degree of fibrosis, and the degree of fibrosis was significantly reduced after curcumin was given; The mRNA and protein levels of Yap protein increased after modeling, but decreased after curcumin treatment.

8. 其他作用 姜黄还具有抗病毒、抗纤维化、抗抑郁、保肝、降血脂、降血糖、保护胃肠道、降低尿酸等作用，可用于治疗皮炎、痤疮、糖尿病、痛风等症。

(8) Other effects *Jiāng huáng* also has antiviral, antifibrotic, antidepressant, hepatoprotective effects, and the functions of lowering blood lipids, lowering blood sugar, protecting the gastrointestinal tract, and reducing uric acid. It can be used to treat dermatitis, acne, diabetes, gout and other symptoms.

【不良反应 / Adverse effects】

犬的临床前毒理学研究显示，姜黄素脂质体 ≥ 20mg/kg 会出现剂量依赖性溶血。

Preclinical toxicology studies of curcumin liposomes in dogs have shown dose-dependent hemolysis at doses greater than or equal to 20mg/kg.

（马秉亮　刘　娟　屈　飞）

题库

第十五章 止咳平喘药
Chapter 15 Antitussive and antiasthmatic medicines

学习目标│Objectives

1.**掌握** 止咳平喘药的主要药理作用及与功效的相关性；半夏、桔梗、川贝母与功效相关的药理作用及药效物质基础。

2.**了解** 浙贝母的主要药理作用；苦杏仁的主要药理作用及不良反应。

1. **Must know** The main pharmacological effects and connection with efficacy of antitussive and antiasthmatic medicines; the efficacy related pharmacological effects and material basis of *Bàn xià, Jié gěng, Chuān bèi mǔ*.

2. **Desirable to know** The main pharmacological effects of *Zhè bèi mǔ*; the main pharmacological effects and adverse reactions of *Kǔ xìng rén*.

第一节 概述
Section 1 Overview

PPT

微课

凡以祛痰、化痰、缓解或制止咳嗽及喘息为主要功效的药物称为止咳平喘药。本类药物药性或温或寒，主要归肺、心、脾、胃及大肠经，具有宣肺祛痰、止咳平喘等功效，主要用于痰证的治疗。

All Chinese materia medica that are mainly used to dispel phlegm, resolve phlegm, relieve and restrain cough, asthma are classified as antitussive and antiasthmatic medicines. These medicines are warm or cold in nature. They majorly enter the meridians of lung, heart, spleen, stomach and large intestine. Their efficacies include ventilating lung to dispel phlegm, relieving cough and dyspnea. Thus, they are used for the treatment of phlegm syndrome.

中医对"痰"的认识有广义与狭义之分。广义的"痰"临床表现复杂，涉及神经系统、心血管系统、纤维组织增生、水液代谢失调、肿瘤等多种病变，分为"有形之痰"和"无形之痰"。无形之痰指停积于脏腑经络之间的各种痰证，如痰浊滞于皮肤经络，可生瘰疬瘿瘤，常见皮下肿块、单纯性甲状腺肿和慢性淋巴结炎等；痰迷心窍，则昏迷、谵妄、心神不宁、精神障碍，常见于脑血管意外、精神分裂症及癫痫等；痰阻胸痹，则胸闷、胸痛、心悸，常见于冠心病、心绞痛、心力衰竭、高血压等。此外，前列腺增生、子宫肌瘤、乳腺增生等，中医亦多辨证为痰证。狭义的"痰"则专指呼吸道咳出的痰，为"有形之痰"，多见于上呼吸道感染、急慢性支气管炎、支气管扩张、肺气肿等肺部疾病。

According to TCM theory, the interpretation of "phlegm" has both a broad and a narrow sense. In its broad sense, phlegm exhibits a variety of clinical manifestations, including proliferation of nervous system, cardiovascular system, fibrous tissue, metabolism disorder of water, tumor and pathophysiological changes. From TCM perspective, there are two types of phlegm: "tangible phlegm" and "intangible phlegm". Intangible phlegm refers to the phlegm syndromes caused by stasis of phlegm in organs and meridians, such as cervical scrofula, clinically common subcutaneous masses, simple goiter, chronic lymphadenitis, etc., are attributed to phlegm stagnated in the skin meridians and collaterals；stupor, delirium, restlessness, mental disorder, clinically common in cerebrovascular accident, schizophrenia, epilepsy, etc., are attributed to phlegm obstructing the heart orifices; chest distress, chest pain, palpitation, clinically common in coronary heart disease, angina, heart failure, hypertension, etc., are attributed to stagnation of phlegm inducing chest impediment. Furthermore, such diseases as prostatic hyperplasia, myoma of uterus and mammary gland hyperplasia are also considered to be caused by stagnation of phlegm from the perspective of traditional Chinese medicine. Phlegm, in the narrow sense, which is defined as "tangible phlegm", specially refers to the phlegm from the respiratory tract, and it is mostly found in lung diseases such as upper respiratory tract infection, acute or chronic bronchitis, bronchiectasis and emphysema.

一般而言，咳嗽有痰者居多，痰又容易引起咳喘，因此，痰、咳、喘三者关系密切，互为因果。目前对于止咳平喘药的药理研究，主要集中在呼吸系统的痰、咳、喘方面。现代研究表明，本类药主要具有以下药理作用。

Generally, cough is usually accompanied with phlegm and excessive phlegm is easy to induce cough and dyspnea. Therefore, phlegm, cough and dyspnea are closely related and cause and effect each other. Nowadays, the pharmacological researches on antitussives and antiasthmatics mainly focus on the phlegm, cough and dyspnea in respiratory system. According to modern pharmacological researches, antitussives and antiasthmatics medicines have the following pharmacological effects.

1. 祛痰　桔梗、皂荚、前胡、川贝母、款冬花、天南星、紫菀、薜菜、满山红、半夏等均有祛痰作用，能增加呼吸道腺体分泌量，一般在给药后 1 小时作用达到高峰，其中以桔梗、前胡、皂荚的作用最强。家兔灌服天南星煎剂后，其增强呼吸道分泌功能可持续 4 小时以上。除薜菜含薜菜素、满山红含杜鹃素外，其他药物的祛痰作用多与其所含皂苷类成分有关。皂苷能刺激咽喉黏膜或胃黏膜，反射性引起轻度恶心，增加支气管腺体分泌，使痰液稀释而易于咳出。杜鹃素祛痰是直接作用于呼吸道黏膜，促进气管黏液纤毛运动，增强呼吸道清除异物的功能并可溶解黏痰，使呼吸道分泌物中酸性黏多糖纤维断裂，唾液酸含量降低，痰液黏度下降而易于咳出。

(1) Dispelling phlegm　*Jié gěng, Zào jiá, Qián hú, Chuān bèi mǔ, Kuǎn dōng huā, Tiān nán xīng, Zǐ wǎn, Hàn cài, Mǎn shān hóng* and *Bàn xià h*ave expectorant effect and increase the secretion of the respiratory tract gland. In general, the efficacies of all these preparations reach the peak within one hour after oral administration. Among them *Jié gěng, Qián hú* and *Zào jiá* exhibit significant pharmacological effects. When taken orally, the effect of *Tiān nán xīng* decoction on increasing the secretion of respiratory fluids could last for more than four hours in rabbits. Apart from rorifone in the *Hàn cài* and farrerol in

Mǎn shān hóng, the dispelling phlegm effect of other medicines could be mainly attributed to saponins they contain. Saponins can stimulate pharyngeal or gastric mucosa, induce mild nausea, increase secretion of bronchial glands, dilute mucus and thus phlegm can be removed more easily through coughing. Unlike saponins, farrerol acts directly on respiratory mucosa. It promotes the movement of mucociliary of trachea, enhances the function of removing foreign matters from respiratory tract and dispel phlegm. Also, it breaks the disulfide bond of acid mucopolysaccharide fiber in respiratory secretions, decreases the viscosity of phlegm and thus make it easy to cough up.

2. **镇咳** 苦杏仁、半夏、百部、桔梗、川贝母、款冬花、紫菀、满山红等均有不同程度的镇咳作用。

(2) Relieving cough Medicines including *Kǔ xìng rén*, *Bàn xià*, *Bǎi bù*, *Jié gěng*, *Chuān bèi mǔ*, *Kuǎn dōng huā*, *Zǐ wǎn* and *Mǎn shān hóng* have varying degrees of effect on relieving cough.

3. **平喘** 川贝母、浙贝母、苦杏仁、蕹菜、枇杷叶、款冬花、洋金花等可通过扩张支气管、改善通气功能而平喘，涉及多方面的作用机制，如浙贝母含浙贝碱能扩张家兔与猫的支气管平滑肌，直接抑制支气管痉挛而缓解哮喘症状；款冬花醚提取物可通过兴奋神经节而平喘，通过抗过敏而抑制组胺所致豚鼠支气管痉挛；洋金花含莨菪类生物碱，平喘作用与阻断 M 受体有关。

(3) Relieving dyspnea Medicines, such as *Chuān bèi mǔ*, *Zhè bèi mǔ*, *Kǔ xìng rén*, *Hàn cài*, *Pí pá yè*, *Kuǎn dōng huā*, *Yáng jīn huā*, have the effect of calming panting by dilating bronchus and improving the ventilatory function. This effect involves various mechanisms. For instance, the peimine in *Zhè bèi mǔ* can dilate the bronchial smooth muscles of rabbits and cats, and prevent bronchospasm to reduce dyspnea symptoms. The ether extract of *Kuǎn dōng huā* has relieving dyspnea effect , which may be related to its effect of exciting the ganglion cells. In addition, it has the effect of anti-allergy, which makes it effective in prohibiting histamine-induced bronchospasm in guinea pigs. The belladonna alkaloid in *Yáng jīn huā* has the effect of relieving dyspnea which is related to its effect of blocking M receptor.

4. **其他作用** 除呼吸系统外，止咳平喘药祛"无形之痰"的功效还与其对心血管系统疾病、神经系统疾病、消化系统疾病以及肿瘤的治疗作用相关。部分止咳平喘药还具有抗菌、抗炎、抗病毒、抗心律失常、抗惊厥、抗肿瘤以及调血脂、镇吐、镇静等作用。

(4) Other effects In addition to the respiratory system, the efficacy of antitussive and antiasthmatic medicines in eliminating "invisible phlegm" is also related to its therapeutic effect on cardiovascular system, nervous system, digestive system diseases and tumors. Some antitussive and antiasthmatic medicines also have antibacterial, antiinflammatory, antiviral, antiarrhythmic, anticonvulsant, antitumor, blood lipid regulating, antiemetic and sedative effects.

常用止咳平喘药的主要药理作用见表 15-1。

The main pharmacological effects of common antitussives and antiasthmatics are summarized in Table 15-1.

表 15-1 常用止咳平喘药的主要药理作用

药物	祛痰	镇咳	平喘	其他药理作用
半夏	+	+	−	镇吐、催吐、抗溃疡、调节胃肠运动、抗肿瘤、抗早孕
桔梗	+	+	−	松弛平滑肌、抗炎、降血糖、降血脂
川贝母	+	+	+	抗菌、抑制胃肠平滑肌、抗溃疡
浙贝母		+	+	兴奋子宫、降血压
苦杏仁	+	+	+	抗炎、增强免疫、泻下、镇痛、抗肿瘤

续表

药物	祛痰	镇咳	平喘	其他药理作用
款冬花	+	+	+	抑制血小板聚集
紫菀	+	+	−	抗菌、抗病毒、抗肿瘤
前胡	+	−	−	抗炎、抗过敏、抗心律失常
葶菜	+	+	+	抗菌
天南星	+	−	−	镇静、镇痛、抗惊厥、抗肿瘤
洋金花	−	+	+	影响中枢神经系统

注："+"表示有明确作用；"−"表示无作用，或未查阅到相关研究文献

第二节　常用药物

Section 2　Commonly used medicines

| 半夏 | *Bàn xià (Pinelliae Rhizoma)* |

【来源 / Origin】

本品为天南星科植物半夏 [*Pinellia ternata* (Thunb.) Breit.] 的干燥块茎。主产于四川、湖北、安徽、江苏等地。一般用姜汁、明矾制过入药，有姜半夏、法半夏、半夏曲等。

Bàn xià is the dried tubers of the *Pinellia ternata* (Thunb.) Breit. The plant is widely cultivated in Sichuan province, Hubei province, Anhui province, and Jiangsu province in China. It's generally used after being baked with ginger juice and alumen. There are *Jiāng Bàn xià*, *Fǎ Bàn xià* and *Bàn xià qǔ*, etc.

【化学成分 / Chemical ingredients】

含有 β–谷甾醇、β–谷甾醇–β–D–葡萄糖苷、胆碱、左旋麻黄碱、毒芹碱、葫芦巴碱、3,4–二羟基苯甲醛及其葡萄糖苷、胡萝卜苷、葡萄糖醛酸苷、鸟嘌呤核苷、甲硫氨酸、尿黑酸、β–氨基丁酸、葡萄糖醛酸、甘氨酸、双（4–羟基苯基）醚、2–氯丙烯酸甲酯、原儿茶酸、3–甲基二十烷、半夏蛋白、多糖等成分。

The tubers of *Bàn xià* contain β-sitosterol, β-sitosterol-β-D-glucoside, choline, L-ephedrine conine, trigonelline, 3,4-dihydroxy benzaldehyde and its glucoside, daucosterol, glucuronide, guanosine, methionine, homogentisate, β-aminobutyric acid, glucuronic acid, glycine, bis (4-hydroxyphenyl) ether, methyl 2-chloroacrylate, protocatechuic acid, 3-methyl eicosane, pinellia protein, polysaccharide, etc.

【药性与功效 / Chinese medicine properties】

味辛，性温，有毒，归脾、胃、肺经。具有燥湿化痰、降逆止呕、消痞散结的功效，外用消肿止痛。用于治疗湿痰证与寒痰证。

In Chinese medicine theory, *Bàn xià* has the nature of pungent, warm, toxic. It can enter the meridians of spleen, stomach and lung. It can dry dampness and resolve phlegm, reduce vomiting and stop vomiting, and eliminate swelling and disperse stagnation; external use can reduce swelling and pain. Clinically it can be used for damp phlegm or cold-phlegm syndrome.

【药理作用 / Pharmacological effects】

1. **镇咳** 作用比可待因弱，比浙贝母强，镇咳部位在中枢，镇咳有效成分为生物碱。

(1) Relieving cough The antitussive effects of *Bàn xià* is weaker than codeine and better than *Zhè bèi mǔ*. The antitussive action site of *Bàn xià* is in the center, and its antitussive active component is alkaloid.

2. **镇吐、催吐** 制半夏具有镇吐作用，镇吐成分为生物碱、甲硫氨酸、葡萄糖醛酸、甘氨酸及左旋麻黄碱，镇吐机制与抑制中枢有关。生半夏具有催吐作用，半夏苷元（3,4- 二羟基苯甲醛葡萄糖苷）具有强烈的黏膜刺激作用，推测是半夏催吐的主要成分。

(2) Antiemetic and emetic Processed *Bàn xià has* antiemetic effects. Its anti-emetic ingredients are alkaloids, methionine, glucuronic acid, glycine and L-ephedrine, and the anti-emetic effect may be related to the inhibition of vomiting center in central nervous system. Raw *Bàn xià* has emetic effects. Pinellia aglycone (3,4-dibydroxy benzaldehyde glucoside) has strong mucosal stimulation, which is considered to be the main ingredient of its emetic effects.

3. **抗溃疡** 半夏能抑制胃液分泌、降低胃液酸度，减少游离酸与总酸含量，抑制胃蛋白酶活性，保护急性胃黏膜损伤并促进其修复，并具有抗炎、镇痛作用。生半夏则因抑制胃肠黏膜细胞前列腺素 E_2（PGE_2）分泌而损伤胃黏膜。

(3) Anti-ulcer *Bàn xià* can inhibit gastric secretion, decrease gastric acidity, reduce the content of free acid and total acids, inhibit pepsin activity, protect acute gastric mucosal injury and promote mucosal repair, and have anti-inflammatory and analgesic effects. Raw *Bàn xià* damages gastric mucosa, which is related to its inhibition of gastric mucosal cell E_2（PGE_2）secretion.

4. **调节胃肠运动** 半夏影响胃肠运动功能比较复杂，生半夏能促进胃肠运动，姜矾半夏和姜煮半夏则抑制胃肠运动。促进胃肠运动作用机制与激动乙酰胆碱（ACh）受体有关，抑制胃肠运动有效成分是麻黄碱。

(4) Regulate gastrointestinal movement *Bàn xià* affects gastrointestinal motor function, and its mechanism is very complex. Raw *Bàn xià* can promote gastrointestinal movement, but *Bàn xià* processed with ginger juice and alum or only with ginger juice can inhibit gastrointestinal movement. The mechanism of promoting gastrointestinal motility is related to the activation of acetyl choline (ACh) receptors. Ephedrine is suggested to be the active ingredient of inhibiting gastrointestinal motility.

5. **抗肿瘤** 体外抗肿瘤试验表明，半夏总生物碱具有抑制红白血病细胞（K562）及人肺癌细胞（A549）增殖的作用；掌叶半夏总蛋白可显著抑制人卵巢癌细胞（SKOV3）增殖，并引起其蛋白质组学的改变；半夏中葫芦巴碱对小鼠肝癌亦有抑制作用；半夏凝集素（PTA）可凝集多种癌细胞，包括人肝癌细胞、小鼠艾氏腹水癌细胞（ECA）和腹水型肝癌细胞（HCA），还是一种鉴别乳房上皮细胞是否恶性化的指示剂；半夏多糖亦具有抗肿瘤和活化多形核白细胞作用。

(5) Anti-tumor Vitro anti-tumor experiments show that, total alkaloids of *Bàn xià* have inhibitory effects on chronic myeloid leukemia cell (K652) and human lung cancer cell (A549) proliferation. Total protein of pinellia pedatisecta schott can significantly inhibit human ovarian cancer cell (SKOV3) proliferation, and cause proteomic changes. Trigonelline in *Bàn xià* can inhibits liver cancer in mice. Pinellia ternata agglutinin（PTA）can agglutinate a variety of cancer cells, including human hepatoma cell, Ehrlich ascites cancer (ECA) cell in mice and ascites hepatocellular carcinoma cells (HCA), and is also an indicator of malignant breast epithelial cells. *Bàn xià* polysaccharides can inhibit tumors and activate polynuclear leukocytes.

6. **其他作用** 半夏还具有一定的镇痛、抗炎、镇静、抗真菌，抗心律失常、抗硅沉着病、降血脂、抗帕金森病等作用，小鼠半夏蛋白皮下注射有明显抗生育和抗早孕作用。

(6) Other effects *Bàn xià* also has analgesic, anti-inflammatory, sedative, antifungal, antiarrhythmic, anti silicosis, antihyperlipidemic and anti-parkinson's disease effects. *Bàn xià* protein administered via subcutaneous injection has obvious anti fertility and anti-early pregnancy effect on mice.

【不良反应 / Adverse effects】

生半夏对口腔、喉头及消化道黏膜有强烈刺激性，人误服可致咽喉肿胀、疼痛、失音、痉挛、流涎、呼吸困难，严重者可致死亡。临床应用半夏多采用生姜和明矾炮制以降低其毒性。

Raw *Bàn xià* is strongly irritative to buccal, laryngeal and gastrointestinal mucosa. Misuse of it will result in swollen throat, pain, aphonia, spasm, salivation, dyspnea and even cause death. In clinical applications, *Bàn xià* is always baked with ginger and alumen to reduce its toxicity.

桔梗 ┊ *Jié gěng*（ Platycodonis Radix ）

【来源 / Origin】

本品为桔梗科植物桔梗 [*Platycodon grandiflorum* (Jacq.) A. DC.] 的干燥根。生用、炒用或蜜炙用。

Jié gěng is the dried root of *Platycodon grandiflorus* (Jacq.) A. DC. It can be used in raw, sauteed or roasted with honey.

【化学成分 / Chemical ingredients】

含多种皂苷类成分，主要为三萜皂苷类，约有 40 种，根据皂苷元母核化学结构变化规律可分为桔梗酸类，如桔梗皂苷 A、桔梗皂苷 B、桔梗皂苷 D；桔梗二酸类，如桔梗二酸 A、桔梗二酸 B、桔梗二酸 C；远志酸类，如远志皂苷 D。此外，还含有白桦脂醇、甲基 –3–O–β–D–吡喃葡萄糖基远志酸甲酯、3–O–β– 昆布二糖基远志酸甲酯、α– 菠菜甾醇、2–O–甲基桔梗苷酸 A 甲酯、α– 菠菜甾醇 –β–D– 葡糖苷等。

Jié gěng contains various saponins, among which triterpenoid saponin is the main component. To date, more than 40 triterpenoid saponins have been reported to exist in *Jié gěng*. Based on how the chemical structures of parent nucleus are changed, saponins are classified as platycodic acid like platycodin A, B, D, platycogenic acid like platycogenic acid A, B, C, and polygala acids like polygalacin D. In addition, it contains botulin, methyl-3-O-β-D-methyl pyranoglucosyl polygalate, 3-O-β-laminandiosylpolygalate methyl ester, α-spinagosterol, 2-O-methyl platycoside A methyl ester, α-borneosterol-β-D-glucoside, etc.

【药性与功效 / Chinese medicine properties】

味苦、辛，性平，归肺经。具有宣肺、利咽、祛痰、排脓的功效。用于咳嗽痰多、咽痛音哑、胸闷不畅、肺痈吐脓等证。

In Chinese medicine theory, *Jié gěng* has the nature of bitter and acrid flavor, neutral in nature, and enters the meridians of lung. It can ventilate lung, soothe the throat, dispel phlegm and expel pus. It can be used for cough with copious phlegm, pharyngalgia and hoarseness, oppression in the chest, pulmonary abscess, vomiting of pus and blood, etc.

【药理作用 / Pharmacological effects】

1. 祛痰　桔梗不同药用部位（根、根皮、叶、茎、花、果）均有显著祛痰作用，野生桔梗与二年栽培品的祛痰作用无明显差别，主要成分为桔梗总皂苷和黑曲霉转化的总桔梗次皂苷。桔梗祛痰强度与氯化铵相似，作用机制主要是其所含的皂苷经口服刺激胃黏膜，反射性增加支气管黏膜分泌，使痰液稀释而被排出。

(1) Dispelling phlegm All of the different medicinal parts (root, rind, leaf, stem, flower and fruit) of *Jié gěng* can dispel phlegm significantly. There are no significant differences in expectorant effects between the wild and two year cultivation. The main components are total platycodin and its secondary saponins transformed by aspergillus niger. The expectorant effect of *Jié gěng* is similar to that of ammonium chloride. The main mechanism of expectorant is that the total platycodin can stimulate the gastric mucosa by oral administration, reflectively increases secretion of bronchial mucosa, the sputum is diluted and discharged.

2. 镇咳　桔梗水提物和桔梗皂苷均有镇咳作用。桔梗水提物腹腔注射能抑制机械刺激豚鼠气管黏膜引起的咳嗽，镇咳率达 60%；桔梗皂苷镇咳的半数有效量（ED_{50}）为 6.4mg/kg，大约是半数致死量（LD_{50}）的 1/4。野生桔梗与二年栽培品的镇咳作用无明显差别。

(2) Relieving cough　Both water extract and platycodin of *Jié gěng* have antitussive effects. Water extract of *Jié gěng* administered by intraperitoneal injection can inhibit cough caused by mechanical stimulation of tracheal mucosa in guinea pigs and antitussive rate was 60%. The median effective dose (ED_{50}) of platycodin for antitussive was 6.4mg/kg, about 1/4 of that of median lethal dose (LD_{50}). There is no significant difference in antitussive effects between the wild and two year cultivation.

3. 松弛平滑肌　桔梗皂苷对离体豚鼠气管和回肠平滑肌均无直接作用，但能竞争性拮抗 ACh 引起的回肠收缩及组胺致回肠收缩和气管收缩。

(3) Relax smooth muscle　Platycodin has no direct effect on trachea and ileum smooth muscle of isolated guinea pigs. However, it can competitively antagonize ACh-induced ileum contractions and histamine-induced ileum contractions and tracheal contractions.

4. 抗炎　对角叉菜胶致大鼠足跖肿胀、醋酸致小鼠扭体反应、大鼠棉球肉芽肿及佐剂性关节炎均有抑制作用，并能抑制过敏性休克小鼠毛细血管通透性，抗炎主要成分为桔梗皂苷，作用机制与调节小鼠腹腔巨噬细胞一氧化氮（NO）的释放有关。桔梗总皂苷能抑制体外培养的肺炎支原体（MP）生长繁殖，减轻慢性支气管炎模型小鼠气道重塑的病理改变，作用机制与清除小鼠肺组织中的炎症因子和自由基含量、抑制基质金属蛋白酶 –9（MMP-9）和金属蛋白酶组织抑制剂 –1（TIMP-1）的表达有关。

(4) Anti-inflammation　It has strong inhibitory effect rats paw edema induced by carrageenan, mice writhing reaction induced by acetic acid, rats cotton ball granuloma and adjuvant arthritis. It can also inhibit the capillary permeability of mice with anaphylactic shock. The saponins is the main anti-inflammatory component, and the mechanism is related to the regulation of nitric oxide (NO) release from peritoneal macrophages. The total saponins from *Jié gěng* can also inhibit the proliferation of mycoplasma pneumonia (MP) *in vitro* experiments and the pathological changes of airway remodeling in mice with chronic bronchitis. The mechanism is related to removal of inflammatory factors and free radicals in the lung tissues of mice and the inhibition of matrix metalloproteinase-9 (MMP-9) and tissue inhibitor of metalloproteinase-1(TIMP-1) expression.

5. 其他作用　桔梗还具有降血糖、降血脂、镇静、镇痛、解热、扩张血管、减慢心率、抗溃疡、利尿、抗肿瘤等作用。

(5) Other effects　*Jié gěng* also has the effects of hypoglycemic, hypolipidemic, sedative, analgesic, antipyretic, expanding blood vessel, slowing heart rate, anti-ulcer, promoting diuresis and inhibiting tumors.

【不良反应 / Adverse effects】

口服桔梗的不良反应少见，常见的有恶心、呕吐，严重者有心烦、乏力、四肢出汗等。桔梗皂苷具有很强的溶血作用，溶血指数为 1∶10 000，故不能静脉注射给药。

Adverse reactions with oral preparations of *Jié gěng* are rare. Nausea and vomiting are common.

Serious adverse reactions include irritability, fatigue, sweating, etc. Platycodin has strong hemolysis with the haemolytic index of 1 : 10 000 *in vitro*, so it can not be administered intravenously.

川贝母 ┊ *Chuān bèi mǔ*（*Fritillariae Cirrhosae Bulbus*）

【来源 / Origin】

本品为百合科植物川贝母（*Fritillaria cirrhosa* D. Don）、暗紫贝母（*Fritillaria unibracteata* Hsiao et K. C. Hsia）、甘肃贝母（*Fritillaria przewalskii* Maxim.）、梭砂贝母（*Fritillaria delavayi* Franch.）、太白贝母（*Fritillaria taipaiensis* P. Y. Li）或瓦布贝母［*Fritillaria unibracteata* Hsiao et K. C. Hsia var. *wabuensis*（S. Y. Tang et S. C. Yue）Z. D. Liu, S. Wang et S. C. Chen］的干燥鳞茎。按性状不同分别习称"松贝""青贝""炉贝"和"栽培品"。主产于四川、云南、甘肃等地。

Chuān bèi mǔ is the dried bulbs of *Fritillaria cirrhosa* D. Don, *Fritillaria unibracteata* Hsiao et K. C. Hsia, *Fritillaria przewalskii* Maxim, *Fritillaria delavayi* Franch., *Fritillaria taipaiensis* P. Y. Li or *Fritillaria unibracteata* Hsiao et K. C. Hsia var. *wabuensis* (S. Y. Tang et S. C. Yue) Z. D. Liu, S. Wang et S. C. Chen. According to different traits, they can be classified as *Song bei*, *Qing bei*, *Lu bei*, and cultivated products. It mainly grows in Sichuan province, Yunnan province, Gansu province, etc., in China.

【化学成分 / Chemical ingredients】

主要成分为生物碱类。川贝母含川贝母碱、西贝母碱、青贝碱、考瑟蔚胺碱、考瑟蔚宁碱、考瑟蔚灵碱、考瑟文宁碱、考辛碱及茄啶；暗紫贝母含 β-谷甾醇、硬脂酸、松贝甲素、蔗糖；甘肃贝母含腺苷、梭砂贝母酮碱、西贝素、胸腺嘧啶核苷、川贝酮；梭砂贝母含梭砂贝母碱、梭砂贝母酮碱、梭砂贝母芬酮碱、西贝素、川贝酮碱。另含皂苷类成分。

The main components are alkaloids. *Chuān Bèi mǔ* contains fritimine, sipeimine, chinpeimine, korseveramine, korseverinine, korseveriline, korsevinine, korsine and solanidine; *Àn zǐ Bèi mǔ* contains β-sitosterol, stearicacid, matsubicin, saccharose; *Gān sù Bèi mǔ* contains adenosine, delavinone, imperialine, thymidine, chuanbeinone; *Suō shā Bèi mǔ* contains hupehenine, delavinone, delafrinone, imperialine and chuanbeinone. It also contains saponins.

【药性与功效 / Chinese medicine properties】

味苦、甘，性微寒，归肺、心经。具有清热润肺、化痰止咳、散结消痈的功效。用于虚劳咳嗽、肺热燥咳、瘰疬、疮肿、乳痈、肺痈等证。

In Chinese medicine theory, *Chuān bèi mǔ* has the nature of bitter and sweet flavor, slightly cold property. It can enter the meridians of lung and heart. It has the efficacies of clearing heat and moistening lung, resolving phlegm and relieving cough, and dissipating mass and resolving carbuncle. Clinically it can be used for syndrome of cough due to asthenia of the viscera, dry cough due to lung heat, cervical scrofula, boil, acute mastitis, lung abscess, etc.

【药理作用 / Pharmacological effects】

1. 祛痰、镇咳　祛痰作用显著，主要成分为川贝总苷；镇咳作用不太稳定，主要成分为川贝总碱。

(1) Resolving phlegm and cough　The expectorant effect of *Chuān bèi mǔ* is significant, and the main component of expectorant is total glycoside; the antitussive effect is not stable, and the main component of antitussive is total alkaloid.

2. 平喘　川贝母具有平喘作用，能显著抑制 ACh 和组胺引起的豚鼠哮喘，平喘主要成分为总生物碱。

(2) Relieving dyspnea　*Chuān bèi mǔ* has antiasthmatic effects. It can inhibit the dyspnea caused by acetylcholine and histamine in guinea pigs. The main component of antiasthmatic is total alkaloid.

3. 抗菌　体外抗菌试验表明，川贝母醇提物对金黄色葡萄球菌与大肠埃希菌有明显抑制作用。

(3) Anti-bacteria　The vitro antibacterial test shows that the alcohol extract of *Chuān bèi mǔ* has obvious suppression on *staphylococcus aureus* and *escherichia coli*.

4. 其他作用　①抗溃疡：川贝母具有松弛胃肠道平滑肌、抗溃疡作用，主要成分为贝母碱，作用机制与抑制胃蛋白酶活性有关。②降血压：静脉注射引起血压下降并伴有短暂性呼吸抑制或心律减慢，主要成分为贝母碱。③抗血小板聚集：主要成分为腺苷。

(4) Other effects　①Anti-ulcer: *Chuān bèi mǔ* has the effects of relaxing gastrointestinal smooth muscle and being anti-ulcer. The main components are alkaloids, and the mechanism may be related to inhibition of pepsin activity. ②Anti-hypertensive: the intravenous injection can lower blood pressure, and is accompanied by transient respiratory suppression or heart rate reduction. ③Anti-platelet aggregation: the main component is adenosine.

浙贝母 ┆ *Zhè bèi mǔ* (*Fritillariae Thunbergii Bulbus*)

【来源 / Origin】

本品为百合科植物浙贝母（*Fritillaria thunbergii* Miq.）的干燥鳞茎。

Zhè bèi mǔ is the dried bulbs of the *Fritillaria thunbergii* Miq..

【化学成分 / Chemical ingredients】

主要成分为浙贝母碱、去氢浙贝母碱、异浙贝母碱和胆碱等生物碱类以及浙贝母苷、贝母醇、胡萝卜素、二萜类化合物和脂肪酸。

The main ingredients of *Zhè bèi mǔ* are alkaloids, such as verticine, isoverticine, verticinone verticinone and so on, peiminoside, propeimine, carotene, diterpenoids and fatty acid.

【药性与功效 / Chinese medicine properties】

味苦，性寒，归肺、心经。具有清热化痰止咳、解毒散结消痈的功效。用于风热咳嗽、痰火咳嗽、肺痈、乳痈、瘰疬、疮毒等。

In Chinese medicine theory, *Zhè bèi mǔ* has the nature of bitter and cold. It can enter the meridians of lung and heart. It has the efficacies of clearing heat and resolving phlegm，relieving cough, detoxification, dissipating mass and resolving carbuncle. Clinically it can be used for cough due to wind heat, cough due to phlegm fire, lung abscess, acute mastitis, cervical scrofula and sodoku.

【药理作用 / Pharmacological effects】

1. 祛痰、镇咳　浙贝母醇提物、浙贝母碱和去氢浙贝母碱均有显著镇咳作用。

(1) Resolving phlegm and cough　The antitussive effect of *Zhè bèi mǔ* is significant, and the main components of antitussive are the alcohol extract of *Zhè bèi mǔ*, verticine, verticinone.

2. 松弛支气管平滑肌　浙贝母碱低浓度对支气管平滑肌有扩张作用，高浓度则有收缩作用。浙贝母醇提物对组胺引起的豚鼠离体支气管收缩有明显松弛作用。

(2) Relaxation of bronchial smooth muscle　Low concentration of verticine can expand bronchial smooth muscle, and high concentration of verticine can shrink it. The alcohol extract of *Zhè bèi mǔ* can evidently slack contraction of isolated bronchi in guinea pigs caused by histamine.

3. 其他作用

(3) Other effects

（1）抗炎　浙贝母对二甲苯致小鼠耳肿胀和角叉菜胶引起的大鼠足跖肿胀均有抑制作用，并能抑制腹腔注射醋酸所致小鼠毛细血管通透性增加。

1) Anti-inflammation   *Zhè bèi mǔ* can inhibit mouse ear swelling caused by xylene and plantar swelling in rats caused by carrageenan. it also can inhibit the increase of capillary permeability in mice caused by intraperitoneal injection of acetic acid.

（2）镇静、镇痛   镇静成分为浙贝母碱和去氢浙贝母碱，二者皮下注射可使小鼠自发活动明显减少；灌胃可使戊巴比妥钠引起的小鼠睡眠率提高，睡眠时间延长。镇痛成分为浙贝母碱和去氢浙贝母碱和浙贝母醇提物，皮下注射可抑制腹腔注射醋酸所引起的小鼠扭体反应，浙贝母醇提物还能抑制热痛刺激引起的甩尾反应。

2) Sedation and analgesia   The main components of sedation are verticine and verticinone, and injecting them subcutaneously can significantly reduce the spontaneous activity of mice. Intragastric administration can increase the sleep rate and sleep time of mice induced by pentobarbital sodium. The main components of analgesia are verticine, verticinone, and subcutaneous injection can inhibit the writhing response of mice induced by intraperitoneal injection of acetic acid. The alcohol extract of *Zhè bèi mǔ* can inhibit the tail flick response caused by thermal pain stimulation.

（3）收缩子宫平滑肌   主要成分为浙贝母碱，已孕子宫比未孕子宫敏感。其收缩子宫作用不被阿托品拮抗，预先使用 α 受体阻滞剂酚苄明能减弱或消除其对子宫的作用。

3) Contraction of uterine smooth muscle   The main component is verticine, and pregnant womb is more sensitive than non-pregnant womb. The contraction of uterus is not antagonized by atropine, and advance use of α-receptor blocker phenacetin can weaken or eliminate the effect on uterus.

（4）逆转肿瘤细胞耐药   浙贝母总生物碱可逆转 A549 细胞对顺铂（DDP）的耐药性，降低 A549/DDP 细胞多药耐药基因 1（MDR1）mRNA 和 A549/DDP 细胞 P-糖蛋白（P-gp）表达。

4) Reversal of drug resistance in tumor cells   Total alkaloids of *Zhè bèi mǔ* can reverse the tolerance of human lung adenocarcinoma cell A549 to cisplatin (DDP), and decrease the expression of multidrug resistance gene1(MDR1) mRNA and P-gp in A549 / DDP cells.

此外，浙贝母碱和去氢浙贝母碱还具有降血压作用；浙贝母碱滴眼能使兔、猫、犬瞳孔扩大；犬静脉注射可抑制涎液分泌。

In addition, the antihypertensive effects of verticine and verticinone are also observed. Eye drops of verticine can dilate pupils of rabbits, cats and dogs, and intravenous injection in dogs can inhibit salivary secretion.

苦杏仁 ┊ *Kǔ xìng rén (Armeniacae Semen Amarum)*

【来源 / Origin】

本品为蔷薇科植物山杏（*Prunus armeniaca* L. var. *ansu* Maxim.*）*、西伯利亚杏（*Prunus sibirica* L.）、东北杏 [*Prunus mandshurica* (Maxim.) Koehne] 或杏（*Prunus armeniaca* L.）的干燥成熟种子。

Kǔ xìng rén is the dried mature seed *Prunus armeniaca* L. var. *ansu* Maxim., *Prunus sibirica* L., *Prunus mandshurica* (Maxim.) Koehne and *Prunus armeniaca* L.

【化学成分 / Chemical ingredients】

主要成分为脂肪油、苦杏仁苷、蛋白质及多种游离氨基酸。脂肪油约占 50%，包括己醛、(E)-2-壬烯醛、(E)-2-己烯醛、(E, E)-2,4-癸二烯醛、柠檬醛、芳樟醇、胆甾醇、环氧 α-松油醇、二氢芳樟醇、异松油烯、硬脂酸、亚麻酸、花生油酸、肉豆蔻酸、棕榈油酸、棕榈酸、γ-癸内酯、γ-十二碳内酯等；苦杏仁苷约占 3%。此外，尚含有苦杏仁苷酶、苦杏仁酶及樱苷酶、玉红黄质、扁桃苷、野樱苷、毛茛黄素、β-紫罗兰酮、扁桃腈等。

The main components of *Kǔ xìng rén* are fatty oil, amygdalin, protein and a variety of free amino acids. About 50% of them is fatty oil, including hexanal, (E)-2-nonenal, (E)-2-hexenal, (E, E)-2,4-decadienal, citral, linalool, cholesterol, epoxy α-terpineol, dihydrolinalool, terpinolene, stearic acid, linolenic acid, peanut oleic acid, myristic acid, palmitoleic acid, palmatic acid, γ-decanolactone and γ-dodecalactone; 3% is amygdalin. It also contains amygdalae, emulsin, pronase, rubixanthin, amygdalin, prunasin, β-ionone, mandelonitrile, and flavoxanthin, etc.

【药性与功效 / Chinese medicine properties 】

味苦，性微温，有小毒，归肺、大肠经。具有降气止咳平喘、润肠通便的功效。用于咳嗽气喘、胸满痰多、肠燥便秘等证。

In Chinese medicine theory, *Kǔ xìng rén* has the nature of medicine bitter, tepid and hypotoxic. It can enter the meridians of lung and large intestine. It has the efficacies of descending Qi, relieving cough and dyspnea, and moistening intestines to relieve constipation. Clinically it can be used for cough, dyspnea, phlegm, intestinal dryness and constipation, etc.

【药理作用 / Pharmacological effects 】

1. **镇咳、平喘、祛痰** 豚鼠苦杏仁炮制品水煎液灌胃有显著的镇咳、平喘作用，作用机制是苦杏仁苷，经本身所含苦杏仁苷酶或肠道微生物酶分解产生微量氢氰酸，抑制呼吸中枢；小鼠苦杏仁水煎液灌胃有显著祛痰作用。

(1) Resolving cough, dyspnea and phlegm Administration of *Kǔ xìng rén* decocted by gavage has an obvious effect on relieving cough and asthma in guinea pig. The mechanism is that *Kǔ xìng rén* has amygdalin which can be resolved by enzyme or gut microbiota, and generate trace hydrocyanic acid which can inhibit the respiratory center. Administration of *Kǔ xìng rén* decote by gavage can have a significant effect on dispelling phlegm.

2. **抗炎** 苦杏仁胃蛋白酶水解物可抑制大鼠棉球肉芽肿、抑制结缔组织增生并延长优球蛋白溶解时间，但不抑制角叉菜胶致大鼠足跖急性肿胀，对佐剂致大鼠关节炎的 Ⅰ 期与 Ⅱ 期损伤也无抑制作用。苦杏仁水溶性部位无上述活性；大鼠苦杏仁蛋白 KR-A 和 KR-B 灌胃有明显抗炎作用，抗角叉菜胶性足跖肿胀的 ED_{50} 分别为 13.9mg/kg 和 6.4mg/kg。

(2) Anti-inflammation The pepsin hydrolysate of *Kǔ xìng rén* can inhibit cotton-ball-induced granuloma of rats and connective tissue hyperplasia, and prolong the dissolution time of euglobulin, but it cannot reduce the hind paw edema induced by carrageenan or development of adjuvant arthritis at stage Ⅰ or stage Ⅱ in rats. The water-soluble components of *Kǔ xìng rén* have no effects mentioned above. Protein KR-A and KR-B of *Kǔ xìng rén* have obvious anti-inflammatory effect, and their values of ED_{50} used to control hind paw edema of rats induced by carrageenan are 13.9mg/kg and 6.4mg/kg, respectively.

3. **增强免疫** 小鼠苦杏仁苷肌内注射可促进有丝分裂原所致脾 T 淋巴细胞增殖，增强小鼠脾脏自然杀伤细胞（NK）活性，提高小鼠肝细胞 Kupffer 的吞噬功能。

(3) Enhance immunity Amygdalin given by intramuscular injection can significantly promote splenic T lymphocyte proliferation induced by mitogen, reinforce activities of splenic natural killer (NK) cells from mice, and facilitate the phagocytic function of hepatic Kupffer cells.

4. **泻下** 苦杏仁富含脂肪油，具有润滑性泻下作用，可润肠通便。

(4) Purgative *Kǔ xìng rén* contains a large amount of fatty oil, which has the effects of lubricating cathartic and can moisten the intestines and relieve constipation.

5. **其他作用**

(5) Other effects

（1）抑制胃蛋白酶活性 苦杏仁苷被酶催化分解形成氢氰酸的同时也产生苯甲醛，可抑制胃蛋白酶活性。

1) Inhibit pepsin activity   Amygdalin is decomposed into hydrocyanic acid and benzaldehyde, which can inhibit pepsin activity.

（2）保肝 苦杏仁水溶性部位的胃蛋白酶水解产物可抑制四氯化碳引起的大鼠谷草转氨酶（AST）、谷丙转氨酶（ALT）水平升高，降低羟脯氨酸含量并抑制肝结缔组织增生；对二甲基亚硝胺诱导的大鼠肝纤维化也有显著改善作用；但对 D–半乳糖胶引起的 AST 和 ALT 水平升高不具有抑制作用。

2) Hepatoprotective effects   The pepsin hydrolysate of the water soluble ingredients of *Kǔ xìng rén* can inhibit the levels of aspartate aminotransferase (AST) and alanine aminotransferase (ALT) of rats, the content of hydroxyproline, and the proliferation of liver connective tissue caused by carbon tetrachloride, and improve the hepatic fibrosis induced by dimethylnitrosamine in rats; but it cannot inhibit the increase of AST and ALT levels caused by D-galactose.

（3）抗肿瘤 体外试验表明，氢氰酸、苯甲醛和苦杏仁苷均有微弱的抗肿瘤作用，氢氰酸与苯甲醛，或苦杏仁苷与 β 葡糖苷酶合用可明显提高抗肿瘤作用。氢氰酸与苯甲醛对癌细胞具有协同杀伤作用；苦杏仁苷可被 β 葡糖苷酶特异性激活从而诱导细胞凋亡。

3) Anti-tumor   The *in vitro* experiment shows that hydrocyanic acid, benzoic acid and amygdalin have slight antineoplastic effects. Combination of hydrocyanic acid and benzoic acid or amygdalin and β-glucosidase can significantly improve the antineoplastic activity. Combination of hydrocyanic acid and benzoic acid can kill the cancer cells. Amygdalin can be activated by β-glucosidase to induce apoptosis.

（4）镇痛 苦杏仁及其胃蛋白酶水解产物、苦杏仁蛋白 KR-A 和 KR-B 具有镇痛作用。

4) Analgesic effects   *Kǔ xìng rén* and its pepsin hydrolysate, as well as proteins KR-A and KR-B have analgesic effects.

【 不良反应 / Adverse effects 】

苦杏仁过量服用（儿童 10~20 粒，成人 40~60 粒）可引起急性中毒，临床表现为头晕乏力、头痛、恶心、呕吐、呼吸急促、紫绀、惊厥、昏迷等，抢救不当可因呼吸或循环衰竭而死亡。每日口服苦杏仁 4 g 持续半月或静脉给药苦杏仁苷连续 1 个月，可见毒性反应，以消化系统损害多见，并可引起心电图 T 波改变及房性期前收缩，停药后上述不良反应均可消失。

Overdose of *Kǔ xìng rén* (10-20 capsules for children, 40-60 capsules for adults) can cause acute poisoning. The clinical manifestations include dizziness, fatigue, headache, nausea，vomiting, tachypnea, cyanosis, convulsions, coma, etc. Improper rescue will cause breathing problems or death due to circulatory failure. Daily oral administration of 4 g of *Kǔ xìng rén* for half a month or intravenous injection of amygdalin for one month, can show toxic reactions, most of which are digestive system damage. It can cause ECG T wave changes and atrial premature beats. All of the above adverse reactions can disappear after withdrawal.

中毒机制：本品含苦杏仁苷，分解后产生氢氰酸可抑制细胞色素氧化酶，也可直接损害延髓呼吸中枢与血管运动中枢，引起呼吸抑制，导致死亡。因苦杏仁苷口服后极易在胃肠道分解产生氢氰酸，故口服比静脉注射毒性大。

Poisoning mechanism: *Kǔ xìng rén* contains amygdalin which is decomposed into hydrocyanic acid can inhibit the activity of cytochrome oxidase and directly damage the respiratory center and vascular motility center of the brain, and cause respiratory depression even death. As amygdalin is more easily decomposed into hydrocyanic acid in the gastrointestinal tract after oral administration, it is more toxic when orally administered than intravenously administered.

　　中毒解救：除常规处理与对症治疗外，主要用亚硝酸钠与硫代硫酸钠解救氢氰酸引起的中毒，可先静脉注射3%亚硝酸钠10ml，使血红蛋白变性，与细胞色素氧化酶竞争氰基，形成氰化高铁血红蛋白，从而使细胞色素氧化酶恢复活性。随后注射25%的硫代硫酸钠50ml，在硫氰化酶的作用下与氰化物反应，形成无毒的硫氰酸盐，迅速从尿液排出体外。

　　Detoxification: In addition to conventional treatment and symptomatic treatment, sodium nitrite and sodium thiosulfate are mainly used for detoxification caused by hydrocyanic acid. First, 10ml of 3% sodium nitrite is injected intravenously to denature hemoglobin, which compete with cytochrome oxidase for cyano groups to form cyanated methemoglobin, thereby restoring the activity of cytochrome oxidase. Then, 50ml of 25% sodium thiosulfate is injected. Sodium thiosulfate reacts with cyanide in the presence of thiocyanation to form a non-toxic thiocyanate, which is quickly excreted from the urine.

题库

（李红艳　屈　飞）

第十六章　安神药
Chapter 16　Tranquilizing medicines

学习目标 ┊ Objectives

　　1. 掌握　安神药的主要药理作用；酸枣仁与功效相关的药理作用、作用机制及药效物质基础。

　　2. 了解　远志、磁石和灵芝的药理作用及药效物质基础。

　　1. Must know　The main pharmacological effects of tranquilizing medicines; the efficacy related pharmacological effects, mechanism of action, and material basis of *Suān zǎo rén*.

　　2. Desirable to know　The main pharmacological effects and material basis of *Yuǎn zhì*, *Cí shí* and *Líng zhī*.

微课

第一节　概述
Section 1　Overview

PPT

　　凡以宁心安神为主要功效，用于治疗心神不安证的药物称为安神药。安神药可分为以下两种。①养心安神药：多味甘，归心、肝经，具甘润滋养之性，有滋养心肝、养阴补血、交通心肾等功效，主要用于阴血不足、心脾两虚、心肾不交等导致的心悸、怔忡、虚烦不眠、健忘多梦等证，代表药有酸枣仁、柏子仁、远志、合欢皮和首乌藤等。②重镇安神药：多性寒，归心、肝、肾经，具质重沉降之性，有重镇安神、平惊定志、平肝潜阳等功效，主要用于心火炽盛、痰火扰心、惊吓等引起的惊悸、失眠及惊痫、癫狂等证，代表药物有朱砂、磁石、琥珀和龙骨等。

All Chinese materia medica that are used to treat disquieted heart spirit by calming heart and tranquilizing mind are classified as tranquilizing medicines. Tranquilizing medicines can be divided into two types: heart-nourishing tranquilizers and settling tranquilizers. The heart-nourishing tranquilizers mainly are sweet flavor and enter heart and liver meridians. Moreover, they have moistening and nourishment nature. So, the heart-nourishing tranquilizers have the efficacy of nourishing heart and liver, nourishing Yin and tonifying blood and restoring coordination between heart and kidney. They are mainly used in the treatment of palpitations, fearful throbbing, deficiency vexation and insomnia, forgetfulness and profuse dreaminess caused by deficiency of Yin and blood, dual deficiency of heart and spleen, or non-interaction of the heart and kidney. This kind of tranquilizing medicines include *Suān zǎo rén*, *Bǎi*

医药大学堂
www.yiyaodxt.com

zǐ rén, *Yuǎn zhì*, *Hé huān pí*, *Shōu wū téng* and so on. The settling tranquilizers are cold in nature and enter heart, liver and kidney meridians. In addition, they have heavy in substance and down-sinking in nature. Therefore, they have the functions of tranquilizing mind with heavy settlers, calming fright and stabilizing mind, pacifying liver and subduing Yang. They are available treatments for fright palpitations, insomnia, fright epilepsy, mania and withdrawal due to intense heart fire, phlegm-fire harassing heart or startle. This class of medicines include *Zhū shā*, *Cí shí*, *Hǔ pò*, *Lóng gǔ* and so on.

心神不安多为外受惊恐、肝郁化火、内扰心神或阴血不足、心神失养所致，表现为惊狂善怒、烦躁不安者，多属实证，据"惊者平之"治则，治宜重镇安神；表现为心悸健忘、虚烦失眠者，多属虚证，根据"虚者补之"治则，治宜养心安神。安神药治疗心神不安证与下列药理作用有关。

Disquieted heart spirit is mainly caused by fright and fear, liver depression transforming into fire, harassing the inner heart spirit, insufficiency of Yin-blood or dystrophy of heart spirit. According to fright treated by calming therapeutic principle, excess pattern patients suffering from fright mania irascibility or agitation should be treated with settling tranquilizers. On the other hand, nourishing tranquilizers are suitable for palpitations forgetfulness, or deficiency vexation and insomnia patients classified as deficiency pattern. The tranquilizing mind function is related to the following pharmacological effects.

1. **镇静**　安神药具有镇静作用。酸枣仁、磁石、琥珀、龙骨、朱砂、远志等均可减少小鼠自发性活动，协同巴比妥类起中枢抑制作用，拮抗苯丙胺的中枢兴奋作用。

(1) Sedative effects　Tranquilizing medicines have sedative effects. *Suān zǎo rén*, *Cí shí*, *Hǔ pò*, *Lóng gǔ*, *Zhū shā* and *Yuǎn zhì* can reduce the spontaneous locomotor activity of mice, and synergistically enhance the inhibition in the central nervous system (CNS) of barbiturates, and antagonize the excitatory effects of CNS of amphetamine.

2. **抗惊厥**　酸枣仁、远志可抑制戊四氮引起的阵挛性惊厥。酸枣仁、琥珀、磁石可对抗士的宁引起的惊厥。琥珀对大鼠听源性惊厥及小鼠电惊厥、龙骨对二甲弗林引起的惊厥、灵芝对烟碱引起的惊厥、朱砂对安钠咖引起的惊厥，均具有抑制作用。

(2) Anticonvulsant effects　Tranquilizing medicines have anticonvulsant effects on different kinds of experimental seizures model, such as inhibition of pentylenetetrazol (PTZ)-induced clonic seizures of *Suān zǎo rén* and *Yuǎn zhì*, strychnine-induced seizures of *Suān zǎo rén*, *Hǔ pò* and *Cí shí*, rat's auditory and mice's electrical stimulation-induced seizures of *Hǔ pò*, dimefline-induced seizures of *Lóng gǔ*, nicotine-induced seizures of *Líng zhī*, caffeine and sodium benzoate-induced seizures of *Zhū Shā*, respectively.

3. **改善睡眠**　大多数安神药能延长戊巴比妥钠所致睡眠时间，并能延长实验动物总睡眠时间，延长非快速动眼睡眠（NREMS）时相的慢波睡眠（SWS），促进机体功能恢复，提高睡眠质量，如酸枣仁、首乌藤、磁石、龙骨等。

(3) Improving sleep effects　Most tranquilizers can increase sleep (NREMS) duration of the mice treated with pentobarbital sodium. Meanwhile, tranquilizers also prolong the total sleep time in experiment animal, especially the slow wave sleep (SWS) duration of non-rapid eye movement sleep (NREMS), and promote a recovery of body function, such as *Suān zǎo rén*, *Shōu wū téng*, *Cí shí* and *Lóng gǔ*.

4. **影响心血管系统**　酸枣仁、远志、灵芝具有抗心律失常、抗心肌缺血和降血压等作用。

(4) Effects on cardiovascular system　The medicines including *Suān zǎo rén*, *Yuǎn zhì* and *Líng zhī*, have antiarrhythmia, anti-myocardial ischemia and lowering blood pressure effects.

常用安神药的主要药理作用见表 16-1。

The main pharmacological effects of commonly used tranquilizing medicines are summarized in Table 16-1.

表 16-1　常用安神药的主要药理作用

药物	镇静	抗惊厥	改善睡眠	其他药理作用
朱砂	+	-	+	镇咳、祛痰、解毒
琥珀	+	+	-	—
磁石	+	+	+	抗炎、止血、镇痛、补血
龙骨	+	+	+	促凝血、收敛、固涩
酸枣仁	+	+	+	增强学习记忆、抗焦虑、镇痛、降血脂、降血压、抗心律失常
远志	+	+	+	增强学习记忆、祛痰、镇咳、保护神经、抗抑郁、兴奋子宫
灵芝	+	+	+	增强免疫、增强学习记忆、延缓衰老、抗肿瘤、降血糖、抗炎、抗过敏、保肝、解毒、抗心肌缺血、抗心律失常

注："+"表示有明确作用；"-"表示无作用，或未查阅到相关研究文献

第二节　常用药物

Section 2　Commonly used medicines

PPT

酸枣仁 ┆ *Suān zǎo rén (Semen Ziziphi Spinosae)*

【来源 / Origin】

本品为鼠李科植物酸枣 [*Ziziphus jujuba* Mill. var. *spinosa* (Bunge) Hu ex H. F. Chou] 的干燥成熟种子。主产于河北、陕西、河南、辽宁等地。生用或炒制。

Suān zǎo rén is the dried mature seed of *Ziziphus jujuba* Mill. var. *spinosa* (Bunge) Hu ex H. F. Chou. It is mainly cultivated in Hebei province, Shaanxi province, Henan province, Liaoning province in China. Raw or stir-fry *Suān zǎo rén* all can be used.

【化学成分 / Chemical ingredients】

主要含有黄酮、三萜、生物碱以及脂肪油等多种成分。皂苷类主要有酸枣仁皂苷 A、酸枣仁皂苷 B、酸枣仁皂苷 B1。酸枣仁中含有约 32% 的脂肪油，其中包含 8 种脂肪酸。此外，酸枣仁还含有阿魏酸、17 种氨基酸、微量元素、磷脂类成分等。

Suān zǎo rén mainly contains flavonoids, triterpenoids, alkaloids and fatty oil. The main saponin components of *Suān zǎo rén* were jujubosides A, jujuboside B and jujuboside B1. *Suān zǎo rén* also contains 32% fatty oil, including eight kinds of fatty acid. In addition, *Suān zǎo rén* contains ferulic acid, seventeen kinds of amino acids, microelements and phospholipids.

【药性与功效 / Chinese medicine properties】

味甘、酸，性平，归心、肝、胆经。具有养心益肝、安神、敛汗的功效。主治心悸失眠、体

医药大学堂
WWW.YIYAODXT.COM

虚多汗等证。

In Chinese medicine theory, *Suān zǎo rén* has sweet and sour in flavor, neutral in nature. It can enter meridians of heart, liver and gallbladder. *Suān zǎo rén* has the efficacies of nourishing heart and boosting liver, tranquilizing mind and constraining sweat. Clinically it can be used for palpitation insomnia, weak health profuse sweating.

【 药理作用 / **Pharmacological activities** 】

1. **镇静**　酸枣仁煎剂、醇提物对小鼠、大鼠、豚鼠、兔、猫、犬均有镇静作用；酸枣仁提取物可减少正常小鼠的活动次数，抑制苯丙胺的中枢兴奋作用，降低大鼠的协调运动；酸枣仁黄酮和皂苷均可减少小鼠自发性活动。

(1) **Sedative effects**　Both *Suān zǎo rén* decoction and ethanol extracts have sedative effects in different animal species, such as mice, rats, guinea pigs, rabbits, cats and dogs. The extracts of *Suān zǎo rén* can also reduce the locomotor activity in normal mice, inhibit amphetamine-type CNS stimulating activity, and lower motor coordination in rats. Both flavonoids and saponins of *Suān zǎo rén* can decrease the spontaneous activity of mice.

2. **抗惊厥**　酸枣仁提取物可延长小鼠出现惊厥的时间及存活时间。酸枣仁皂苷能显著降低戊四氮引起的惊厥率；酸枣仁黄酮也可拮抗咖啡因诱发的小鼠精神运动性兴奋，降低小鼠惊厥的发生率。抗惊厥的药效物质基础主要是酸枣仁皂苷、黄酮和生物碱。

(2) **Anticonvulsant effects**　The extract from *Suān zǎo rén* prolong latency and survival time of seizure mice. Saponins of *Suān zǎo rén* can significantly decrease the incidence of PTZ-induced seizures. Total flavone of *Suān zǎo rén* can also antagonize caffeine-induced psychomotor stimulation and reduce the seizure incidence in mice. Saponins, flavones and alkaloids may be the active ingredients of anticonvulsant effect.

3. **改善睡眠**　酸枣仁能延长戊巴比妥钠阈剂量的小鼠睡眠时间，增加戊巴比妥钠阈下剂量的入睡动物数和睡眠时间；酸枣仁煎剂可使大鼠慢波睡眠的总时间明显增加，发作频率也增加，每次发作的持续时间亦趋延长，慢波睡眠的脑电波幅度明显增大；酸枣仁的不饱和脂肪酸部位有镇静作用，对戊巴比妥钠引起的小鼠睡眠，可明显缩短潜伏期，延长睡眠时间，随着用药时间的延长，其作用越明显，无耐受现象。

(3) **Improving sleep effects**　*Suān zǎo rén* prolong sleep duration of the mice treated with pentobarbital sodium threshold dosage, and increase the sleep ratio of the mice treated with pentobarbital sodium under subthreshold dosage, respectively. Moreover, *Suān zǎo rén* decoction can significantly increase the total time, duration and number of slow wave sleep episodes, which is associated with high-amplitude slow waves in rats. In the pentobarbital-induced sleep experiment. Unsaturated fatty acids in *Suān zǎo rén* show a reduction latency of and increasement duration of pentobarbital-induced sleep in a dose-time dependent manner, and no tolerance is observed.

4. **抗抑郁**　对慢性应激抑郁大鼠模型，酸枣仁可通过降低大鼠前额叶 5- 羟色胺（5-HT）和多巴胺（DA）的含量而发挥抗抑郁作用。通过对行为绝望小鼠抑郁模型的研究，发现酸枣仁皂苷和黄酮具有一定的抗抑郁作用。

(4) **Antidepressant effects**　Reduction levels of serotonin (5-HT) and dopamine (DA) can be observed in chronic stress model of depression in rats after administration of *Suān zǎo rén*. Experiments have also shown that saponins and flavonoids of *Suān zǎo rén* has antidepressant effects in behavioral despair test in mice.

5. **抗焦虑**　运用高架十字迷宫诱发动物焦虑状态，研究不同给药剂量的抗焦虑作用，表明酸枣仁具有抗焦虑作用，其作用机制涉及对中枢神经递质、免疫细胞因子、下丘脑–垂体–肾上腺轴的整体调控，提高相关脑区的单胺类递质的含量，增强 γ–氨基丁酸（GABA）受体的 mRNA 表达，脑组织中白细胞介素–lβ 和糖皮质激素受体（GR）的表达，避免焦虑症伴有的高皮质酮状态可能导致神经元损伤等作用。

(5) Antianxiety effects *Suān zǎo rén* in different dosages can attenuate anxiety-like behavioral response in the elevated plus maze, and its mechanism of action involves comprehensive regulation on central neurotransmitters, neuromodulation, immune cytokines and hypothalamus-pituitary-adrenal axis, that is an increase in monoaminergic neurotransmitters in related brain regions, higher levels of γ-aminobutyric acid (GABA) receptor mRNA and interleukin-1β (IL-lβ) and glucocorticoid receptor (GR) expression, prevention of neuronal damage correlated with higher corticosterone levels and so on.

6. 增强学习记忆　酸枣仁可缩短正常小鼠在复杂水迷宫内由起点抵达终点的时间，减少错误次数；延长记忆获得障碍及记忆再现障碍模型小鼠的首次错误出现时间，减少错误发生率，改善小鼠学习记忆能力。酸枣仁油可改善用跳台法和避暗法评价的小鼠学习记忆能力，延长小鼠的错误潜伏期，减少错误次数。

(6) Improving learning and memory effects In complex maze test, *Suān zǎo rén* not only shorten escape latency time and the number of errors in normal mice, but also prolong latency of the first onset of error and reduce the error rates in impaired memory acquisition and retrieval mice. After administration with *Suān zǎo rén* oil, mice also exhibit prolonged the latency of the first onset of error and reduced number of errors in step-down test or step-through test.

远志 ┊ *Yuǎn zhì* (*Radix Polygalae*)

【来源 / Origin】

本品为远志科植物远志（*Polygala tenuifoia* Willd.）或卵叶远志（*Polygala sibirica* L.）的干燥根。主产于河北、山西、陕西、吉林、河南等地。

Yuǎn zhì is the dried root of *Polygala tenuifoia* Willd. or *Polygala sibirica* L.. It is mainly cultivated in Hebei province, Shanxi province, Shaanxi province, Jilin province, Henan province in China.

【化学成分 / Chemical ingredients】

主要含三萜皂苷类如远志皂苷 A~G、远志寡糖酯 A~C、3,6′–二芥子酰基蔗糖、3,4,5–三甲氧基肉桂酸、远志醇、山酮类化合物、生物碱等。

Yuǎn zhì mainly contains triterpenoid saponins, such as onjisaponin A, B, C, D, E, F, G. *Yuǎn zhì* also contains tenuifoliside A, B, C, 3,6′-disinapoyl sucrose, 3,4,5-trimethoxy cinnamic acid, polygalitol, polygalaxanthone, alkaloids, etc.

【药性与功效 / Chinese medicine properties】

味苦、辛，性微温，归心、肾、肺经。具有宁心安神、祛痰开窍、消散痈肿的功效。主治惊悸、失眠健忘、癫痫发狂、咳嗽痰多、痈疽疮毒、乳房肿痛等证。

In Chinese medicine theory, *Yuǎn zhì* has bitter and pungent in flavor, warm in nature. It can enter meridians of heart, kidney and lung. *Yuǎn zhì* has the efficacies of calming heart and tranquilizing mind, dispelling phlegm and opening the orifices, and dispersing welling-abscess swelling. Clinically it can be used for fright palpitation, insomnia and amnesia, epilepsy and mania, cough and copious phlegm, welling-and flat-abscesses and sore-toxin, painful swollen breast.

【药理作用 / Pharmacological effects】

1. 镇静 远志可通过与戊巴比妥钠协同作用发挥对小鼠中枢神经系统的抑制作用，远志寡糖酯 A、远志寡糖酯 C 是镇静作用的物质基础；在体内肠道细菌的作用下，远志寡糖酯 A 能转化成具有镇静活性的 3,4,5– 三甲氧基肉桂酸而产生持续的镇静作用；远志皂苷在体内通过拮抗 DA 和 5-HT 受体发挥镇静作用。

(1) Sedative effects *Yuǎn zhì* has synergistic CNC inhibition with sodium pentobarbital, and tenuifoliside A and C are suggested to be the active ingredients. Tenuifoliside A can be converts into 3,4,5-trimethoxy cinnamic acid under the action of intestinal bacteria, which exhibits long-term sedation. In addition, experiment show that saponins from *Yuǎn zhì* exhibit sedative effects due to the DA and 5-HT receptor antagonism.

2. 抗惊厥 远志醇提物对戊四氮致小鼠惊厥模型具有显著的抗惊厥作用。

(2) Anticonvulsant effects The ethanol extracts from *Yuǎn zhì* have significantly anticonvulsant effects in the mice model of PTZ-induced seizures.

3. 改善睡眠 对电刺激剥夺睡眠大鼠，远志可使其觉醒期缩短，总睡眠时间延长，慢波睡眠 1 期睡眠延长。

(3) Improving sleep effects *Yuǎn zhì* can shorten wake time, prolong the total sleep time and the time spent in SWS1 stage in sleep deprived rats by electrical stimulation.

4. 抗抑郁 远志对慢性轻度不可预见性应激结合孤养的抑郁有对抗作用。远志中的 3,6′– 二芥子酰基蔗糖对药物诱发的抑郁模型有抗抑郁作用，其抗抑郁活性与增强 5-HT 和肾上腺素能神经功能有关。

(4) Antidepressant effects *Yuǎn zhì* has an antagonistic effect on depression-like behaviors in chronic mild unpredictable stress combined with solitary model. 3,6′-disinapoyl sucrose, an active component of *Yuǎn zhì*, also has antidepressant effect on drug-induced depression model, and the mechanisms are associated with strengthening 5-HT and adrenergic nerves function.

5. 增强学习记忆 远志皂苷能在学习的获得、巩固、再现阶段提高学习记忆障碍模型小鼠跳台和水迷宫成绩，改善学习记忆能力。远志皂苷能提高 β– 淀粉样肽和鹅膏蕈氨酸引起的痴呆大鼠的学习记忆能力，升高脑内 M 受体密度，增强胆碱乙酰基转移酶（ChAT）活性，抑制脑内乙酰胆碱酯酶（AChE）活性。远志皂苷可通过调节 Bax/Bcl-2 的比值，阻止细胞色素 C（Cyt C）的释放，降低 Caspase-3 的表达，对抗 Aβ1-40 诱导的海马神经细胞凋亡，进而改善阿尔茨海默病大鼠的学习记忆能力。远志糖苷 B 能改善东莨菪碱诱导的小鼠和大鼠记忆损害，增强中枢胆碱能系统活性。

(5) Improving learning and memory effects Saponins from *Yuǎn zhì* can improve learning and memory by enhancing the performance of jumping test and water maze test at the stages of acquisition, consolidation and retrieval. *Yuǎn zhì* saponins also enhance learning and memory in rat models of dementia induced by co-injection of beta-amyloid with ibotenic acid, and the effect is related to increasing acetylcholine receptor density and inhibiting acetylcholinesterase (AChÈ) in the brain, enhancing acetylcholine transferase (ChAT) activity. The mechanism of *Yuǎn zhì* saponins improving the learning and memory ability in rat models in Alzheimer's disease is related to its effects of regulating Bax/ Bcl-2 ratio, inhibiting cytochrome C (Cyt C) release, reducing the expression of Caspase-3 and preventing Aβ1-40 induced hippocampal neuronal apoptosis. Scopolamine-induced memory impairment in rats and mice may be susceptible to attenuation with tenuifoliside B treatments by activating central cholinergic system.

6. 保护神经 远志可通过提高糖尿病周围神经病变大鼠尾部感觉神经传导速度，降低坐骨神经醛糖还原酶活性、上调坐骨神经神经丝蛋白表达，发挥对坐骨神经保护作用；远志预处理对糖尿病大鼠坐骨神经损伤也具有预防作用。

(6) Neuroprotective effects　*Yuǎn zhì* has therapeutic and preventive effect on sciatic nerve in the peripheral nerves of the diabetic rats. The therapeutic effect is associated with accelerating caudal sensory nerve conduction velocity, inhibiting sciatic nerve aldose reductase activity, up-regulating sciatic nerve neurofilament proteins expression.

7. 祛痰、镇咳　远志提取物可促进呼吸道黏液上皮细胞黏蛋白黏液素 5AC 的分泌，但不能刺激其生成，较长时间使用可使痰液减少。远志具有镇咳作用。

(7) Expectorant and antitussive effects　The extract of *Yuǎn zhì* can promote the secretion of mucin 5AC in airway epithelial cells, but cannot stimulate its synthesis. So, it is necessary for long-term administration to decrease sputum. *Yuǎn zhì* also has antitussive effects.

磁石 ┊ *Cí shí* (*Magnetitum*)

【来源 / Origin】

本品为氧化物类矿物尖晶石族磁铁矿。分布于河北、山东、江苏、湖北、广东、福建、四川、云南等地。

Cí shí is a mineral of magnetitum of oxide mineral of family spinella. It is mainly distributed in Hebei province, Shandong province, Jiangsu province, Hubei province, Guangdong province, Fujian province, Sichuan province and Yunnan province in China.

【化学成分 / Chemical ingredients】

主含四氧化三铁（Fe_3O_4），其中含铁不得少于 50%。

The main content of *Cí shí* is Fe_3O_4, in which the percentage of iron is less than 50%.

【药性与功效 / Chinese medicine properties】

味咸，性寒，归肝、心、肾经。具有镇惊安神、平肝潜阳、聪耳明目、纳气平喘的功效。用于惊悸失眠、头晕目眩、视物昏花、耳鸣耳聋、肾虚气喘。

In Chinese medicine theory, *Cí shí* has salty in flavor and cold in nature. It can enter meridians of liver, heart and kidney. *Cí shí* has the efficacies of settling fright and tranquilizing mind, calming liver and subduing Yang, sharpening hearing and brightening the eyes, and promoting Qi absorption and calming panting. Clinically it can be used for fright palpitation and insomnia, dizzy head and vision, clouded flowery vision, ringing in the ears and deafness, and kidney deficiency and panting.

【药理作用 / Pharmacological activities】

1. 镇静　磁石水煎剂可显著减少小鼠自发活动，具有镇静作用。

(1) Sedative effects　*Cí shí* decoction can produce sedation and reduction in spontaneous activity of mice.

2. 抗惊厥　磁石混悬液具有拮抗戊四氮诱发小鼠惊厥的作用，且生磁石作用优于煅磁石。

(2) Anticonvulsant effects　*Cí shí* suspension have anticonvulsant effects in PTZ-treated mice, especially raw *Cí shí* is more effective comparing to calcined.

3. 改善睡眠　磁石水煎液能明显增加阈下剂量戊巴比妥钠小鼠的入睡率，缩短阈剂量戊巴比妥钠小鼠的入睡时间并延长其睡眠时间。磁石水煎液还能延长大鼠的总睡眠时间和 SWS2 时间。

(3) Improving sleep effects　*Cí shí* decoction can increase the sleep ratio of sodium pentobarbital-treated mice with under subthreshold dosage, and prolong sleep duration and shorten sleep latency of sodium pentobarbital-treated mice with threshold dosage. It also can prolong the total time spent in sleep and SWS2 stage in rats.

灵芝 ┊ *Líng zhī* (*Ganoderma*)

【来源 / Origin】

本品为多孔菌科真菌赤芝 [*Ganoderma lucidum*（Leyss. ex Fr.）Karst.] 或紫芝（*Ganoderma sinense* Zhao. Xu et Zhang）的干燥子实体。主要分布于浙江、福建、广东、江西、湖南、安徽、贵州、黑龙江、吉林等地。

Líng zhī is the dried sporophore of *Ganoderma lucidum* (Leyss. ex Fr.) Karst. or *Ganoderma sinense* Zhao. Xu et Zhang. It is mainly cultivated in Zhejiang province, Fujian province, Guangdong province, Jiangxi province, Hunan province, Anhui province, Guizhou province, Heilongjiang province and Jilin province in China.

【化学成分 / Chemical ingredients】

含有多种化学成分，包括多糖类、三萜类、甾醇类、蛋白类、多肽类、生物碱、挥发油和微量元素等。

Líng zhī contains abundant ingredients, including polysaccharides, triterpenes, sterols, proteins, peptides, alkaloids, volatile oils and trace elements, etc.

【药性与功效 / Chinese medicine properties】

味甘，性平，归心、肺、肝、肾经。具有补气安神、止咳平喘的功效。用于心神不宁、失眠心悸、肺虚咳喘、虚劳短气、不思饮食。

In Chinese medicine theory, *Líng zhī* has sweet in flavor and neutral in nature. It can enter meridians of heart, lung, liver and kidney. *Líng zhī* has the efficacies of supplement Qi and tranquilizing mind, and suppressing cough and calming panting. Clinically it can be used for disquieted heart spirit, insomnia and fright palpitations, lung deficiency and panting, deficiency taxation and shortness of breath, and no thought of food and drink.

【药理作用 / Pharmacological activities】

1. 镇静　灵芝及灵芝孢子粉的水提物均可显著减少小鼠自主活动次数，表现出镇静作用。

(1) Sedative effects　The water extract of *Líng zhī* or spore powder of *Líng zhī* all decrease the locomotor activity in mice, and exert sedative effect.

2. 抗惊厥　灵芝孢子粉可拮抗戊四氮诱发的癫痫发作，主要通过调节免疫、促进神经细胞修复、抗自由基生成、抑制细胞凋亡等途径减轻癫痫神经损伤。

(2) Anticonvulsant effects　The spore powders of *Líng zhī* have an inhibitory effect on PTZ-induced seizures in rat. It exerts multiple mechanism against seizures nerve injury, such as immune regulation, promoting nerve cell repair, resisting free radical production, and inhibiting apoptosis and so on.

3. 改善睡眠　灵芝及灵芝孢子粉的水提物均可延长戊巴比妥钠引起的小鼠睡眠时间和增加入睡发生率。灵芝水提物可延长自由活动大鼠和巴比妥诱导大鼠的总睡眠时间和非快速动眼睡眠持续时间，TNF-α 和 GABA 能神经元参与其改善睡眠作用。

(3) Improving sleep effects　The water extract of *Líng zhī* or spore powder of *Líng zhī* all can prolong sleep time and increase the number of sleeping in mice treated with pentobarbital sodium. Moreover, the water extract of *Líng zhī* can also increase the total sleep time and the time spent in NREMS. The improving sleep effects are attributed to modulation of cytokines such as TNF-α and GABAergic neuron involvement.

4. 增强学习记忆　灵芝水煎液可以增强小鼠的学习能力。灵芝醇提物可提高记忆障碍小鼠模型脑内的乙酰胆碱水平，改善其学习记忆能力。灵芝孢子粉能提高戊四氮癫痫大鼠的学习记忆能力，其作用与降低海马及皮质 Caspase-3 表达有关。灵芝三萜类化合物对 D– 半乳糖衰老小鼠和自然衰老大鼠的学习记忆能力下降均具有改善作用，其作用与改善脑内能量代谢和抗氧化作用有关。灵芝多糖能提高 Aβ 诱导的阿尔茨海默病大鼠的学习记忆能力，其作用与抗细胞凋亡、抑制海马 IL-6 表达、升高海马的突触数量和突触素表达以及抗氧化作用有关。

(4) Improving learning and memory effects *Líng zhī* decoction can enhance the ability of learning in mice. The ethanol extracts from *Líng zhī* can improve memory deficits in some mice models by increasing acetylcholine contents in brain. The spore powders of *Líng zhī* also improve learning and memory of PTZ-induced seizures rats, and the effect is related to reducing the expression of Caspase-3. Triterpenes, the active ingredients of *Líng zhī* extract, have inhibition effect on learning and memory deficits of D-galactose aging mice and natural aging rat. Regulating energy metabolism in brain and antioxidative ability are involved in the effect of triterpenes. Moreover, polysaccharides have a potential nootropic effects in Aβ-induced Alzheimer's disease rats, and the effect is related to inhibiting cell apoptosis and hippocampal IL-6 expression, enhancing the number of synapses and synaptophysin expression in hippocampus, and antioxidative effect.

5. 抗肿瘤　灵芝对体外多种肿瘤细胞表现出不同程度的抑制作用。抗肿瘤的药效物质基础主要是三萜和多糖。灵芝抗肿瘤作用与调节免疫功能、抑制细胞增殖、诱导细胞凋亡、抑制肿瘤转移和血管生成有关。

(5) Anti-tumor effects *Líng zhī* exert different degrees of inhibitive effect on a variety of tumor types *in vitro*. Both triterpenes and polysaccharides of *Líng zhī* are the active ingredients of anti-tumor effects. The potential mechanisms are related to regulating immune, inhibiting cell proliferation, inducing apoptosis, preventing tumor metastasis and angiogenesis.

（黄莉莉　屈　飞）

题库

第十七章　平肝息风药
Chapter 17　Liver-pacifying and wind-extinguishing medicines

学习目标 | Objectives

1.**掌握**　平肝息风药的主要药理作用；天麻和钩藤与功效相关的药理作用、作用机制及药效物质基础。

2.**了解**　牛黄、地龙和羚羊角的主要药理作用、不良反应和药效物质基础。

1. **Must know**　The main pharmacological effects of liver-pacifying and wind-extinguishing medicines; the efficacy related pharmacological effects, mechanism, and material basis of *Tiān má, Gōu téng*.

2. **Desirable to know**　The efficacy related pharmacological effects, adverse effect, and material basis of *Dì lóng, Niú huáng* and *Líng yáng jiǎo*.

第一节　概述
Section 1　Overview

PPT

微课

　　凡以平肝潜阳、息风止痉为主要功效的药物称为平肝息风药。本类药物药性多寒或平，入肝经。具有平肝潜阳、息风止痉、清泄肝火、通络止痛等功效，主要用于肝阳上亢或肝风内动所呈现的证候。

　　Herbs with the major efficacy to pacify the liver to subdue Yang or extinguish wind to arrest convulsions are called liver-pacifying and wind-extinguishing medicinals. They are mostly cold or neutral in nature, all entering liver meridian. Liver-pacifying and wind-extinguishing medicines has the effects of pacify the liver to subdue Yang, extinguishing wind to arrest convulsions, clearing and draining liver-heat and fire, freeing the collateral vessels to relieve pain, etc. It is mainly used for the syndrome of ascendant hyperactivity of liver Yang or internal stirring wind.

　　本类药物可分类为平肝潜阳药和息风止痉药。平肝潜阳药以贝壳类和矿石类药物居多，质重沉降，性味多咸寒或苦寒，用于肝肾阴虚导致肝阳上亢引起的头晕目眩、头痛、耳鸣、烦躁、发怒、失眠多梦等症状，如石决明、珍珠母、牡蛎等。息风止痉药主要包括昆虫和其他动物类药物，性多偏寒凉，用于肝阳化风、热极生风、血虚生风等所致的眩晕、抽搐、颈背僵硬、震颤、四肢痉挛，如地龙、全蝎、蜈蚣、僵蚕、牛黄、羚羊角等。

The herbs in this chapter can be classified into liver-pacifying and subduing Yang, as well as, wind-extinguishing and convulsions-relieving medicines. The former mainly consists of shells and minerals. The minerals medicines are heave and lowering in property. They are mostly bitter and salty in flavor, cold in nature. They are mainly used to treat liver-kidney Yin deficiency due to ascendant hyperactivity of liver Yang with symptoms of dizziness, dizzy vision, headache, tinnitus, irritability, tendency to anger, insomnia and dream-disturbed sleep, etc. such as *Shí jué míng*, *Zhēn zhū mǔ*, *Mǔ lì*, etc. Extinguishing wind and arresting convulsion medicinals are mostly cold in nature, and applicated in suppressing liver Yang transforming into wind and indicated for extreme heat engendering and wind, blood deficiency engendering wind, with the symptoms of dizziness, convulsions, stiff nape, trembling, spasms of the limbs. They mostly includes insect and other animal source products, such as *Dì lóng*, *Quán xiē*, *Wú gōng*, *Jiāng cán*, *Niú huáng*, *Líng yáng jiǎo*, etc.

肝风内动是肝阴不足，肝阳上亢和高热所致，主要表现为头痛、头晕、视物模糊、耳鸣、烦躁不安、心悸不安和抽搐。这些症状与西医学中高血压病的表现相似。肝风内动也可导致震颤、痉挛抽搐、肢体麻木、偏瘫、失语，在脑血管意外及其后遗症和癫痫等病中最常见。温热病时可见热极生风，病变过程可出现惊厥、抽搐甚至角弓反张。热极生风的症状常见于小儿惊厥、乙型脑炎、流行性脑脊髓膜炎、破伤风和其他急性传染病等。平肝息风药治疗肝阳上亢或肝风内动病症与下列药理作用有关。

Internal stirring wind can be raised from the liver Yin deficiency, liver Yang ascendant and high fever. It may manifest itself in headache, dizziness, blurred vision, tinnitus, irritability, palpitations with anxiety and muscle twitches. In accordance with the modern medicinal theory, these symptoms are common in hypertension. The progression of internal stirring wind may lead to tremors, tonic-clonic spasm of the extremities, sudden loss of consciousness, hemiplegia, aphasia. Those are seen most frequently in cerebrovascular accident and its sequelae, epilepsy, etc. Extreme heat engendering wind, can occur in any disease with high fever, and usually manifest itself in convulsion, hyperspasmia and opisthotons. The syndromes of extreme heat engendering wind are observed commonly in infantile convulsion, encephalitis B, epidemic cerebrospinal meningitis, tetanus, and other acute infectious disease. The effect of liver-pacifying and wind-extinguishing medicines on the treatment of ascendant hyperactivity of liver Yang and internal stirring wind is related to the following pharmacological effects.

1. **镇静、抗惊厥**　本类药物大多具有不同程度的镇静和抗惊厥作用，如天麻、钩藤、羚羊角、地龙、僵蚕、全蝎、牛黄、牡蛎、赭石等能减少动物的自主活动。在抑制中枢神经系统方面与戊巴比妥钠、硫喷妥钠、水合氯醛产生协同作用，并能抵抗戊四氮、咖啡因、苯丙氨酸和电刺激引起的惊厥。

(1) **Sedation and anti-convulsion**　Most medicinals have sedative and anticonvulsant effects in different degrees, such as *Tiān má*, *Gōu téng*, *Líng yáng jiǎo*, *Dì lóng*, *Jiāng cán* , *Quán xiē*, *Niú huáng*, *Mǔ lì* and *Zhě shí*, which can reduce animal activities independently; produce synergistic effect with sodium pentobarbital, sodium thiopental, chloral hydrate, on inhibiting central nervous system (CNS), and resist convulsions caused by the pentrazol, caffeine, strychnine, and electrical stimulation.

2. **降血压**　本类药物大多具有降血压作用。天麻、钩藤、羚羊角、地龙、全蝎、蜈蚣、天麻钩藤饮等降血压主要与中枢神经系统抑制相关的不同机制有关。如天麻、钩藤能扩张外周血管，降低外周阻力，其降压作用与抑制血管运动中枢有关。

(2) Anti-hypertension Most medicinals have anti-hypertensive effects. *Tiān má*, *Gōu téng*, *Líng yáng jiǎo*, *Dì lóng*, *Quán xiē*, *Wú gōng*, and *Tiān má gōu téng yǐn* lower blood pressure through different mechanisms mostly related to CNS inhibition. Such as *Tiān má* and *Gōu téng* can dilate peripheral blood vessels and decrease total peripheral resistance. Its hypotensive effect is related to the inhibition of vasomotor centers.

3. 抗血栓 天麻、钩藤、地龙、蒺藜、全蝎等均有不同程度抑制血小板聚集、抗血栓形成的作用。其中，地龙的抗血栓形成作用尤为显著，地龙提取物可使血液黏度和血小板聚集性降低。地龙中含有纤溶酶样物质，具有促进纤溶作用，能直接溶解纤维蛋白和血块。

(3) Anti-thrombosis *Tiān má*, *Gōu téng*, *Dì long*, *Jí lí* and *Quán xiē* show different effects on anti-platelet aggregation and anti-thrombosis. Among them, the anti-thrombotic effect of *Dì lóng* is particularly significant. *Dì lóng* extract can reduces the blood viscosity and platelet aggregation. *Dì lóng* contains plasmin-like substance, which can promote fibrinolysis and can directly dissolve fibrin and blood clots.

4. 解热、镇痛 羚羊角、地龙、牛黄均具有解热作用。羚羊角、天麻、地龙、蜈蚣和全蝎均具有不同的镇痛作用。

(4) Antipyretic and analgesic effects *Líng yáng jiǎo*, *Dì lóng* and *Niú huáng* have antipyretic effects. *Líng yáng jiǎo*, *Tiān má*, *Dì lóng*, *Wú gōng*, and *Quán xiē* have different analgesic effects.

常用平肝息风药的主要药理作用见表 17-1。

The main pharmacological effects of commonly used liver-pacifying and wind-extinguishing medicines are summarized in Table 17-1.

表 17-1 常用平肝息风药的主要药理作用

类别	药物	镇静	抗惊厥	降血压	抗血栓	解热	镇痛	其他药理作用
息风止痉	天麻	+	+	+	+	–	+	增加脑血流量、改善记忆、延缓衰老、保护脑神经细胞、抗心肌缺血
	钩藤	+	+	+	+	–	–	减缓心率、降低心肌收缩力、钙阻滞
	牛黄	+	+	+	–	+	+	抗病毒、抗炎、利胆、保肝、镇咳、平喘、祛痰、抗氧化、兴奋子宫、抗脑缺血
	羚羊角	+	+	+	–	+	+	抗病毒
	地龙	+	+	+	+	+	+	平喘、抗肿瘤、增强免疫、兴奋子宫
	全蝎	+	+	+	+	–	+	抗肿瘤
	蜈蚣	–	+	+	–	–	+	抗炎、抗肿瘤、解痉
	僵蚕	+	+	+	–	–	–	抑菌、抗肿瘤、降血糖
平肝潜阳	罗布麻叶	+	–	+	–	–	–	降血脂、抗血小板聚集、利尿
	石决明	+	–	+	–	+	–	抗菌、抗氧化
	珍珠母	+	–	+	–	–	–	抗氧化、抗衰老、抗肿瘤、抗胃溃疡
	牡蛎	+	+	–	–	–	+	抗炎、抗胃溃疡
	赭石	+	–	–	–	–	–	促进红细胞生成、促进肠蠕动
	蒺藜	–	–	+	+	–	+	抗肿瘤、利尿、抗脑缺血、抗菌、降血糖

注："+"表示有明确作用；"–"表示无作用，或未查阅到相关研究文献

微课

第二节 常用药物

Section 2 Commonly used medicines

PPT

天麻 ┊ *Tiān má (Rhizoma Gastrodiae)*

【来源 / Origin】

本品为兰科植物天麻（*Gastrodia elata* Bl.）的干燥块茎。主产于四川、云南、贵州等地。冬春二季采集，生用或蒸煮。

Tiān má derives from the dried rhizome of *Gastrodia elata* Bl., family of Orchidaceae. The medicinal material is mainly produced in the areas of Sichuan, Yunnan, Guizhou Province, etc. Collected in winter and spring. the crude or boiled one is used.

【化学成分 / Chemical ingredients】

主要含酚类化合物及其苷类、固醇、有机酸等。酚类成分主要包括天麻素、天麻苷元（对羟基苯甲醇）、香草醇、香兰素等，还含有糖类化合物（蔗糖、杂多糖、天麻多糖）、黏液质、微量元素和含氮化合物等。其中，天麻素含量高，是主要的活性成分，其含量为 0.33%~0.67%。

The chemical ingredients of *Tiān má* include phenolic components and their glycosides, sterols, organic acids, etc. Phenols mainly include gastrodin (4-hydroxymethylphenyl-β-D-glucopyranoside), gastrodigenin (4-hydroxybenzyl alcohol), vanillyl alcohol (4-hydroxy-3-methoxybenzyl alcohol), vanillin and so on. It also contains carbohydrates (sucrose, heteropolysaccharides, gastrodia polysaccharides), phlegmatic temperament, trace elements and nitrogen compounds. Among them, gastrodin has a high content and is considered as the major active component, and its content is about 0.33% ~ 0.67%.

【药性与功效 / Chinese medicine properties】

味甘，性平，归肝经。具有息风止痉、平抑肝阳、祛风通络的功效。用于小儿惊风、癫痫抽搐、破伤风、头痛眩晕、手足不遂、肢体麻木、风湿痹痛等证。

In Chinese medicine theory, *Tiān má* has the nature of sweet, and neutral. It can enter the meridian of liver. *Tiān má* can extinguish wind to arrest convulsions, repress the liver Yang, and dispel wind to free the collateral vessels. It is used for infantile convulsion, epilepsy and convulsions, tetanus, headache, dizziness, hemiplegia, numb limbs and tense tendons, arthralgia due to wind-dampness, etc.

【药理作用 / Pharmacological effects】

1. 镇静、催眠 天麻的镇静作用明确。天麻粉、天麻水煎剂、天麻素及其苷元、香草醇等口服均能减少小鼠自发性活动，延长巴比妥钠所致小鼠睡眠时间，对抗咖啡因引起的中枢兴奋作用。天麻素可透过血脑屏障，在脑组织中以较高速度降解为天麻苷元，天麻苷元为脑内苯二氮䓬受体的配基，作用于苯二氮䓬受体，从而产生镇静、抗惊厥等中枢抑制作用。此外，天麻的镇静、催眠作用还与其降低脑内多巴胺（DA）和去甲肾上腺素（NA）含量有关。

(1) Sedation and hypnosis *Tiān má* have sedative and hypnotic effects. *Tiān má* powder, *Tiān má* decoction, gastrodin, gastrodigenin and vanillyl alcohol can decrease the frequency of spontaneous activity of mice as well as increase the sleeping time of mice induced by sodium pentobarbital. Besides, they can also antagonize the excitatory effect on central nervous system(CNS) caused by caffeine.

医药大学堂
WWW.YIYAODXT.COM

Gastrodin decomposes to gastrodigenin and subsequently, gastrodigenin combines with benzodiazepine receptor competitively after passing through blood brain barrier to generate the effect of sedation and hypnosis. In addition, *Tiān má* can decrease dopamine (DA) and noradrenaline (NA) content to show its sedative and hypnosis effects.

2. 抗惊厥、抗癫痫　天麻及其共生蜜环菌、香兰素、天麻素及其苷元、香草醇均能抑制戊四氮所致小鼠惊厥，延长惊厥潜伏期，降低死亡率。天麻能抑制脑癫痫样放电。香草醇在不产生中枢镇静作用的剂量下能显著改善脑电波，产生抗癫痫作用。

(2) Anti-convulsion and anti-epileptic effects　*Tiān má* and its symbiotic armillaria mellea, vanillin, gastrodin, gastrodigenin and vanillyl alcohol have effect on anti-convulsion caused by pentylenetetrazol. It can prolong the latency of convulsion and reduce mortality. *Tiān má* suppresses epilepsy-like discharges in the brain. At doses without central sedation, vanillyl alcohol can significantly improve brain waves and show antiepileptic effects.

3. 抗眩晕　口服天麻醇提物或天麻多糖能改善旋转诱发的小鼠食欲缺乏症状，并能对抗旋转后小鼠自主活动的降低。天麻苷元能竞争性抑制地西泮等药物与其受体结合，抑制神经冲动向前庭外侧多突触神经元传导，阻断或减弱脑干网状结构上行传递系统功能，从而产生抗眩晕的作用。

(3) Anti-vertigo effects　*Tiān má* alcohol extract or gastrodia polysaccharide administered orally can improve the symptoms of anorexia in mice induced by rotation, and can antagonize the reduction of mouse autonomy after rotation. Gastrodigenin can competitively inhibit the binding of diazepam to receptors, and inhibit the conduction of nerve impulses to lateral vestibular polysynaptic neurons, and block or weaken the function of the brainstem reticular structure upstream transmission system to show anti-vertigo effect.

4. 抗炎、镇痛　天麻对多种炎症反应有抑制作用。能降低毛细血管通透性，直接对抗 5- 羟色胺（5-HT）和前列腺素 E_2（PGE_2）所致炎症反应。天麻呈剂量依赖性对多种实验性疼痛有抑制作用。

(4) Anti-inflammation and analgesic effects　*Tiān má* inhibits various inflammations, and reduces capillary permeability, directly inhibits inflammation caused by 5-hydroxytryptamine (5-HT) and Prostaglandin E_2(PGE_2). *Tiān má* inhibits different experimental pains in a dose-dependent manner.

5. 降血压　天麻、天麻素对多种实验动物有降压作用。天麻能降低外周阻力，使血压迅速下降。天麻素降低收缩压的作用比降低舒张压和平均压更明显。在增强中央动脉顺应性方面，天麻优于其他扩血管药，使主动脉、大动脉等血管弹性增强，从而增强血管对血压的缓冲能力。天麻多糖也有明显的降压作用。

(5) Anti-hypertension　Both *Tiān má* and gastrodin have shown anti-hypertensive effect on many animal models. *Tiān má* can decrease total peripheral resistance and show fast hypotensive activity with duration of several hours. Gastrodin reduces contracting pressure more significantly than diastolic pressure and mean pressure. Gastrodin is superior to other vasodilators in enhancing the central artery compliance, the vascular elasticity of aorta and arteries, among others, and improve the buffering capacity of blood vessels on blood pressure. In addition, gastrodia polysaccharide also has a significant anti-hypertensive effect.

6. 抑制血小板聚集、抗血栓　天麻提取物、天麻素、天麻苷元和天麻多糖均有抑制血小板聚集和抗血栓作用。它们可以降低花生四烯酸诱发的急性肺血栓栓塞症小鼠的死亡率、扩张血管以改善微循环。

(6) Inhibition of platelet aggregation and anti-thrombosis Gastrodin and gastrodigenin have inhibitive action on platelet aggregation. They can decrease the mortality of mice with acute pulmonary thromboembolism induced by arachidonic acid. Moreover, blood vessel can be dilated to improve microcirculation.

7. 抗心肌缺血 体内和体外试验均表明，天麻和天麻素均能拮抗心肌缺血，减慢心率，减少心肌耗氧量。天麻提取物或天麻注射液能对抗垂体后叶素或冠脉结扎致实验性心肌缺血，缩小心肌梗死面积，降低血清丙二醛（MDA）含量。天麻素可使体外培养的心肌组织心率加快，心肌收缩力加强，具有促进细胞能量代谢的作用。天麻抗心肌缺血的作用机制与其抗自由基产生、改善细胞能量代谢相关。天麻素是其抗心肌缺血的主要活性成分。

(7) Anti-myocardial ischemia Both *in vivo* and *in vitro* experiments indicate that *Tiān má* and gastrodine are able to resist myocardial ischemia, slow the heart rate and reduce myocardial oxygen consumption. *Tiān má* extract or *Tiān má* injection can prevent experimental myocardial ischemia caused by hypophysin or coronary ligation, reduce the area of myocardial infarction, and reduce the amount of malondialdehyde (MDA) in the serum. Gastrodin can increase the heart beat frequency of cultured myocardial tissue *in vitro*, strengthen the contractility of myocardium, and promote energy metabolism of cells. The mechanism of *Tiān má*'s anti-myocardial ischemia is related to its resistance to free radical production and improvement of cell energy metabolism. Gastrodin is the main active ingredient of anti-myocardial ischemia.

8. 保护脑神经细胞 天麻和天麻素通过不同机制对神经细胞具有保护作用。天麻素能够显著减少乳酸脱氢酶的泄漏，从而维持神经细胞膜的流动性，减少乳过氧化物酶的产生，增强脑中Na^+-K^+-ATP 酶的活性，并改善能量代谢。天麻素的脑保护作用与其对抗兴奋毒性、抗自由基、保护细胞膜、抑制一氧化氮合酶（NOS）活性、抗细胞凋亡和改善能量代谢等相关。

(8) Protection of nerve cell *Tiān má* and gastrodin have protective effect on nerve cells through different mechanisms. Gastrodin is able to produce a significant reduction in the leakage of lactate dehydrogenase to maintain nerve cell membrane fluidity, reduce the production of lactoperoxidase, augment the activity of Na^+-K^+-ATPase in brain, and improve energy metabolism. This protective action of *Tiān má* on brain nerve cells is related to its resistance to excitotoxicity, anti-free radicals, protection of cell membranes, inhibition of nitric oxide synthase (NOS) activity, anti-apoptosis and improvement of energy metabolism.

9. 其他作用 天麻可以改善衰老大鼠的学习记忆能力，并对东莨菪碱、亚硝酸钠、乙醇所致记忆的获得、巩固和再现障碍等小鼠模型具有保护作用。实验表明，天麻可通过清除自由基、抗氧化损伤而延缓衰老。

(9) Other effects *Tiān má* can improve the study and memory ability of aging rats, protect the mice from memory acquisition, consolidation and reproduction impairment induced by scopolamine, sodium nitrite and ethanol. Many experiments have shown that *Tiān má* can postpone senility by improving the ability of free radical scavenging and resisting oxidative damage.

【不良反应 / Adverse effects】
服用大剂量天麻可能出现心律失常、胸闷气促、口干咽燥、恶心、呕吐、大便干结及皮肤瘙痒等皮肤过敏性反应。天麻肌内注射后，有些患者会出现口干、头晕、胃部不适。

Taking large doses of *Tiān má* may cause arrhythmia, chest distress, breathlessness, dry mouth and throat, nausea, emesis, pruritus and skin allergic reactions, etc., vomiting and dry stool. Some patients can experience the symptoms of xerostomia, dizziness, stomach discomfort after *Tiān má* intramuscular injection.

钩藤 ┊ *Gōu téng* (*Ramulus Uncariae Cum Uncis*)

【来源 / Origin】

本品为茜草科植物钩藤［*Uncaria rhynchophylla* (Miq.) Miq. ex Havil.］、大叶钩藤（*Uncaria macrophylla* Wall.）、毛钩藤（*Uncaria hirsuta* Havil.）、华钩藤［*Uncaria sinensis* (Oliv.) Havil.］或无柄果钩藤（*Uncaria sessilifructus* Roxb.）的干燥带钩茎枝。主产于广西、江西、浙江等地。春秋二季采收，晒干生用。

Gōu téng is the dried hooked stem of *Uncaria rhynchophylla* (Miq.) Miq. ex Havil., *Uncaria macrophylla* Wall., *Uncaria hirsuta* Havil., *Uncaria sinensis* (Oliv.) Havil., or *Uncaria sessilifructus* Roxb., family of Rubiaceae. The plant is widely cultivated in Guangxi, Jiangxi, Zhejiang province, etc.

【化学成分 / Chemical ingredients】

主要含生物碱类、黄酮、三萜类等。生物碱中主要成分有钩藤碱、异钩藤碱、去氢钩藤碱、异去氢钩藤碱、毛钩藤碱、柯诺辛、硬毛帽柱木碱、硬毛帽柱木因碱等，总生物碱含量约为0.22%，其中钩藤碱含量约占总碱的34.5%~51%。此外，还含有甾醇类、多酚类（如儿茶素、表儿茶素）、糖苷类化合物。

Gōu téng contains alkaloids, triterpenoids, flavonoids and saponins, etc. Alkaloids mainly contains rhynchophylline, isorhynchophylline, corynoxeine, isocorynoxeine, corynoxine, hirsutine and hirsuteine. The content of total alkaloid is 0.22%, of which rhynchophylline content is 34.5%~51%. In addition, it also contains sterols, polyphenols (such as catechinic acid and epicatechin) and glycosides.

【药性与功效 / Chinese medicine properties】

味甘，性微寒，归肝、心经。具有清热平肝、息风止痉的功效。用于治疗肝风内动、惊痫抽搐、高热惊厥、妊娠子痫、头痛眩晕等证。

In Chinese medicine theory, *Gōu téng* has the nature of sweet and cool. It can enter the meridians of liver and pericardium. *Gōu téng* can clear heat and pacify liver, extinguish wind and arrest convulsion. It is used for internal stirring wind, epilepsy and convulsions, febrile convulsions, pregnancy eclampsia, headache and dizziness, etc. *Gōu téng* is a common medicine for the treatment of live-wind stirring inside with convulsions.

【药理作用 / Pharmacological effects】

1. **镇静、抗癫痫** 灌服钩藤水提物或异钩藤碱能抑制小鼠自发性活动，且随着剂量增加，钩藤的镇静作用增强，并能对抗咖啡因的中枢兴奋作用。这一作用与其调节不同脑区单胺类递质如DA和NA及5-HT的释放有关；腹腔注射钩藤醇提液能抑制毛果芸香碱致癫痫家兔大脑皮质电活动，减少癫痫发作次数，缩短发作持续时间，延长发作间隔时间。

(1) Sedation and anti-epileptic effects After oral administration of *Gōu téng* decoction or isorhynchophylline, it can dose-dependent reduce the locomotor activity, and antagonize the excitatory effect of caffeine on CNS. The sedative effect may be due to the regulation of the release of monoamine transmitters such as DA, NA, and 5-HT in different brain regions. Intraperitoneal injection of *Gōu téng* extract can inhibit the electrical activity of cerebral cortex in epilepsy rabbits induced by pilocarpine, reduce the number of seizures, shorten the duration, and prolong the interval between seizures.

2. **降血压** 钩藤煎剂、钩藤总碱、异钩藤碱、钩藤碱对血压正常或高血压动物均有明显的降压作用，降压的同时有负性心率作用。钩藤碱和异钩藤碱是其降压的主要活性成分。异钩藤碱的降压作用强于钩藤碱，且在降压的同时不减少肾血流量。钩藤或钩藤碱降压作用呈现三相变化，先降压，继之快速升压，然后持续下降。钩藤降压起效温和而且缓慢，重复给药无快速耐受现象。钩藤降压机制是抑制血管运动中枢，扩张外周血管，降低外周阻力，阻滞交感神经和神经节，抑制神经末梢递质的释放。钩藤碱扩张动脉还与钙拮抗相关。钩藤碱能抑制动脉平滑肌的外钙内流和内钙释放。

(2) Anti-hypertension *Gōu téng*, total alkaloids, isorhynchophylline and rhynchophylline have shown significantly anti-hypertension effect on normotensive or hypertensive animals, it has negative heart rate effect as well. Isorhynchophylline and rhynchophylline are the main active ingredients. Isorhynchophylline has a stronger anti-hypertensive effect than that of rhynchophylline, and does not reduce renal blood flow while reducing blood press. *Gōu téng* or rhynchophylline can induce a three-phase changes in blood pressure, in other words, the blood pressure decreases first, then increases rapidly, and finally decreases continuously. The anti-hypertensive effect of *Gōu téng* is mild and slow, and there is no rapid tolerance phenomenon when repeated administration. Inhibition of the vasomotor center and inhibition of sympathetic nerves and ganglia are main anti-hypertensive mechanisms that lead to peripheral vasodilatation and resistance decrease. The anti-hypertensive effect works through the inhibition of vasomotor center; dilation of peripheral blood vessels; and suppression of the release of the transmitters in the nerve terminals. Inhibition of intracellular Ca^{2+} release is also involved in vasodilatation. Rhynchophylline can inhibit external calcium influx and internal calcium release from arterial smooth muscle.

3. 抑制血小板聚集和抗血栓形成 钩藤碱可抑制花生四烯酸、胶原、二磷酸腺苷（ADP）等诱导的血小板聚集，抗血栓形成。钩藤碱抑制血小板聚集和抗血栓形成的机制与抑制血小板释放花生四烯酸，减少血栓素 A_2（TXA_2）合成相关。钩藤碱对血小板释放的其他活性物质也有一定的抑制作用。

(3) Inhibition of platelet aggregation and anti-thrombosis Rhynchophylline inhibit platelet aggregation induced by arachidonic acid, collagen, and adenosine diphosphate, and inhibit thrombosis. This mechanisms are related to inhibiting platelet release of arachidonic acid, reducing thromboxane A_2 (TXA_2) synthesis. In addition, rhynchophylline also has a certain inhibitory effect on the release of other active substances from platelets.

4. 保护神经细胞 钩藤总碱灌服给药对大鼠脑缺血再灌注损伤有保护作用，该作用与抑制自由基产生、增强超氧化物歧化酶、抗氧化损伤、钙拮抗、舒张脑血管、抑制血小板聚集等有关。钩藤中的氧化吲哚碱如钩藤碱、异钩藤碱、去氢钩藤碱、吲哚碱如硬毛帽柱木碱、硬毛帽柱木因碱以及部分酚性成分如儿茶素、表儿茶素等均对脑神经细胞有保护作用。

(4) Protection of nerve cell *Gōu téng* total alkaloids administered intragastrically has protective effect on cerebral ischemia-reperfusion injury in rats, and this effect is related to inhibition of free radical production, enhancement of superoxide dismutase antioxidant damage, calcium antagonist, relaxation of cerebral blood vessels, and inhibition of platelet aggregation and so on. Oxindole alkaloids in *Gōu téng* such as hynchophylline, isorhynchophylline and corynoxeine, indole alkaloids such as hirsutine, hirsuteine and some phenolic ingredients catechinic acid and epicatechin have protective effects on brain nerve cells.

5. 解痉 钩藤碱、异钩藤碱、去氢钩藤碱均能不同程度地抑制乙酰胆碱引起的小鼠离体肠管收缩。钩藤碱对缩宫素引起的大鼠离体子宫收缩有抑制作用。钩藤总碱灌胃或注射能抑制组胺引起的豚鼠哮喘。

(5) Antispasmolysis Rhynchophylline, isorhynchophylline, and corynoxeine can produce an antispasmodic action on the isolated intestinal smooth muscle caused by acetylcholine. Rhynchophylline also relieves oxytocin-induced contractions of uterus smooth muscle in rats. Intragastric administration or injection of *Gōu téng* total alkaloids can inhibit histamine-induced asthma in guinea pigs.

【不良反应 / Adverse effects】

有老年高血压患者服用治疗量钩藤总碱出现心动过缓、头晕、皮疹等个案病例报告，停药后可自行恢复。

After taking therapeutic amount of *Gōu téng* total alkaloids, several elderly hypertensive patients can experience bradycardia, dizziness, rash and spanomenorrhea, which can be eliminated after withdrawl.

牛黄 | *Niú Huáng* (*Calculus Bovis*)

【来源 / Origin】

本品又称天然牛黄、西黄，为牛科动物牛（*Bos taurus domesticus* Gmelin）的胆囊或胆管结石。主产于中国西北、东北、河南、河北、江苏等地。现以牛胆汁或猪胆汁为原料，经化学合成得到牛黄代用品，称为人工牛黄。研末冲服或入丸散用。

Niú huáng is the stones in the gallbladder or bile ducts of *Bostaurus domesticus* Gmelin, family Bovidae, and called natural cow-bezoare. It is produced in northwest and northeast of China, Henan, Hebei and Jiangsu Provinces. The artificial cow-bezoare is synthesized from cow-bile or pig bile. The stones are collected and ground into powder for oral use, or used in pills. It is also known as *Xī huáng*.

【化学成分 / Chemical ingredients】

主要含有胆汁酸、胆色素、胆固醇、氨基酸、脂肪酸及无机元素等。胆汁酸主要为胆酸（CA）和去氧胆酸（DCA）及少量的鹅去氧胆酸（CDCA）和熊去氧胆酸（UDCA）等。胆红素（bilirubin）包括游离胆红素、胆红素钙、胆红素酯等。还含牛磺酸、胆甾醇、麦角甾醇、卵磷脂、脂肪酸、维生素 D、水溶性肽类成分，以及铜、铁、镁、锌等。

Chemical ingredients of *Niú huáng* include bilirubin, bile acids, amino acid, fatty acid, and mineral. Bile acids are a mixture of steroids, mainly including cholic acid (CA), deoxycholic acid (DCA), and a small quantity of chenodeoxycholic acid (CDCA) and ursodeoxycholic acid (UDCA). Bilirubin includes free bilirubin, bilirubin calcium, bilirubin esters, etc. It also contains taurine, cholesterol, ergosterol, lecithin, fatty acid, vitamin D, water-soluble peptide SMC, as well as copper, iron, magnesium, zinc and so on.

【药性与功效 / Chinese medicine properties】

味苦，性凉，归心、肝经。具有清心、豁痰、开窍、凉肝、息风、解毒的功效。用于治疗热病神昏、中风痰迷、惊痫抽搐、癫痫发狂、咽喉肿痛、口舌生疮、痈肿疔疮等证。

In Chinese medicine theory, *Niú huáng* has the nature of bitter and cool. It can enter the meridians of heart and liver. *Niú huáng* has the effects of removing heat from the heart, eliminating phlegm, inducing resuscitation, removing heat from the liver, checking endogenous wind and clearing away toxins. It is used for coma in a febrile disease, apoplexy and mental confusion due to phlegm, epilepsy induced by terror and convulsion, epileptic madness, sore and swollen throat, canker sores in the mouth and on the tongue, and carbuncles, boils and other pyogenic skin infections.

【药理作用 / Pharmacological effects】

1. **影响中枢神经系统**　牛黄对中枢神经系统表现为兴奋和抑制的双重作用。牛黄能增加中枢抑制药的镇静作用，也可拮抗中枢兴奋药的兴奋作用。牛磺酸是其镇静和抗惊厥的主要物质基础。

(1) **Effects on the central nervous system**　*Niú huáng* shows dual effects of excitement and

inhibition on the central nervous system. *Niú huáng* can both increase the sedative effects of central inhibitors and antagonize the excitatory effects of central stimulants. Taurine is the effective component of *Niú huáng* for its sedation and anti-convulsions.

（1）镇静　牛黄中去氧胆酸和胆酸可拮抗中枢神经兴奋作用，并与吗啡、巴比妥钠等中枢抑制药产生协同作用。牛磺酸具有中枢抑制作用，可减少小鼠自主活动，增强阈下剂量戊巴比妥钠对小鼠的催眠作用，能使戊巴比妥钠所致的小鼠睡眠时间延长。人工牛黄也有镇静作用。

1) Sedation　*Niú huáng* has sedative activity. Deoxycholic acid and cholic acid in *Niú huáng* can antagonize central nervous system excitement, and synergize with central inhibitory drugs such as morphine and sodium barbiturate. Taurine has central inhibitory effect, can reduce the locomotor activity, and increase the hypnotic effect of the mice treated with pentobarbital sodium under subthreshold dose, and prolong the sleep duration of the mice treated with pentobarbital sodium above threshold dose respectively. The artificial cow-bezoare also has sedative effect.

（2）抗惊厥　牛黄可拮抗咖啡因、可卡因或戊四氮诱导的小鼠惊厥，延长惊厥潜伏期，降低惊厥强度，减少发作次数。牛磺酸对多种因素所致的惊厥有抑制作用，牛磺酸是其镇静和抗惊厥的主要物质基础。人工牛黄与天然牛黄有相似的抗惊厥活性。

2) Anti-convulsion　*Niú huáng* has effect on anti-convulsion. *Niú huáng* can antagonize convulsions induced by caffeine, cocaine or pentylenetetrazol in mice, prolong convulsion latency, reduce the intensity of seizures, and reduce the number of seizures. Taurine has inhibitory effect on convulsions caused by various factors, and it is the main active ingredient for its sedative and anticonvulsant effects. Artificial cow-bezoare has similar anticonvulsant activity to natural cow-bezoare.

2. 抗病毒　牛黄对流行性乙型脑炎病毒有直接杀灭作用。皮下感染流行性乙型脑炎病毒24小时后小鼠灌服牛黄，对小鼠有保护作用，天然牛黄作用比人工牛黄作用强。

(2) Anti-virus　*Niú huáng* has direct killing effect on encephalitis B virus. 24 hours after subcutaneous infection with encephalitis B virus, mice were given *Niú huáng*, which had a protective effect on mice. The effect of natural cow-bezoare is stronger than that of artificial cow-bezoare.

3. 解热　牛黄具有解热作用。牛黄可抑制 2,4 – 二硝基苯酚等引起发热模型大鼠体温升高，且能降低正常大鼠的体温。牛磺酸是其解热的主要有效成分。牛磺酸可通过血脑屏障，进入下丘脑体温调节中枢，通过调节中枢 5-HT 系统或儿茶酚胺，使产热减少、散热增加而起解热作用。

(3) Anti-pyretic effects　*Niú huáng* has an anti-pyretic effect. *Niú huáng* can inhibit body temperature rise febrile model rats caused by 2,4-dinitrophenol, and it can reduce the temperature of normal rats. Taurine is the main effective ingredient for its anti-pyretics. The anti-pyretic effect of taurine is related to its reducing heat production and increasing heat dissipation by penetrating the blood-brain barrier and enter the hypothalamic thermoregulatory center.

4. 抗炎　牛黄对实验性急性和慢性炎症均有抑制作用。牛黄可减轻二甲苯致小鼠耳郭肿胀及角叉菜胶致大鼠足跖肿胀，抑制胸膜炎大鼠白细胞的趋化和游走，抑制小鼠棉球肉芽肿的形成。其作用机制与抑制炎症组织中致炎物质 PGE_2 的生成及抗自由基、抗氧化相关。

(4) Anti-inflammation　*Niú huáng* inhibits experimental acute and chronic inflammation. *Niú huáng* can reduce the auricle swelling in mice induced by 2,4-DNP and the swelling of the plantar in rats caused by carrageenan, and inhibit the chemotaxis and migration of leukocytes and the formation of cotton ball granuloma in mice. Its mechanism of action is related to inhibiting the production of the inflammatory substance prostaglandin E_2 (PGE_2) in inflammatory tissues, as well as anti-free radicals and antioxidants.

5. **利胆、保肝**　牛黄可松弛大鼠胆道括约肌，促进胆汁分泌。牛磺酸对 CCl_4 所致的小鼠肝损伤有保护作用，可预防脂肪肝。熊去氧胆酸可对抗炔雌醇诱导的肝细胞损伤。牛黄主要成分胆汁酸盐能促进脂肪、类脂肪及脂溶性维生素的吸收，预防胆结石的形成。

(5) Hepatoprotective and choleretic effects　*Niú huáng* have hepatoprotective and choleretic effects. *Niú huáng* relaxes biliary sphincter and promotes bile secretion in rats. Taurine has a protective effect on liver injury caused by carbon tetrachloride (CCl_4) in mice, and can prevent fatty liver. Ursodeoxycholic acid is effective against ethinyl estradiol-induced hepatocyte damage. Bile salts can promote the absorption of fats, lipids and fat-soluble vitamins, and prevent the formation of gallstones.

6. **降压**　牛黄具有显著而持久的降压作用。去氧胆酸、胆红素、牛磺酸等有不同程度的降压作用。牛黄降压作用与扩张血管、抗肾上腺素有关。

(6) Anti-hypertension　*Niú huáng* is able to produce a slow and everlasting anti-hypertension action. Deoxycholic acid, bilirubin, and taurine have different levels of hypotensive effects which is related to dilation of blood vessels and anti-adrenaline.

7. **祛痰、镇咳、平喘**　牛黄可使小鼠支气管酚红的分泌量增加，并对氨水刺激引起的小鼠咳嗽有抑制作用。牛黄中的胆酸也具有化痰、镇咳和平喘作用。

(7) Dispelling phlegm, relieving cough and asthma　*Niú huáng* have effects on dispelling phlegm, relieving cough and asthma. *Niú huáng* can increase the secretion of bronchial phenol red in mice, and can inhibit the cough induced by ammonia in mice. The cholic acid in *Niú huáng* also has dispelling phlegm, relieving cough and calming panting effects.

8. **其他作用**

(8) Other effects

（1）影响免疫系统　牛黄能增强机体免疫系统的功能。天然牛黄能提高脂多糖诱导的淋巴细胞转化，增强小鼠巨噬细胞的吞噬能力。熊去氧胆酸和鹅去氧胆酸也能增强机体特异性免疫和非特异性免疫功能。

1) Effects on the immune system　*Niú huáng* can enhance the function of the body's immune system. Natural cow-bezoare can increase lipopolysaccharide-induced lymphocyte transformation and enhance phagocytic capacity of mouse phagocytes. Both ursodeoxycholic acid and chenodeoxycholic acid can enhance the body's specific and non-specific immune functions.

（2）抗氧化　牛黄具有抗氧化作用，其主要有效成分是胆红素。胆红素能清除自由基，抑制脂质过氧化，对生物大分子和细胞膜结构及功能有保护作用。胆红素是机体抵抗脂质过氧化、清除自由基的一种天然抗氧化剂。

2) Anti-oxidation　*Niú huáng* has antioxidant effect, and its main active ingredient is bilirubin. Bilirubin can scavenge free radicals, inhibit lipid peroxidation, and protect the structure and function of biological macromolecules and cell membranes. Bilirubin is a natural antioxidant that resists lipid peroxidation and scavenges free radicals.

（3）脑保护　牛黄具有保护脑血管的作用。牛磺酸能对抗氧化应激和缺血再灌注损伤，还可减少患阿尔茨海默病的风险，是脑保护作用的主要有效成分。

3) Cerebral protection　*Niú huáng* has protective effect on cerebral blood vessels. Taurine is resistant to oxidative stress and ischemia-reperfusion injury and reduces the risk of Alzheimer's disease. Taurine is the main active ingredient for brain protection.

地龙 ┆ *Dì lóng* (*Lumbricus, Earthworm*)

【来源 / Origin】

本品为钜蚓科动物参环毛蚓〔*Pheretima aspergillum* (E. Perrier)〕、通俗环毛蚓（*Pheretima vulgaris* Chen）、威廉环毛蚓〔*Pheretima guillelmi* (Michaelsen)〕或栉盲环毛蚓（*Pheretima pectinfera* Michaelsen）的干燥体。前一种主产于广东、广西、福建等地，习称"广地龙"；后三种各地均产，习称"沪地龙"。夏秋二季捕捉，晒干，生用或鲜用。

The source is from the dry body with the organs removed of *Pheretima aspergillum* (E.Perrier), *Pheretima vulgaris* Chen, *Pheretima guillelmi* (Michaelsen) or *Pheretima pectinfera* Michaelsen, family of Megascolecidae. The former sort is mainly produced in Guangdong, Guangxi and Fujian Provinces, called *Guǎng dì lóng*, and the latter three kinds are produced in all parts of the country, called *Hù dì lóng*. They are caught in spring and summer, dried in the sun for or use when fresh.

【化学成分 / Chemical ingredients】

主要有蚯蚓解热碱（lumbrofebin）、蚯蚓素（lumbritin）、蚯蚓毒素（terrestro-lumbrilysin）、蚓激酶（lumbrokinase）和类血小板活化因子（platelet-like activating factor）；另有18种氨基酸（如亮氨酸和谷氨酸）、多肽、脂肪酸（如月桂酸和琥珀酸）、黄嘌呤、次黄嘌呤，以及钙、镁、铁、锌等微量元素。

Dì lóng primarily contains lumbrifebin, lumbritin, terrestro-lumbrilysin, lumbrokinase and platelet-like activating factor. Besides, it also contains 18 kinds of amino acid (e. g., leucine and glutamic acid), peptide, fatty acids (e. g., lauric acid and succinic acid), xanthine, hypoxanthine and trace elements (e. g., Ca, Mg, Fe and Zn).

【药性与功效 / Chinese medicine properties】

味咸，性寒，归肝、脾、膀胱经。具有清热息风、通络、平喘、利尿的功效。用于壮热惊痫抽搐、肺热哮喘、热痹关节红肿热痛、屈伸不利及中风后遗症等。

In Chinese medicine theory, *Dì lóng* has the nature of salty and cold. It can enter the meridians of liver, spleen and urinary bladder. It has the effect of clearing away heat to check endogenous wind, dredge meridians, relieve asthma, promote diuresis. It is applied for high fever with convulsion and spasm, and heat in the lung with bronchial asthma. It is used for Bi-syndrome of heat-type with reddish, swelling, feverish and painful joints, unsmooth movement of joints, and sequela of wind stroke.

【药理作用 / Pharmacological effects】

1. 解热 地龙粉灌胃给予内毒素诱导的家兔发热可明显降低发热家兔的体温。蚯蚓解热碱和地龙水解后的氨基酸是地龙解热作用的主要有效成分，其机制为调节体温中枢、使散热增加，因而体温下降。

(1) Anti-pyretic effects *Dì lóng* has an antipyretic effect. *Dì lóng* powder can significantly reduce the body temperature of endotoxin-induced febrile rabbits after intragastric administration of *Dì lóng* powder. Lumbrifebin and *Dì lóng* hydrolyzed amino acids are the main active ingredients for this antipyretic action. The mechanism for fever-relieving is attributed to central thermoregulation, and increases heat dissipation and decreases body temperature.

2. 镇静、催眠 地龙水煎液灌胃可明显降低小鼠的自主活动，显著增加阈下剂量戊巴比妥钠小鼠的入睡率，延长阈上剂量戊巴比妥钠小鼠的睡眠时间。

(2) Sedation and hypnosis *Dì lóng* has sedative and hypnotic activity. It can significantly reduce the the locomotor activity, and increase the sleep ratio of the mice treated with pentobarbital sodium under subthreshold dose, and prolong the sleep duration of the mice treated with pentobarbital sodium above threshold dose respectively.

3. 抗惊厥　地龙水煎液灌胃能明显拮抗戊四氮诱导的小鼠惊厥。小鼠腹腔注射 20g/kg 地龙乙醇提取液，其抗电惊厥的效果与 20mg/kg 苯巴比妥钠相当，但不能拮抗士的宁引起的惊厥，故认为其抗惊厥的作用部位在脊髓以上的中枢神经。琥珀酸是地龙抗惊厥作用的主要有效成分。

(3) Anti-convulsion　*Dì lóng* has anti-convulsive effect. After oral administration of *Dì lóng* decoction, it has been found effective for pentylenetetrazol-induced convulsions in mice. Intraperitoneal injection of 20g/kg *Dì lóng* ethanol extract to mice, its anti-convulsant effect is equivalent to 20mg/kg sodium phenobarbital, but it is ineffective for strychnine-induced convulsion. Therefore, it is speculated that *Dì lóng*'s anticonvulsant action site is in the central nerve above the spinal cord. Succinic acid is the main active ingredient of the anti-convulsant effect of *Dì lóng*.

4. 抗血栓　地龙提取液可使血液黏度和血小板聚集性降低，红细胞变形能力增强、刚性指数降低。地龙中含有纤溶酶样物质，可促进纤溶，激活纤溶酶原，能直接溶解纤维蛋白和血凝块。从地龙提取液中已分离多种纤溶酶和纤溶酶原激活物，如蚓激酶，具有溶栓作用。蚓激酶能降低纤溶酶原的含量，抑制纤维蛋白原生成纤维蛋白，并可直接降解纤维蛋白；还能间接激活纤溶酶原形成纤溶酶，起到纤溶酶原激活物的作用。蚓激酶可刺激血管内皮细胞释放纤溶酶原激活物，增强纤溶酶原激活物活性。地龙抗血栓作用与增强纤溶酶活性及抗凝活性、改善血液流变性相关。

(4) Anti-thrombosis　*Dì lóng* has an anti-thrombotic effect. *Dì lóng* extract can reduce blood viscosity and platelet aggregation, enhance the deformability of red blood cells, and reduce the rigidity index. *Dì lóng* contains plasmin-like substance, which has the functions of promoting fibrinolysis and activating plasminogen, and can directly dissolve fibrin and blood clots. A variety of plasmin and plasminogen activators, such as lumbrokinase, have been isolated from *Dì lóng* extracts and have a thrombolytic effect. Lumbrokinase can reduce the content of fibrinolytic zymogen, inhibit fibrinogen production of fibrin, and can directly degrade fibrin. It can also indirectly activate plasminogen to form plasmin, which acts as a plasminogen activator. Lumbrokinase can stimulate vascular endothelial cells to release plasminogen activator and enhance plasminogen activator activity. The antithrombotic effect of *Dì lóng* is related to the enhancement of plasmin activity, anticoagulant activity and improvement of blood rheology.

5. 镇咳、平喘　地龙能扩张支气管，缓解支气管痉挛。地龙对组胺、毛果芸香碱引起的支气管收缩有对抗作用，可使肺灌流量增加。腹腔注射地龙水煎液能降低致敏性哮喘豚鼠支气管洗液中细胞总数、白蛋白含量及白三烯水平，尤其能抑制嗜酸性粒细胞增多，并阻止该细胞激活。地龙平喘的作用机制是通过阻滞组胺受体和抑制平滑肌肌动蛋白的表达，进而抑制气管重建。平喘的主要有效成分是琥珀酸、黄嘌呤和次黄嘌呤。

(5) Relieving cough and asthma　*Dì lóng* can dilate the bronchi, relieve bronchospasm, and has the effect of relieving cough and asthma. *Dì lóng* can antagonize bronchoconstriction caused by histamine and pilocarpine by increase in pulmonary flow volume. Intraperitoneal injection of *Dì lóng* decoction, can reduce the total number of cells, albumin content, and leukotriene levels in bronchial washes of sensitized asthma guinea pigs, and can especially inhibit eosinophils. The mechanism of action of *Dì lóng*'s antiasthma is to inhibit tracheal remodeling by blocking histamine receptors and inhibiting smooth muscle actin expression. The main active ingredients of asthma are succinic acid, xanthine and hypoxanthine.

6. 降血压　地龙能产生缓慢而持久的降压作用。静脉注射地龙水煎剂可引起大鼠血压明显下降，预先使用特异性血小板活化因子受体阻断剂可显著抑制地龙的降压作用。单次或多次静脉注射地龙降压蛋白可明显降低自发性高血压大鼠的血压。类血小板活化因子和地龙多肽是地龙降血压的主要成分。

(6) Anti-hypertension *Dì lóng* is able to produce a slow and everlasting anti-hypertension. Intravenous injection *Dì lóng* decoction caused a significant decrease in blood pressure in rats. Pre-administration of specific platelet activating factor (PAF) receptor blocker can significantly inhibit the anti-hypertensive effect of *Dì lóng*. Single or multiple intravenous injections of *Dì lóng* anti-hypertensive protein can significantly reduce blood pressure in spontaneously hypertensive rats. Platelet-like activating factor and earthworm peptides are the main components of *Dì lóng's* blood pressure.

【不良反应 / Adverse effects】

地龙对子宫有刺激作用，导致痉挛性收缩，因此孕妇使用这种药物时应格外谨慎。注射地龙可能会引起过敏反应。蚯蚓毒素和蚯蚓热解碱具有毒性，蚯蚓素无毒性或副作用。

Dì lóng has stimulation to uterus, leading to spasmodic contraction, so the application of this drug to pregnant women should be very careful. Besides, the injection of *Dì lóng* may induce anaphylactic reaction. Lumbrofebin and terrestro-lumbrilysin are toxic, while lumbritin has no side effects.

羚羊角 | *Líng yáng jiǎo* (*Cornu Saigae Tataricae*)

【来源 / Origin】

本品为牛科动物赛加羚羊（*Saiga tatarica* Linnaeus）的角。主产于新疆、青海等地。全年均可捕捉，捕得后切取角，用时磨成粉末、锉末或镑为薄片。

Líng yáng jiǎo is from the horn of *Saiga tatarica* Linnaeus, family of Bovidae. The medicinal material is mainly produced in the areas of Xinjiang Uygur Autonomous region, Qinghai province and others in China. The animal is caught all year round. After capture of the animal, the horn is cut, and when it is used, it can be prepared as juice, slices or powder.

【化学成分 / Chemical ingredients】

主要含有角蛋白、胆固醇、磷脂类等。其中角蛋白含量最多，角蛋白水解后可得18种氨基酸及多肽类物质。磷脂类成分包括卵磷脂、脑磷脂等。

Líng yáng jiǎo mainly contains keratin, cholesterin, phospholipids, etc. The major content is keratin, which can hydrolyze to 18 kinds of amino acids and peptides. Phospholipids mainly consists of lecithin and encephain, etc.

【药性与功效 / Chinese medicine properties】

味咸，性寒，归肝、心经。具有平肝息风、清肝明目、清热解毒的功效。主治高热惊痫、神昏惊厥、子痫抽搐、癫痫发狂、头痛眩晕、目赤翳障、痈肿疮毒等。

In Chinese medicine theory, *Líng yáng jiǎo* has the nature of salty and cold. It can enter the meridians of liver, heart and has the effect of calming the liver to check endogenous wind, clearing away from the liver to improve acuity of vision and removing blood stasis and clearing away toxins. It is used for epilepsy due to high fever, loss of consciousness, eclampsia and convulsion, epileptic and madness, headache and dizziness, conjunctivitis and nebula, carbuncles and sores.

【药理作用 / Pharmacological effects】

1. **镇静、催眠** 羚羊角口服液可降低小鼠自主活动次数，协同阈下剂量戊巴比妥钠起催眠作用，明显缩短阈剂量异戊巴比妥钠引起的小鼠睡眠潜伏期，延长小鼠睡眠时间。小鼠腹腔注射羚羊角注射液，能延长戊巴比妥钠的睡眠时间，小鼠腹腔注射羚羊角醇提取液、水煎剂均能延长硫喷妥钠的睡眠时间。

(1) Sedation and hypnosis *Líng yáng jiǎo* has sedative and hypnotic activity. *Líng yáng jiǎo* oral solution can reduce the locomotor activity, increase the sleep ratio of the mice treated with pentobarbital sodium under subthreshold dose. It can also decrease the latent period and prolong the sleep duration of the mice treated with pentobarbital sodium above threshold dose respectively. Intraperitoneal injection of *Líng yáng jiǎo* injection can prolong the sleep duration of the mice treated with pentobarbital sodium, and intraperitoneal injection of *Líng yáng jiǎo* aqueous and ethanol extracts can prolong the sleep duration of the mice treated with pentothal sodium.

2. **抗惊厥** 口服羚羊角口服液和腹腔注射羚羊角水煎液可明显拮抗戊四氮引起的小鼠惊厥和电惊厥。

(2) Anti-convulsion *Líng yáng jiǎo* has obvious effect on anti-convulsion. Oral administration of *Líng yáng jiǎo* oral solution and intraperitoneal injection of aqueous extract can significantly antagonize pentylenetetrazol-induced convulsions and electrical convulsions in mice.

3. **解热** 静脉注射羚羊角水煎剂和醇提液、水解液、注射液均对人工发热兔具有明显的解热作用。羚羊角煎剂灌服酵母致热家兔，可降低发热家兔的体温。

(3) Anti-pyretic effects Intravenous injection of *Líng yáng jiǎo* aqueous extract, ethanol extract, hydrolysate and injection have obvious antipyretic effect on fever rabbits. *Líng yáng jiǎo* aqueous extract could alleviate yeast-induced pyrexia in rabbits.

4. **降血压** 静脉注射羚羊角水煎剂可降低麻醉猫的血压，切断两侧迷走神经后，降压作用有所下降，说明其降压作用可能与中枢神经系统有关。

(4) Anti-hypertension *Líng yáng jiǎo* has anti-hypertensive effect. Intravenous injection of *Líng yáng jiǎo* decoction can reduce blood pressure in anesthetized cats, after cutting off the vagus nerve on both sides, its hypotensive effect decreased, indicating that this effect may be related to the central nervous system.

题库

（王艳艳　王　宁）

第十八章　开窍药
Chapter 18　Resuscitative medicines

学习目标 | Objectives

1. **掌握**　开窍药的基本药理作用；麝香和冰片与功效相关的药理作用、药效物质基础。

2. **了解**　石菖蒲的主要药理作用和药效物质基础；苏合香、蟾酥与功效相关的药理作用。

1. **Must know**　The main pharmacological effects of resuscitative medicines; the efficacy related pharmacological effects, mechanism, and material basis of *Shè xiāng*, *Bīng piàn*.

2. **Desirable to know**　Pharmacological effects and material basis of *Shí chāng pǔ*; the efficacy related pharmacological effects of *Sū hé xiāng* and *Chán sū*.

微课

第一节　概述
Section 1　Overview

PPT

　　凡以开窍醒神为主要作用的药物称为开窍药。本类药物具有通关、开窍、醒神的功效，主要用于邪气壅盛、蒙蔽心窍所致的窍闭证。窍闭证因其病因不同，又有寒闭、热闭之分。

All Chinese materia medica that are used to resuscitate the consciousness are classified as resuscitative medicines. The medicines in the category mainly open the orifices and resuscitate the consciousness, which is mainly applied in the block syndrome when heart is attacked by pathogenic factors. Because of its different etiology, block syndrome can be divided into cold block and heat block.

　　寒闭乃风、痰、癖等浊邪合而为患，其中痰湿偏盛，风夹痰湿，上蒙清窍，表现为神昏的基础上多无明显热象，可见中风、中寒、气郁、痰厥等证；热闭表现为神昏的基础上有明显热象，常见于温病闭证神昏，其关键在于热毒。热闭临床多见于严重的全身感染如流行性脑脊髓膜炎、乙型脑炎引起的高热昏迷、谵语、抽搐等症状。寒闭伴有面青、脉迟、苔白等症状，多见于脑血管意外、中毒等引起的昏迷、神志不清等。现代药理研究表明，开窍药开窍醒神的作用与下列药理作用有关。

Cold block syndromes refer to the pathological changes and syndromes that are caused by that the combination of wind, phlegm, obturation and other turbid pathogens may block the orifices. The clinical

医药大学堂
WWW.YIYAODXT.COM

feature of cold block is dizziness without obvious heat symptoms, such as stroke, apoplexy, Qi depression, phlegm syncope and so on. The clinical feature of heat block syndromes refers to dizziness with heat symptoms, such as febrile disease. The key of heat block lies in pyretic pathogen. The symptoms of heat block have the similarities with serious systemic infections, such as epidemic cerebrospinal meningitis, encephalitis B. The symptoms of cold block have the similarities with cerebrovascular accident and poisoning. The resuscitative function of resuscitative medicines may involve following pharmacological effects.

1. **影响中枢神经系统**　开窍药常因药物及其成分，以及给药途径、用药剂量、动物种属及机体功能状态不同而表现出对中枢神经系统的兴奋或抑制作用。麝香、苏合香、冰片、石菖蒲的作用特点是小剂量兴奋中枢，大剂量抑制中枢。

(1) Effect on central nervous system　Resuscitative medicines often show excitement or inhibitory effects on the central nervous system due to different drugs and their components, as well as different routes of administration, dosages, animal species and functional status of the body. It is universally considered that resuscitative medicines excites central nervous system with low dosage and suppressed with high dosage, such as *Shè xiāng*, *Sū hé xiāng*, and *Shí chāng pǔ*.

2. **改善学习记忆**　开窍药一般具有益智作用，可改善动物的学习记忆能力。麝香酮可明显拮抗痴呆小鼠的学习记忆功能减退，并可升高血清超氧化物歧化酶（SOD）活力，降低脑组织中升高的丙二醛（MDA）含量，抑制单胺氧化酶（MAO）活力。石菖蒲的挥发油类成分如β- 细辛醚、α- 细辛醚对各型记忆障碍模型均有不同程度的改善作用。

(2) Improve learning and memory　Resuscitative medicines have a nootropic effect, which can improve the learning and memory function of animals. Muscone significantly antagonizes learning and memory dysfunction in dementia mice. Increase serum superoxide dismutase (SOD) activity, reduce elevated malondialdehyde (MDA) content in brain tissue, and inhibit monoamine oxidase (MAO) activity. The volatile oil components of *Shí chāng pǔ*, such as β-asarone and α-asarone, are able to improve various types of memory impairment models.

3. **抗脑缺血**　麝香能减轻缺血性神经元损伤，减轻脑细胞超微结构损害。冰片可通过增加缺血脑组织的血氧供应，明显改善脑水肿，抑制脑皮质和海马神经细胞凋亡。麝香、冰片、苏合香中的有效成分易通过血脑屏障，发挥抗脑缺血作用。

(3) Anti-cerebral ischemia　*Shè xiāng* is able to relieve ischemic neuronal damages and ultra-microstructure damages of brain cells. *Bīng piàn* can inhibit neuronal apoptosis in cerebral cortex and hippocampus by increasing the blood and oxygen supply of ischemic brain tissue and significantly ameliorate brain edema. The effective compositions in *Shè xiāng*, *Bīng piàn* and *Sū hé xiāng* can easily pass through the blood-brain barrier and play an anti-cerebral ischemic role.

4. **抗心肌缺血**　麝香、苏合香、冰片可增加缺血心肌血流量，降低心肌耗氧量，扩张冠脉，增加冠脉血流量，可减轻缺血所致的心肌损伤。蟾酥能改善心肌能量代谢，减轻心肌损伤。

(4) Anti-myocardial ischemia　*Shè xiāng*, *Sū hé xiāng*, *Bīng piàn* are able to increase ischemic myocardial blood flow, reduce myocardial oxygen consumption, expand coronary artery and increase coronary blood flow, and relieve myocardial injury caused by ischemia.

5. **抗炎**　麝香对炎症的早、中、晚期均有明显效果，尤其是对早、中期的作用较强，抗炎机制可能与兴奋神经-垂体-肾上腺皮质系统有关。冰片具有拮抗前列腺素（PG）和抑制炎症介质释放的作用，还可以有效抑制脑缺血再灌注损伤时炎症细胞因子的表达，减少白细胞浸润，降低脑缺血再灌注损伤的程度。蟾酥醇提物对脂多糖（LPS）诱导小鼠腹腔巨噬细胞分泌的炎症因子有明显抑制作用。

(5) Anti-inflammation *Shè xiāng* has obvious effects on the early, middle and late stages of inflammation, especially on the early and middle stages. The anti-inflammatory mechanism may be related to the excitation of the hypothalamic-pituitary-adrenal axis. In addition, *Bīng piàn* antagonizes PG and inhibits the release of inflammatory mediators. It can also effectively inhibit the expression of inflammatory cytokines, inhibit leukocyte infiltration and decrease cerebral ischemia-reperfusion injury. The alcohol extract of *Chán sū* can significantly inhibit the secretion of inflammatory factors by mouse peritoneal macrophages induced by lipopolysaccharide (LPS).

常用开窍药的主要药理作用见表 18-1。

The main pharmacological effects of commonly used resuscitative medicines are summarized in Table 18-1.

表 18-1　常用开窍药主要药理作用

药物	对中枢神经系统的影响	抗脑缺血	抗心肌缺血	抗炎	其他药理作用
麝香	+	+	+	+	抑制血小板聚集、兴奋子宫、抗肿瘤、降血脂
苏合香	+	+	+	−	抑制血小板聚集、抗血栓
冰片	+	+	+	+	抗菌、镇痛、促吸收、抗生育
石菖蒲	+				改善学习记忆、抗抑郁、抗病原微生物、松弛肠胃和气管平滑肌、抗心律失常
蟾酥	+			+	局部麻醉、镇痛、强心、升压、抑制血小板聚集、抗休克、抗肿瘤

注："+"表示有明确作用；"−"表示无作用，或未查阅到相关研究文献

第二节　常用药物

Section 2　Commonly used medicines

PPT

麝香 ┆ *Shè xiāng* (*Moschus*)

【来源 / Origin】

本品为鹿科动物林麝（*Moschus berezovskii* Flerov）、马麝（*Moschus sifanicus* Przewalski）或原麝（*Moschus moschiferus* Linnaeus）成熟雄体香囊中的干燥分泌物。主产于四川、西藏、云南、陕西、甘肃、内蒙古等地。

Shè xiāng is the dry secretion of mature male sachet of *Moschus berezovskii* Flerov, *Moschus sifanicus* Przewalski or *Moschus moschiferus* Linnaeus, which is produced in Sichuan province, Tibet Autonomous region, Yunnan province, Shaanxi province, Gansu province, Inner Mongolia Autonomous region and so on.

【化学成分 / Chemical ingredients】

含有大环酮类化合物、吡啶类化合物、甾体类化合物、多肽类化合物、脂肪酸、无机化合物等。其中，麝香酮是大环酮类主要成分。

Shè xiāng contains a variety of chemical ingredients, including macrocyclic ketones, pyridines, steroids, polypeptides, fatty acids, inorganic compounds and so on. Muscone is the main component in macrocyclic ketones.

【药性与功效 / Chinese medicine properties】

性辛、温，味苦，归心、脾、肝经。具有开窍醒神、活血通经、止痛、催产的功效。主治热病神昏、中风痰厥、气郁暴厥、中恶昏迷、癥瘕经闭、难产死胎、心腹暴痛、痈肿瘰疬、咽喉肿痛等。

Shè xiāng is pungent, warm, bitter. It can enter the meridians of heart, spleen and liver. *Shè xiāng* can resuscitate the consciousness, promote blood circulation and menstruation, ease pain and expedite child delivery, which is always applied in coma of febrile disease, apoplectic phlegm syncope, Qi depression syncope, coma, menstrual block, dystocia and fetal death, severe pain in heart and abdomen, carbuncle swelling, sore throat and so on.

【药理作用 / Pharmacological effects】

1. 影响中枢神经系统　麝香对中枢神经系统表现为兴奋和抑制的双重作用。小鼠腹腔注射麝香能缩短巴比妥类药物引起的睡眠时间，麝香对巴比妥麻醉家兔具有唤醒作用。腹腔注射麝香还可抑制小鼠自发性活动，麝香灌胃能明显抑制戊四氮引起的惊厥。麝香酮是其调节中枢神经系统作用的主要物质基础。麝香酮可迅速通过血脑屏障进入中枢发挥作用。麝香酮还可激活肝微粒体转化酶，加速肝内戊巴比妥钠等物质代谢而失活。

(1) **Effects on central nervous system**　The mice treated *Shè xiāng* by intraperitoneal infection can shorten the sleep time caused by barbiturates and wake up rabbits anesthetized with barbiturates. Moreover, oral administration of *Shè xiāng* can significantly inhibit convulsion caused by pentylenetetrazol. Muscone is the main effective component for central nervous system.

2. 改善学习记忆　麝香酮明显改善东莨菪碱所致痴呆模型大鼠的学习记忆能力。

(2) **Improve learning and memory**　Muscone significantly improves scopolamine-induced dementia model rats and improves learning and memory abilities.

3. 抗脑缺血　麝香能降低脑组织含水量、减轻脑水肿、缩小脑梗死面积、改善脑微循环、增加脑血流量、减轻脑组织病理损伤。

(3) **Anti-cerebral ischemia**　*Shè xiāng* is capable of decreasing the moisture content of brain tissue, alleviating brain edema, reducing the area of cerebral infarction, improving cerebral microcirculation, increasing cerebral blood flow and reducing the pathological injury of brain tissue.

4. 抗心肌缺血　麝香能改善垂体后叶素致大鼠心肌缺血心电图的病理变化，抑制心肌酶活性的升高。此外，麝香还有强心的作用，使心脏收缩力增强，心输出量增加，扩张冠脉血管。

(4) **Anti-myocardial ischemia**　Man-made *Shè xiāng* is capable of anti-myocardial ischemia. *Shè xiāng* can improve the pathological changes of rat ischemic myocardial ECG induced by posterior pituitary and inhibit the increase of myocardial enzyme activity. In addition, musk also has a heart-strengthening effect, which increases the contractility of the heart, increases cardiac output, and dilates the coronary vessels.

5. 抗血小板聚集　麝香酮可抑制二磷酸腺苷（ADP）诱导的血小板聚集率，使血浆凝块不能正常收缩，明显延长家兔凝血时间。

(5) **Anti-platelet aggregation**　Muscone inhibit ADP-induced platelet aggregation, affect the function of platelet contractile protein, prevent plasma clots from contracting normally, and significantly prolong the clotting time of rabbits.

6. 抗炎　麝香对炎症的早、中、晚三期均有抑制作用，尤其对早、中期作用较强。麝香多肽类物质是其抗炎的主要物质基础，其抗炎机制可能与兴奋下丘脑–垂体–肾上腺皮质系统相关。其抗炎作用还与抑制溶酶体酶释放、抑制白细胞趋化相关。

(6) Anti-inflammation *Shè xiāng* has a suppressive impact on the early, middle and late period of inflammation, especially in the early and middle period. The polypeptides of *Shè xiāng* are the main material basis of its anti-inflammation. This anti-inflammatory mechanism may be related to the excitation of the hypothalamic-pituitary-adrenal axis. In addition, its anti-inflammatory effect is also related to the release of lysosomal enzymes and inhibiting chemotaxis of white blood cells.

【不良反应 / Adverse effects】

可引起头晕、头胀、恶心、食欲减退。有过量服用引起中毒的个案病例报告，表现为面色潮红、口腔及咽部黏膜溃烂充血、牙龈出血、鼻出血、瞳孔散大、抽搐、昏迷、呼吸困难，有死亡病例报告。

The main composition in *Shè xiāng* is muscone, which is noxious in an inappropriate way. It has a stimulating effect on the digestive tract mucosa. In some severe cases, it can cause respiratory center paralysis, heart failure, extensive visceral bleeding and death.

冰片 ¦ *Bīng piàn (Bomel)*

【来源 / Origin】

本品为龙脑香科常绿乔木植物龙脑香（*Dryobalanops aromatica* Gaertn. F.）树脂的加工品，或龙脑香的树干经蒸馏冷却而得到的结晶，又称龙脑冰片。由菊科多年生植物艾纳香［*Blumea balsamifera* (L.)DC.］升华物经加工而成，又称艾片。主产于东南亚地区，我国台湾有引种。现多用松节油、樟脑等经化学方法合成制得，为人工冰片。

Bīng piàn is processed products of resin or crystals obtained from the trunk of *Dryobalanops aromatica* Gaertn. F. which is an evergreen arbor plant of the family dipterocarpacae, called *Longnao Bingpian*. Processed sublimate of *Blumea balsamifera* (L.)DC. which belongs to composite family, called *Aipian*. It is mainly from Southeast Asia and Taiwan province of China. Turpentine and camphor are mostly used to synthesize artificial borneol.

【化学成分 / Chemical ingredients】

龙脑冰片主要含有右旋龙脑；艾片主要含有左旋龙脑；人工合成的冰片主要含有龙脑和异龙脑。冰片还含有萜类成分，包括 P–榄香烯、石竹烯等倍半萜成分和齐墩果酸、积雪草酸、龙脑香二醇酮等三萜化合物。

Bīng piàn mainly contains borneol. *Longnao Bingpian* mainly contains D-borneol, *Aipian* mainly contains L-borneol and synthetic borneol mainly contains borneol and isoborneol. *Bīng piàn* also contains terpenoids as well, including P-elemene, caryophyllene and other sesquiterpenoids, oleanolic acid, asiatic acid, borneol diol ketone and other triterpenoids.

【药性与功效 / Chinese medicine properties】

味辛、苦，性微寒，归心、脾、肺经。具有开窍醒神、清热止痛的功效。主治热病神昏、惊厥、中风痰厥、气郁暴厥、中恶昏迷、胸痹心痛、目赤、口疮、咽喉肿痛、耳道流脓。

Bīng piàn is pungent, bitter and slightly cold. It can enter the meridians of heart, spleen and lung. It is able to clear heat for resuscitation and relieve pain. It is applied to treat febrile disease, unconsciousness, apoplexy, phlegm syncope, Qi depression, chest impediment, heart pain, red eye and aphtha.

【药理作用 / Pharmacological effects】

1. 抗脑缺血　冰片改善脑缺血区细胞能量代谢，抗自由基损伤，减轻炎症反应，从而使脑组织免受损伤。

(1) Anti-cerebral ischemia *Bīng piàn* improves the energy metabolism of cells in the ischemic area of the brain, resists free radical damage and reduces the inflammatory response, thereby protecting brain tissue from damage.

2. **中枢抑制**　龙脑、异龙脑均能延长戊巴比妥引起的睡眠时间延长，与戊巴比妥产生协同作用。

(2) Central inhibition Both borneol and isoborneol can prolong the sleep time caused by pentobarbital and have a synergistic effect with pentobarbital.

3. **促进其他药物通过血脑屏障**　冰片能提高血脑屏障对顺铂、卡马西平、丙戊酸钠、磺胺嘧啶等药物的通透性。

(3) Promotion of other drugs through the blood-brain barrier *Bīng piàn* can improve the permeability of drugs such as cedar, carbamazepine, valproate, and sulfadiazine to the blood-brain barrier.

4. **促进吸收**　冰片可使小鼠皮肤角质细胞疏松、细胞间隙增大、毛囊口孔径加宽进而促进药物透皮吸收。冰片可促进川芎嗪透过鼻黏膜吸收，还可促进葛根素、丹参素等通过角膜吸收，该作用与其改善角膜上皮细胞膜磷脂分子排列有关。冰片还可促进秋水仙碱、川芎嗪在小肠的吸收，提高生物利用度。

(4) Promotion of absorption *Bīng piàn* is capable of loosing the keratinocytes, enlarging the intercellular space, widing the pore size of the hair follicle and promoting the drug transdermal absorption. *Bīng piàn* can promote the absorption of Ligustrazine through the nasal mucosa, puerarin and danshensu through the cornea. *Bīng piàn* can also promote the absorption of colchicine and ligustrazine in the small intestine and improve the bioavailability.

5. **抗炎、镇痛**　龙脑与异龙脑均能抑制蛋清所致大鼠足跖肿胀，可拮抗炎症介质释放。冰片延长热刺激引起小鼠疼痛反应时间，减少化学刺激引起的小鼠扭体次数。

(5) Anti-inflammatory and analgesia Both borneol and isoborneol are able to inhibit the paw swelling induced by albumen, inhibit the release of inflammatory mediators. *Bīng piàn* prolonged the pain response time and reduced the number of writhing induced by chemical stimulation.

【不良反应 / Adverse effects】

局部应用有轻微刺激性，外用偶致过敏反应。

Slight irritation; occasionally allergic reaction caused by external use.

石菖蒲 ┆ *Shí chāng pú (Grassleaf Sweetflag Rhizome)*

【来源 / Origin】

本品为天南星科植物石菖蒲（*Acortw tatarinowii* Schott.）的干燥根茎。主要分布于四川、浙江、江苏等地。秋冬二季采挖，晒干，生用。

Shí chāng pú is the dried rhizome of *Acortw tatarinowii* Schott., belonged to family of Araceae, mainly distributed in Sichuan province, Zhejiang province and Jiangsu province, and harvested in autumn and winter dried in the sun and directly used for Chinese medicinal preparation.

【化学成分 / Chemical ingredients】

主要含多种挥发油，挥发油中的主要有效成分为 β-细辛醚、α-细辛醚、石竹烯、α-葎草烯、石菖醚、细辛醚等。此外，还含有氨基酸、有机酸和糖类。

Shí chāng pú mostly contains a variety of volatile oil. The main effective components are β- asarone, α-asarone, caryophyllene, α-humulus, acorus calamus, asarone, etc. It contains amino acids, organic acids and sugars likewise.

【药性与功效 / **Chinese medicine properties**】

味辛、苦，性温，归心、胃经。具有开窍豁痰、醒神益智、化湿开胃的功效。用于治疗神昏癫痫、健忘失眠、耳鸣耳聋、脘痞不饥、噤口下痢。

Shí chāng pú is pungent, bitter and warm. It can enter the meridians of heart and stomach. It is capable of opening the orifices, eliminating phlegm, awakening the mind and benefiting the intellect, removing dampness and appetizing the stomach. It is used to treat the syndromes of dizziness and epilepsy, forgetfulness and insomnia, tinnitus and deafness, dysentery.

【药理作用 / **Pharmacological effects**】

1. 影响中枢神经系统　石菖蒲具有镇静、抗惊厥、抗癫痫、改善学习记忆、抗抑郁的作用。石菖蒲提取物或挥发油对中枢神经系统有抑制作用，可降低单胺类神经递质的含量。石菖蒲挥发油、水提液、醇提物有抗惊厥作用。石菖蒲水溶性成分可调节癫痫大鼠脑内兴奋性与抑制性氨基酸的平衡。石菖蒲总挥发油和α-细辛醚对各种类型记忆障碍模型均有不同程度的改善作用，提高学习记忆能力，该作用与保护神经元、降低兴奋性氨基酸的含量、改善胆碱能神经功能、抗自由基损伤、调节神经生长因子等相关。石菖蒲水提液、水提醇沉液和醇提物等均具有抗抑郁作用。

(1) Effects on central nervous system　*Shí chāng pú* is capable of sedation, anti-convulsion, antiepileptic, improving memory and anti-depression. The extract or volatile oilcan inhibit the central nervous system，which reduce the content of monoamine neurotransmitter. The volatile oil, water extract and alcohol extract have anticonvulsant effects. Water soluble components keep the balance between the excitatory and inhibitory of amino acids in the brain of epileptic rats. The total volatile oil and α-asarone improve the abilities on learning and memory from various types of memory impairment models, which is related to protecting neurons, reducing excitatory amino acid content, improving cholinergic nerve function, antagonizing lesion of free radicals and regulating nerve growth factor. The antidepressant effects of water extract, alcohol precipitation and alcohol extract were all found.

2. 解痉　石菖蒲水提液、总挥发油、β-细辛醚、α-细辛醚对家兔离体肠管自发性收缩幅度均有抑制作用，可拮抗乙酰胆碱（ACh）及氯化钡引起的肠管痉挛，且呈剂量依赖性，能增强肠管蠕动及肠道推进功能；对气管平滑肌具有解痉作用。这些作用以总挥发油的作用最强，其次为α-细辛醚和β-细辛醚。

(2) Spasmolysis　Water extract of *Shí chāng pú*, total volatile oil, β-asarone and α-asarone are able to inhibit the spontaneous contraction of isolated intestine. Antagonize the spasm of intestine caused by acetylcholine (ACh) and barium chloride (BaCl$_2$) in a dose-dependent manner, and enhance the peristalsis and intestinal propulsion function. They have antispasmodic influences on smooth muscle of trachea, the most important of which are total volatile oil, followed by α-asarone and β-asarone.

3. 影响心血管系统　石菖蒲具有抗心律失常、抗动脉粥样硬化、抗心肌缺血、抗血栓的作用。腹腔注射石菖蒲挥发油可抑制乌头碱、肾上腺素和氯化钡等诱发的心律失常。石菖蒲挥发油降低动脉粥样硬化动物的血脂，改善高黏血症实验动物的血液流变学异常。高剂量β-细辛醚可以抑制阿尔茨海默病大鼠内皮素-1（ET-1）mRNA表达水平的升高，提高一氧化氮含量，降低心肌组织损伤程度和坏死率；石菖蒲挥发油中β-细辛醚能使豚鼠冠状动脉扩张。

(3) Effects on cardiovascular system　*Shí chāng pú* possesses the effects of anti-arrhythmia, anti-atherosclerosis, anti-myocardial ischemia and anti-thrombus. The volatile oil inhibit the arrhythmia induced by aconitine, adrenaline and barium chloride, reduce the blood lipid of atherosclerotic animals and improve the hemorheology of experimental animals with hyperviscosity. High dose of β-asarone can inhibit the increase of endothelin-1 (ET-1) mRNA expression, increase the content of nitric oxide and reduce the degree of myocardial injury and necrosis in Alzheimer's disease rats. β-asarone in volatile oil of *Shí chāng pú* can dilate the coronary artery of guinea pigs.

4. 抗菌 石菖蒲对常见致病菌如真菌、结核分枝杆菌、葡萄球菌等有抑制作用。

(4) Anti-bacterial *Shí chāng pú* can inhibit common pathogenic bacteria such as fungi, *Mycobacterium tuberculosis* and *Staphylococcus*.

【不良反应 / Adverse effects】

有发热、头昏、恶心、呕吐及大剂量内服导致皮肤潮红、血尿和血压升高的个案病例报告。

Overdose is able to result in poisoning, such as fever, nausea, vomiting, dizziness, severe convulsion and convulsion, and finally die of compulsory convulsion.

苏合香 ┆ *Sū hé xiāng (Styrax)*

【来源 / Origin】

本品为梅科植物苏合香树（*Liquidam barorientalis* Mill.）的树干渗出的香树脂经加工精制而成的半流动性浓稠液体。主产于印度、索马里、叙利亚和土耳其等地区，我国广西、云南也有栽培。我国产苏合香与进口苏合香药材的作用基本相同，可替代使用。

Sū hé xiāng is the semi-fluidity thick liquid made by processing and refining the incense resin exudate from the trunk of *Liquidam barorientalis* Mill.. It is mostly from in India, Somalia, Syria and Turkey and so on. It is also cultivated in Guangxi province and Yunnan province of China. The effect of *Sū hé xiāng* from China is basically the same as that from foreign countries, which can be replaced.

【化学成分 / Chemical ingredients】

主要含有树脂和油状液体，树脂由树脂酯和树脂酸类组成，油状液体主要由芳香族类和萜类化合物组成，苏合香中尚含有一些不饱和脂肪酸。

Sū hé xiāng mainly contains resin and oily liquid. The resin is composed of resin esters and resin acids, while the oily liquid is mainly composed of aromatic and terpenoid compounds. *Sū hé xiāng* also contains some unsaturated fatty acids.

【药性与功效 / Chinese medicine properties】

味辛，性温，归心、脾经。具有开窍、温散止痛的功效。主治中风痰厥、胸腹冷痛、惊痫和猝然昏倒等。

Sū hé xiāng is pungent, warm. It can enter the meridians of heart and spleen. It is able to open the orifices, warm and relieve pain. Thus, *Sū hé xiāng* is often used for apoplectic phlegm syncope, chest and abdominal pain, epilepsy and sudden fainting and so on.

【药理作用 / Pharmacological effects】

1. 影响中枢神经系统 苏合香挥发油能缩短戊巴比妥钠睡眠持续时间，减少印防己毒素及士的宁导致的惊厥次数，对惊厥潜伏期有延长趋势，能降低惊厥导致的死亡率。对中枢神经系统兴奋性有较强的双向调节作用，在生理、病理不同情况下，既能镇静、抗惊厥，又可兴奋中枢神经系统。

(1) Effect on central nervous system *Sū hé xiāng* can shorten the sleep duration of pentobarbital sodium, reduce the number of convulsions caused by bitterness and strychnine, prolong the latent period of convulsions and reduce the mortality caused by convulsions. It has a strong bi-directional regulating effect on the central nervous system. Under different physiological or pathological conditions, it can be not only sedation, anti-convulsion, but also excite central nervous system.

2. **抗心肌缺血** 苏合香可通过改善心功能、减少心肌梗死面积、减缓心肌细胞坏死、降低心肌酶活性，有效防治大鼠心肌缺血损伤。

(2) Anti-myocardial ischemia *Sū hé xiāng* prevent myocardial ischemic injury in rats by improving cardiac function, reducing myocardial infarction size, slowing myocardial cell necrosis and reducing myocardial enzyme activity.

3. **抗血栓** 苏合香能提高血小板内环磷酸腺苷（cAMP）含量，使血栓长度缩短、重量减轻，抑制血栓素合成酶。苏合香还能明显延长血浆复钙时间，降低纤维蛋白原含量，促进纤溶酶活性。桂皮酸是其抗血栓的主要物质基础。

(3) Anti-thrombosis *Sū hé xiāng* can increase the content of cAMP in platelets, shorten the length and weight of thrombosis, inhibit thromboxane synthetase. *Sū hé xiāng* can also significantly prolong plasma recalcification time, reduce fibrinogen content and promote plasmin activity. Cinnamic acid is the main active ingredient on its anti-thrombosis.

4. **抗脑缺血** 苏合香能减轻缺血再灌注大鼠的脑水肿程度，对脑缺血损伤有一定保护作用，可能与减少氧化应激损伤、改善脑血管血流动力状态、调节脑内氨基酸水平、降低兴奋性氨基酸毒性、抑制脑细胞凋亡、降低脑缺血性神经元损伤相关。

(4) Anti-cerebral ischemia *Sū hé xiāng* can reduce the degree of brain edema and protect the brain from ischemia-reperfusion injury, which may be related to reducing oxidative stress injury, improving the blood dynamic state of cerebral vessels, regulating the level of amino acids in the brain, reducing the toxicity of excitatory amino acids, inhibiting the apoptosis of brain cells, and reducing the damage of cerebral ischemic neurons.

蟾酥 | *Chán sū* (Toad Venom)

【来源 / Origin】

本品为蟾蜍科动物中华大蟾蜍（*Bufo bufo gargarizans* Cantor）或黑眶蟾蜍（*Bufo melanostictus* Schneider）的干燥分泌物。多于夏、秋二季捕捉蟾蜍，洗净，挤取耳后腺和皮肤腺的白色浆液，加工，干燥。

Chán sū is the dry secretion of *Bufo bufo gargarizans* Cantor or *Bufo melanostictus* Schneider. Usually, they are caught in summer and autumn for processing. After washing, squeeze the white slurry from the posterior ear gland and skin gland.

【化学成分 / Chemical ingredients】

较为复杂，主要化学成分是蟾毒配基类及其酯类、蟾毒色胺类、甾醇类及其他化合物。华蟾毒配基有华蟾毒精、蟾毒它灵、华蟾毒灵、蟾毒灵、蟾毒配基等。此外，还含吲哚衍生物、蟾蜍色胺、蟾蜍特尼定等。

The chemical components of *Chán sū* are complex. The main chemical components are toad venom ligands and their esters, toad venom tryptamines, sterols and other compounds. The Chinese toad poison matching base includes the Chinese toad poison essence, the toad poison other spirit, the Chinese toad poison spirit, the toad poison spirit, the toad poison matching base and so on. In addition, there are indole derivatives such as Bufo tryptamine and Bufo tenidine.

【药性与功效 / Chinese medicine properties】

味辛，性温，有毒，归心经。具有解毒、止痛、开窍醒神的功效。用于痈疽疔疮、咽喉肿痛、中暑神昏、痧胀腹痛吐泻。

Chán sū is pungent, warm and poisonous. It can enter the meridian of heart. It is used for carbuncle, sore throat, heat stroke, dizziness, and diarrhea.

【药理作用 / Pharmacological effects】

1. **强心**　表现为促进心肌收缩峰和舒张峰同时增大，在一定阈值内低浓度蟾酥使心肌收缩力增强，并使心肌细胞内 Na^+ 浓度增高，从而使 Ca^{2+} 通过 Na^+-Ca^{2+} 交换通道进入心肌细胞，继而使血压上升，这是蟾酥用以强心的基础。蟾酥强心成分中蟾毒配基作用较强，其次为蟾毒灵和华蟾毒灵。蟾酥还具有增加心肌供氧量等作用。

(1) Cardiotonic effects　The cardiotonic effect of toad venom is to promote the contraction and relaxation peak of the heart muscle at the same time. In a certain threshold, the low concentration of toad venom can increase the contractile force of the heart muscle, and increase the concentration of Na^+ in the heart muscle cells, so that Ca^{2+} can enter the heart muscle cells through the Na^+ - Ca^{2+} exchange channel, and then increase the blood pressure, which is the basis of toad venom medicine to strengthen the heart. Among the components of *Chán sū*, cinobufagin has a strong coordination effect, followed by bufalin and cinobufagin.

2. **调节血压**　不同剂量的蟾酥对血压具有双重调节作用，小剂量蟾酥可增强离体蟾蜍心脏的收缩力，大剂量可减慢麻醉猫、犬、兔、蛙的心率。蟾酥中的蟾毒配基能导致高血压，蟾酥的水溶性成分具有降血压的作用。

(2) Regulating blood pressure　Different dosages of *Chán sū* has dual regulating effect on blood pressure. Low dose of *Chán sū* can enhance the contractility of isolated toad heart, while large dose can slow the heartbeat of anesthetized cat, dog, rabbit and frog. Moreover, there is a substances called bufogenin in *Chán sū* promoting hypertension. Rather, the water-soluble components of *Chán sū* have the effect of lowering blood pressure.

3. **影响神经系统**　蟾酥能直接抑制神经纤维动作电位的形成和传导，产生神经阻滞的麻醉作用。其调节作用呈现先增强后抑制的趋势，在短时间内可以增强神经元兴奋性，长时间作用反而抑制神经元兴奋性。

(3) Effects on central nervous system　*Chán sū* directly inhibit the formation and conduction of nerve fiber action potential and produce the anesthetic effect of nerve block. It is showed that the regulation trend of *Chán sū* is first enhancement and then inhibition, which can enhance the excitability of neurons in a short time, but inhibit the excitability of neurons in a long time.

4. **镇痛与麻醉**　蟾酥具有良好的镇痛作用。蟾酥内含有的蟾毒配基类物质是发挥局部麻醉作用的主要活性成分。

(4) Analgesia and anaesthesia　*Chán sū* has analgesic effect. The main active components of local anesthesia are the lipotoad venom ligands contained in toad venom.

5. **抗肿瘤**　蟾酥提取物可抑制肿瘤细胞生长，具有诱导肿瘤细胞凋亡的作用。

(5) Anti-tumor　*Chán sū* is capable of inhibiting the growth of tumor cells and inducing apoptosis of tumor cells.

【不良反应 / Adverse effects】

蟾酥主要对心脏有毒性作用，中毒症状主要出现在用药后 30~60 分钟。

Chán sū is mainly toxic to the heart, and the toxic symptoms mainly occur 30-60 minutes after the application.

题库

医药大学堂
WWW.YIYAODXT.COM

（韩　岚　汪　宁）

第十九章 补益药
Chapter 19 Chinese tonics

学习目标 | Objectives

1. **掌握** 补益药的主要药理作用；人参、甘草、黄芪、当归、鹿茸、淫羊藿、熟地黄与功效相关的药理作用、作用机制及药效物质基础。

2. **了解** 何首乌、冬虫夏草、白术、白芍、党参、北沙参、麦冬、枸杞子的主要药理作用及药效物质基础；常用补益药的不良反应。

1. **Must know** The main pharmacological effects of tonics; the efficacy related pharmacological effects, mechanism, and material basis of *Rén shēn*, *Gān cǎo*, *Huáng qí*, *Dāng guī*, *Lù róng*, *Yín yáng huò*, and *Shú dì huáng*.

2. **Desirable to know** Pharmacological effects and material basis of *Hé shǒu wū*, *Dōng chóng xià cǎo*, *Bái zhú*, *Bái sháo*, *Dǎng shēn*, *Běi shā shēn*, *Mài dōng*, and *Gǒu qǐ zǐ*; the adverse effects of commonly used tonics.

第一节 概述
Section 1 Overview

凡以补虚扶弱、纠正人体气血阴阳虚衰为主要功效，临床用于治疗虚证的药物，称为补益药。气、血、阴、阳是中医对人体物质组成和功能的高度概括，当机体物质不足或功能低下时则产生虚证。补益药根据主要功效的不同，可分为补气药、补血药、补阴药、补阳药四类，分别主治气虚证、血虚证、阴虚证和阳虚证。

Tonics refer to the single herbs that can relieve deficiency and improve the visceral function, supplement Qi, blood, Yin and Yang, and mainly treat deficiency syndrome. Qi, blood, Yin and Yang are related to essential substances and body functions in Chinese medicine theory. According to their efficacy, the tonics can be divided into four categories, including Qi tonics, blood tonics, Yin tonics and Yang tonics, indicated for Qi deficiency syndrome, blood deficiency syndrome, Yin deficiency syndrome and Yang deficiency syndrome, respectively.

气虚证是指人体的元气耗损，功能失调，脏腑功能减退，抗病能力下降的病理变化，主要表现为脾气虚和肺气虚。现代研究认为，脾气虚证是以消化系统分泌、吸收和运动功能障碍为主的全身性适应调节和营养代谢失调的一种疾病状态，与西医学中功能性消化不良、慢性胃炎、溃疡病及慢性腹泻等诸多消化系统慢性疾病相似。肺气虚证则表现为肺换气功能障碍、全身氧代谢障碍、免疫功能低下，出现咳、痰、喘及呼吸道炎症反应。补气药主要用于治疗气虚证，其最主要的功效是益气健脾，并兼具其他不同功效。常用补气药有人参、党参、黄芪、白术、甘草等。

Qi deficiency syndrome refers to the pathological changes of the loss of original Qi, disorders of Zangfu function (namely internal organ function), and decrease of body defense function against diseases. Qi deficiency mainly includes spleen Qi deficiency and lung Qi deficiency. The present research suggests that the spleen Qi deficiency is a disease state with systemic adaptation and nutritional metabolism disorders mainly due to digestive system secretion, absorption and motor dysfunction, which are similar with various chronic disease of digestive systems, such as functional dyspepsia, chronic gastritis, ulcer disease, diarrhea. Lung Qi deficiency syndrome is manifested as pulmonary ventilation dysfunction, systemic oxygen metabolism disorders, immunocompromised function, cough, sputum, asthma, and respiratory inflammation. The main action of Qi tonics is tonifying Qi and invigorating the spleen. Commonly used Qi tonifying medicines include *Rén shēn*, *Dǎng shēn*, *Huáng qí*, *Bái zhú*, *Gān cǎo*, etc.

血虚证是由于血液不足或血液的濡养功能减退而出现的病理状态，可见面色萎黄、嘴唇及指甲苍白、头晕目眩、心悸、神疲乏力、手足麻木、屈伸不利以及月经量少色淡、经期延后甚至闭经等症状。血虚证涵盖了西医学多种疾病如贫血、心血管疾病、神经衰弱以及妇科疾病。常用补血药有当归、熟地黄、白芍、阿胶、龙眼肉等。

Blood deficiency syndrome is a pathological condition due to the deficiency of blood or the decrease of the nourishing function of blood. The major symptoms include pale complexion, pale lips and nails, dizziness, palpitation, fatigue, limb numbness, poor flexion and extension, and less menstruation, color, delayed menstruation and even amenorrhea. Blood deficiency syndrome covers a variety of diseases such as anemia, cardiovascular disease, neurasthenia and gynecological diseases. Commonly used blood tonics include *Dāng guī*, *Shú dì huáng*, *Bái sháo*, *Lóng yǎn ròu*, etc.

阴虚证是指机体精、血、津液等物质亏耗，阴气不足，不能制阳，阳气相对亢盛，出现阴虚内热、阴虚火旺和阴虚阳亢的各种证候。阴虚可见于五脏六腑，常见肺阴虚、胃阴虚、肝阴虚和肾阴虚，但一般以肾阴亏虚为主，常见五心烦热、骨蒸潮热、消瘦、盗汗、咽干口燥、腰膝酸软、头晕耳鸣、记忆力减退、性欲减退、遗精、早泄等症状。补阴药具有滋养阴液、生津润燥等功效，主要治疗阴虚证。常用补阴药有沙参、麦冬、天冬、枸杞子等。

Yin deficiency syndrome refers to the deficiency of essence, blood, body fluid and other substances in the body. Yin deficiency occurs in all organs, commonly observed as lung Yin deficiency, stomach Yin deficiency, liver Yin deficiency and kidney Yin deficiency, and it is mainly characterized by kidney Yin deficiency. The common symptoms of kidney Yin deficiency include vexing heat in the chest, palms and soles, osteopyrexia and fever, weight loss, night sweating, dry throat and tongue, sore waist and knees, dizziness and tinnitus, memory loss, loss of libido, spermatorrhea, premature ejaculation, etc. The drug or prescription that has the effects of nourishing Yin fluid, invigorating body and moistening dryness, and treating Yin deficiency syndrome called Yin tonics. Commonly used Yin tonics include *Shā shēn*, *Mài dōng*, *Tiān dōng*, etc.

阳虚证是指机体阳气虚损，功能减退或衰弱，热量不足之证。肾阳虚可见畏寒肢冷、腰膝酸软或冷痛、阳痿早泄、宫冷不孕、白带清稀、夜尿增多及脉沉苔白等。肾阳虚诸证与西医学中性功能障碍、遗精阳痿、慢性支气管哮喘、风湿性关节炎等病症相似。补阳药能补人体之阳气，主要用于治疗阳虚证。常用补阳药有鹿茸、淫羊藿、补骨脂、菟丝子、巴戟天等。

Yang deficiency refers to Yang Qi deficiency, hypofunction and heat deficiency of the body. As kidney Yang is the primordial Yang of the body, kidney Yang deficiency is dominant in Yang deficiency. Kidney Yang deficiency commonly manifested as aversion to cold, sore or cold pain in waist and knees, impotence, premature ejaculation, uterine cold infertility, leucorrhea, increased nocturia, deep pulse and white tongue coating. The syndrome of kidney Yang deficiency is similar to various diseases such as sexual dysfunction, spermatorrhea impotence, chronic bronchial asthma, rheumatoid arthritis and etc. Yang tonics can be used to tonify the Yang Qi of the body and indicated for Yang deficiency syndrome. Commonly used Yang tonics include *Lù róng*, *Yín yáng huò*, *Bǔ gǔ zhǐ*, *Tù sī zǐ*, *Bā jǐ tiān*, etc.

补虚药的主要药理作用如下。

The pharmacological effects of tonic medicines are as following.

1. 调节机体免疫功能 中医辨证为虚证患者，常有免疫功能低下，补虚药通过提高人体正气，恢复免疫功能，从而抵抗外邪，促使疾病恢复。补虚药对免疫系统的调节作用主要包括以下几方面。

(1) Regulating immune system function Hypoimmunity is common in patients with weakness syndrome. The tonics is indicated for improving immune function and can be used to treat hypoimmunity, cancer and infectious diseases. Some tonics exerts bidirectional immunologic regulation activity on cellular immunity, humoral immunity and immune function of reticuloendothelial system, which depend on the status of the body. The mechanisms of tonics on the immune system are follows.

（1）提高非特异性免疫功能 ①增加胸腺、胰腺等免疫器官的重量。②增强巨噬细胞和中性粒细胞的吞噬作用。如人参、党参、当归、枸杞子等可以增强巨噬细胞的吞噬作用。③促进自然杀伤细胞（NK 细胞）和淋巴因子激活的杀伤细胞（LAK 细胞）的功能。④增加放疗和化疗引起的白细胞减少。如人参、黄芪、熟地黄和枸杞子可以增加白细胞减少症患者外周血白细胞的数量。

1) Regulating non-specific immunity function ①Increasing the weight of immune organs such as thymus and pancreas. ②Enhancing the phagocytosis of macrophages and neutrophils. Tonics such as *Rén shēn*, *Dǎng shēn*, *Dāng guī*, and *Gǒu qǐ zǐ* could enhance the phagocytosis of macrophage. ③Promoting the functions of natural killer cells and lymphokine-activated killer cells. ④Increasing peripheral white blood cell count against leukopenia caused by radiotherapy and chemotherapy. *Rén shēn*, *Huáng qí*, *Shú dì huáng* and *Gǒu qǐ zǐ* could increase the number of peripheral blood leucocytes in patients with leukopenia reduction sickness.

（2）提高细胞免疫功能 ①通过增加外周血 T 淋巴细胞计数来增强 T 淋巴细胞的功能，并促进 T 淋巴细胞的转化和增殖。例如，淫羊藿可增加外周血 T 淋巴细胞，黄芪和枸杞子可以促进红细胞受体 C_3b（RBC-C_3b）玫瑰花环和红细胞免疫复合物玫瑰花环的形成。②增强 B 淋巴细胞的增殖反应，刺激抗体的产生，刺激体内各种免疫活性细胞的成熟、分化和繁殖，并诱导细胞因子的产生和细胞因子受体的表达。

2) Regulating cellular immunity ①Enhancing the function of T cells by increasing peripheral blood T lymphocyte count, and promoting T lymphocyte transformation and proliferation. *Yín yáng huò* could increase T cells in peripheral blood. *Huáng qí* and *Gǒu qǐ zǐ* could raise the formation of erythrocyte acceptor C_3b (RBC-C_3b) rosette and erythrocyte immune complexes rosette. ②Enhancing B lymphocyte proliferation response and stimulating the production of antibody, stimulating the maturation, differentiation and reproduction of various immune active cells in the body, and inducing the production of cytokines and the expression of cytokine receptors.

（3）调节体液免疫功能 ①促进抗体形成。如人参、冬虫夏草、肉苁蓉等均能促进免疫球蛋白 G（IgG）和 IgA 及 IgM 的产生。②增加脾脏抗体形成细胞的数量。

3) Regulating humoral immunity ①Tonics could promote the formation of antibody. *Rén shēn*,

Dōng chóng xià cǎo and *Ròu cóng róng* could promote the production of immunoglobulin G (IgG)、IgA and Ig M. ②Tonics could increase the number of spleen antibody forming cells.

2. 调节内分泌系统功能 多数补虚药可兴奋下丘脑、垂体，促进肾上腺皮质激素、性激素、甲状腺激素的释放。也有少数药具有激素样作用，在调节机体物质代谢和抗炎、抗应激作用中起重要作用。

(2) Regulating the endocrine system Most tonics could stimulate hypothalamus and pituitary, and then promote the release of adrenocortical hormone, sex hormone and thyroid hormone. Some tonics also have hormone-like effects, and play an important role in regulating material metabolism, anti-inflammation and anti-stress process.

（1）对下丘脑–垂体–肾上腺皮质轴功能的影响 肾阳虚患者多数伴有下丘脑–垂体–肾上腺皮质轴功能减退，补气药人参、黄芪、甘草，补血药熟地黄、当归、何首乌，补阴药玄参、生地黄、知母，补阳药巴戟天、淫羊藿、鹿茸等均可促进肾上腺皮质激素的合成和释放。

1) Enhancing the function of hypothalamus-pituitary-adrenocortical axis Most patients with kidney Yang deficiency experience degradation of hypothalamic-pituitary-adrenocortical axis function. The Qi tonifying drugs (e. g., *Rén shēn*, *Huáng qí*, *Gān cǎo*), blood tonifying drugs (e. g., *Shú dì huáng*, *Dāng guī*, *Hé shǒu wū*), Yin tonifying drugs (e. g., *Xuán shēn*, *Shēng dì huáng*, *Zhī mǔ*), and Yang tonifying drugs (e. g., *Bā jǐ tiān*, *Yín yáng huò* and *Lù róng*) could promote the synthesis and release of adrenocortical hormone.

（2）对下丘脑–垂体–性腺轴功能的影响 临床阳虚患者常有性功能低下、性激素水平降低，鹿茸、淫羊藿、人参等均有兴奋下丘脑–垂体–性腺轴功能的作用。少数补虚药具有性激素样作用，如淫羊藿流浸膏具有雄激素样作用，鹿茸中的雌二醇具有雌激素样作用。

2) Enhancing the function of hypothalamus-pituitary-gonadal axis The patients with clinical Yang deficiency often have low sexual function and the level of sex hormone is low. The tonics, such as *Lù róng*, *Yín yáng huò* and *Rén shēn* could enhance the function of hypothalamus-pituitary-gonadal axis. Some tonics also manifest sex hormone-like effect, for example, *Yín yáng huò* fluid extract has androgen-like effect, and estradiol in *Lù róng* has estrogenic-like effect.

（3）对下丘脑–垂体–甲状腺轴功能的影响 人参具有调节下丘脑–垂体–甲状腺轴功能的作用，能防治甲状腺素引起的小鼠"甲亢"和6–甲硫氧嘧啶导致的"甲减"。

3) Enhancing the function of hypothalamus-pituitary-thyroid axis *Rén shēn* could regulate the thyroid axis function, and prevent hypothyroidism caused by 6-methylthiouracil in mice.

3. 影响物质代谢 补虚药与物质代谢及能量代谢关系密切。一方面，补虚药含有大量营养物质，可补充营养、纠正营养缺失；另一方面，补虚药可影响物质代谢过程。

(3) Effects on metabolism of substances The tonics are closely related to material metabolism and energy metabolism. On the one hand, the tonics contain a variety of beneficial ingredients to supply nutrition and resolve the deficiency syndrome. On the other hand, tonics can affect the process of substance metabolism.

（1）对核酸和蛋白质代谢的影响 人参中的蛋白质合成促进因子及人参皂苷对生发活动旺盛的组织（如睾丸、骨髓等）的 DNA 和 RNA 及蛋白质的生物合成有促进作用；黄芪能促进血清和肝脏蛋白质的更新。

1) Effects on nucleic acid and protein metabolism The protein synthesis inducer and ginsenosides in *Rén shēn* could promote the biosynthesis of DNA, RNA, and proteins in tissues testes, bone marrow, and etc. *Huáng qí* could promote the renewal of serum and liver proteins.

（2）对糖代谢的影响　人参、地黄、淫羊藿等具有调节血糖作用；枸杞子可降糖，对抗糖尿病大鼠视网膜组织氧化损伤。某些补虚药具有双向调节血糖的作用，如黄芪多糖能明显对抗肾上腺素引起的小鼠血糖升高和苯乙双胍致小鼠实验性低血糖；人参对四氧嘧啶或链脲佐菌素引起的小鼠高血糖有明显的降低作用，对注射胰岛素而降低的血糖又有回升作用。

2) Effects on glucose metabolism　Some tonics, such as *Rén shēn*, *Dì huáng* and *Yín yáng huò* could reduce the blood sugar level. *Gǒu qǐ zǐ* could reduce the blood sugar level and antagonize the oxidative damage of retinal tissue in diabetic rats. Some tonics showed bidirectional effect on glucose metabolism regulation, such as *Rén shēn* and *Huáng qí*.

（3）对脂质代谢的影响　很多补虚药可改善脂质代谢，如人参、当归、何首乌、枸杞子可降低高脂血症家兔血清胆固醇和甘油三酯的含量，并能减少脂质在主动脉壁的沉着。

3) Effects on lipid metabolism　Many tonics could improve lipid metabolism, such as *Rén shēn*, *Dāng guī*, *Hé shǒu wū*, *Gǒu qǐ zǐ* could reduce the contents of serum cholesterol and triglycerides in hyperlipidemic rabbits, and reduce the deposition of lipids in the aortic wall.

4. 调节中枢神经系统功能　补虚药对中枢神经系统功能的影响，主要表现在对于学习记忆能力的改善作用，如人参、黄芪、党参、何首乌、枸杞子等可显著提高正常小鼠的学习记忆能力，改善学习记忆过程的三个阶段，即记忆获得、记忆巩固和记忆再现。其作用的主要环节包括调节大脑皮质的兴奋与抑制过程；调节神经递质合成、贮存、释放；提高脑组织抗氧化酶活性，抗氧自由基损伤；改善大脑的血氧和能量供应；增加脑内蛋白质合成，促进大脑发育。

(4) Improving nervous function　The effects of tonics on the function of the central nervous system mainly manifested as the regulation of learning and memory activities. Tonics including *Rén shēn*, *Huáng qí*, *Dǎng shēn*, *Hé shǒu wū*, and *Gǒu qǐ zǐ* could increase the learning and memory activities of normal mice and improve the three phrases of improving learning and memory including memory acquisition, memory consolidation and memory reproduction. The potential mechanisms include: regulating the process of excitation and inhibition of the cerebral cortex; regulating the synthesis, storage, and release of neurotransmitters; increasing the antioxidant enzyme activity of the brain tissue, and protecting against free radical damage; improving blood oxygen and energy supply to the brain; increasing protein synthesis in the brain, and promoting the brain development.

5. 影响心血管系统功能　补虚药对心血管功能的影响比较广泛而且复杂，主要包括以下几方面。①正性肌力：如人参、党参、黄芪、生脉散、参附汤等均具有强心、升压、抗休克的作用。②调节血压：如人参及生脉散均显示双向调节血压作用，升压或降压作用与剂量及机体状态有关，黄芪、刺五加、淫羊藿、当归、杜仲等有扩张血管和降压的作用。③抗心肌缺血：如人参、党参、当归、淫羊藿、补骨脂、麦冬、女贞子等能扩张冠脉、增加冠脉血流量，改善心肌血氧供应，提高心肌抗缺氧能力，缩小心肌梗死面积。④抗心律失常：如人参可降低心肌细胞自律性，改善传导速度，消除折返，延长动作电位时程和有效不应期，改善心脏泵血功能，促进窦性心律恢复。

(5) Effects on cardiovascular system　The effects of tonics on cardiovascular function are diverse and complex, including the followings. ①Positive inotropic effect: *Rén shēn*, *Dǎng shēn* and *Huáng qí* could improve heart function, boost blood pressure in patients with circulatory failure and relieve shock symptoms. ②Regulation of blood pressure: *Rén shēn* could regulate blood pressure bidirectionally. *Huáng qí*, *Yín Yáng Huò*, *Dāng guī* could reduce blood pressure and dilate blood vessel. ③Anti-myocardial

ischemic effect: *Rén shēn*, *Dǎng shēn*, *Dāng guī*, *Yín yáng huò*, *Mài Dōng*, *Nǚ zhēn zǐ* manifested anti-myocardial ischemic effect by dilating coronary arteries, increasing coronary blood flow and improving myocardial oxygen supply, as well as increasing myocardial anti-hypoxia capacity, and reducing the area of myocardial infarction. ④Anti-arrhythmic effect: *Rén shēn* has anti- arrhythmic actions.

6. **影响血液系统功能**　补血药、补气药促进造血作用明显，如人参、党参、黄芪、当归等对实验性急性失血性贫血、缺铁性贫血、溶血性贫血等有一定的提升造血功能作用，还能有效地修复化学药品及射线对造血组织的损伤，促进骨髓造血干、祖细胞增殖，升高骨髓造血祖细胞集落形成单位数量。

(6) Effects on hematopoietic system　Blood tonics and Qi tonics exhibit remarkable ability to improve the hematopoietic function. The tonics such as *Rén shēn*, *Dǎng shēn*, *Huáng qí* and *Dāng guī* could improve hemopoietic function of experimental acute hemorrhagic anemia, iron deficiency anemia and hemolytic anemia, it can also effectively repair the damage of chemicals and radiation on hematopoietic tissue, promote the proliferation of bone marrow hematopoietic stem cells, and increase the number of colony forming units of bone marrow hematopoietic progenitor cells.

7. **影响消化系统功能**　多数补气药可调节胃肠运动。如人参、党参、黄芪和当归等均能促进小肠吸收功能，调节胃肠平滑肌运动，并有抗溃疡、保护胃黏膜的作用。

(7) Digestive system　Most Qi tonics an regulate gastrointestinal motility. For example, *Rén shēn*, *Dǎng shēn*, *Huáng qí*, and *Dāng guī* can promote the absorption function of the small intestine, regulate the movement of gastrointestinal smooth muscle, and have the effect of anti-ulcer and protecting gastric mucosa.

8. **抗肿瘤**　人参、刺五加、黄芪、甘草、大枣、白术、党参、当归、枸杞子、补骨脂、冬虫夏草、鹿茸、天冬、女贞子和龟甲等对实验性动物肿瘤有不同程度的抑制作用。

(8) Anti-tumor　The tonics such as *Rén shēn*, *Cì wǔ jiā*, *Huáng qí*, *Gān cǎo*, *Dà zǎo*, *Bái zhú*, *Dǎng shēn*, *Dāng guī*, *Gǒu qǐ zǐ*, *Bǔ gǔ zhǐ*, *Dōng chóng xià cǎo*, *Lù róng*, *Tiān dōng*, *Nǚ zhēn zǐ*, and *Guī jiǎ* could inhibit the tumor growth in animal models.

9. **延缓衰老**　自由基参与许多疾病的病理生理过程，自由基介导的自由基连锁反应具有病理损害作用。许多补虚药都有延缓衰老的作用，抗氧化损伤是其重要途径之一。例如，人参和黄芪可以清除自由基，提高超氧化物歧化酶（SOD）的活性；鹿茸能显著降低衰老小脑和肝组织中的丙二醛（MDA）含量。

(9) Anti-aging　Free radicals participate in the pathophysiology of various of diseases, and free radical-mediated free radical chain reactions can lead to pathological damage. The antioxidant damage activity was the potential mechanism for anti-aging action of many tonics. For example, *Rén shēn* and *Huáng qí* could scavenge free radicals and increase the activity of superoxide dismutase (SOD). *Lù róng* could significantly reduce the malondialdehyde (MDA) content in the brain and liver tissues of aging mice.

常用补益药的主要药理作用见表 19-1。

The main pharmacological effects of commonly used tonic medicines are summarized in Table 19-1.

表 19-1 常用补益药的主要药理作用

类别	药物	增强非特异性免疫	增强细胞免疫	增强体液免疫	增强下丘脑-垂体-肾上腺轴	增强下丘脑-垂体-性腺轴	抗心肌缺血	扩张血管	调节血压	强心	改善学习记忆	延缓衰老	降血脂	降血糖	促进蛋白质合成	改善消化功能	抗肿瘤	促进造血功能	其他药理作用
补气药	人参	+	+	+	+	+	+	+	+	+	+	+	+	+	+	+	+	+	抗应激、抗心律失常、抗氧化
	党参	-	+	+	+	-	+	+	+	+	+	+	+	+	+	+	-	+	抗应激、镇静、催眠、保肝
	黄芪	+	+	+	+	+	+	+	+	+	+	+	+	+	+	+	+	+	保肝、抗氧化、利尿、抗病毒、抗应激
	甘草	+	+	-	+	-	-	+	+	-	+	+	-	+	+	+	-	+	解毒、祛痰镇咳、抗心律失常、抗炎、抗病原微生物
	白术	+	+	+	-	-	-	+	-	-	+	+	-	+	-	+	-	-	抗应激、抗氧化
补血药	当归	+	+	+	+	+	+	+	+	-	+	+	+	-	-	+	+	+	抗氧化、抗子宫收缩
	白芍	+	+	+	-	-	-	+	-	+	+	-	-	-	+	-	-	+	调节子宫平滑肌、抗炎、镇痛
	何首乌	+	+	+	-	-	-	-	-	-	+	+	+	-	-	-	-	+	保肝、镇静、镇痛
	熟地黄	+	+	+	+	-	-	-	-	-	+	+	-	+	+	-	+	+	抗炎、镇痛、润肠通便、抗骨质疏松
补阳药	鹿茸	+	+	+	+	+	-	-	-	+	+	+	-	-	-	+	-	+	抗甲状腺功能、抗氧化
	淫羊藿	+	+	+	+	+	+	+	+	+	+	+	-	-	-	-	+	-	促进骨生长、抗炎、抗氧化
	冬虫夏草	+	+	+	+	+	+	+	+	+	+	+	+	+	+	-	+	-	促进骨生长、抗炎、抗氧化
补阴药	枸杞子	+	+	+	-	-	-	-	-	-	+	+	+	+	+	+	+	-	平喘、肾保护、保肝
	北沙参	+	+	+	-	-	-	-	-	+	+	+	+	-	-	-	+	-	保肝、抗疲劳、抗突变、抗氧化
	麦冬	+	-	-	-	-	+	+	-	+	-	+	-	+	-	-	-	-	镇咳平喘、抗炎、保肺、纤维化、镇静、抗心律失常

注："+"表示有明确作用；"-"表示无作用，或未查阅到相关研究文献

第二节　常用药物
Section 2　Commonly used medicines

PPT

微课

| 人参 | *Rén shēn (Radix Ginseng)* |

【来源 / Origin】

本品为五加科植物人参（*Pannax ginseng* C. A. Mey.）的干燥根。主产于吉林、黑龙江、辽宁省。多于秋季采挖，洗净经晒干或烘干，切片或粉碎用。

Rén shēn is the dried root of *Pannax ginseng* C. A. Mey., family of Araliaceae. It is widely cultivated in Jinlin province, Heilongjiang province and Liaoning province and harvested in Autumn. Slices or crush of the dried foot is used for Chinese medicinal preparation after washing and drying in the sun.

【化学成分 / Chemical ingredients】

主要含有多种皂苷类成分，根据其苷元结构可分成人参二醇类、人参三醇类和齐墩果酸类皂苷。人参二醇类主要有 Ra_{1-3}、Rb_{1-3}、Rc、Rd、Rg_3 等；人参三醇类主要有 Re、Rf、Rg_1、Rg_2、Rh_1 等；齐墩果酸类有 Ro。此外，尚含有人参多糖、寡糖、单糖、多肽类化合物、氨基酸、蛋白质、酶、有机酸、生物碱、挥发油、微量元素等。

Rén shēn mainly contains a variety of ginsenosides, which can be divided into panaxadiol, panaxatriol and oleanolic acid according to their aglycone structure. Panaxadiols mainly include Ra_{1-3}, Rb_{1-3}, Rc, Rd, Rg_3, etc. Panaxatriols mainly include Re, Rf, Rg_1, Rg_2, Rh_1, etc. Oleanolic acids include Ro. Furthermore, *Rén shēn* also contains polysaccharides, monosaccharides, ologosaccharides, polypeptide, amino acids, proteins, enzymes, organic acids, alkaloids, volatile oil, trace elements, etc.

【药性与功效 / Chinese medicine properties】

味甘、微苦，性微温，归肺、脾、心经。具有大补元气、补脾益肺、生津和安神益智等功效。主治元气虚极欲脱、脉微欲绝、脾虚食少便溏、肺虚咳喘、心悸怔忡、失眠多梦、气津两伤、口渴、内热消渴、肾虚阳痿、久病虚羸等证。

In Chinese medicine theory, *Rén shēn* has the nature of sweet, slightly bitter and warm. It can enter the meridians of lung, spleen and heart. *Rén shēn* can powerfully tonify primordial Qi, invigorate spleen and benefit lung, engender fluid, tranquilize mind and improve intelligence. Clinically, it can be used for collapse of primordial Qi, weak pulse, poor appetite and loose stool due to spleen deficiency, cough and asthma due to lung deficiency, palpitation, insomnia and excessive dreaming during sleep, consumptive thirst, kidney deficiency and impotence, and body deficiency due to long-term chronic diseases.

【药理作用 / Pharmacological effects】

1. 对中枢神经系统的影响

(1) Effects on central nervous system function

（1）抗脑缺血损伤　人参皂苷能减少大鼠脑缺血或脑缺血再灌注引起脑梗死面积，减轻神经症状评分，抑制神经细胞凋亡，促进星形胶质细胞增殖。人参皂苷抗脑缺血损伤的作用机制如下。①抗氧化作用。②抗炎。③抑制兴奋性氨基酸、减轻细胞内钙超载。④促进神经干细胞（NSCs）的增殖和分化。⑤改善脑组织能量代谢。

1) Anti-cerebral ischemia injury　*Rén shēn* has the effect of anti-cerebral ischemia injury.

Ginsenosides can alleviate the infarct area of brain tissue, decrease neurological scores, inhibit neuron apoptosis, and promote the profiliation of astrocytes in rates with cerebral ischemia or cerebral ischemia and reperfusion. The mechanisms of ginsenosides on anti-cerebral ischemia injury are mainly as follows. ①Anti-oxidation. ②Anti-inflammation. ③Inhibiting the release of excitatory amino acids and reducing intracelluar Ca^{2+} overload. ④Promoting the proliferation and differentiation of neural stem cells (NSCs). ⑤Improving the energy metabolism of brain tissue.

（2）改善学习记忆　人参 20% 醇提物对氢溴酸樟柳碱所引起的学习记忆获得障碍、蛋白质合成抑制剂环己酰亚胺诱导的记忆巩固障碍以及 40% 乙醇诱导的记忆再现障碍均有改善作用。人参皂苷被认为是其改善学习记忆的活性成分。研究发现，人参皂苷（Rg₁ 和 Rb₁ 等）能改善脑缺血、应激及阿尔茨海默病引起的认知障碍。人参改善学习记忆的作用机制如下。①促进脑内物质代谢，增加蛋白质、核酸等的合成。②提高脑内乙酰胆碱水平和单胺类神经递质的活性。③促进神经细胞发育和提高突触可塑性。④减少神经细胞凋亡和坏死。⑤增加脑血流量，改善脑能量代谢。⑥促进神经干细胞的增殖和迁移。

2) Learning and memory improvement　*Rén shēn* can improve the learning and memory function. 20% alcohol extract of *Rén shēn* improve memory acquisition disorder caused by anisodine hydrobromide and memory consolidation disorder induced by cycloheximide, and antagonize the deficits of memory retrieval induced by 40% ethanol. Ginsenosides are suggested to be the active ingredients for the learning and memory improvement. Ginsenoside (Rg_1, Rb_1, etc.) can improve learning and memory impairment induced by multi-factor, such as cerebral ischemia, stress, and Alzheimer's disease. The main mechanisms are related with the following actions. ①Promoting the metabolism of substances in the brain, increasing the synthesis of protein and nucleic acid. ②Enhancing the level of acetylcholine (ACh) and monoamine neurotransmitters(DA, NA) in the brain. ③Promoting the development of nerve cells and the plasticity of synapses. ④Reducing the apoptosis and necrosis of nerve cells. ⑤Increasing the cerebral blood flow, improving the metabolism of brain energy. ⑥Promote the proliferation and migration of NSCs.

（3）调节中枢神经系统功能　人参通过对大脑皮质的兴奋和抑制作用的调节，改善神经活动过程，提高大脑的工作效率。人参对中枢有兴奋和抑制作用与其成分和剂量有关。一般小剂量表现为兴奋作用，大剂量表现为抑制作用；人参皂苷 Rg 类有兴奋作用，Rb 类有抑制作用。

3) Regulating central nervous system function　*Rén shēn* can improve the process of nerve activity and the working efficiency of brain by regulating the excitation and inhibition of cerebral cortex. The excitatory and inhibitory effects of *Rén shēn* on the central nervous system are related to its composition, dosage and the status of the body. In general, the small dosage of *Rén shēn* has the excitatory effects, while the large dosage of *Rén shēn* shows the inhibitory effects; Ginsenoside Rg has excitatory effects while ginsenoside Rb has inhibitory effects.

2. 对机体免疫功能的影响

(2) Effects on immunological function

（1）提高非特异性免疫功能　人参超微粉、人参提取物、人参皂苷、人参多糖能提高正常小鼠的胸腺指数，增强 NK 细胞活性，提高小鼠碳粒廓清速率。人参超微粉可增加环磷酰胺诱导的免疫低下小鼠的白细胞数目和脾匀浆乳酸脱氢酶（LDH）、酸性磷酸酶（ACP）活性。人参总皂苷、人参多糖可提高巨噬细胞、单核巨噬细胞系统的吞噬功能。

1) Enhancing non-specific immunity　Superfine powder and extract of *Rén shēn*, ginsenosides and polysaccharides in *Rén shēn* can increase the thymus index and the activity of NK cell, enhance the carbon clearance rate of normal mice. *Rén shēn* superfine powder can increase the number of leukocytes

and the activity of LDH and acid phosphatase(ACP) in spleen of immunocompromised mice induced by cyclophosphamide. Ginsenosides and polysaccharides can increase the phagocytic function of macrophages and reticuloendothelial system.

（2）提高特异性免疫功能　人参能增强机体的细胞免疫。体内外试验显示，人参皂苷、人参多糖灌胃可明显增强刀豆素 A（Con A）和脂多糖（LPS）刺激小鼠淋巴细胞的转化。人参也能增强体液免疫。人参超微粉可增加磷酰胺诱导的免疫低下的血清中 IL-2、IL-4、IgG、IgM 水平。人参多糖、人参皂苷灌胃能增加正常小鼠血清溶血素和补体水平。

2) Enhancing specific immunity　Rén shēn can enhance the cellular immunity. Ginsenosides, polysaccharides of Rén shēn administered orally can significantly enhance the lymphocyte transformation stimulated by concanavalin A (Con A) and lipopolysaccharide (LPS) in vivo and in vitro. Rén shēn can also enhance the humoral immunity. Rén shēn superfine powder can increase the levels of IL-2, IL-4, IgG and IgM in serum of immunocompromised rats induced by cyclophosphoramide. Ginsenosides and polysaccharides of Rén shēn administered orally can also increase the serum hemolysin and complement level in normal mice.

3. 对内分泌系统的影响

(3) Effects on endocrine system function

（1）增强下丘脑-垂体-肾上腺功能　人参皂苷可增加正常和切除一侧肾上腺大鼠的肾上腺重量，降低肾上腺内维生素 C 含量和胆固醇含量，增加尿中 17- 羟皮质类固醇含量，增加血浆中皮质类固醇激素水平，提示人参能促进肾上腺皮质激素的合成与释放。该作用可能与其促进垂体前叶分泌促肾上腺皮质激素（ACTH）有关。

1) Enhancing hypothalamus-pituitary-adrenal function　Rén shēn can increase the weight of adrenal gland, decrease the contents of vitamin C and cholesterol in adrenal gland, increase the content of 17 hydroxy corticosteroids in urine, and increase the level of corticosteroids in plasma, suggesting that ginsenosides can promote the synthesis and release of corticosteroids, which may be related to the ACTH secretion in anterior pituitary.

（2）增强下丘脑-垂体-性腺功能　人参能促进垂体分泌促性腺激素，加快大鼠、小鼠性成熟。给予出生后 6~7 周的雌性小鼠人参乙醇提取物，可使动情间期缩短，动情期延长，并且子宫和卵巢重量增加，黄体酮分泌增加。人参也可使家兔附睾中精子数增多，提高精子活动能力，延长精子体外生存时间。

2) Enhancing hypothalamus-pituitary-sexual gland function　Rén shēn can increase the gonad function. Rén shēn can promote the secretion of gonadotropin in the pituitary and accelerate the sexual maturity of rats and mice. Ethanol extract of Rén shēn was administered orally to female mice 6-7 weeks after birth, which can shorten the diestrus, prolong the estrus, increase the weight of uterus and ovary, and promote the secretion of lutein hormone. Rén shēn also increase the number of sperm in rabbit epididymis, improve sperm motility and prolong the survival time of sperm in vitro.

4. 对心血管系统的影响

(4) Effects on cardivascular system function

（1）改善心肌缺血　人参制剂及人参皂苷等对垂体后叶素、异丙肾上腺素引起的心肌缺血有改善作用。Rb₁、Rg₁、Rh₃、Re 等均可减轻心肌缺血再灌注损伤后的心肌组织梗死面积、心肌超微结构损伤。人参皂苷改善心肌缺血及缺血再灌注损伤的机制主要如下。①改善能量代谢过程、促进三磷酸腺苷和磷酸肌酸等能量合成。②抗氧化，减轻心肌细胞膜脂质过氧化。③减轻心肌细胞内钙超负荷、抑制心肌细胞凋亡。④促进冠状动脉侧支血管生成。⑤扩张血管，增加血液流通，减轻或逆转心室重构等。

1) Anti-myocardial ischemia   *Rén shēn* preparation and ginsenosides can improve myocardial ischemia induced by pituitrin and isoproterenol. Rb_1, Rg_1, Rh_3 and Re can attenuate infarction area and ultrastructural damage of myocardium after myocardial ischemia and reperfusion. The mechanisms of ginsenosides improving myocardial ischemia and reperfusion injury are mainly as follows. ①Improving energy metabolism process and promoting energy synthesis (ATP and creatine phosphate). ②Antioxidation can reduce lipid peroxidation of myocardial cell membrane. ③Reducing calcium overload in myocardial cells and inhibiting apoptosis of myocardial cells. ④Promoting collateral circulation of coronary arteries. ⑤Dilating blood vessels, increasing blood flow, alleviating or reversing ventricular remodeling.

（2）扩张血管，调节血压   人参能扩张冠状血管、脑血管、椎动脉、肺动脉，增加相关器官的血流量。扩张血管的主要成分是人参皂苷 Re、Rg_1、Rb_1 等。人参皂苷具有升压和降压的双向调节作用，与机体的功能状态和使用剂量等因素有关。小剂量可使麻醉动物血压升高，大剂量使血压降低。人参皂苷可能通过调节内皮细胞一氧化氮合酶（NOS）表达，诱导 NO 产生，阻滞钙离子通道，松弛血管平滑肌，产生扩张血管、降低血压的作用。

2) Dilating vessels and regulating blood pressure   *Rén shēn* can dilate coronary, cerebrovascular, vertebral and pulmonary arteries, which can increase blood flow to these organs. The main components of vasodilation are ginsenoside Re, Rg_1, Rb_1, etc. Ginsenosides have the two-directional regulation, raising blood pressure or reducing blood pressure, which is related to the functional status of the body and the dosage being used. Small doses of *Rén shēn* raise blood pressure in anesthetized animals while large doses of *Rén shēn* decrease it. The effect of ginsenosides on dilating blood vessels and reducing blood pressure maybe related with the expression of nitric oxide synthase in endothelial cells, inducing the production of NO, blocking the calcium channel, relaxing vascular smooth muscle.

（3）抗心律失常   人参对缺血性心律失常、缺血再灌注心律失常、期前收缩、心动过速、心室颤动、心室扑动与室性停搏等多种心律失常有明显的改善作用。人参抗心律失常作用的成分是人参皂苷 Re、Rb、Rh、Rg、Ro 等，人参三醇苷对心肌电生理的影响与胺碘酮相似，可延长离体豚鼠乳头状肌细胞动作电位时程和有效不应期。人参皂苷抗心律失常的作用机制可能与阻滞心肌细胞膜 Ca^{2+} 通道和 K^+ 通道有关。

3) Anti-arrhythmia   *Rén shēn* has significant improvement on ischemic arrhythmia, ischemia-reperfusion arrhythmia, ventricular premature beat, tachycardia, ventricular fibrillation, ventricular flutter and ventricular arrest. The anti-arrhythmic active components of ginsenosides include Re, Rb, Rh, Rg, Ro, etc. Ginsenosides have similar effects on myocardial electrophysiology as amiodarone, which can prolong the action potential duration and effective refractory period of isolated papillary myocyte of pig guinea. The anti-arrhythmic mechanisms of ginsenosides may be related to the blocking of Ca^{2+} and K^+ channels in the myocardial cell membrane.

（4）强心、抗休克   人参具有强心作用，表现为增加动物心肌收缩力，增加左心室最大上升速率。主要活性成分为人参皂苷，其中人参三醇型皂苷的强心作用优于人参二醇型皂苷，多糖成分起强心协同作用。其强心作用机制与促进儿茶酚胺的释放及抑制心肌细胞膜 Na^+-K^+-ATP 酶活性有关。

4) Enhancing cardiac function and anti-shock   *Rén shēn* has a strong cardiotonic effects, which is manifested by the increase of the contractility of the myocardium and the maximum ascending rate of the left ventricle in animals. The main active ingredients are ginsenosides, and panaxatriol is better than

panaxadiol. Polysaccharides have synergistic effects on cardiotonic action. The mechanism of cardiotonic action is related to promoting the release of catechinolamine and inhibiting the activity of Na^+-K^+-ATPase in myocardial cell membrane.

人参注射液、人参皂苷 Re 对多种原因诱导的休克有防治作用，可延长休克动物的存活时间，提高存活率，增加失血性循环衰竭动物心脏收缩力和频率，能增加内毒素致休克大鼠平均动脉压，增加肾血流量，可能与调节 NO/NOS 系统功能有关。

Rén shēn injection, ginsenoside Re have prevention and treatment to the shock induced by a variety of reasons. They can prolong survival time, improve the survival rate, increase myocardial contraction and frequency in animal with hemorrhagic circulation failure, increase the mean arterial pressure of shock rats induced by the endotoxin, increase renal blood flow, which may be related to regulating function of NO/NOS system.

5. 对血液系统的影响

(5) Effects on hematological system

（1）对造血功能的影响　人参能刺激骨髓造血功能。人参总皂苷灌胃能增加 ^{60}Co-γ 射线致贫血小鼠的外周血小板、白细胞和血红蛋白含量，提高骨髓粒单系祖细胞、红系祖细胞、巨核系祖细胞的集落形成率。体外试验表明，人参总皂苷也能显著促进小鼠骨髓造血细胞的增殖，促进小鼠造血祖细胞（粒单系祖细胞、红系祖细胞、巨核系祖细胞等）的集落形成。

1) Promoting hematopoietic function　*Rén shēn* can stimulate the hematopoietic function of bone marrow. Total ginsenosides form *Rén shēn* administered orally to the anemia mice induced by ^{60}Co-γ rays irradiation can increase the contents of peripheral platelets, white blood cells and hemoglobin, and the colony forming unit of granulocyte-monocyte progenitor cells, erythroid progenitor cells and megakaryocyte progenitor cells. Total ginsenosides form *Rén shēn* also promote the proliferation of bone marrow hematopoietic cells from mice and enhance the colony forming unit of granulocyte-monocyte progenitor cells, erythroid progenitor cells and megakaryocyte progenitor cells *in vitro*.

（2）抑制血小板聚集　人参总皂苷及其单体 Rb_1、Rg_1、Re 等可抑制 ADP 引起的体外血小板聚集作用。大鼠尾静脉注射 Rg_2 能明显延长体内血栓的形成时间，抑制大鼠 ADP 诱导的血小板聚集率。人参皂苷对血小板聚集的抑制作用与其升高血小板中 cAMP 含量、抑制血小板内 Ca^{2+} 浓度有关。

2) Inhibiting platelet aggregation　Ginsenosides and Rb_1, Rg_1 and Re could inhibit platelet aggregation induced by ADP *in vitro*. Rat tail vein injection with Rg_2 can significantly prolong the time of thrombosis formation and inhibit the platelet aggregation in rats induced by ADP. The inhibitory effects of ginsenosides on platelet aggregation maybe related to the increase of cAMP content in platelets and the inhibition of elevated Ca^{2+} concentration in platelets.

6. 对物质代谢的影响

(6) Effects on the metabolism of substance

（1）调节糖代谢　人参水提物能对抗肾上腺素和高糖高脂引起的血糖升高，还能对抗注射胰岛素诱导的低血糖反应，故人参对血糖具有双向调节作用。人参多肽被认为是胰岛素样物质。人参皂苷（如 Rh_2、Rg_1、Re 等）和人参多糖对多种糖尿病动物的高血糖也有降低作用。

1) Regulating of blood glucose　The water extract of *Rén shēn* can prevent the increase of blood glucose induced by adrenaline, high fat and high sugar. It can also resist hypoglycemia induced by insulin injection, so *Rén shēn* has dual direction regulating effects on blood glucose. Ginseng polypeptides are considered insulin-like substances. Ginsenosides (e. g., Rh_2, Rg_1, Re, etc.), polysaccharides can also lower

the blood glucose level of diabetic animals.

（2）调节脂质代谢　人参水提物、人参皂苷能降低高脂血症小鼠肝系数，血液中甘油三酯（TG）、谷丙转氨酶（ALT）、低密度脂蛋白胆固醇（LDL-C）水平，增加高密度脂蛋白胆固醇（HDL-C）水平，减少脂变肝细胞数目和胞质中脂滴数量，抑制动脉粥样硬化斑块的形成，减轻氧化损伤。人参降血脂作用可能与其加速胆固醇随胆汁经肠道的排出、调节脂质代谢相关基因（FAS、LPL、SREBP-1c 等）表达、激活脂蛋白酯酶和脂质代谢酶活性有关。

2) Reducing lipid and anti-atherosclerosis　*Rén shēn* water extract and ginsenosides can reduce liver coefficient, TG, ALT and LDL-C levels in blood, increase HDL-C level in the blood, reduce the number of lipotropic hepatocytes and lipid droplets in the cytoplasm, inhibit the formation of atherosclerotic plaque, reduce oxidative damage in hyperlipidemia mice. The effects of *Rén shēn* on reducing blood lipids maybe related to accelerating the excretion of cholesterol from the intestine along with bile, regulating the expression of genes related to lipid metabolism (FAS, LPL, SREBP-1c, etc.), and activating lipoprotein esterase and lipid metabolic enzyme activities.

（3）调节核酸和蛋白质代谢　人参皂苷能促进骨髓细胞 DNA、RNA、蛋白质合成，肝肾组织细胞 RNA、蛋白质合成和血清蛋白质合成。口服人参皂苷促进大鼠肝细胞核 RNA 的合成与其激活 RNA 聚合酶的活性有关。从人参中得到的一种蛋白质合成促进因子（prostisol），含有多种人参苷（Rb$_1$、Rb$_2$、Rg$_1$ 等），也能促进正常大鼠核酸、蛋白质的合成。

3) Promoting synthesis of nucleic acids and proteins　Ginsenosides can promote DNA, RNA and protein synthesis in bone marrow cells, RNA, protein synthesis in liver and kidney tissues and protein synthesis in serum. Ginsenosides promote the synthesis of RNA of liver cell nucleus in rats, which are related to the activation of RNA polymerase. Prostisol, a protein synthesis promoter obtained from *Rén Shēn*, contains a variety of ginsenosides (Rb$_1$, Rb$_2$, Rg$_1$, etc.), which can also promote the synthesis of nucleic acid, protein.

7. 延缓衰老　人参总皂苷具有延长动物寿命、促进培养细胞增殖和延长其存活时间，抑制衰老脑组织中皮质神经元密度的降低等作用。人参皂苷 Rg$_1$ 能延缓造血干细胞、神经干细胞的衰老。人参皂苷抗衰老作用主要有以下几方面。①抗氧化作用。②降低细胞膜流动性。③调节免疫系统，减轻炎症反应。④调节脑内神经递质含量与代谢酶活性，如乙酰胆碱（ACh）含量、单胺氧化酶 B 活性等。⑤调节衰老基因（P21、Cyclin、CDK2 等）的表达。

(7) Delaying senescence　The ginsenosides from *Rén shēn* can prolong the life-span of animals, promote the proliferation and survival time of cultured cells, and inhibit the decrease of cortical neuron density in senescent brain tissue. Ginsenoside Rg$_1$ can delay the senescence of hematopoietic stem cells and neural stem cells. The main anti-aging effects of ginsenosides include the followings. ①Antioxidation. ②Reducing cell membrane fluidity. ③Regulating the immune system to reduce inflammation. ④Regulating the content of neurotransmitter and related metabolic enzyme activity in the brain, such as the content of acetylcholine, the activity of monoamine oxidase B. ⑤Regulating the expression of aging genes (P21, Cyclin, CDK2, etc.).

8. 抗应激　人参能增强机体对物理、化学和生物学等多种有害刺激的非特异性抵抗能力，维持机体内环境稳定，增强机体的适应性，这一现象称为"适应原样作用"。人参可降低低温、高温、缺氧等条件下动物的死亡率。人参抗应激作用与其对神经-内分泌-免疫系统及物质代谢的调节有关，特别是兴奋垂体-肾上腺皮质系统功能。

(8) Anti-stress　*Rén Shēn* can enhance the body's non-specific resistance to physical, chemical, biological and other harmful stimuli, maintain the stability of the internal environment of the body, enhance the adaptive ability of the body, this phenomenon is known as the "adapt to primordial effects". *Rén shēn* can reduce animal mortality under low temperature, high temperature, hypoxia, etc. The anti-stress effect of *Rén shēn* is related to the regulation of neuro-endocrine-immune system and substance metabolism, especially the excitation of pituitary-adrenal cortex system function.

9. **抗肿瘤**　人参皂苷 Rh_2、Rg_3、人参多糖、挥发油等均具有抗肿瘤作用。该作用与提高 NK 细胞杀伤活性、诱导肿瘤细胞凋亡、调整机体免疫功能和抑制肿瘤细胞代谢等作用有关。

(9) Anti-tumor　Ginsenoside Rh_2, Rg_3, polysaccharides and volatile oil of *Rén shēn* have anti-tumor effects which is associated with increasing the activity of NK cell, inducing tumor cell apoptosis, regulating immune function and inhibiting tumor cell metabolism.

10. **抗疲劳**　人参水煎液、人参皂苷、人参多糖能延长小鼠负重游泳的力竭游泳时间，改善限制性应激和电场刺激引起的小鼠精神性疲劳症状。人参抗疲劳的作用可能与其抗氧化、调节糖代谢、减少乳酸堆积、调节中枢神经递质稳态有关。

(10) Anti-fatigue　*Rén shēn* decoction, ginsenosides, and polysaccharides can prolong the exhausted swimming time of mice, and improve the mental fatigue symptoms caused by restrictive stress and electrical stimulation. The anti-fatigue effect of *Rén shēn* may be related to antioxidation, regulating glucose metabolism, reducing lactic acid accumulation, and regulating central neurotransmitter homeostasis.

【不良反应 / Adverse effects】

长期服用人参或服用过量，可出现皮疹、失眠、血压升高、头痛、心悸等不良反应。出血是人参中毒的特征。儿童服用人参可引起早熟。

Taking *Rén shēn* for a long time or taking overdose can cause skin rash, insomnia, high blood pressure, headache, palpitation, edema, etc. Bleeding is a poisoning characteristic of *Rén shēn*. *Rén shēn* can cause sexual precocity in children.

黄芪 ┊ *Huáng qí* (Radix Astragali seu Hedysar)

【来源 / Origin】

本品为豆科植物蒙古黄芪 [*Astragalus memeranaceus*（Fisch.）Bge. var. mongholicus (Bge.) Hsiao] 或膜荚黄芪 [*Astragalus memeranaceus*（Fisch.）Bge.] 的根。主产于内蒙古、山西、黑龙江等地。多于初秋采挖，晒干，切片，生用或蜜炙用。

Huáng qí is the dried root of *Astragalus membranceus* (Fisch.) Bge. var. mongholicus (Bge.) Hsiao, or *Astragalus membranceus* (Fisch.) Bge., family of Fabaceae. It is widely cultivated in Inner Mongolia Autonomous region, Shanxi province and Heilongjiang province, etc., and harvested in early autumn. After drying in the sun, slices is directly used for Chinese medicinal preparation or is processed with honey for application.

【化学成分 / Chemical ingredients】

主要含有黄芪多糖、黄酮、三萜皂苷（黄芪皂苷 I~IV）成分。此外还有生物碱、氨基酸、葡萄糖醛酸及多种微量元素等。

Huáng qí mainly contains polysaccharides, flavonoids, triterpenes (astragaloside I-IV). The others are alkaloids, amino acid, glucuronic acid and some trace elements.

【药性与功效 / Chinese medicine properties】

味甘，性微温，归脾、肺经。具有补气健脾、升阳举陷、益卫固表、利水消肿、托毒生肌的功效。主治气虚乏力、食少便溏、中气下陷、久泻脱肛、便血崩漏、表虚自汗、痈疽难溃、久溃不敛、血虚萎黄、内热消渴等证。

In Chinese medicine theory, *Huáng qí* has the nature of sweet, slightly warm. It can enter the meridians of lung and spleen. *Huáng qí* can tonify Qi and invigorate spleen, elevate Yang and raise the drooping, replenish defence and consolidate the exterior, induce diuresis to alleviate edema, express toxin to promote granulation. Clinically it can be used for Qi deficiency and lack of strength, poor appetite, loose stool, sinking of middle Qi, chronic diarrhea, rectocele, bloody stool, metrorrhagia and metrostaxis, spontaneous sweating due to exterior deficiency, carbuncle or gangrene, blood deficiency and shallow yellow, consumptive thirst due to internal heat, etc.

【药理作用 / Pharmacological effects】

1. 增强机体免疫功能

(1) Enhancing immune function

（1）提高非特异性免疫功能　黄芪提取物、黄芪多糖、黄芪皂苷可提高小鼠胸腺和脾脏重量，增强巨噬细胞吞噬功能和 NK 细胞的活性，诱导白细胞介素产生。黄芪注射液能提高腹透患者腹腔巨噬细胞噬菌率、吞噬指数、杀菌率和巨噬细胞分泌 TNF-α 水平，也能直接活化小鼠中性粒细胞，改善老龄小鼠胸腺超微结构的改变。

1) Enhancing non-specific immunity　*Huáng qí* decoction, polysaccharides and astragaloside can increase the weight of thymus and spleen of mice, enhance the phagocytosis of macrophages and the activity of NK cells, and induce interleukin production. *Huáng qí* injection can increase phagocytosis index, sterilizing rate and TNF-α secretion of macrophages in abdomen of patients with abdominal dialysis.

（2）提高细胞免疫功能　黄芪可促进正常人、慢性炎症患者的淋巴母细胞转化，也能促进小鼠淋巴细胞对羊红细胞的玫瑰花环形成和 B 细胞增殖。黄芪注射液可降低患者 CD8$^+$ T 细胞亚群，升高 CD4$^+$ / CD8$^+$ T 细胞亚群比例，使免疫功能恢复正常。黄芪多糖可以明显增加环磷酰胺致免疫抑制小鼠外周血血清中 CD3$^+$ T 细胞亚群、CD4$^+$ T 细胞亚群和 CD4$^+$/CD8$^+$ T 细胞亚群比值，降低 CD8$^+$ T 细胞百分含量，增加淋巴细胞的转化率。

2) Enhancing cell-mediated immunity　*Huáng qí* can promote the transformation of lymphocytes in normal people and patients with chronic inflammation, and also enhance the percentage of erythrocyte rosette forming cells and B-cell proliferation in mice. *Huáng qí* injection can reduce the number of CD8$^+$ T-cells, increase the value of CD4$^+$ / CD8$^+$ T -cells, restore the normal immune function of patients. Astragalus polysaccharides can significantly increase the number of CD3$^+$T- cell and CD4$^+$T-cell, decrease the percentage of CD8$^+$T-cell, increase the value of CD4$^+$/CD8$^+$ T-cell and the lymphocyte transformation rate in peripheral blood serum of immunosuppressive mice induced by cyclophosphamide.

（3）提高体液免疫功能　黄芪水煎液可以促进绵羊红细胞免疫后小鼠 IgG 抗体的产生，增加脾溶血空斑数。黄芪注射液可以增加易感冒患者体内 IgG 和 IgA 及 IgM 抗体数量，增加老年人的补体水平。黄芪多糖可以增加环磷酰胺、荷瘤及放射损伤致免疫低下小鼠血清 IgG 水平，可以增强可的松致免疫功能低下动物的细胞免疫和体液免疫、补体水平及补体介导的免疫复合物溶解活性，使免疫器官组织的超微结构恢复正常。

3) Enhancing humoral immunity　*Huáng qí* decoction can promote IgG antibody production and increase the number of plaque forming cell (PFC) in mice immunized by sheep red blood cell. *Huáng qí* injection can increase the number of IgG, IgA and IgM antibodies in susceptible patients and increase the complement level in old people. Astragalus polysaccharides can increase the IgG level in serum of immunodeficiency mice induced by cyclophosphamide, tumor and radiation, and it also can increase the cell-mediated and humoral immune, complement and complement-mediated immune complex dissolution

activity, restore the injured ultrastructure of immune organs to normal in immunodeficiency animal induced by hydrocortisone.

（4）增强红细胞免疫功能　黄芪水煎液能提高老年人、严重烧伤及急性白血病、慢性肾炎等患者的红细胞免疫功能，明显增加红细胞 C3b 受体花环率。黄芪注射液、黄芪多糖也能增强荷瘤小鼠红细胞免疫功能。

4) Enhancing erythrocyte immunity　*Huáng qí* decoction can significantly increase E-C3bRR to improve the erythrocyte immune function of the aged and patients with severe burn, acute leukemia, chronic nephritis. *Huáng qí* injection and polysaccharide also enhance erythrocyte immune function of tumor-bearing mice.

2. 对心血管系统的影响

(2) Effects on cardiovascular system

（1）改善心功能　黄芪具有强心作用，可增强心肌收缩力，增加心输出量，改善中毒或疲劳衰竭心脏的功能，延缓左心室重构。黄芪多糖能改善心肌梗死犬心肌收缩功能、增加冠脉流量、减小心肌梗死面积；能明显对抗垂体后叶素致大鼠急性心肌缺血时的 ST 段抬高和 T 波上升；还能对抗 $BaCl_2$、氯仿诱发小鼠心律失常。黄芪改善心功能的作用与减少心肌细胞内钙离子超载、保护线粒体和溶酶体、抗氧化损伤、稳定心肌细胞膜等作用有关。

1) Improving cardiac function　*Huáng qí* enhances myocardial contractility, increases the cardiac output, improves heart failure induced by toxicity or fatigue and delays the left ventricular remodeling. Astragalus polysaccharides can improve the myocardial contraction, increase the blood flow of coronary artery, decrease the myocardial infarction area in dog with myocardial infarction; antagonize the increase of ST segment and T wave elevation of acute myocardial ischemia mice induced by hypophysin; and protect against $BaCl_2$ or chloroform-induced arrhythmia in mice. The improvement of *Huáng qí* on cardiac function is related to reducing calcium overload in myocardial cells, protecting mitochondria and lysosomes, preventing oxidative damage and stabilizing the of myocardial cell membrane.

（2）扩张血管，调节血压　黄芪可以扩张冠状血管、外周血管，降低外周血管阻力，产生降压作用。黄芪降压的主要成分为黄芪皂苷Ⅳ和 γ– 氨基丁酸。但当动物血压降低至休克时，黄芪又可以升高血压并保持稳定。

2) Dilating blood vessels and regulating blood pressure　*Huáng qí* can dilate coronary vessels and peripheral blood vessels, reduce peripheral resistance，which can decrease blood pressure in many animals. Astragaloside Ⅳ and γ -GABA are the main components for lowering blood pressure. However, *Huáng qí* can increase the blood pressure and sustain stability in shock model animals.

3. 对血液系统的影响　黄芪煎剂能促进骨髓造血细胞 DNA 合成，促进射线损伤动物的造血干细胞增殖和向红系与粒系细胞分化，增加环磷酰胺、失血等多种原因致贫血动物的外周血红细胞和白细胞数量、血红蛋白含量及骨髓有核细胞数量，促进各类血细胞的形成、发育及成熟过程。黄芪能降低老年大鼠血浆纤维蛋白原含量，抑制红细胞聚集，还能增加人红细胞膜流动性，增加膜蛋白 α– 螺旋的含量，保护红细胞膜。黄芪注射液能改善红细胞的变形力、降低全血黏度、红细胞聚集指数，抑制血小板聚集，抑制体外血栓形成。

(3) Effects on hematological system　*Huáng qí* decoction can promote DNA synthesis of bone marrow hematopoietic cell, promote the proliferation of hematopoietic stem cells and differentiation into erythrocytes and granulocytes in radiation-damaged animals, increase the number of red blood cells and white blood cells, hemoglobin and bone marrow nucleated cells in peripheral blood, promote the formation, development and mature process of all kinds of blood cells in anemia animals induced by cyclophosphamide or the loss of blood. *Huáng qí* can reduce fibrinogen content in plasma and inhibit erythrocyte aggregation in aged rats. It can also increase the fluidity of erythrocyte membrane, increase the content of membrane protein α-helix, and protect erythrocyte membrane. *Huáng qí* injection can improve erythrocyte deformability, reduce blood viscosity and erythrocyte aggregation index, inhibit platelet aggregation in rabbit with blood stasis syndrome, and inhibit thrombosis *in vitro*.

4. 对消化系统的影响

(4) Effects on digestive system

（1）抗溃疡　黄芪乙醇提取物可减轻胃幽门结扎、吲哚美辛致胃溃疡鼠的溃疡面积和溃疡指数，增强西咪替丁对胃黏膜的保护作用。

1) Anti-ulcer　*Huáng qí* alcohol extract can reduce the area and index of gastric ulcer in rats caused by ligation of pylorus or indomethacin, and enhance the protective effects of cimetidine on gastric mucosa.

（2）保肝　黄芪可提高四氯化碳引起肝损伤小鼠血清总蛋白及白蛋白、肝糖原水平，降低血清转氨酶水平，保护肝细胞膜。黄芪也可以减轻白蛋白诱发的免疫性损伤大鼠的肝纤维化程度及超微结构的病理改变，减少总胶原及 Ⅰ 型胶原、Ⅱ 型胶原、Ⅴ 型胶原在肝内的沉积。

2) Hepatoprotection　*Huáng qí* can increase total serum protein, albumin and liver glycogen level, decrease the activity of serum aminotransferase and protect the membrane of hepatocyte in liver-injury mice caused by carbon tetrachloride. *Huáng qí* can also alleviate the liver fibrosis and the pathological changes of the ultrastructure, reduce total collagen and Ⅰ, Ⅱ, Ⅴ type collagen deposition in the liver of immunity-injury rats induced by albumin.

5. 对物质代谢的影响　黄芪水煎液能促进小鼠血清和肝脏蛋白质合成。黄芪多糖能促进小鼠脾脏蛋白及核酸合成。黄芪对正常小鼠血糖无明显影响，能对抗葡萄糖负荷、肾上腺素引起的小鼠血糖升高和苯乙双胍引起的低血糖反应，但对胰岛素引起的低血糖无明显影响。黄芪水煎液和多糖还能降低高脂血症小鼠血清 TG、TC、LDL-C 含量。

(5) Effects on metabolism of substance　*Huáng qí* decoction can promote the protein synthesis in serum and liver of mice. Astragalus polysaccharides can promote the synthesis of protein and nucleic acid in spleen. *Huáng qí* has no significant effect on the blood glucose of normal mice and insulin-induced hypoglycemia, but can antagonize high glucose in mice caused by glucose load, adrenaline and hypoglycemia caused by phenformin. *Huáng qí* decoction and polysaccharides can also reduce serum TG, TC and LDL-C levels in hyperlipidemia mice.

6. 抗氧化、延缓衰老　黄芪水煎液能明显提高小鼠血清 SOD 活性，降低小鼠肝组织中 MDA 含量，升高肝内谷胱甘肽（GSH）水平。黄芪总皂苷、总黄酮、总多糖能降低小鼠肝组织中脂质过氧化物含量，具有清除氧自由基作用。

(6) Anti-oxidation and anti-aging　*Huáng qí* decoction could significantly increase the activity of SOD in serum, decrease the content of MDA and increase the activity of GSH in the liver. The total saponins, total flavonoids and total polysaccharides of *Huáng qí* can reduce the content of lipid peroxides in the liver of mice, indicating that they have the effects of scavenging oxygen free radicals.

黄芪能延长人胚肺二倍体细胞的寿命，延长果蝇和家蚕的平均寿命。黄芪还可以增强小鼠学习记忆能力。黄芪抗衰老作用与其抗氧化、提高免疫功能、改善血液流变学和物质代谢等作用有关。

Huáng qí can prolong the life-span of human embryonic lung diploid cell, fruit fly and silkworm. *Huáng qí* can also enhance the ability of learning and memory in mice. The anti-aging effect of *Huáng qí* is related to its anti-oxidation, improving immune function, improving hemorheology and metabolism of substance.

7. 利尿和保护肾功能 黄芪水提物可增加健康人和盐水负荷大鼠的尿量,但大剂量反而减少动物的尿量。黄芪可有效减轻糖尿病肾病患者和大鼠的肾脏损伤,有效减少蛋白尿。黄芪水提物、黄芪多糖和黄芪皂苷均可减轻慢性肾炎、肾病综合征和肾衰竭动物的肾脏病理变化,改善肾功能。

(7) Diuresis and renal protection The water extract of *Huáng qí* could increase micturition of healthy people and salt-loaded rats, but the high-dose of *Huáng qí* extract can reduce micturition of animals. *Huáng qí* can effectively reduce the kidney injury and effectively reduce proteinuria of diabetic nephropathy patients and rats. *Huáng qí* water extract, polysaccharides and astragaloside can reduce the renal pathological changes and improve renal function in chronic nephritis, nephrotic syndrome and renal failure animals.

8. 抗病毒 黄芪多糖、黄芪皂苷Ⅳ、黄芪总黄酮可抑制柯萨奇病毒、乙肝病毒、疱疹、新城疫病毒、流感病毒等多种病毒的增殖,降低其致病性。黄芪抗病毒作用与其增强机体免疫能力、诱导机体内合成干扰素、增强抗病毒蛋白数量有关。

(8) Anti-virus *Huáng qí* polysaccharides, astragaloside Ⅳ, and total flavonoids can inhibit the proliferation of Coxsackie virus, hepatitis B virus, herpes, newcastle disease virus, and influenza virus, reduce their pathogenicity. Anti-viral effects of *Huáng qí* are related to the enhancement of immunity to induce the synthesis of interferon and the enhancement of antiviral protein.

9. 其他作用 黄芪及所含多种成分具有抗肿瘤作用,减少荷瘤小鼠的死亡率,延长生存期。黄芪注射液具有类雌激素样作用,促进大鼠离体子宫收缩。黄芪还具有抗骨质疏松、抗疲劳、抗应激等作用。

(9) Other effects *Huáng qí* and its various components have anti-tumor effects, which can reduce the mortality of tumor-bearing mice and prolong survival. *Huáng qí* injection has estrogen-like effect, which can promote contractions of uterus of rat in vitro. *Huáng qí* also has anti-osteoporosis, anti-fatigue, anti-stress.

【不良反应 / Adverse effects】

使用黄芪后偶见皮肤瘙痒、荨麻疹、发热、腹胀等症状。

Skin itching, urticaria, fever, abdominal distension are occasionally appeared in patients using *Huáng qí*.

党参 ┆ *Dǎng shēn (Radix Codonopsis)*

【来源 / Origin】

本品为桔梗科植物党参 [*Codonopsis pilosula*(Franch.)Nannf.]、素花党参 [*Codonopsis pilosula* Nannf. var. *modesta*(Nannf.)L. T. Shen] 或川党参 [*Codonopsis tangshen* Oliv.] 的干燥根。主要分布于山西、陕西、甘肃等地。秋季采挖,洗净晒干,切厚片,生用。

Dǎng shēn is the dried root of *Codonopsis pilosula* (Franch.) Nannf., *Codonopsis pilosula* Nannf. var. *modesta* (Nannf.) L.T. Shen, or *Codonopsis tangshen* Oliv., family of Campanulaceae. It is widely cultivated in Shanxi province, Gansu province, Shaanxi province, etc., and harvested in autumn. It is dried and cutted into thick slice for application.

【化学成分 / Chemical ingredients】

主要含有苷类,包括党参苷、党参炔苷等;糖类,包括葡萄糖、菊糖、多糖等;生物碱类,包括党参碱(codonopsine)及党参次碱(codonopsinine)等。此外,尚含有挥发油、黄酮、植物甾醇、三萜、倍半萜内酯、氨基酸及微量元素等。

Dǎng shēn mainly contains saponins, including tangshenoside, lobotyolin, etc., saccharides including glucose, inulin, polysaccharides, etc., alkaloids including codonopsine, codonopsinine, etc. *Dǎng shēn* aslo contains volatile oil, flavonoids, sterols, triterpene, sesquiterpene lactones, amino acids and trace elements, etc.

【 药性与功效 / Chinese medicine properties 】

味甘，性平，归脾、肺经。具有补中益气、健脾益肺的功效。主治脾肺虚弱、食少便溏、虚喘咳嗽、气短心悸、内热消渴等证。

In Chinese medicine theory, *Dǎng shēn* has the nature of sweet and neutral. It can enter the meridians of spleen and lung. *Dǎng shēn* can tonify middle and replenish Qi, invigorate spleen and replenish lung. Clinically it can be used for spleen and stomach deficiency, poor appetite and loosing stool, deficiency-type dyspnea and cough, shortness of Qi and palpitation, consumptive thirst due to interior heat, etc.

【 药理作用 / Pharmacological effects 】

1. 对消化系统的影响

(1) Effects on digestive system

（1）调节胃肠运动　党参水煎液可使正常小鼠胃内容物残留率增高，也可以拮抗阿托品延缓胃排空作用。党参水煎醇沉液能部分对抗束缚水浸应激引起的胃蠕动增加和胃排空加快。党参水煎液可以明显减慢正常小鼠胃肠内容物的推进速度，拮抗阿托品和去甲肾上腺素引起的小肠推进抑制作用，但不影响异丙肾上腺素的抑制作用。党参水煎醇沉液还可以对抗乙酰胆碱引起的离体豚鼠回肠收缩。

1) Regulating gastrointestinal motility　*Dǎng shēn* decoction can increase the residual rate in stomach of normal mice, antagonize the effect on delayed gastric emptying induced by atropine. The water extraction and alcohol-precipitation liquid of *Dǎng shēn* can partly resist the increase of gastric peristalsis and gastric emptying caused by stress. *Dǎng shēn* decoction can obviously slow down the propulsion of gastrointestinal contents in normal mice, antagonize the inhibition of intestinal propulsion caused by atropine and noradrenaline, but has no effect on the inhibition of of intestinal propulsion induced by isoproterenol. The water-extraction and alcohol-precipitation liquid of *Dǎng shēn* can resist the contraction of isolated guinea pig ileum caused by acetylcholine.

（2）抗胃溃疡　党参对应激、幽门结扎、吲哚美辛、阿司匹林等多种因素致大鼠胃溃疡有改善作用。党参抗胃溃疡的主要作用环节如下。①抑制胃酸分泌、降低胃蛋白酶活性。②促进胃黏液分泌、增强胃黏液–碳酸氢盐的屏障保护作用。③促进胃肠上皮细胞增殖，保护和修复胃黏膜。④调节胃肠激素水平和胃肠运动功能。

2) Anti-ulcer　*Dǎng shēn* can improve gastric ulcer induced by various reasons, such as stress, pylorus ligation, indomethacin, and aspirin. The related mechanisms of *Dǎng shēn* in anti-ulcer are mainly as follows. ①Inhibiting the secretion of gastric acid, reducing the activity of pepsin. ②Increasing the secretion of gastric mucosa and the protection of mucous-bicarbonate barrier. ③Promoting the proliferation of gastrointestinal epithelial cells, protecting and repairing gastric mucosa. ④Regulating the level of gastrointestinal hormones and gastrointestinal motility.

2. 增强免疫功能　党参水提物和醇提物灌胃可以增强小鼠腹腔巨噬细胞数量和吞噬活性。党参水煎液可以促进 Con A 诱导的小鼠脾淋巴细胞 DNA 合成，促进环磷酰胺诱导的小鼠淋巴细胞转化，增加抗体产生细胞功能，提高抗体滴度，并能促进体外培养的淋巴细胞有丝分裂。党参多糖是其增强免疫功能的主要有效成分，能促进正常小鼠的抗体生成，也能促进绵羊红细胞和卵清蛋白诱导的小鼠抗体生成，促进 ^{60}Co-γ 射线照射后小鼠内源性脾结节生成。

(2) Enhancing immune system function　The water extract and alcohol extract of *Dǎng shēn* administered orally can enhance the number and phagocytosis of peritoneal macrophages in normal mice. *Dǎng shēn* decoction can promote DNA synthesis of lymphocytes in spleen of mice induced by Con A. It can also promote lymphocyte transformation and increase the titer of antibody in immunosuppressed mice induced by cyclophosphamide. Furthermore, it can increase the mitosis of lymphocytes *in vitro*. Polysaccharides from *Dǎng shēn* are the main active components to enhance the immune function. It can enhance the antibody production in normal mice and mice treated with sheep red blood cells and ovalbumin, and promote the formation of endogenous spleen colony.

3. 对血液系统的影响

(3) Effects on hematological system

（1）促进造血　党参水浸膏和醇浸膏皮下注射、党参粉口服，可增加红细胞数量、降低白细胞数量，口服比皮下注射作用明显，且切除脾脏后作用降低，提示党参有影响脾脏促红细胞生成作用。党参水煎液还可促进环磷酰胺致免疫低下小鼠的骨髓造血功能，升高白细胞和红细胞数量。党参多糖能显著升高溶血性血虚小鼠外周血中血红蛋白含量，促进 ^{60}Co-γ 射线照射小鼠脾结节形成，但对骨髓造血功能 DNA 合成无明显促进作用，提示党参能促进脾脏代偿造血功能。

1) Promoting hematopoietic function　Subcutaneous injection of *Dǎng shēn* water extract, alcohol extract, and oral administration of *Dǎng shēn* powder can increase the number of red blood cells and reduce the number of white blood cells. The effects of oral administration is more obvious than that of subcutaneous injection. This effect can be blocked by splenectomy, suggesting that *Dǎng shēn* can affect the erythropoiesis of spleen. *Dǎng shēn* decoction also can promote the bone marrow hematopoietic function of immunosuppressed mice induced by cyclophosphamide, which can increase the number of red blood cells and white blood cells. Polysaccharides from *Dǎng shēn* can significantly elevate the content of hemoglobin in the peripheral blood of hemolysis blood- deficiency mice and increase the formation of spleen colony, but has less effect on DNA synthese in the blood-deficiency mice induced by ^{60}Co-γ ray, suggesting that *Dǎng shēn* can promote the compensatory hematopoiesis of spleen.

（2）改善血液流变学　党参水煎醇沉液静脉注射可以降低家兔全血黏度，缩短红细胞电泳时间，抑制体外血栓形成。党参注射液还可以抑制 ADP 诱导的家兔血小板聚集。党参醚提液可以提高大鼠纤溶酶活性，显著降低血小板聚集和血浆血栓素 B_2（TXB$_2$）水平。

2) Improving hemorheology　The water-extraction and alcohol-precipitation liquid of *Dǎng shēn* injected intravenously can reduce the whole blood viscosity, shorten the electrophoresis time of red blood cells in rabbits, and inhibit the formation of thrombus *in vitro*. *Dǎng shēn* injection can also inhibit ADP-induced platelet aggregation *in vitro*. The ether extract of *Dǎng shēn* can increase the activity of fibrinolytic enzyme, significantly inhibit platelet aggregation and decrease plasma thromboxane B_2 level.

（3）调节血脂　党参总皂苷可降低高脂血症大鼠血清甘油三酯、胆固醇、低密度脂蛋白胆固醇含量，增加 NO 和高密度脂蛋白胆固醇含量。

3) Regulating blood lipid　Total saponins of *Dǎng shēn* can reduce the contents of triglyceride (TG), cholesterol (TC) and low density lipoprotein cholesterol (LDL-C), increase the contents of NO and high density lipoprotein (HDL-C) in serum of hyperlipidemic rats.

4. 对心血管系统的影响

(4) Effects on cardiovascular system

（1）强心、抗休克　党参口服液可以增强冠心病患者左心室收缩功能，增加心输出量，对心率无明显影响。党参提取物静脉注射能明显增加麻醉猫心输出量而不影响心率。党参注射液可使失血性休克家兔的动脉血压回升，延长家兔存活时间。

1) Enhancing cardiac function and anti-shock　*Dǎng shēn* oral liquid can increase left ventricular systolic function and cardiac output in patients with coronary heart disease, but has no significant effect on heart rate. Intravenous injection of *Dǎng shēn* extract can significantly increase cardiac output of anesthetized cats without affecting heart rate. *Dǎng shēn* injection can increase the arterial blood pressure and prolong the survival time of rabbits with hemorrhagic shock.

（2）调节血压　党参水提物和醇提物静脉注射均能显著降低麻醉家兔和犬的血压。党参降压的作用与其扩张外周血管有关。党参也可升高失血性休克家兔的动脉血压。

2) Regulating blood pressure　*Dǎng shēn* water extract and alcohol extract injected intravenously can significantly reduce the blood pressure of anesthetized rabbits and dogs, which is related to its vasodilation. *Dǎng shēn* injection can also increase arterial blood pressure in rabbits with hemorrhagic shock.

（3）抗心肌缺血　党参水提醇沉液十二指肠给药可显著抑制冠状动脉左前降支结扎引起的心肌缺血犬的左心室舒张终末期压力增高，改善心肌的舒张功能，减少冠状动脉灌注阻力，改善左心室心肌的血流供应。党参注射液静脉给药可对抗异丙肾上腺素和垂体后叶素引起的大鼠心肌缺血。

3) Anti-cardiac ischemia　The water-extraction and alcohol precipitation liquid of *Dǎng shēn* administered through duodenum can significantly inhibit the increase of left ventricular end diastolic pressure (LVEDP), improve the diastolic function of myocardium, reduce the perfusion resistance of coronary artery, and increase the blood flow of left ventricular myocardium in myocardial ischemia dogs caused by ligation of left anterior descending coronary artery. *Dǎng shēn* injection administered intravenously can antagonize myocardial ischemia in rats induced by isoproterenol or pituitrin.

5. 对中枢神经系统的影响

(5) Effects on central nervous system

（1）改善学习记忆　党参醇提物、党参多糖、党参总碱对东莨菪碱致小鼠学习记忆获得障碍、亚硝酸钠引起的小鼠记忆巩固障碍和40%乙醇引起的小鼠记忆再现障碍均有改善作用。党参水提物灌胃可显著增加氢溴酸东莨菪碱致记忆障碍小鼠在 Morris 水迷宫空间探索实验中的穿台次数和平台停留时间，党参醇提物能明显缩短小鼠在定位航行中到达平台的潜伏期。

1) Learning and memory improvement　The alcohol extract of *Dǎng shēn*, *Dǎng shēn* polysaccharide, total alkaloids of *Dǎng shēn* can reduce the impairment of acquisition of memory in mice induced by scopolamine, the disruption of consolidation of memory induced y sodium nitrite, and the memory reproduction disorder induced by 40% alcohol. The water extract of *Dǎng shēn* can significantly increase the number of crossing platform and the residence time in platform area for the mice induced by scopolamine in the spacial probe test of Morris water maze, while the alcohol extract of *Dǎng shēn* can significantly shorten the latency of reaching the platform in the navigation test.

（2）镇静、催眠、抗惊厥　党参水提物和醇提物腹腔注射均能显著减少小鼠的自主活动，协同小剂量氯丙嗪起镇静作用。党参水提物腹腔注射能延长阈下剂量戊巴比妥钠诱导的小鼠睡眠时间。党参水提物和醇提物腹腔注射能延长印防己毒素、戊四氮致小鼠惊厥的潜伏期，延长死亡时间。

2) Sedation, hypnosis and anti-convulsion　Intraperitoneal injection of *Dǎng shēn* water extract and alcohol extract can significantly reduce the spontaneous activity of mice, and enhance the sedative effect of low dose of chlorpromazine. Intraperitoneal injection of *Dǎng shēn* water extract also can prolong the sleep time of mice induced by subthreshold dose of pentobarbital sodium. Furthermore, Intraperitoneal injection of *Dǎng shēn* water extract and alcohol extract can prolong the latency of convulsion and death

time of mice caused by picrotoxin, pentetrazol.

6. 其他作用　党参水提物和党参多糖具有延缓 D- 半乳糖诱导动物衰老的作用。党参水提物能减轻四氯化碳诱导的小鼠肝损伤。党参多糖能通过兴奋垂体-肾上腺皮质功能，增强机体对有害刺激的抵抗能力。

(6) Other effects　The water extract and polysaccharide of *Dǎng shēn* can delay aging of mice induced by D-galactose. The water extract of *Dǎng shēn* has hepatoprotection against the liver injury of mice induced by CCl$_4$. *Dǎng shēn* polysaccharides can enhance the resistance to harmful stimulation by stimulating pituitary-adrenal cortex function.

【不良反应 / Adverse effects 】

大量使用党参可能会引起心前区不适、心律不齐、晕眩、烦躁等症状，停药后可自行恢复正常。

High dose of *Dǎng shēn* can cause chest discomfort, arrhythmia, dizziness, dysthemia, etc., which can disappear after discontinuation.

甘草 ┊ *Gān cǎo (Radix Glycyrrhizae)*

【来源 / Origin 】

本品为豆科植物乌拉尔甘草（*Glycyrrhiza uralensis* Fisch.）、胀果甘草（*Glycyrrhiza infalta* Bat.）或光果甘草（*Glycyrrhiza glabra* L.）的干燥根及根茎。主要分布于新疆、内蒙古、甘肃等地。春、秋二季采收，秋季为佳。除去须根，晒干，切片生用或蜜炙用。

Gān cǎo is the dried root and rhizome of *Glycyrrhiza uralensis* Fishch., *Glycyrrhiza infalta* Bat., and *Glycyrrhiza glabra* L., family of Fabaceae. It is widely cultivated in Xinjiang Autonomous region, Inner Mongolia Autonomous region, and Gansu province, etc., and harvested in spring and autumn, autumn is the better. After drying in the sun, slice is directly used or baked with honey for Chinese medicinal preparation.

【化学成分 / Chemical ingredients 】

主要成分有三萜皂苷类和黄酮类。三萜皂苷类主要包括甘草酸（glycyrrhizic acid)［又称甘草甜素（glycyrrhizin)］、甘草次酸（glycyrrhetinic acid）。黄酮类包括甘草苷（liquiritin）、异甘草苷（isoliquritin）、新甘草苷（neoliquritin)、甘草素（liquiritigenin）和异甘草素（isoliquiritigenin）等。此外，甘草还含有异黄酮类的 FM100、甘草酸单胺（monoammonium glycyrrhizate）、甘草利酮（licoricone）、阿魏酸（ferulaic acid)、多种氨基酸、多糖及微量元素。

Gān cǎo mainly contains triterpene glycosides and flavonoids. Triterpene glycosides include glycyrrhizin (glycyrrhizic acid) and glycyrrhetinic acid. Flavonoids include liquiritin. isoliquritin, neoliquritin, liquiritigenin and isoliquiritigenin (2,4,4-trihydroxychalcone). The others are isoflavone FM100, monoammonium glycyrrhizate, licoricone, ferulaic acid, amino acid, polysaccharide, and some trace elements.

【药性与功效 / Chinese medicine properties 】

味甘，性平，归心、肺、脾、胃经。具有补脾益气、清热解毒、祛痰止咳、缓急止痛、调和诸药的功效。主治脾胃虚弱、心悸气短、咳嗽痰多、脘腹及四肢挛急疼痛、热毒疮疡、咽喉肿痛等证。

In Chinese medicine theory, *Gān cǎo* has the nature of sweet and neutral. It can enter the meridians of heart, lung, spleen and stomach. *Gān cǎo* can tonify spleen and replenish Qi, clear heat and remove toxin, resolve phlegm and relieve cough, relax tension to relieve pain, and harmonize properties of various herbs. Clinically it can be used for spleen-stomach weakness, palpitation, shortness of breath, cough, abundant phlegm, spasmotic pain of abdomen, arm and leg, sores due to heat toxin, sore throat.

【药理作用 / Pharmacological effects】

1. 肾上腺皮质激素样作用 甘草浸膏、甘草酸、甘草次酸均具有去氧皮质酮或类醛固酮样作用，能减少多种实验动物的尿量及 Na^+ 排出，增加 K^+ 排出。甘草、甘草酸还具有糖皮质激素样作用，能使大鼠胸腺萎缩、肾上腺重量增加，血液中嗜酸性粒细胞和淋巴细胞减少，尿中 17– 羟皮质酮增加。甘草具有皮质激素样作用机制如下。①促进皮质激素合成。②甘草次酸与皮质激素的结构相似，可直接产生皮质激素样作用。③竞争性抑制肝脏对皮质激素的灭活，间接提高皮质激素的水平。

(1) Adrenal cortex hormone-like effects *Gān cǎo* extract, glycyrrhizin and glycyrrhetinic acid all have deoxycorticosterone-like or aldosterone-like effects, which can reduce the urine volume and Na^+ excretion, increase the K^+ excretion of various experimental animals. Glycyrrhizin and glycyrrhizin also have glucocorticoid-like effects, which can cause atrophy of thymus, increase adrenal gland weight, decrease eosinophil and lymphocyte in blood and increase 17-hydroxycorticosterone in urine. The mechanisms of the corticosteroid-like effects of *Gān cǎo* are mainly as follows. ①Promoting the synthesis of corticosteroids. ②Glycyrrhetinic acid is similar to corticosteroids in structure, which can directly produce corticosterin-like effects. ③Competitively inhibit inactivation of corticosteroids in liver, indirectly increase the level of corticosteroids in the blood.

2. 对消化系统的影响

(2) Effects on digestive system

（1）解痉 甘草煎液、甘草流浸膏、异甘草素等黄酮类成分可抑制乙酰胆碱、氯化钡、组胺引起的肠管痉挛性收缩，对胃肠道平滑肌有解痉作用。

1) Spasmolysis *Gān cǎo* decoction, *Gān cǎo* extract, isoglycyrrhizin and other flavonoids have the antispasmodic effect on gastrointestinal smooth muscle. They can inhibit the spasmodic contraction of intestine induced by acetylcholine, $BaCl_2$ and histamine.

（2）抗溃疡 甘草浸膏、甘草酸、甘草次酸及其衍生物、甘草黄酮、FM100、甘草多糖等具有减轻动物胃溃疡的作用。甘草抗溃疡作用机制如下。①降低胃液和胃酸分泌。②直接吸附胃酸，降低胃液酸度。③刺激胃黏膜上皮细胞合成和释放内源性前列腺素，增强黏膜屏障的保护作用。④促进消化道上皮细胞再生，促进溃疡面愈合。

2) Anti-ulcer *Gān cǎo* water extract, glycyrrhizin, glycyrrhetinic acid and its derivatives, glycyrrhizin flavone, FM100, polysaccharides can alleviate gastric ulcer in animals. Related machanisms are mainly as follows. ①Inhibiting the secretion of gastric juice and gastric acid. ②Directly adsorbing gastric acid to reduce the acidity of gastric juice. ③Stimulating gastric epithelial cells to synthesize and release endogenous prostaglandins which enhance the protection of the mucosal barrier. ④Promoting the regeneration of digestive tract epithelial cells to accelerate the healing of ulcer.

（3）保肝 甘草浸膏及甘草酸、甘草次酸等甘草黄酮类能减轻 CCl_4、对乙酰氨基酚等多种因素导致的动物肝损伤，可恢复肝糖原水平、降低血清 ALT 水平，减少肝内 MDA 含量，减轻肝脏变性坏死程度，减轻肝纤维组织的增生和间质炎症反应。甘草酸对乙型肝炎病毒有抑制作用，可促使乙肝表面抗原（HBsAg）转阴。甘草酸二铵有抗炎、保护肝细胞膜和改善肝功能作用。

3) Hepatoprotection *Gān cǎo* extract, glycyrrhizin, glycyrrhetinic acid and flavonoids can alleviate liver injury in animals induced by CCl_4, paracetamol and other factors. They can recover liver glycogen level, reduce ALT level in serum and MDA content in liver, alleviate liver degeneration and necrosis degree, and reduce liver fibrosis proliferation and intermesenchymal inflammation. Glycyrrhizic acid

has inhibitory effect on HBV, which can promote the conversion of HBsAg to negative. Diammonium glycyrrizinate can inhibit inflammation，protect hepatocyte membrane, and improve liver function.

3. **对免疫系统的影响** 甘草水提物、甘草酸、甘草素、甘草多糖等具有增强或抑制机体免疫功能的作用。甘草酸能提高小鼠碳粒廓清指数，增强巨噬细胞的吞噬功能和 NK 细胞活性，提高 Con A 诱导人脾细胞干扰素 - γ（IFN- γ）的水平和淋巴细胞分泌 IL-2 的能力，降低抗原特异性抗体水平，抑制迟发型超敏反应，具有增强非特异性免疫及细胞免疫、抑制体液免疫的作用。甘草次酸能增强正常小鼠的 1 型辅助 T 细胞（Th1）型免疫反应，但降低 LPS 诱导白细胞介素 –12、MHC Ⅰ/Ⅱ、CD86、CD80 水平，抑制 Th1 型免疫反应。

(3) Effects on immune system *Gān cǎo* extract, glycyrrhizin, liquiritigenin and polysaccharides have the function of enhancing or inhibiting the immune function. Glycyrrhizic acid can increase the index of carbon clearance, the phagocytosis of macrophages and NK cell activity in mice; enhance the ability of lymphocyte to secrete IL-2 and IFN - γ levels in human spleen cells induced by Con A; decrease the specific antibody level and inhibit delayed type hypersensitivity, indicating that glycyrrhizic acid can enhance the function of non-specific immunity and cellular immunity, while inhibit the humoral immunity. Glycyrrhetinic acid can enhance Th1 type immune response in normal mice, but reduce the LPS- induced interleukin-12, MHC Ⅰ/Ⅱ, CD86, CD80 level and inhibit Th1 immune response.

4. **解毒** 甘草对食物及药物等中毒（敌敌畏、喜树碱、水合氯醛、士的宁、乌拉坦、可卡因、苯、砷、汞等）均有一定的解毒作用。甘草解毒的主要成分为甘草酸。甘草解毒作用机制如下。①通过物理、化学方式沉淀或吸附毒物以减少吸收。②甘草酸水解生成葡萄糖醛酸可以与毒物的羧基、羟基结合，减少毒物的吸收。③甘草次酸具有皮质激素样作用，可提高机体耐受毒物的能力。④诱导机体肝微粒体细胞色素 P450 蛋白表达，增强肝脏对毒物的代谢。

(4) Detoxification *Gān cǎo* has a detoxification to various toxins (e. g., dichlorvos, camptothecin, chloral hydrate, strychnine, urethane, cocaine, benzene, arsenic, mercury). Glycyrrhizin is the main active ingredient. The mechanisms of *Gān cǎo*'s detoxification are mainly as follows. ①*Gān cǎo* can reduce the absorption of toxins by physical and chemical precipitation. ②Glucuronic acid, drived from hydrolysis of glycyrrhizin, can combine with the carboxyl and hydroxyl groups of toxins to reduce the absorption of toxins. ③Glycyrrhetinic acid has the corticosteroids-like effects, which can enhance the tolerance to toxins. ④*Gān cǎo* can induce the expression of cytochrome P450 protein in liver microsomes to enhance the metabolism of toxins in liver.

5. **镇咳、祛痰** 甘草能促进咽喉和支气管黏膜分泌，使痰易于咳出，发挥祛痰作用。甘草浸膏片口内含化后能覆盖在发炎的咽部黏膜上，缓和炎症刺激，达到镇咳作用。甘草次酸、甘草黄酮、甘草流浸膏可以减轻氨水和二氧化硫引起的小鼠咳嗽，并有祛痰作用。

(5) Anti-tussive and expectorant effects *Gān cǎo* can promote the secretion of mucosa in the throat and bronchial to easy expectorate phlegm. The *Gān cǎo* extract buccal tablet can relieve inflammation and cough by covering the inflamed pharyngeal mucosa. Glycyrrhetinic acid, flavounoids and liquid extract of *Gān cǎo* can exert anti-tussive and expectorant effects in mice caused by ammonia and sulfur dioxide.

6. **抗心律失常** 炙甘草提取液腹腔注射对氯仿诱发的小鼠心室纤颤、乌头碱诱发的大鼠心律失常、肾上腺素诱发的家兔心律失常、氯化钡和毒毛花苷 K 诱发的豚鼠心律失常均有抑制作用，能减慢心率。甘草总黄酮可延长乌头碱诱发的小鼠心律失常潜伏期、减少氯仿诱发的小鼠心室纤颤阳性率，拮抗毒毛花苷 G 诱发的豚鼠室性期前收缩、心室纤颤和室性心动过速。

(6) Anti-arrhythmia *Zhì Gān cǎo* extract administered by intraperitoneal injection, can inhibit ventricular fibrillation of mice induced by chloroform, arrhythmia of rats induced by aconitine, arrhythmia of rabbits induced by adrenaline, arrhythmia of guinea pigs induced by $BaCl_2$ and strophanthin K. Total flavonoids of *Gān cǎo* could prolong the latency of arrhythmia induced by aconitine in mice, reduce the positive rate of ventricular fibrillation induced by chloroform in mice, and antagonize the ventricular premature beat, ventricular fibrillation and ventricular tachycardia induced by ouabain in guinea pigs.

7. 抗炎　甘草对醋酸诱发的腹腔毛细血管通透性增加、巴豆油诱发的小鼠耳郭肿胀、大鼠棉球肉芽肿、甲醛性大鼠足跖肿胀、角叉菜胶性大鼠关节炎均有抑制作用。甘草抗炎的主要成分有甘草三萜皂苷类（甘草酸、甘草酸单铵盐和甘草次酸及其衍生物等）和甘草黄酮类（甘草素、异甘草素、甘草苷、异甘草苷、FM100 等）。抗炎作用与其具有肾上腺皮质激素样作用有关，能减少趋化因子和促炎症因子的表达，抑制类固醇代谢酶而发挥抗炎作用。

(7) Anti-inflammation　*Gān cǎo* can inhibit capillary permeability in abdomen induced by acetic acid and the ear swelling induced by croton oil in mice, decrease the cotton ball granuloma of rats, and alleviate foot swelling induced by formaldehyde and carrageenan arthritis in rats. Triterpene glycosides (glycyrrhizic acid, monoammonium glycyrrhizate, glycyrrheinic acid and its derivatives, etc.) and flavonoids (liquiritigenin, isoliquiritigenin, liquiritin, isoliquiritin, FM100, etc.) are the main active components. The anti-inflammation of *Gān cǎo* is related to its adrenal corticosteroid-like effects, which can reduce the expression of chemokines and pro-inflammatory cytokines, inhibit the activity of steroid-metabolizing enzymes.

8. 抗病原微生物　甘草次酸对结核分枝杆菌、大肠埃希菌、金黄色葡萄球菌、阿米巴原虫及阴道滴虫等有抑制作用。甘草酸、甘草皂苷、甘草黄酮等均有不同程度的抗人类免疫缺陷病毒（HIV）的作用，黄酮类成分最为明显。甘草酸、甘草次酸、甘草多糖对水疱性口腔病毒、牛痘病毒、带状疱疹病毒、腺病毒、单纯疱疹病毒、甲型流感病毒等均有抑制作用。

(8) Anti-bacteria and anti-virus　Glycyrrhetinic acid have inhibitory effects on *mycobacterium tuberculosis*, *escherichia coli*, *staphylococcus aureus*, amoeba and trichomonas vaginalis. Glycyrrhizin, *Gān cǎo* glycosides and *Gān cǎo* flavonoids can inhibit human immunodeficiency virus (HIV), and the effect of flavonoids is the best. Glycyrrhizic acid, glycyrrhetinic acid, and *Gān cǎo* polysaccharides have inhibitory effects on vesicular stomatitis virus, vaccinia virus, varicella-zoster virus, adenovirus, herpes simplex virus, influenza A virus.

9. 其他作用　甘草酸、甘草黄酮能降低高脂饲料喂养的动物血脂水平。甘草次酸可降低实验性动脉粥样硬化大鼠血清 TC 和 TG 及 β– 脂蛋白的水平。甘草还有抗肿瘤、抑制血小板聚集、抗氧化、抗抑郁等作用。

(9) Other effects　Glycyrrhizic acid and *Gān cǎo* flavonoids can reduce blood lipid levels in animals fed with high-fat diet. Glycyrrhetinic acid can reduce the level of serum TC, TG and β-lipoprotein in experimental atherosclerosis rats. *Gān cǎo* also has anti-tumor, inhibition of platelet aggregation, antioxidation and anti-depression effects.

【不良反应 / Adverse effects 】

患者长期大量服用甘草制剂，可出现肾上腺皮质功能亢进，表现为高血压、水肿、低血钾、头痛、眩晕、心悸等类醛固酮增多症。

Taking large dose of *Gān cǎo* for a long time may cause hypercortisolism, such as hypertension, oedema, hypokalemia, headache, dizziness, palpitations and other aldosteronism.

白术 ┊ *Bái zhú* (Rhizoma Atractylodis Macrocephalae)

【来源 / Origin】

本品为菊科植物白术（*Atractylodes macrocephala* Koidz.）的干燥根茎。冬季下部叶枯黄、上部叶变脆时采挖。

Bái zhú is the dried rhizome of *Atractylodes macrocephala* Koidz., family of Compositae. *Bái zhú* is excavated when the lower leaves are yellow and the upper leaves become brittle in winter.

【化学成分 / Chemical ingredients】

主要含有挥发油、内酯类、多糖等。挥发油主要包括苍术醇 (atractylol)、苍术酮（atratylon）等；内酯类主要包括白术内酯Ⅰ（atractylenolide Ⅰ）、白术内酯Ⅱ（atractylenolide Ⅱ）、白术内酯Ⅲ（atractylenolide Ⅲ）、8β-乙氧基白术内酯Ⅲ（8β-ethoxyactylenolide Ⅲ）等；多糖类主要包括白术多糖 PM、甘露聚糖 Am-3、果糖 (fructose)、菊糖（synanthrin）等。

Bái zhú mainly contains volatile oils, lactones, and polysaccharides. The volatile oils mainly include atractylol and atratylon. The lactones mainly include atractylenolide Ⅰ, atractylenolide Ⅱ, atractylenolide Ⅲ, and 8β-ethoxyactylenolide Ⅲ. The polysaccharides mainly include atractylodes polysaccharide PM, mannan Am-3, fructose, and synanthrin.

【药性与功效 / Chinese medicine properties】

味苦、甘，性温，归脾、胃经。具有健脾益气、燥湿利水、止汗、安胎的功效。用于治疗脾虚食少、泄泻、汗出、胎动不安等。

In Chinese medicine theory, *Bái zhú* has the nature of bitter, sweet and warm. It can enter the meridians of the spleen and stomach. *Bái zhú* can invigorate spleen and replenish Qi, dry dampness and induce diuresis, check sweating and prevent miscarriage. It is indicated for spleen deficiency and loss of appetite, diarrhea, spontaneous sweating, and threatened miscarriage.

【药理作用 / Pharmacological effects】

1. 对消化系统的影响

(1) Effects on digestive system

（1）调整胃肠运动　白术水煎液对家兔离体肠管活动的影响与肠管所处功能状态有关。白术可兴奋正常状态的肠管，也可兴奋肾上腺素致抑制状态的肠管，抑制受乙酰胆碱作用处于兴奋状态的肠管。白术水煎液可促进小鼠胃排空及小肠推进功能，推测其兴奋肠运动的作用主要是通过兴奋 M 胆碱能受体而产生的。白术挥发油可抑制肠管的自发运动，并可拮抗氯化钡的兴奋肠管作用，挥发油中的杜松脑拮抗乙酰胆碱的作用较强。

1) Regulating gastrointestinal motility　The effects of *Bái zhú* water decoction on the activity of isolated rabbit intestine are related to the functional state of the intestine. *Bái zhú* can stimulate the intestine in the normal state, as well as the intestine inhibited by adrenaline. However, it could inhibit the intestine that was stimulated by acetylcholine. *Bái zhú* water decoction could promote gastric emptying and intestinal propulsion in mice. The potential mechanism is related to the excitation of M-cholinergic receptor. The volatile oil of *Bái zhú* could inhibit the spontaneous movement of intestines and antagonize the excitatory effect of barium chloride, and the juniper in the volatile oil manifested strong anticholinergic properties.

（2）抗溃疡　白术丙酮提取物灌胃给药，对盐酸–乙醇所致大鼠胃黏膜损伤有抑制作用；经十二指肠给药对幽门结扎大鼠胃液分泌量有抑制作用，降低胃液酸度，减少胃酸及胃蛋白酶的排出量。

2) Anti-ulcer   When orally administered with acetone extract of *Bái zhú*, gastric mucosal injury induced by hydrochloric acid-ethanol could be alleviated in rats. When transduodenal administered, it could inhibit gastric juice secretion and reduce gastric juice acidity and gastric acid and pepsin excretion in pyloric ligation rats.

（3）抗肝损伤　白术水煎液可防治四氯化碳致小鼠肝损伤，减轻肝糖原减少以及肝细胞变性坏死，使升高的 ALT 下降。

3) Anti-liver injury   *Bái zhú* water decoction showed prevention effect on liver injury induced by carbon tetrachloride in mice. *Bái zhú* decoction could inhibit the reduction of liver glycogen and hepatocyte degeneration and necrosis, decrease the ALT levels.

2. 抑制子宫收缩　白术安胎的功效与其抑制子宫收缩作用有关。白术醇提物与石油醚提取物对未孕小鼠离体子宫的自发性收缩，缩宫素、益母草引起的子宫兴奋性收缩有抑制作用。白术醇提取物还能拮抗缩宫素引起豚鼠在体妊娠子宫的紧张性收缩。

(2) Inhibiting uterine contraction   The miscarriage prevention effect of *Bái zhú* was related to its inhibiting activity on uterine contraction. The alcohol extract and petroleum ether extract of *Bái zhú* could inhibit the spontaneous contraction of isolated uterus of non-pregnant mice, as well as the excitatory contraction of the uterus induced by oxytocin and motherwort. The alcohol extract of *Bái zhú* could also antagonize the tension contraction of pregnant guinea pig uterus induced by oxytocin.

3. 提高免疫功能　白术能显著增强白细胞吞噬金黄色葡萄球菌的能力。白术水煎剂可增加环磷酰胺致免疫功能低下小鼠外周血白细胞总数，提高巨噬细胞吞噬功能，减缓小鼠胸腺萎缩，促进溶血素生成，促进小鼠抗体产生和淋巴细胞转化，促进骨髓增殖，提高白细胞介素 –1 的表达。白术醇提物可提高氢化可的松和环磷酰胺致免疫低下小鼠的脾和胸腺指数、增强单核巨噬细胞的吞噬功能，增强迟发型超敏反应。白术挥发油可增强二硝基氯苯（DNCB）所致小鼠的迟发型超敏反应，提高小鼠腹腔巨噬细胞 EA 花环率，增强巨噬细胞的吞噬能力。白术多糖在一定的浓度范围内能单独激活或协同 Con A、PHA 促进正常小鼠淋巴细胞转化，并提高 IL-2 分泌的水平。

(3) Improving immune function   *Bái zhú* could obviously enhance the ability of leukocytes to engulf *Staphylococcus aureus*. *Bái zhú* decoction could increase the total number of leukocytes in peripheral blood of immunocompromised mice induced by cyclophosphamide. It could increase the phagocytic function of macrophages, slow down the thymus atrophy, promote the production of hemolysin, and promote the production of antibodies and lymphocyte transformation in mice. In addition, it could enhance the phagocytosis of macrophages and promote bone marrow proliferation and increase the expression of interleukin-1. The alcohol extract of *Bái zhú* could increase the spleen and thymus index and promote the phagocytosis of mononuclear phagocytes and enhance the delayed-type hypersensitivity in immunocompromised mice induced by hydrocortisone and cyclophosphamide. *Bái zhú* volatile oil could enhance the delayed-type hypersensitivity of mice induced by dinitrochlorobenzene (DNCB) and increase the EA rosette rate of peritoneal macrophages, and enhance the phagocytosis of macrophages. In a certain concentration range, the lymphocyte transformation could be activated by polysaccharide of *Bái zhú*.

4. 抗应激　白术具有抗疲劳和增强肾上腺皮质功能的作用。白术水煎液能增加体重，增强体力，延长游泳时间。

(4) Anti-stress   *Bái zhú* showed anti-fatigue and enhancing adrenocortical activities. *Bái zhú* decoction could increase body weight and enhance physical strength and prolong swimming time.

5. 抗氧化　白术可抑制脂质过氧化，降低组织脂质过氧化物的含量。白术水煎液可提高老龄小鼠全血 GSH-Px 的活力，降低红细胞中 MDA 含量。白术及白术多糖均能提高小鼠脑及肝的 SOD 活力，降低脑、肝 MDA 含量。白术多糖可提高 D–半乳糖致衰老大鼠大脑皮质神经细胞抗氧化物酶的活性，降低自由基代谢产物的含量，减少 DNA 损伤，具有一定的抗衰老作用。白术可预防运动应激性胃溃疡，保护机制可能与降低大鼠胃组织中自由基含量、增强 SOD 活性和提高 HSP70 的表达有关。

(5) Anti-oxidation *Bái zhú* could inhibit lipid peroxidation and reduce the content of lipid peroxides in tissues. *Bái zhú* decoction could increase the activity of GSH-Px in whole blood of aged mice and decrease the content of MDA in erythrocytes. Both *Bái zhú* and *Bái zhú* polysaccharides could increase the SOD activity of brain and liver and decrease the content of MDA in brain and liver. *Bái zhú* polysaccharide could increase the activity of antioxidant enzymes and reduce the content of free radical metabolites and reduce DNA damage in cerebral cortical neurons of aging rats induced by D-galactose, which related to its anti-aging effect. *Bái zhú* could prevent gastric ulcer induced by stress. The protective mechanism of *Bái zhú* might be related to reducing the content of free radicals, increasing the activity of SOD and increasing the expression of HSP70 in gastric tissue of rats.

6. 抗肿瘤 白术水煎液、白术挥发油乳剂可抑制小鼠肉瘤 S_{180}，促进肿瘤细胞凋亡及坏死，降低小鼠肉瘤 S_{180} 凋亡相关基因 *Bcl-2* 的表达，抑制 Lewis 肺癌小鼠肿瘤生长，延长 H_{22} 肝癌小鼠平均生存天数。白术挥发油能明显阻止癌性恶病质鼠体重下降，增加其摄食量，延缓肿瘤生长。

(6) Anti-tumor *Bái zhú* decoction and *Bái zhú* volatile oil emulsion could inhibit sarcoma S_{180} in mice and promote tumor cell apoptosis and necrosis. *Bái zhú* decoction and *Bái zhú* volatile oil emulsion could reduce the expression of apoptosis-related gene *Bcl-2* in sarcoma S_{180} and inhibit tumor growth in Lewis lung cancer mice, and prolong the average survival time of H_{22} hepatoma mice. *Bái zhú* volatile oil could obviously prevent the weight loss of cancerous cachexia mice, and increase the food intake and delay tumor growth.

7. 抗肝损伤 白术多糖可降低自体移植肝脏缺血再灌注大鼠血清 ALT 和 AST、总胆红素、直接胆红素和 MDA 含量，提高 SOD 活性，减轻肝脏病理损伤。白术内酯 I 可降低卡介苗联合脂多糖致免疫性肝损伤小鼠的肝、脾指数，改善肝组织病理学变化，降低血清 ALT 和 AST 含量。

(7) Anti-liver injury *Bái zhú* polysaccharide could reduce the contents of serum alanine aminotransferase, aspartate aminotransferase, total bilirubin, direct bilirubin and MDA in liver autotransplantation ischemia-reperfusion rat. It could also increase the activity of SOD and reduce the pathological injury of liver. Atractylodes I could reduce the liver and spleen index of mice with immune liver injury induced by BCG combined with lipopolysaccharide and improve the pathological damage of liver tissue, and reduce the contents of ALT and AST in serum.

8. 其他作用 白术可促进红系造血祖细胞生成。白术及白术多糖均能提高小鼠学习记忆能力。白术内酯类化合物可抑制二甲苯致小鼠耳肿胀。

(8) Other effects *Bái zhú* could promote the formation of erythroid hematopoietic progenitors. Both *Bái zhú* and its polysaccharide could improve the abilities of learning and memory in mice. Atractylodes could inhibit xylene-induced ear swelling in mice.

当归 ┆ *Dāng guī (Radix Angelicae Sinensis)*

【来源 / Origin】

本品为伞形科植物当归 [*Angelica sinensis* (Oliv.) Diels] 的干燥根。主要分布于甘肃、陕西、四川、云南、湖北等地。秋末采挖，除尽芦头、须根，用微火熏干或硫黄烟熏，切片生用，或经酒拌、酒炒用。

Dāng guī is the dried root of *Angelica sinensis* (Oliv.) Diels, family of Umbelliferae. It is widely cultivated in Gansu province, Shaanxi province, Sichuan province, Yunnan province and Hubei province, etc. and harvested in late autumn. It is dried with slight fire or sulfur after removing the basel part of the stem and fibrous root. Slices are directly used for Chinese medicinal preparation or fried with wine for application.

【化学成分 / Chemical ingredients】

主要含有挥发油，以藁本内酯（ligustilide）为主，还有正丁烯酰内酯（n-butylidene phthalide）、当归酮、月桂烯等。此外，尚含有阿魏酸（ferulic acid）、琥珀酸（succinic acid）等有机酸，以及多糖、维生素、氨基酸及无机元素等。

Dāng guī mainly contains volatile oils, including ligustilide, n-butylidene phthalide, angelic ketone, myrcene, etc. The others are ferulic acid, succinic acid, polysaccharide, vitamins, amino acid, inorganic elements, etc.

【药性与功效 / Chinese medicine properties】

味甘、辛，性温，归肝、心、脾经。具有补血活血、调经止痛、润肠通便的功效。主治血虚萎黄、心悸失眠、月经不调、经闭痛经、虚寒腹痛、风寒痹痛、跌打损伤、痈疽疮疡等证。

In Chinese medicine theory, *Dāng guī* has the nature of sweet, pungent and warm. It can enter the meridians of liver, heart and spleen. *Dāng guī* can tonify blood and activate blood, regulate menstruation and relieve pain, moisten intestines to relieve constipation. Clinically it can be used for blood deficiency and shallow yellow, palpitation, insomnia, menstrual irregularities, amenorrhea, dysmenorrheal, abdomen pain due to deficiency-cold, numbness and pain due to wind-cold, traumatic injury, carbuncle and ulcer, etc.

【药理作用 / Pharmacological effects】

1. 对血液系统的影响

(1) Effects on hematologic system

（1）促进造血功能　当归能升高外周血红细胞、白细胞数量和血红蛋白含量，当化疗药物、射线照射引起外周血细胞减少和骨髓造血功能抑制时，其作用更明显。当归多糖是其促进造血功能的主要药效物质基础。当归多糖皮下注射能提高苯肼和 ^{60}Co-γ 射线诱导的贫血小鼠的粒单系祖细胞和晚期红系祖细胞的生成率。当归多糖不能降低骨髓造血细胞对射线的敏感性，但能提升射线照射致贫血小鼠造血功能的恢复速度。

1) Promoting hematopoietic function　*Dāng guī* can increase the number of red blood cells, white blood cells and hemoglobin content, This effect is more obvious when chemotherapy drugs and radiation exposure cause peripheral blood cell reduction and inhibit marrow hematopoietic function. Olysaccharides form *Dāng guī* are one of the main effective components in promoting hematopoietic function. The subcutaneous injection of polysaccharide from *Dāng guī* can promote the production rate of granulocyte-monocyte and late-stage erythroid progenitor cells in anemic mice induced by phenylhydrazine and ^{60}Co-γ ray. Polysaccharides from *Dāng guī* can not inhibit the sensitivity of bone marrow hematopoietic cells to radiation, but can promote the recovery of hematopoietic function in anemic mice induced by radiation exposure.

（2）抗凝血、抑制血小板聚集及抗血栓形成　当归水煎液能延长大鼠血浆凝血酶时间及凝血活酶时间。当归能改善脑血栓患者血液流变学特性，降低血液黏度和血浆纤维蛋白原含量，缩短红细胞及血小板电泳时间，延长凝血酶原时间。静脉注射阿魏酸钠可抑制 ADP、胶原及凝血酶诱导的血小板聚集。阿魏酸钠抑制血小板聚集作用与其抑制血小板释放反应，升高血小板内 cAMP/cGMP 比值，以及抑制血小板膜磷脂酰肌醇磷酸化过程等环节有关。当归注射液和阿魏酸钠还能调节 PGI_2/TXA_2 平衡而抑制血小板聚集。当归和阿魏酸钠能抑制大鼠动静脉旁路血栓的形成，减轻血栓重量。当归抗血栓形成作用于其抗凝血、抑制血小板聚集、增加纤溶酶活性、改善血液流变学及微血管状态等有关。

2) Anti-coagulation, anti-paltelet aggregation and anti-thrombosis　*Dāng guī* decoction can prolong the thrombin time and thromboplatin time. *Dāng guī* can improve the hemorheological characteristics of patients with cerebral thrombosis, reduce the blood viscosity and plasma fibrinogen content, shorten the electrophoresis time of red blood cells and platelets, and prolong the prothrombin time. Intravenous injection of sodium ferulate can inhibit platelet aggregation induced by ADP, collagen or thrombin. The inhibition of platelet aggregation by sodium ferulate is related to the inhibition of platelet release, the increase of cAMP/cGMP ratio and the inhibition of phosphatidylinositol phosphorylation. *Dāng guī* injection and sodium ferulate can also inhibit platelet aggregation by regulating the balance of PGI_2/TXA_2. *Dāng guī* and ferulic acid sodium can inhibit the formation of arterio-venous loop thrombus in rats and reduce the weight of thrombus. The related mechanisms of anti-thrombotic effect of *Dāng guī* include: anticoagulation, inhibition of platelet aggregation, increase of fibrinolytic enzyme activity, improvement of hemorheology and microvascular state.

（3）降血脂、抗动脉粥样硬化　当归注射液可降低高脂饲料饲养的家兔血中甘油三酯水平，减少主动脉斑块面积和血清 MDA 含量。阿魏酸可降低高脂血症大鼠血清胆固醇水平，对 TG 和磷脂水平无明显影响，其降低胆固醇的作用机制与抑制肝脏合成胆固醇的限速酶甲羟戊酸 –5– 焦磷酸脱羧酶（MDD），减少肝脏内胆固醇的合成，进而降低血浆胆固醇含量有关。降低血脂和抗氧化减少血管内皮损伤是当归抗动脉粥样硬化的主要作用机制。

3) Reducing blood lipid and anti-atherosclerosis　*Dāng guī* injection can reduce the level of TG in blood, the area of aortic plaque and the content of MDA in serum of hyperlipidaemia rabbits. Ferulic acid can reduce the serum cholesterol level of hyperlipidemia rats, but has no significant effect on TG and phospholipid level. Ferulic acid inhibit the mevalonate-5-pyrophosphate decarboxylase (rat-limiting enzyme for synthesis of cholesterol) activity, lead to reduce the synthesis of cholesterol in the liver, and then reduce the content of plasma cholesterol. Reducing blood lipid, antioxidation and alleviating vascular endothelial damage are involved in anti- atherosclerosis of *Dāng guī*.

2. 对心血管系统的影响

(2) Effects on cardiovascular system

（1）抗心肌缺血　当归挥发油、阿魏酸能拮抗垂体后叶素引起的小鼠急性心肌缺血损伤。静脉滴注当归注射液可缩小结扎冠状动脉左前降支引起的犬急性心肌梗死的梗死区面积，改善缺血性心电图。离体大鼠心脏缺血再灌注研究显示，当归水煎液及阿魏酸钠能明显减轻心肌超微结构损伤，改善心功能。

1) Anti-myocardial ischemia　*Dāng guī* volatile oils and ferulic acid can resist acute myocardial ischemia injury in mice caused by pituitrin. Intravenous infusion of *Dāng guī* injection can reduce the infarct area of acute myocardial infarction and ischemic electrocardiogram (ECG) of dogs induced by ligation of left anterior descending branch of coronary artery. *Dāng guī* decoction and ferulic acid sodium can significantly alleviate the damage of myocardial ultrastructure and improve the cardiac function of isolated rat heart after ischemia-reperfusion.

（2）抗心律失常　当归水提物、乙醇提取物可拮抗强心苷、肾上腺素和 $BaCl_2$ 等诱发的动物心律失常。当归醇提液静脉注射可预防乌头碱诱发的大鼠心律失常。当归注射液腹腔注射对大鼠心肌缺血再灌注引发的心律失常有保护作用。当归总酸对氯仿–肾上腺素、乌头碱、$BaCl_2$等诱发的动物心律失常有保护作用。

2) Anti-arrhythmia *Dāng guī* water extract and ethanol extract can antagonize the arrhythmia induced by cardiac glycoside, adrenaline or $BaCl_2$. Intravenous injection of *Dāng guī* alcohol extract can prevent aconitine-induced arrhythmia in rats. *Dāng guī* injection can alleviate the arrhythmia induced by myocardial ischemia-reperfusion in rats. Total organic acid of *Dāng guī* has protective effect against the arrhythmia induced by chloroform, adrenaline, aconitine, or $BaCl_2$, etc.

（3）扩张血管 当归对外周血管、冠状血管、脑血管及肺血管均有扩张作用，能降低血管阻力，降低血压，增加血流量。给麻醉犬股静脉注射当归注射液，可增加股动脉血流量，大剂量能对抗去甲肾上腺素引起的血管痉挛及血流量减少。当归挥发油、藁苯内酯、正丁烯酞内酯及阿魏酸钠是其扩张血管作用的重要活性成分。

3) Vasodilation *Dāng guī* can dilate peripheral vessels, coronary vessels, cerebral vessels and pulmonary vessels, reduce vascular resistance and blood pressure, and increase blood flow. *Dāng guī* injection can increase the blood flow of femoral artery in anesthetized dogs. High dose of *Dāng guī* injection can resist the vasospasm and decrease of blood flow caused by noradrenaline. The volatile oil of *Dāng guī*, ligustilide, butylene lactone and sodium ferulate are the important active components of vasodilation.

3. 对子宫平滑肌的影响 当归挥发油类成分能抑制肾上腺素、垂体后叶素或组胺引起的多种动物离体子宫平滑肌收缩，当归水溶性或醇溶性成分则可引起多种在体动物或离体动物及人的子宫平滑肌收缩增强、张力增高或节律加快，产生兴奋作用。当归对在体子宫平滑肌的作用与其所处状态有关。当归可通过抑制子宫平滑肌的收缩而缓解痛经，也可通过兴奋子宫平滑肌减轻伴有子宫收缩不全的出血。

(3) Effects on uterine smooth muscle The volatile oils of *Dāng guī* can inhibit the contraction of uterine smooth muscle isolated from normal and different stage of pregnancy animals induced by adrenaline, pituitrin or histamine. However, the water-soluble or alcohol-soluble components of *Dāng guī* can enhance the contraction, tension or rhythm of the smooth muscle of uterus of various animals *in vivo* or *in vitro*. *Dāng guī* has different regulating effect on uterine smooth muscle according to the its functional state. *Dāng guī* can relieve dysmenorrhea by inhibiting the contraction of uterine smooth muscle, also it can improve metrorrhagia accompanied by incomplete uterine contraction by exciting the uterine smooth muscle.

4. 增强机体免疫功能 当归、当归多糖及阿魏酸钠静脉注射均能提高单核细胞对刚果红的廓清率。当归多糖能提高单核巨噬细胞的吞噬功能，对抗环磷酰胺对小鼠腹腔巨噬细胞功能的抑制。当归多糖腹腔注射还可对抗皮质激素所致的小鼠免疫抑制，增加胸腺和脾脏重量，对抗外周血中白细胞数量下降。

(4) Enhancing immune function Intravenous injection of *Dāng guī*, *Dāng guī* polysaccharide and sodium ferulate can increase the clearance rate of monocyte to Congo red. *Dāng guī* polysaccharide can increase the phagocytosis of monocyte macrophage to resist the inhibition of cyclophosphamide. The intraperitoneal injection of *Dāng guī* polysaccharide also antagonized the corticosteroids-induced immunosuppression, which increase the weight of thymus and spleen, and inhibit reduction of leukocytes in peripheral blood.

小鼠皮下注射当归多糖可提高 E 花环形成率及 α– 醋酸萘酯酶染色阳性率。当归多糖能促进

Con A 活化的小鼠胸腺细胞增殖，直接激活参与抗体反应的 T 淋巴细胞，明显促进牛血清蛋白诱导小鼠产生迟发型超敏反应。当归水煎液能促进小鼠绵羊红细胞抗体溶血素 IgM 的产生。当归多糖腹腔注射还能增加溶血空斑形成细胞数，增加 IgM 数量。

Subcutaneous injection of *Dāng guī* polysaccharide can increase the formation rate of E-rosette and the positive rate of α-naphthylacetase staining. *Dāng guī* polysaccharide can promote the proliferation of mouse thymocytes activated by Con A, directly activate T lymphocytes involved in antibody response, and obviously promote the delayed-type hypersensitivity induced by bovine serum protein. *Dāng guī* decoction can promote the production of IgM in serum of mice immunized with sheep erythrocytes. Intraperitoneal injection of *Dāng guī* polysaccharide can also increase the number of haemolytic plaque forming cells and IgM level.

5. 抗炎、镇痛　当归水煎液对多种致炎剂引起的急、慢性炎症有抑制作用，对大鼠摘除双侧肾上腺后仍有抗炎作用，但不能拮抗组胺的致炎作用。当归水煎液和乙酸乙酯提取物均能降低冰醋酸引起的小鼠扭体反应，提高小鼠热板致痛的痛阈，镇痛作用维持时间长，但镇痛作用不如吗啡。

(5) Anti-inflammation and analgesia　*Dāng guī* decoction can inhibit acute and chronic inflammation caused by a variety of inflammatory agents (formadehyde, croton oil, cotton ball, etc.). It still has anti-inflammation after bilateral adrenalectomy, but it can't antagnize the histamine-induce inflammation. The *Dāng guī* decoction and the ethyl acetate extract can reduce the writhing response of mice induced by acetic acid, increase the pain threshold of mice caused by hot plate. The analgesic effect of *Dāng guī* can maintain for a long time, but it is not as good as analgesic effect of morphine.

6. 其他作用　当归还有保肝、抗损伤等作用。

(6) Other effects　*Dāng guī* has the effects of hepatoprotection, anti-radiation damage, etc.

【不良反应 / Adverse effects】

当归注射液静脉滴注可引起过敏反应。

infusion of *Dāng guī* injection can cause allergic reaction.

何首乌 ⋮ *Hé shǒu wū (Radix Polygoni Multiflori)*

【来源 / Origin】

本品为蓼科植物何首乌（*Polygonum multiflorum* Thunb.）的块根。主产于陕西南部、甘肃南部、华东、华中、华南、四川、云南及贵州等地。秋后茎叶枯萎后或次年发芽前采收其块根，去两端，切片，晒干为生首乌；如用黑豆煮汁拌蒸，晒后为黑色，为制首乌。

Hé shǒu wū is the dried root of *Polygonum multiflorum* Thunb., family of Polygonaceae. It is widely cultivated in south of Shaanxi province and Gansu province, Sichuan province, Yunnan province, and Guizhou province, etc., and harvested when the stem and leaf withered after autumn or before germination next year. It is dried and sliced after removing the ends, which is called *Fresh shǒu wū*. If steamed with black bean sauce, it will be black after drying, which is called *Processed shǒu wū*.

【化学成分 / Chemical ingredients】

主要含有磷脂、蒽醌类、葡糖糖苷类化合物。磷脂主要为卵磷脂，蒽醌类以大黄酚和大黄素含量最多，葡糖糖苷类主要为二苯乙烯苷（2,3,5,4′-tetrahydroxystilbene-2-O-β-D-glucoside)。还含有 β–谷甾醇、没食子酸及多种微量元素等。

Hé shǒu wū mainly contains phospholipids, anthraquinones and glucosides. Phospholipids are mainly lecithin. Anthraquinones main include chrysophanol, emodin, physcion and rhein, etc., chrysophanol and emodin are the most abundant ingredients. The main glusoside is 2,3,5,4′-tetrahydroxystilbene-2-O-β-D-glucoside (stilbene glycoside). The others are β-sitosterol, gallic acid, and trace elements, etc.

【药性与功效 / Chinese medicine properties】

味苦、甘、涩，性微温，归肝、肾经。生首乌具有解毒、截疟、润肠通便之功效，主治瘰疬疮痈、皮肤瘙痒、血虚肠燥便秘等证；制首乌具有补肝肾、益精血、强筋骨、乌须发的功效，主治血虚萎黄、失眠健忘、腰酸足软、须发早白、头晕目眩、耳鸣耳聋、遗精、崩漏带下等证。

In Chinese medicine theory, *Hé shǒu wū* has the nature of bitter, sweet, astringent and slightly warm. It can enter the meridians of liver and kidney. *Fresh shǒu wū* can remove toxin, prevent malaria, moisten intestines to relieve constipation. Clinically it can be used for scrofula, carbuncle, constipation and intestinal dryness due to blood deficiency, etc. *Processed shǒu wū* can tonify liver and kidney, replenish essence and blood, strengthen sinew and bone, make the hair and beard black. Clinically it can be used for blood deficiency and shallow yellow, insomnia and amnesia, soreness in waist and knee, white beard and hair, dizziness and blurred vision, tinnitus, deafness, seminal emission, metrorrhagia and metrostaxis, leukorrhea, etc.

【药理作用 / Pharmacological effects】

1. 延缓衰老　何首乌能延长老年鹌鹑半数死亡时间和果蝇的平均寿命，延迟大鼠二倍体皮肤成纤维细胞的老化。何首乌能明显增强老年小鼠脑和肝组织中 SOD 活性，降低 MDA 含量，增加脑内单胺类神经递质 5– 羟色胺（5-HT）、去甲肾上腺素（NE）、多巴胺（DA）水平，抑制 MAO-B 活性。何首乌乙醇浸膏可以提高老年大鼠外周淋巴细胞 DNA 损伤的修复能力。

(1) Delay-aging　*Hé shǒu wū* can prolong median dead time of old quail and the mean life-span of fruit fly, and postpone the aging of diploid fibroblasts of rat skin. *Hé shǒu wū* can obviously enhance SOD activity in brain and liver, reduce MDA content, increase monoamine neurotransmitter (5-HT, NE, DA) level in brain, and inhibit MAO-B activity in the brain of aged mice. Ethanol extract of *Hé shǒu wū* can improve the DNA repairment of peripheral lymphocytes in aged rats.

2. 改善学习记忆　何首乌浸膏及何首乌多糖、二苯乙烯苷能改善 D– 半乳糖、Aβ$_{1-40}$ 诱导痴呆模型动物的学习记忆能力，与降低突触体内 Ca^{2+} 浓度、提高海马区神经元线粒体功能有关。二苯乙烯苷还能减少 SAMP8 鼠脑内 β 淀粉样蛋白前体（APP）和早老蛋白（PS-1）的表达，促进 ACh 合成并减少乙酰胆碱的分解，促进单胺类神经递质的合成，提高学习记忆能力。

(2) Learning and memory improvement　*Hé shǒu wū* extract, polysaccharide, protein and stilbene glycoside can improve the learning and memory ability of dementia model animals induced by D-galactose or Aβ$_{1-40}$, which is related to the decrease of Ca^{2+} concentration in synapse and the improvement of mitochondrial function of hippocampal neurons. Stilbene glycoside can also decrease the expression of APP and PS-1, promote the synthesis of ACh, reduce the decomposition of ACh, and promote the synthesis of monoamine neurotransmitters in the brain, improve the learning and memory ability of SAMP8 mice.

3. 降血脂、抗动脉粥样硬化　何首乌水提取物、何首乌多糖及二苯乙烯苷等能降低高脂血症大鼠血清 TC 和 TG 含量，提高 HDL-C/TC 比值。二苯乙烯苷还可以抑制细胞内 TC 的合成，升高低密度脂蛋白受体的表达。何首乌降脂的作用机制主要如下。①何首乌多糖、二苯乙烯苷、蒽醌类成分可以抑制脂肪酶活性。②何首乌能与胆固醇结合形成不易吸收的大分子聚合物，减少胆固醇的吸收；蒽醌类物质可以加速胆汁酸从肠道中排出。③二苯乙烯苷通过调节 3– 羟基 –3– 甲基戊二酰辅酶 A 还原酶 (HMG-CoA) 及 7α– 羟化酶的活性，抑制内源性胆固醇的合成。

(3) Reducing blood lipid and anti-atherosclerosis　*Hé shǒu wū* water extract, polysaccharide and stilbene glycoside can reduce the content of serum TC and TG, increase the ratio of HDL-C/TC in hyperlipidemic rats. Stilbene glycoside can also inhibit the synthesis of TC and increase the expression of LDL receptor in Bel-7402 cells. The mechanisms for reducing blood lipid of *Hé shǒu wū* are as follows. ①Polysaccharide, stilbene glycoside and anthraquinones can inhibit the activity of lipase. ②*Hé shǒu wū* can combine with cholesterol to form macromolecular polymer which reduce cholesterol absorption; anthraquinones can accelerate bile acid excretion from intestine. ③Stilbene glycoside inhibit the synthesis of endogenous cholesterol by regulating the activity of 3-hydroxy-3-methylglutaryl CoA (HMG-CoA) reductase and 7 α-hydroxylase.

何首乌总苷可以通过降低 ApoE-/- 小鼠主动脉壁细胞间黏附分子（ICAM-1）与血管细胞黏附分子（VCAM-1）的表达，抑制 ApoE-/- 小鼠主动脉壁粥样斑块的形成，与其降血脂、抗炎、抗氧化、抑制血管平滑肌细胞增殖与迁移有关。

Hé shǒu wū total glycosides can inhibit the formation of atherosclerotic plaques on the aortic wall of ApoE-/-mice by reducing the expression of ICAM-1 and VCAM-1, which is associated with reducing blood lipid, anti-inflammation, anti-oxidation, and inhibiting the proliferation and migration of vascular smooth muscle cells.

4. 增强免疫系统功能　何首乌煎剂能增加正常小鼠胸腺重量，也能对抗免疫抑制剂泼尼松龙和环磷酰胺引起的老年小鼠脾、胸腺萎缩，提高脾巨噬细胞的吞噬率和吞噬指数。何首乌水煎醇提物皮下注射能增强正常小鼠脾脏抗体形成数，也能增强 Con A 诱导的小鼠胸腺和脾脏 T 淋巴细胞、B 淋巴细胞免疫功能，对 T 淋巴细胞的作用更为显著。何首乌多糖、蒽醌苷是其增强免疫功能的主要活性成分。

(4) Enhancing immune system function　The *Hé shǒu wū* decoction can increase the weight of thymus of normal mice. It also can resist the atrophy of spleen and thymus, increase the phagocytic ratio and phagocytic index of spleen macrophage of aged mice caused by immunosuppressant prednisolone and cyclophosphamide. Subcutaneous injection of *Hé shǒu wū* extract can enhance the number of antibody formation in the spleen of normal mice. *Hé shǒu wū* extract also can promote the immune function of T and B lymphocytes in the thymus and spleen of mice induced by Con A, and the immune function of T lymphocytes is more sensitive to *Hé shǒu wū* extract. Polysaccharides and anthraquinone glycosides are the main active components for the immune enhancement of *Hé shǒu wū*.

5. 影响血液系统　何首乌提取液腹腔注射可以增加小鼠骨髓造血干细胞、粒单系祖细胞和红系祖母细胞数量，增加外周血网织红细胞比例。

(5) Effects on hematological system　Intraperitoneal injection of *Hé shǒu wū* extract can increase the number of bone marrow hematopoietic stem cells, progenitors of granulocyte and macrophages (CFU-GM) and progenitor of erythroid (CFU-E and BFU-E). It can also elevate the percentage of reticulocytes in peripheral blood.

6. 抗炎、镇痛　何首乌乙醇提取物能抑制二甲苯致小鼠耳肿胀和角叉菜胶致大鼠足肿胀，降低醋酸引起的小鼠腹腔毛细血管通透性，大剂量能减轻醋酸引起的小鼠扭体反应，具有一定的抗炎镇痛作用。

(6) Anti-inflammation and analgesia　The ethanol extract of *Hé shǒu wū* can inhibit xylene-induced the ear swelling of mice and carrageenan-induced the paw edema of rats. It also reduce the permeability of capillaries in abdomen of mice caused by acetic acid, and the high dose of *Hé shǒu wū* extract can decrease the writing response of mice induced by acetic acid. These effects indicate *Hé shǒu wū* has anti-inflammatory and analgesic effects.

7. 促进肠管运动 何首乌生用，其所含蒽醌类成分如大黄酚、大黄素能促进小鼠肠平滑肌运动，具有润肠通便作用。

(7) Promoting intestines movement *Fresh shǒu wū* can promote the smooth muscle movement of mouse intestine because it contain anthraquinones such as chrysophanol and rhubarb, indicating it can moisten intestines to relieve constipation.

8. 抗骨质疏松 何首乌水提液能减少去势小鼠的骨胶原、骨钙、骨磷的流失，增加骨碱性磷酸酶水平。何首乌乙醇提取液能减轻糖皮质激素诱导的骨质疏松大鼠的骨微结构的恶化，增加骨密度。二苯乙烯苷也有抗骨质疏松的作用。

(8) Anti-osteoporotic effect The water extract of *Hé shǒu wū* can promote the activity of bone alkaline phosphatase, inhibit the loss of organic and mineral content in the bone, and improve bone morphological features of osteoporotic femur in ovariectomied rat. The ethanol extract of *Hé shǒu wū* can inhibit the deterioration of femoral microstructure in osteoporotic rats induced by prednisone, and increase bone mineral density. Stilbene glycoside also has anti-osteoporosis effect.

9. 其他作用 何首乌具有肾上腺皮质激素样作用，可提高摘除双侧肾上腺小鼠的抗应激能力。此外，何首乌还具有抗肿瘤、抗诱变、抗氧化、减慢心率、扩张冠状动脉、抗心肌缺血等作用。

(9) Other effects *Hé shǒu wū* has adrenocortical hormone-like effects which can enhance the anti-stress ability of mice with bilateral adrenalectomy. In addition, *Hé shǒu wū* has anti-tumor, anti mutation, anti-oxidation, decreasing heart rate, relaxing coronary artery, anti-myocardial ischemia effects.

【不良反应 / Adverse effects】

部分患者服用何首乌后出现大便稀薄或伴有腹痛、恶心呕吐等消化道反应。个别患者服用大量何首乌后出现肢体麻木感、皮疹等。长期大剂量服用何首乌可引起肝肾毒性，与服用时间和剂量、所含蒽醌类成分、炮制方法及特异性体质等有关。

Hé shǒu wū causes gastrointestinal responses, such as thin stool, abdominal pain, nausea and vomiting in some patients. Taking high dose of *Hé shǒu wū* causes rash and numbness of limb in individuals. *Hé shǒu wū* can cause the hepatotoxicity, which is related to the time and dose of administration, the anthraquinones, the processing method and idiosyncrasy.

熟地黄 ┊ *Shú dì huáng (Radix Rehmanniae Preparata)*

【来源 / Origin】

本品为玄参科植物地黄（*Rehmannia glutinaosa* Libosch.）的干燥块根经炮制而成。地黄主要分布于辽宁、河北、河南、山东、山西、陕西、甘肃、内蒙古、江苏、湖北等省区。通常与酒、陈皮、砂仁等辅料一起反复蒸晒至内外色黑油润。切片或炒炭用。

Dì huáng is the dried root of *Rehmannia glutinosa* Libosch., family of Scrophulariaceae. It is widely cultivated in Liaoning province, Hebei province, Henan province, Shandong province, Shanxi province, Shaanxi province, Gansu province, Inner Mongolia Autonomous region, Jiangsu province and Hubei province, etc., and harvested in autumn. It is usually repeatedly steamed with wine, *Citri Reticulatae Pericarpium*, or *Amomi Fructus* until it is black and oily moisten inside and outside, which is called *Shú dì huáng*. Slice is directly used or fried into charcoal for Chinese medicinal preparation.

【化学成分 / Chemical ingredients】

主要含梓醇（catalpol）、地黄素（rehmannin）、桃叶珊瑚苷（aucubin）、地黄苷（rehmannioside）A~D、益母草苷（leonuride）等，此外，尚含有单糖、低聚糖、多糖、氨基酸及微量元素等。与生地黄比较，熟地黄所含单糖量增加，而梓醇含量减少。

Shú dì huáng mainly contains catalpol, rehmannin, aucubin, rehmannioside A, B, C, D, leonuride, etc. The others are monosaccharides, oligosaccharides, polysaccharides, amino acid and trace elements, etc. Compared with *Dì huáng*, the content of monosaccharides is increased while the content of catalpol is decreased in *Shú dì huáng*.

【药性与功效 / Chinese medicine properties】

味甘，性微温，归肝、肾经。具有滋阴补血、益精填髓之功效。主治肝肾阴虚、腰膝酸软、骨蒸潮热、遗精盗汗、内热消渴、血虚萎黄、心悸怔忡、月经不调、崩漏下血、眩晕、耳鸣、须发早白等证。

In Chinese medicine theory, *Shú dì huáng* has the nature of sweet, and slightly warm. It can enter the meridians of live and kidney. *Shú dì huáng* can nourish Yin and blood, supplement essence and replenish marrow. Clinically it can be used for liver-kidney Yin deficiency, soreness in waist and knee, steaming bone fever, seminal emission, night sweat, consumptive thirst due to interior heat, blood deficiency and shallow yellow, palpitation, menstrual irregularities, metrorrhagia and metrostaxis, dizziness, tinnitus, white beard and hair, etc.

【药理作用 / Pharmacological effects】

1. 增强免疫功能 熟地黄可增强猕猴细胞免疫功能。熟地黄醚提物能对抗氢化可的松引起的小鼠血中 T 淋巴细胞减少。地黄多糖能提高正常小鼠 T 淋巴细胞增殖能力，促进 IL-2 分泌，呈免疫增强作用。

(1) Regulating immune system function *Shú dì huáng* can enhance the cellular immune function of macaque. The ether extract of *Shú dì huáng* can reverse the inhibition of T lymphocyte in the blood of mice caused by hydrocortisone. Polysaccharide of *Shú dì huáng* can increase the proliferation of T lymphocytes of normal mice, promote the secretion of IL-2 *in vitro* and *in vivo*, and which enhance immune function.

2. 降血糖 地黄低聚糖腹腔注射可降低四氧嘧啶型糖尿病大鼠血糖水平，增加肝糖原含量。地黄低聚糖对正常大鼠血糖无明显影响，但可部分预防葡萄糖及肾上腺素引起的高血糖。

(2) Reducing blood glucose The intraperitoneal injection of *Dì huáng* oligosaccharide can reduce the blood glucose level and increase the content of glycogen in the liver of diabetic rats induced by tetraoxypyrimidine. *Dì huáng* oligosaccharide has no obvious effect on blood glucose of normal rats, but it can partly prevent hyperglycemia caused by glucose and adrenaline.

3. 促进造血功能 地黄多糖腹腔注射可促进正常小鼠骨髓造血干细胞增殖，粒单系祖细胞集落形成和早、晚期红系祖细胞的增殖分化。给予放血加环磷酰胺诱导的气血双虚小鼠熟地黄多糖灌胃，可以提高小鼠外周血红细胞、白细胞、血小板、血红蛋白含量及血清粒-巨噬细胞集落因子含量。

(3) Promoting hematopoietic function The intraperitoneal injection of *Dì huáng* polysaccharide can promote the proliferation of hematopoietic stem cells, the formation of granulocyte progenitor cells and the proliferation and differentiation at early and late stage of erythroid progenitor cells in normal mice. Oral administration of *Shú dì huáng* polysaccharide can increase the content of red blood cells, white blood cells, platelets, hemoglobin and serum granulocyte macrophage colony factor in Qi-blood deficiency mice induced by bleeding and cyclophosphamide.

4. 抗甲状腺 熟地黄水煎剂可降低 T_3 所致甲亢型阴虚模型大鼠血浆中 T_3 水平，明显减少饮水量及尿量，缓解体重减轻。

(4) Anti-thyroid function *Shú dì huáng* decoction can decrease T_3 level in the plasma, reduce amount of drink and urine, and alleviate the weight loss of Yin deficiency model rats with hyperthyroidism caused by T_3.

5. **抗氧化** 熟地黄水提液能提高小鼠红细胞膜 Na^+-K^+-ATP 酶活性，降低心肌脂质过氧化物含量，提高 GSH-Px 的活性。熟地黄多糖可提高 D– 半乳糖诱发的亚急性衰老模型血 SOD、过氧化氢酶（CAT）及 GSH-Px 活性，降低血浆、脑匀浆及肝匀浆 LPO 水平。

(5) Anti-oxidation The water extract of *Shú dì huáng* can increase the Na^+-K^+- ATPase activity of erythrocyte membrane, decrease the content of LPO and increase the activity of GSH- Px in myocardium of mice. *Shú dì huáng* polysaccharide can increase the activities of SOD, CAT and GSH-Px in the plasma and decrease the LPO level in plasma, brain homogenate and liver homogenate of aged model mice induced by D-galactose.

6. **改善学习记忆** 熟地黄水煎液可以改善 $AlCl_3$ 和谷氨酸单钠毁损下丘脑弓状核大鼠的学习记忆能力，能延长大鼠跳台潜伏期、减少错误次数，缩短水迷宫实验寻台时间。熟地黄改善学习记忆作用与调节动物脑内谷氨酸和 γ– 氨基丁酸平衡，抑制胆碱酯酶活性，提高海马区 N– 甲基 –D– 天冬氨酸受体（NMDA-R）和 γ– 氨基丁酸受体（γ-GABA-R）、生长因子及 *c-fos* 基因的表达有关。

(6) Learning and memory improvement The decoction of *Shú dì huáng* can improve the learning and memory deficits of rats induced by $AlCl_3$ or by monosodium glutamate damage hypothalamus arcuate nucleus, which can prolong the latency of jumping platform and reduce the number of errors in the step-down test, and shorten the time of searching platform in water maze. The effects of *Shú dì huáng* on learning and memory is related to regulating the balance between glutamate and γ-GABA and inhibiting cholinesterase activity in the brain, increasing the expression of N-methyl-D-aspartate receptor, γ-GABA receptor, growth factor and *c-fos* gene in hippocampus.

7. **其他作用** 熟地黄还有抗溃疡、抗突变等作用。

(7) Other effects *Shú dì huáng* also has the effects of anti-ulcer, anti-mutation, etc.

白芍 ┆ *Bái sháo (Radix Paeoniae Alba)*

【来源 / Origin】

本品为毛茛科植物芍药（*Paeonia lactiflora* Pall.）的根。主要分布于浙江、安徽、四川等地。夏秋二季采挖，除去支根和皮，沸水浸或略煮，晒干，用时润透切片，生用，酒炒用或清炒用。

Bái sháo is the dried root of *Paeonia lactiflora* Pall., family of Ranunculaceae. It is widely cultivated in Zhejiang province, Anhui province, and Sichuan province, etc., and harvested in summer and autumn. It is dried in the sun after removing fibrous root and scarfskin and soaking in boiling water. Moistened slices are directly used for Chinese medicinal preparation or fried with wine or without wine for application.

【化学成分 / Chemical ingredients】

主要含芍药苷（paeoniflorin）、羟基芍药苷（hydroxypaeoniflorin）、牡丹酚芍药花苷（paeonolide）、芍药内酯苷（albiflorin）、苯甲酰芍药苷（benzoylpaeoniflorin）等。还含有挥发油、脂肪油、淀粉、鞣质、蛋白质及三萜类成分。

Bái sháo mainly contains paeoniflorin, hydroxypaeoniflorin, paeonolide, albiflorin, benzoylpaeoniflorin, etc. The others are volatile oil, fat oil, starch, tannin, protein and triterpenes, etc.

【药性与功效 / Chinese medicine properties】

味苦、酸，性微寒，归肝、脾经。具有养血敛阴、柔肝止痛、平抑肝阳的功效。主治肝血亏虚、眩晕心悸、月经不调、崩中漏下、胸胁疼痛、痢疾腹痛、手足挛急疼痛、自汗、盗汗等证。

In Chinese medicine theory, *Bái sháo* has the nature of bitter, sour and slightly cold. It can enter the meridians of liver and spleen. *Bái sháo* can nourish blood to astringe Yin, emolliate liver to relieve pain, stabilize liver-Yang. Clinically it can be used for liver blood deficiency, dizziness and palpitation, menstrual irregularities, metrorrhagia and metrostaxis, pain in chest and hypochondrium, dysentery and abdomen pain, spasmodic pain of hand and foot, spontaneous sweating or night sweat, etc.

【药理作用 / Pharmacological effects】

1. 对血液系统的影响　白芍水煎液、白芍总苷具有明显抑制血小板聚集、降低血栓湿重，延长血栓形成时间等作用。白芍醇提取物能延长急性血瘀证大鼠活化部分凝血酶原时间、凝血酶时间，降低血小板黏附率。白芍总苷还可以提高红细胞变形能力，降低血细胞比容和血黏度，改善血液流变学。

(1) Effects on hematologic system　*Bái sháo* decoction and total saponins can significantly inhibit platelet aggregation, reduce wet weight of thrombus and prolong thrombus formation time. *Bái sháo* alcohol extract can prolong the time of APTT and TT and reduce the adhesion rate of platelets in acute blood stasis rats. Total glycosides of *Bái sháo* also can enhance erythrocyte deformability and reduce hematocrit and blood viscosity, which improve hemorheology.

2. 保肝　白芍水提物可以减轻 D– 半乳糖胺诱导的肝细胞变性坏死程度，降低血清 ALT 含量。白芍醇提物可以预防或逆转黄曲霉毒素 B_1 引起的大鼠轻度急性肝损伤，降低血清乳酸脱氢酶及其同工酶活性。白芍总苷可减轻 D– 半乳糖胺或 CCl_4 引起的鼠肝脏病理形态变化和血浆 ALT 含量，提高血清白蛋白及肝糖原含量。

(2) Hepatoprotection　Water extract of *Bái sháo* can alleviate the degree of degeneration and necrosis of hepatocyte, and decrease the content of alanine transaminase in serum induced by D-galactosamine. The alcohol extract of *Bái sháo* can reduce the activity of lactate dehydrogenase and its isoenzyme in serum, and prevent or reverse the mild acute liver injury caused by aflatoxin B_1 in rats. total glycosides of *Bái sháo* can reduce the pathomorphological changes and GPT content in plasma, increase the content of albumin in serum and glycogen in liver of rat caused by D-galactosamine or CCl_4.

3. 镇静、抗惊厥　白芍注射液能抑制小鼠自发性活动，延长戊巴比妥钠引起的小鼠睡眠时间。白芍总苷可延长正常大鼠慢波睡眠持续时间，促进咖啡因致失眠大鼠的睡眠参数恢复。白芍总苷可剂量依赖性地对抗电刺激、士的宁引起的小鼠惊厥，但对戊四氮致小鼠惊厥无影响。

(3) Sedation and anticonvulsion　*Bái sháo* injection can inhibit the spontaneous activity of mice, prolong the sleep time of mice caused by pentobarbital sodium. Total glycosides of *Bái sháo* can prolong the duration of slow wave sleep in normal rats and promote the recovery of sleep parameters in caffeine-induced insomnia rats. Total glycosides of *Bái sháo* could antagonize the convulsion of mice induced by electricity or strychnine in a dose-dependent manner, but it has no effect on the convulsion of mice caused by pentylenetetrazol.

4. 抗炎、镇痛　白芍水提物和白芍总苷能减轻二甲苯诱导的小鼠耳肿胀、蛋清诱导的大鼠足肿胀和棉球肉芽肿。白芍总苷可抑制胶原性关节炎大鼠滑膜细胞的过度增殖，改善滑膜细胞超微结构的病理变化，也能抑制佐剂性关节炎大鼠滑膜细胞过度分泌 IL-1 和 TNF 及 PGE_2。白芍总苷还能抑制大鼠慢性非细菌性前列腺炎、慢性盆腔炎、脓毒症的炎症反应。

(4) Anti-inflammation and analgesia　*Bái sháo* water extract and total saponins can reduce ear swelling induced by xylene, paw swelling induced by egg-white and cotton ball granuloma. Total

glycosides of *Bái sháo* can inhibit the excessive proliferation of synovial cells, and improve the pathological changes of ultrastructure of synovial cells in collagen-induced arthritis (CIA) rats. It also can inhibit the excessive secretion of IL-1, TNF and PGE$_2$ in synovial cells in rats with adjuvant arthritis. In additoin, It can alleviate inflammation of chronic non-bacterial prostatitis, chronic pelvic inflammatory disease and sepsis in rats.

白芍水提物、醇提物能显著提高光热法致痛小鼠的痛阈，延长醋酸诱导的小鼠扭体反应的潜伏期，减少扭体次数。白芍总苷及芍药苷、芍药内酯具有一定的镇痛作用。白芍总苷能加强吗啡的镇痛作用，但白芍总苷的镇痛作用不能被纳洛酮阻断，提示其镇痛作用与阿片受体无关。

Water extract and alcohol extract of *Bái sháo* could significantly enhance the pain threshold of mice induced by photothermal method, prolong the latency of writhing and reduce the number of writhing of mice induced by acetic acid. Total glycosides of *Bái sháo*, paeoniflorin and paeoniolactone also have analgesic effect.

5. 调节平滑肌运动　芍药和芍药苷能对抗氯化钡引起的肠管收缩。芍药苷能抑制豚鼠小肠自发收缩，降低肠管张力，还能对抗缩宫素引起的子宫平滑肌收缩。白芍总苷可延长豚鼠离体结肠收缩时间、增强收缩幅度，而阿托品可以阻断该作用，提示白芍总苷可能有兴奋 M 受体的作用。

(5) Effects on smooth muscle motility　*Bái sháo* and paeoniflorin can inhibit the contraction of intestine caused by barium chloride. Paeoniflorin can inhibit the spontaneous contraction of small intestine smooth muscle isolated from guinea pig, reduce the tension of small intestine, and also can antagonize the contraction of uterine smooth muscle caused by oxytocin. Total glycosides of *Bái sháo* can prolong the contraction time and increase the contraction amplitude of isolated colon of guinea pig, but atropine can block this effect, suggesting that total glycosides *of Bái sháo* maybe exert the excitation of M receptor.

6. 抗心肌缺血　白芍水提物能延长异丙肾上腺素引起的心肌缺血小鼠存活时间，对抗垂体后叶素引起的大鼠缺血性心电图改变，增加心肌营养性血流量。白芍总苷能缩小急性心肌缺血犬的心肌梗死面积，降低血清磷酸激酶和乳酸脱氢酶活性，减轻脂质过氧化反应对心肌细胞膜的损伤；改善冠状动脉结扎缺血再灌注大鼠心功能，减少心肌梗死面积、心肌细胞内质网应激及凋亡。

(6) Anti-myocardial ischemia　*Bái sháo* water extract can prolong the survival time of mice with myocardial ischemia induced by isoproterenol. It can also increase the myocardial blood flow and reverse the electrocardiogram changes of rats with myocardial ischemia caused by pituitrin. Total glycosides of *Bái sháo* can reduce the area of myocardial infarction, the activity of phosphocreatine kinase and lactate dehydrogenase in serum, and the damage of lipid peroxidation to myocardial cell membrane in dogs with acute myocardial ischemia. It can also improve the cardiac function of the ischemia-reperfusion rat induced by coronary artery ligation through attenuating the myocardial infarction area, endoplasmic reticulum stress and apoptosis.

7. 调节免疫功能　白芍水煎液能提高小鼠腹腔巨噬细胞的吞噬率和吞噬指数，增加环磷酰胺致小鼠外周血减少的 T 淋巴细胞数量，促进脾细胞抗体生成。白芍总苷具有免疫调节作用，低浓度时促进细胞免疫功能，高浓度时抑制细胞免疫功能。白芍总苷对佐剂性关节炎大鼠脾 B 淋巴细胞增殖及 LPS 诱导的小鼠 B 淋巴细胞增殖均有抑制作用，也能促进 Con A 诱导小鼠脾淋巴细胞的增殖，对抗环磷酰胺引起的抗体减少，但对正常小鼠的抗体生成和地塞米松引起的抗体生成抑制无影响。

(7) Regulating immune system function　*Bái sháo* decoction can increase the percentage and index of phagocytosis of peritoneal macrophages in mice, reverse the decrease of T lymphocytes in peripheral blood caused by cyclophosphamide, and promote the production of antibody in spleen cells. Total glycosides of *Bái sháo* has immunomodulatory effects, which can promote cellular immune function in low concentration, and inhibit cellular immune function in high concentration. Total glycosides of *Bái sháo* can inhibit the proliferation of B lymphocytes in the spleen of rats with adjuvant arthritis and mice induced by LPS. It also promotes the proliferation of spleen lymphocytes in mice induced by Con A, and reverse the reduction of antibody caused by cyclophosphamide, while it has no effect on the production of antibody of normal mice and inhibtion of antibody production caused by dexamethasone.

8. **其他作用** 白芍可延长缺氧、高温应激条件下动物存活时间；减轻应激性胃溃疡和幽门结扎致胃溃疡。白芍及白芍总苷对多种因素致肾脏功能降低有一定的改善作用。白芍总苷还具有减轻大鼠全脑和局灶性脑缺血损伤、改善学习记忆障碍和抗抑郁等作用。

(8) Other effects *Bái sháo* can prolong the survival time of animals under hypoxia and high temperature stress, relieve stomach ulcer caused by pyloric ligation or stress. *Bái sháo* and total glycosides of *Bái sháo* have nephroprotection against various factors-induced renal dysfunction. Total glycosides of *Bái sháo* can also alleviate the whole brain and focal cerebral ischemia injury, improve learning and memory deficits and inhibit the depression in rats.

【不良反应 / Adverse effects】

白芍总苷可引起类风湿关节炎患者出现腹泻、腹痛症状。罕见乳腺增生和疱疹。

Bái sháo total saponins can cause diarrhea, abdominal pain in rheumatoid arthritis patients. The rare adverse effects are hyperplasia of mammary glands and herpes.

枸杞子 ┊ *Gǒu qǐ zǐ (Fructus Lycii)*

【来源 / Origin】

本品为茄科植物宁夏枸杞（*Lycium barbamm* L.）的干燥成熟果实。主要分布于宁夏、甘肃、新疆等地。夏秋二季果实为橙红色时采收，置阴凉处晾至果皮起皱再晒至外皮干硬，果肉柔软，生用。

Gǒu qǐ zǐ is the dried ripe fruit of *Lycium barbamm* L., family of Solanaceae. It is widely cultivated in Ningxia Autonomous region, Gansu province, Xinjiang Autonomous region and harvested in summer and autum when the color of fruit is red-orange. It was placed in the shade until the skin is wrinked and then dried in the sun until the outer skin is hard but the fruit is soft, which can be directly used for Chinese medicinal preparation.

【化学成分 / Chemical ingredients】

主要含甜菜碱（betanie）、枸杞多糖、莨菪亭（scopoletin）、氨基酸、维生素 B_1、维生素 B_2、维生素 C、胡萝卜素及多种微量元素等。

Gǒu qǐ zǐ mainly contains betaine, polysaccharides, scopoletin, amino acid, vitamin B_1, B_2, and C, carotene, and trace elements, etc.

【药性与功效 / Chinese medicine properties】

味甘，性平，归肝、肾经。具有滋补肝肾、益精明目的功效。主治虚劳精亏、腰膝酸痛、眩晕耳鸣、内热消渴、血虚萎黄、目昏不明等证。

In Chinese medicine theory, *Gǒu qǐ zǐ* has the nature of sweet and neutral. It can enter the meridians of liver and kidney. *Gǒu qǐ zǐ* can tonify liver and kidney, replenish essence to improve vision. Clinically it can be used for essence-deficiency due to consumptive disease, aching pain in waist and knee, dizziness and tinnitus, consumptive thirst due to interior heat, blood deficiency and shallow yellow, blurred vision, etc.

【药理作用 / Pharmacological effects】

1. 增强机体免疫功能　枸杞子能增加小鼠脾脏和胸腺重量，提高小鼠腹腔巨噬细胞吞噬指数和吞噬率，升高小鼠血清中卵清蛋白抗体和 IL-2 水平；增强 Con A 诱导的小鼠脾 T 淋巴细胞的 DNA 和蛋白质合成；还能促进小鼠 B 淋巴细胞活性，促进 B 淋巴细胞增殖分化，升高小鼠血清 IgG 和 IgM 及补体 C4 水平。枸杞多糖是其增强免疫功能的主要活性成分。枸杞多糖可明显对抗环磷酰胺及 ^{60}Co 照射所致的小鼠白细胞数目减少，拮抗环磷酰胺对巨噬细胞 Fc 和 C_3b 受体的数量和活性的抑制作用。枸杞多糖腹腔注射能增加小鼠外周血 T 淋巴细胞数量，拮抗环磷酰胺对小鼠脾脏 T 淋巴细胞和 NK 细胞的免疫抑制作用，还能拮抗环磷酰胺的抑制抗体形成作用。

(1) Regulating immune system function　Water extract of *Gǒu qǐ zǐ* can increase the weight of spleen and thymus gland, the phagocytic index and phagocytic rate of macrophages in abdomen and IgG and IL-2 level in serum of mice. It can also enhance DNA and protein synthesis of Con A-induced T lymphocytes in mouse spleen. Furthermore, it can promote the proliferation and differentiation of B lymphocytes, and increase IgG, IgM and complement C4 levels in serum of mice. *Gǒu qǐ zǐ* polysaccharides, the main active ingredients in *Gǒu qǐ zǐ*, can significantly increase the number of white blood cells in mice with leukopenia caused by cyclophosphamide or ^{60}Co irradiation. It can also antagonize the inhibition of cyclophosphamide on the number and activity of macrophages Fc and C_3b receptors. Intraperitoneal injection of *Gǒu qǐ zǐ* polysaccharides can increase the number of T lymphocytes in peripheral blood of normal mice. Oral administration of *Gǒu qǐ zǐ* polysaccharides can increase the number of T lymphocytes and the activity of NK cells in spleen of normal mice and immunosuppressed mice by cyclophosphamide. In addition, *Gǒu qǐ zǐ* polysaccharides can also antagonize the inhibition of cyclophosphamide on antibody formation.

2. 延缓衰老　枸杞子水提物和枸杞多糖能延长二倍体成纤维细胞和果蝇的寿命。枸杞子醇提取物能减少 D– 半乳糖致衰老小鼠心、肝、脑组织脂褐质含量，增强红细胞 SOD 活性，提高小鼠学习记忆能力。枸杞多糖具有直接清除羟自由基的作用，能抑制自发或羟自由基引发的脂质过氧化反应。枸杞多糖不仅能抑制老年小鼠和 D– 半乳糖致衰老小鼠骨髓中 *c-myc* 基因表达，也能降低 D– 半乳糖致衰老大鼠肝脏修复酶 8– 羟基鸟嘌呤糖苷酶表达，减少 DNA 损伤和细胞凋亡。枸杞子延缓衰老作用与其抗氧化、提高机体免疫功能、提高 DNA 修复能力、抑制细胞凋亡等有关。

(2) Anti-aging　The water extract of *Gǒu qǐ zǐ* and *Gǒu qǐ zǐ* polysaccharides can prolong the life-span of diploid fibroblasts and fruit flies. The alcohol extract *Gǒu qǐ zǐ* can reduce the content of lipofuscin in heart, liver and brain, enhance the activity of SOD and GSH-Px in erythrocyte, and improve the learning and memory ability of aging mice induced by D-galactose. *Gǒu qǐ zǐ* polysaccharides can directly scavenge hydroxyl free radical to inhibit lipid peroxidation. It can not only inhibit *c-myc* gene expression in bone marrow of normal aging mice and D-galactose-induce aging mice, but also reduce the expression of 8-hydroxyguanine glycosidase in liver, reduce DNA damage and cell apoptosis of aging mice induced by D-galactose. Anti-oxidation, improving the immune function, enhancing the ability of DNA repairment, and inhibiting apoptosis are involved in the anti-aging effect of *Gǒu qǐ zǐ*.

3. 降血糖　枸杞子水提取物、枸杞多糖灌胃可降低正常大鼠和小鼠，以及肾上腺素、四氧嘧啶、STZ 致糖尿病大鼠和小鼠的血糖。其降血糖作用可能与促进胰岛素分泌、增加肝糖原含量、清除氧自由基减轻胰岛 B 细胞的氧化损伤、增加胰岛素敏感性和抑制 α 葡糖苷酶的活性有关。

(3) Reducing blood glucose　The water extract of *Gǒu qǐ zǐ* and polysaccharides from *Gǒu qǐ zǐ* can reduce the blood glucose of normal mice and rats and the diabetic mice and rats induced by adrenalin, alloxan or STZ, which maybe related with promoting the secretion of insulin, increasing the content of liver glycogen, scavenging free radical to reduce the oxidative damage of pancreatic B cells, enhancing insulin sensitivity and inhibiting α-glucosidase activity.

4. 保肝　枸杞子水浸液、枸杞多糖能轻度抑制四氯化碳致肝损伤小鼠肝细胞内的脂肪沉积，促进肝细胞再生。甜菜碱被认为是枸杞子保肝的主要成分，在体内起到甲基供应体的作用。枸杞多糖保肝机制可能是阻止内质网的氧化损伤，促进蛋白质合成及解毒，增强肝细胞的再生，恢复肝功能。

(4) Hepatoprotection　The water extract of *Gǒu qǐ zǐ* and polysaccharides of *Gǒu qǐ zǐ* could slightly inhibit the fat deposition in liver and promote the regeneration of hepatocyte of liver injury mice caused by CC1₄. Betaine is suggested to be the main active ingredient of *Gǒu qǐ zǐ* for the hepatoprotection, which can supply a methyl in the body. The hepatoprotection of polysaccharides of *Gǒu qǐ zǐ* maybe related with preventing the oxidative damage of endoplasmic reticulum, promoting protein synthesis and detoxification, enhancing the regeneration of liver cell to restore the liver function.

5. 抗肿瘤　枸杞多糖能显著抑制人肝癌细胞 Bel-7402、人宫颈癌 Hela 细胞、人前列腺癌 PC-3 细胞的生长和小鼠白血病细胞 L_{1210} 的代谢增殖，延长腹水型（U14 小鼠宫颈癌、肉瘤 S_{180}）荷瘤小鼠的生存时间，提高荷瘤鼠胸腺指数、巨噬细胞吞噬功能，促进脾细胞抗体形成、淋巴细胞转化反应。枸杞多糖通过诱导肿瘤细胞凋亡、增强机体免疫功能、抑制肿瘤血管生成而抑制肿瘤生长和转移。

(5) Anti-cancer　*Gǒu qǐ zǐ* polysaccharides could inhibit the proliferation and metabolism of human liver cancer cell Bel-7402, cervix cancer Hela cell, human prostate cancer cell PC-3 and mouse leukemic cell L_{1210}. It can extend the survival time of ascitic type (cervical cancer U14 in mice, fibre sarcoma S_{180}) tumor-bearing mice, increase the thymus index, the phagocytosis of macrophage, antibody formation in spleen, and transformation of lymphocyte in tumor-bearing mice. *Gǒu qǐ zǐ* polysaccharides inhibit the proliferation and metastasis of tumor which is related with inducing tumor cell apoptosis, enhancing immune function, and inhibiting tumor angiogenesis.

6. 其他作用　枸杞子提取液和枸杞多糖还有降血脂、改善肾功能、抗缺氧、抗疲劳、抗辐射损伤、抗生殖系统损伤等作用。

(6) Other effects　*Gǒu qǐ zǐ* extract and polysaccharide also have the effects of reducing blood lipid, improving renal function, anti-hypoxia, anti-fatigue, anti-radiation damage, anti-reproductive system damage, etc.

【不良反应 / Adverse effects】

枸杞子偶见引起皮肤潮红、瘙痒和荨麻疹等过敏症状。

Gǒu qǐ zǐ can cause erubescence, pruritus and urticaria occasionally.

麦冬　｜　*Mài dōng (Radix Ophiopogonis)*

【来源 / Origin】

本品为百合科植物麦冬 [Ophiopogon japonicus (Thunb.) Ker-Gawl.] 的块根。主要分布于四川、浙江、江苏等地。夏季采收，反复暴晒去掉须根，干燥，生用。

Mài dōng is the dried root of *Ophiopogon japonicus* (Thunb.) Ker-Gawl., family of Liliaceae. It is widely cultivated in Sichuan province, Zhejiang province, Jiangsu province, etc., and harvested in summer. It is dried by repeated expose to the blazing sun and removing the fibrous root for application.

【化学成分 / Chemical ingredients】

主要含多种甾体皂苷、β–谷甾醇、豆甾醇、黄酮类化合物、多糖、氨基酸和维生素等。

Mài dōng mainly contains steroid saponin, β-sitosterol, stigmasterol, flavonoids, polysaccharides, amino acid, and vitamin, etc.

【药性与功效 / Chinese medicine properties】

味甘、微苦，性微寒，归心、肺、胃经。具有养阴润肺、益胃生津、清心除烦的功效。主治肺燥干咳、失眠多梦、健忘、心悸怔忡、津伤口渴、内热消渴、肠燥便秘等证。

In Chinese medicine theory, *Mài dōng* has the nature of sweet, slightly bitter and slightly cold. It can enter the meridians of heart, lung and stamach. *Mài dōng* can nourish yin and moisten lung, benefit stomach and promote fluid production, clear heart to relieve restlessness. Clinically it can be used for dry cough due to lung dryness, insomnia and dreamful sleep, amnesia, palpitation, thirst due to fluid consumption, consumptive thirst due to interior heat, intestinal dryness and constipation, etc.

【药理作用 / Pharmacological effects】

1. 对心血管系统的作用

(1) Effects on cardiovascular system function

（1）抗心肌缺血　麦冬总皂苷、总氨基酸可以减轻异丙肾上腺素诱导的大鼠心肌缺血，降低血清磷酸激酶的水平和心电图 ST 段变化；减小冠状动脉结扎引起的心肌梗死面积、心肌酶谱水平及心肌超微结构变化。麦冬总皂苷及多糖可增加小鼠心肌营养血流量。麦冬多糖可对抗垂体后叶素、冠脉结扎致大鼠 ST 段升高。麦冬抗心肌缺血的作用与降低心肌细胞脂质过氧化和改善脂肪酸代谢有关。

1) Anti-myocardial ischemia　*Mài dōng* total saponins and amino acids can reduce the level of creatine phosphokinase in serum and the change of ST segment in ECG, which alleviate myocardial ischemia of rats induced by isoproterenol. They also reduce the area of myocardial infarction, the level of myocardial enzyme spectrum and myocardial ultrastructural changes in rats with coronary artery ligation. *Mài dōng* total saponins and polysaccharides can increase the myocardial nutritional blood flow in mice. *Mài dōng* polysaccharide can resist the ST segment elevation caused by pituitrin or coronary artery ligation. The anti-myocardial ischemia effect of *Mài dōng* is related to the decrease of lipid peroxidation and the improvement of fatty acid metabolism.

（2）抗心律失常　麦冬水提物和麦冬总皂苷对 $BaCl_2$、乌头碱及冠状动脉结扎诱发的心律失常有明显的抑制作用，可能与减少心肌细胞的 Na^+ 和 Ca^{2+} 内流、增加有效不应期（ERP）/动作电位时程（APD）比值、减慢心率和传导有关。

2) Anti-arrhythmia　*Mài dōng* extract and *Mài dōng* total saponins can significantly prevent the arrhythmia induced by $BaCl_2$, aconitine and coronary artery ligation, which may be related to the reduction of influx of Na^+ and Ca^{2+} in cardiomyocytes, the increase of ERP / APD, the slowing heart rate and conduction.

2. 调节免疫功能　麦冬多糖可以增加幼鼠的胸腺和脾脏重量，增强小鼠单核巨噬细胞系统的吞噬能力和血清溶血素水平，对抗环磷酰胺和 ^{60}Co-γ 照射引起的小鼠白细胞减少。麦冬多糖还可以对抗乙酰胆碱和组胺混合液诱导的正常豚鼠和卵蛋白致敏豚鼠的支气管平滑肌收缩，抑制致敏豚鼠哮喘的发生。

(2) Enhancing immune system function　*Mài dōng* polysaccharide can increase the weight of thymus and spleen of infancy mic, enhance the phagocytosis of reticulo endothelial system of mice, and reverse the decrease of leukocyte in serum of mice caused by cyclophosphamide or ^{60}Co- γ irradiation.

3. 降血糖　麦冬水提物、醇提物可以降低正常家兔的血糖水平，也可降低四氧嘧啶致糖尿病家兔的血糖，并促使胰岛细胞恢复，增加肝糖原。麦冬多糖可阻止小肠对葡萄糖的吸收而起到降糖作用。

(3) Reducing blood glucose *Mài dōng* water extract and alcohol extract can reduce the blood glucose level of normal rabbits, and also can reduce the blood glucose, promote the recovery of islet cells and increase the glycogen of liver in diabetic rabbits induced by alloxan. The *Mài dōng* polysaccharide can prevent the absorption of glucose from small intestine.

4. 抗衰老　麦冬水提物可增加 D– 半乳糖致衰老大鼠红细胞 SOD 活性，降低血清 MDA 含量，降低血液黏度。麦冬多糖能够剂量依赖性地延长家蚕及果蝇的寿命，降低 D– 半乳糖致衰老小鼠脑内单胺氧化酶 B（MAO-B）活性，增加血清溶血素，提高衰老小鼠的体液免疫功能。

(4) Anti-aging　The water extract of *Mài dōng* can increase SOD activity in erythrocyte, decrease MDA content in serum, and reduce blood viscosity in aging rats induced by D-galactose. *Mài dōng* polysaccharide can prolong the life-span of silkworm and fruit fly with a dose-dependence. *Mài dōng* polysaccharide also reduce the activity of monoamine oxidase (MAO-B) in the brain and increase the serum hemolysin, and improve the humoral immune function of aging mice caused by D-galactose.

5. 镇静　麦冬煎剂能延长阈下催眠剂量戊巴比妥钠的睡眠时间，增强氯丙嗪的镇静作用，拮抗咖啡因诱导的小鼠兴奋作用。

(5) Sedation　*Mài dōng* decoction can prolong the sleeping time of subthreshold dose of pentobarbital sodium, as well as enhance the sedative effect of chlorpromazine. It also antagonize the excitation of mice induced by caffeine.

6. 其他作用　麦冬注射液可提高小鼠耐缺氧能力。麦冬粉对白色葡萄球菌、大肠埃希菌有抑制作用。

(6) Other effects　*Mài dōng* injection can enhance the tolerance to hypoxia. Powder of *Mài dōng* has inhibitory effect on *Staphylococcus albicans* and *Escherichia coli*.

【不良反应 / Adverse effects】

有报道服用麦冬出现恶心、呕吐、心悸、烦躁、全身瘙痒、红斑、谵妄等过敏症状。

Mài dōng occasionally causes nausea, vomiting, palpitation, rash, pruritus, delirium, etc.

北沙参　*Běi shā shēn (Radix Glehniae)*

【来源 / Origin】

本品为伞形科植物珊瑚菜（*Glehnia littoralis* Fr. Schmidt ex Miq.）的根。主要分布于山东、江苏、福建等地。夏秋两季采挖，沸水烫后，去外皮，干燥，或洗净后直接干燥。

Běi shā shēn is the dried root of *Glehmia littoralis* Fr. Schmidt ex. Miq., family of Umbelliferae. It is widely cultivated in Shandong province, Jiangsu province, Fujian province, etc., and harvested in summer and autumn. It is dried after removing the skin with boiling water or directly dried after washing.

【化学成分 / Chemical ingredients】

主要含有挥发油、糖苷、香豆素类成分〔欧前胡素（imperatorin）、异欧前胡素（isoimperatorin）等〕、磷脂、淀粉、多糖、佛手苷内酯（5-methoxypsoralen）、氨基酸及微量元素等。

Běi shā shēn mainly contains volatile oil, glycosides, coumnrins (imperatorin, isoimperatorin, etc.), phospholipids, starch, polyschride, 5-methoxypsoralen, amino acid and trace elements, etc.

【药性与功效 / Chinese medicine properties】

味甘、微苦，性微寒，归肺、胃经。具有养阴清肺、益胃生津的功效。主治少痰干咳、咯血、咽干音哑、口干多饮、饥不欲食、大便干结、胃痛、胃胀、干呕等证。

In Chinese medicine theory, *Běi shā shēn* has the nature of sweet, slightly bitter and slightly cold. It can enter the meridians of lung and stomach. *Běi shā shēn* has nourish Yin and clear Lung, benefit stomach and promote fluid production. Clinically it can be used for dry cough with less sputum, hemoptysis, dry throat and hoarseness, dry mouth and more drinking, hunger without appetite, constipation, stamachache, gastric distention, retching, etc.

【药理作用 / Pharmacological effects】

1. 调节免疫功能　北沙参水提物能增加小鼠脾脏、胸腺重量，增强小鼠腹腔巨噬细胞的吞噬能力和 NK 细胞杀伤能力，提高环磷酰胺致免疫低下小鼠外周血 T 淋巴细胞数量。北沙参多糖可以促进甲状腺素和利血平致阴虚小鼠迟发型超敏反应和脾脏抗体生成细胞数量。北沙参多糖对羊红细胞致敏小鼠脾脏抗体空斑形成反应和 IgM 数量、二硝基氯苯致鼠耳迟发型超敏反应、PHA和 Con A 及美洲商陆（PWM）诱导的人正常淋巴细胞增殖均有抑制作用。

(1) Regulating immune system function　The water extract of *Běi shā shēn* can increase the weight of spleen and thymus, enhance the phagocytosis of peritoneal macrophages and killing activity of NK cells in mice. It also increases the number of T lymphocytes in peripheral blood of immunocompromised mice caused by cyclophosphamide. *Běi shā shēn* polysaccharide can promote the delayed hypersensitivity and the number of antibody forming cells in spleen of Yin deficiency mice induced by thyroxine and reserpine. Moreover, *Běi shā shēn* polysaccharide has inhibitory effects on spleen antibody plaque forming cell response and IgM level in serum of mice induced by SRBC sensitization, delayed-type hypersensitivity of rat ear induced by DNCB, and proliferation of normal human lymphocyte induced by PHA, Con A and PWM.

2. 抗肿瘤　北沙参水提醇沉液对肺癌细胞 A_{549} 和肝癌细胞 HepG2 有一定的抑制作用。北沙参香豆素类成分异欧前胡素对肺癌细胞 A_{549} 和人卵巢癌细胞 SK-OV-3 有明显的抑制增殖作用，佛手苷内酯对肝癌、胃癌细胞株有明显的抑制作用。

(2) Anti-tumor　The water extraction and alcohol precipitation of *Běi shā shēn* has inhibitory effect on lung cancer cells A_{549} and liver cancer cells HepG2. Isoimperatorin, a component of coumarins, can inhibit the proliferation of lung cancer cells A_{549} and human ovarian cancer cells SK-OV-3. The other component of coumarins named bergamolide had the inhibitory effect on the liver cancer cells and stomach cancer cells.

3. 镇咳、祛痰　北沙参醇提物可显著延长氨水引咳小鼠的咳嗽潜伏期，还能减少气管酚红分泌，有明显的镇咳祛痰作用。

(3) Anti-tussive and expectorant effect　*Běi shā shēn* alcohol extract can significantly prolong the latency of cough in mice induced by ammonia, and reduce the secretion of phenol red in trachea of mice, indicating it has anti-tussive and expectorant effects.

4. 解热、镇痛　北沙参根乙醇提取物能轻度降低正常家兔体温，也能降低伤寒疫苗引起的发热家兔的体温。北沙参可以提高家兔牙髓电刺激阈值，有镇痛作用。

(4) Antipyretic effect and analgesia　The ethanol extract of *Běi shā shēn* can slightly decrease the body temperature of normal rabbits and fever rabbits caused by typhoid vaccine. It can increase the electrical stimulation threshold of dental pulp of rabbit, which has analgesic effect.

5. 保肝　北沙参乙醇提取物能降低 CCl_4 致肝损伤大鼠肝组织中 MDA 含量，提高 SOD 和CAT 活性，改善肝小叶变性、坏死的范围和程度。

(5) Hepatoprotection　The ethanol extract of *Běi shā shēn* can reduce the content of MDA, increase the activity of SOD and CAT in the liver, and alleviate the degeneration and necrosis of liver lobular in rats caused by CCl_4.

6. 抗肺纤维化　予博来霉素诱导的肺纤维化大鼠北沙参水提物连续灌胃 4 周，可以降低大鼠血清纤连蛋白和层连蛋白含量，减轻肺纤维化的病理变化。

(6) Anti-pulmonary fibrosis　Intragastrical administration of *Běi shā shēn* extract for 4 weeks can decrease the contents of fibronectin and laminin in serum, alleviate the pathological changes of pulmonary fibrosis of rats induced by bleomycin.

7. 其他作用　北沙参水提物还有抗氧化、抗突变等作用。

(7) Other effects　The water extract of *Běi shā shēn* also has the effects of antioxidation, antimutation, etc.

【不良反应 / Adverse effects】

北沙参对少数人群有致敏性和刺激性，可引起过敏性皮炎。

Běi shā shēn has anaphylaxis and irritation in a few cases, which can cause the allergic dermatitis.

鹿茸　┆　*Lù róng* (Cornu Cervi Pantotrichum)

【来源 / Origin】

本品为鹿科动物梅花鹿（*Cervus nippon* Temminck）或马鹿（*Cervus elaphus* Linnaeus）的雄鹿未骨化密生茸毛的幼角。夏、秋二季锯取鹿茸，经加工后，阴干或烘干。

Lù róng is the hairy, non-ossificying young born of male deer or stag of *Cervus nippon* Temminck or *Cervus. elaphus* Linnaeus, vertebrae of the family Cervidae.

【化学成分 / Chemical ingredients】

含多种氨基酸，以甘氨酸含量最高；还含有胆固醇、卵磷脂、脑磷脂、神经磷脂、次黄嘌呤、雌二醇、雄激素以及多胺、多糖、多肽、脂肪酸等。此外，鹿茸中还含有大量的无机元素，如氮、钙、磷、硫、镁、钠、钾，以及锰、锌、铜、铁、硒、钼、镍、钛、钡、钴、锶等多种微量元素。

Lù róng contains a variety of amino acids, the highest content of glycine, but also contains cholesterol, lecithin, brain lecithin, neurolecithin, hypoxanthine, estradiol, androgen, polyamines, polysaccharides, peptides, fatty acids and etc. In addition, *Lù róng* also contains a large number of inorganic elements, such as nitrogen, calcium, phosphorus, sulfur, magnesium, sodium, potassium, as well as manganese, zinc, copper, iron, selenium, molybdenum, nickel, titanium, barium, cobalt, strontium and other trace elements.

【药性与功效 / Chinese medicine properties】

味甘、咸，性温，归肾、肝经。具有壮肾阳、益肾精血、强筋骨、调冲任、托疮毒的功效。用于肾阳不足、精血亏虚、阳痿滑精、宫冷不孕、羸瘦、神疲、畏寒、眩晕、耳鸣、耳聋、腰脊冷痛、筋骨痿软、崩漏带下、阴疽不敛。

In Chinese medicine theory, *Lù róng* has the nature of sweet, salty and warm. It can enter the meridians of kidney and liver. It can warm kidney-Yang, reinforce kidney essence and blood, strengthen muscles and bones, recuperate Chong pulse and Ren pulse, and promote sepsis excretion and new muscle regeneration. It is indicated for kidney-Yang deficiency syndrome and insuffciency of essence and blood syndrome, impotence and spermatorrhea, uterus coldness infertility, emaciation, fatigue, aversion to cold, dizziness, tinnitus, deafness, cold lumbago, weakness of muscles and bones, metrostaxis and vaginal discharge, and Yin gangrene without healing.

【药理作用 / Pharmacological effects】

1. 性激素样作用　鹿茸兼有雄激素和雌激素样作用，鹿茸中性激素成分主要是雌二醇、睾酮。鹿茸可提高去卵巢大鼠子宫和阴道指数，升高血清雌二醇水平；雄鼠交配前给药可提高受孕

295

率；增加肾阳虚不育大鼠精子总数，增加附睾质量及系数，升高大鼠血浆睾酮、附睾顶体酶水平等。鹿茸乙醇提取液可使大鼠睾丸精原细胞数目增多，生精细胞层数增多。鹿茸乙醇提取物可使老化小鼠血浆睾酮含量明显增加，但对正常小鼠血浆睾酮含量的影响不明显。鹿茸的雄激素作用并非介导内源性雄激素的生成，可能通过诱导颌下腺内生理活性物质的活性产生，进而介导雄激素及各种类固醇激素与甲状腺激素的调节，从而产生雄激素样作用。此外，鹿茸可兴奋垂体–性腺轴，促进雄性激素和生长素分泌。

(1) Sex hormone-like effects *Lù róng* has both androgen-like and estrogen-like effects, and the main sex hormone components of *Lù róng* are estradiol and testosterone. *Lù róng* could increase the uterine and vaginal index and the level of serum estradiol in ovariectomized rats. When administered to male rats before mating, *Lù róng* could increase the pregnancy rate. It could also increase the total number of sperm, the quality and coefficient of epididymis, the levels of plasma testosterone and epididymal acrosin in infertile rats with kidney-Yang deficiency. The ethanol extract of *Lù róng* could increase the number of spermatogonia and the layers of spermatogenic cells in rat testis. The ethanol extract of *Lù róng* could significantly increase the content of plasma testosterone in aging mice, but showed no obvious effect on the content of plasma testosterone in normal mice. *Lù róng* could induce the production of physiologically active substances in the submandibular gland, and then mediate the regulation of androgens, various steroids and thyroid hormones, and manifest androgen-like effects. In addition, *Lù róng* could stimulate the pituitary gland axis and promote the secretion of androgen and auxin.

2. 促进核酸和蛋白质合成 饲喂含有鹿茸的饲料可使小鼠、大鼠体重显著增加，加速未成年小鼠的生长发育。鹿茸促进 ^{14}C–亮氨酸和 ^{14}C–尿嘧啶核苷参与老化小鼠肝和肾组织的蛋白质和 RNA 的合成，鹿茸促进核酸和蛋白质合成的有效成分主要为多胺类物质，机制可能与激活 RNA 聚合酶有关。

(2) Promoting nucleic acid and protein synthesis Feeding the food containing *Lù róng* could significantly increase the body weight of mice and rats, and accelerate the growth of immature mice. *Lù róng* could promote ^{14}C-leucine and ^{14}C-uracil nucleoside incorporation into the protein and RNA synthesis of liver and kidney tissues of aging mice. The polyamines, such as putrescine and spermidine are suggested to be the active ingredients. The mechanism might be related to the activation of RNA polymerase.

3. 调节骨代谢 鹿茸可提高去卵巢致骨质疏松大鼠股骨部位骨密度，升高血清碱性磷酸酶、骨形成蛋白 –2 和骨钙素水平；上调骨关节炎大鼠关节软组织 Smad2、Smad3 及转化生长因子 β1 的基因和蛋白表达。鹿茸中至少含有 4 种参与局部调节骨生长的活性因子。鹿茸多肽可加速骨折大鼠骨痂形成，促进骨折愈合；抑制关节炎家兔软骨细胞凋亡，延缓软骨破坏和退变，还可抑制软骨细胞过度氧化应激反应。

(3) Improving the bone metabolism *Lù róng* could increase the bone mineral density of femur, and increase the levels of serum alkaline phosphatase, bone morphogenetic protein-2 and osteocalcin in ovariectomized rats. *Lù róng* could up-regulate the gene and protein expression of Smad2, Smad3, and transforming growth factor-β1 in joint soft tissue of osteoarthritis rats. At least four active factors were involved in local regulation of bone growth. The polypeptide of *Lù róng* could accelerate callus formation and promote fracture healing in fracture rats. The polypeptide also could inhibit chondrocyte apoptosis in arthritic rabbits, delay cartilage destruction and degeneration, and inhibit excessive oxidative stress of chondrocytes.

4. 提高免疫功能 鹿茸片具有增强免疫力作用，可提高小鼠单核巨噬细胞碳廓清能力。鹿茸

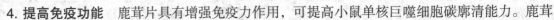

水提物可增强甲氨蝶呤致免疫功能低下小鼠的迟发型免疫反应，增加脾细胞中的玫瑰花环细胞数量，升高红细胞凝集素和红细胞溶血素。

(4) Regulating immune system function　*Lù róng* tablet could enhance immune function and improve the carbon clearance ability of monocytes and macrophages in mice. The aqueous extract of *Lù róng* can enhance the delayed immune response of immunocompromised mice induced by methotrexate, increase the number of rosette cells of spleen cells, and increase erythrocyte agglutinin and hemolysin.

5. 增强造血功能　用含鹿茸饲料饲育小鼠，能增加小鼠的红细胞数、网织红细胞数及血红蛋白含量。健康成年家兔饲喂鹿茸粉或注射鹿茸浸出物，其红细胞数、血红蛋白含量、网织红细胞数均增加。鹿茸精注射液能改善乙酰苯肼所致溶血性贫血小鼠和肾脏大部分（5/6）切除所致肾性贫血大鼠的骨髓造血功能，加速红细胞和血红蛋白的生成。

(5) Improving hematopoietic function　*Lù róng* is able to increase the number of red blood cells, reticulocyte and hemoglobin content in mice. When healthy adult rabbits were fed with *Lù róng* powder or injected with *Lù róng* extract, the number of red blood cells, hemoglobin and reticulocyte were increased. *Lù róng* injection could promote bone marrow hematopoiesis in mice with hemolytic anemia caused by acetylphenylhydrazine and rats with renal anemia caused by nephrectomy, and accelerate the production of red blood cells and hemoglobin.

6. 抗氧化、延缓衰老　鹿茸及鹿角胶可提高衰老大鼠肝和血清中 SOD、GSR、CP 水平，降低肝 MAO 活性，降低肝 MDA 和 LPF 含量。鹿茸可提高老龄鼠血清 SOD 活性，降低血清、垂体和肾上腺组织的 LPO 浓度。鹿茸提取物可提高环磷酰胺免疫抑制小鼠清除自由基的能力，降低细胞脂质过氧化水平和生物膜受损程度，对老化小鼠脑和肝组织中 MDA 含量也有明显降低作用，但对正常小鼠影响不明显。

(6) Anti-oxidation and anti-aging　*Lù róng* and antler glue could increase the levels of SOD, GSR and CP of liver and serum in aging rats, and decrease the activity of MAO of liver and the content of MDA and LPF of liver. *Lù róng* could increase the activity of serum SOD and decrease the concentration of LPO in serum, pituitary and adrenal tissue of aged rats. The extract of *Lù róng* could improve the free radical scavenging ability of immunosuppressive mice induced by cyclophosphamide, and reduce the level of cell lipid peroxidation and the damage degree of biofilm, and significantly reduce the content of MDA in brain and liver tissue of aging mice, but had no obvious effect on normal mice.

7. 抗应激　鹿茸具有抗疲劳、耐缺氧、耐高温、耐低温等多种抗应激作用。鹿茸提取物、鹿茸胶原酶解物、鹿茸多肽均显示抗疲劳作用。鹿茸水提物能明显延长小鼠负重游泳时间，降低小鼠血中乳酸和尿素氮的含量，提高小鼠体内肝糖原和肌糖原储备量及运动后乳酸脱氢酶的活力。鹿茸多肽可增加小鼠肝糖原和肌糖原的含量，降低代谢产物 LA、MDA、BUN 的水平，提高 LDH、SOD、GSH-Px 活性，加速自由基的清除，增强小鼠的抗氧化能力，提高小鼠的运动能力。

(7) Anti-stress　*Lù róng* is indicated for a variety of stress conditions, such as fatigue, hypoxia, high temperature, low temperature and etc. *Lù róng* extract, *Lù róng* collagenase hydrolysate and *Lù róng* polypeptide all showed anti-fatigue effect. The water extract of *Lù róng* could significantly prolong the swimming time of weight-bearing mice, reduce the contents of blood lactic acid and urea nitrogen, increase the reserve of liver glycogen and muscle glycogen and the activity of lactate dehydrogenase after exercise. *Lù róng* polypeptide could increase the content of liver glycogen and muscle glycogen, accelerate the scavenging of free radicals, enhance the antioxidation ability of mice, and improve the exercise ability in mice.

8. 调节中枢神经系统　鹿茸提取物对东莨菪碱及亚硝酸钠造成的学习记忆障碍小鼠的学习记

忆能力均有改善作用。鹿茸多肽可改善东莨菪碱所致的大鼠学习记忆障碍，作用机制与提高脑组织 ACh 含量、降低 AChE 活性以及改善过度氧化应激有关。鹿茸多肽局部应用可促进损伤坐骨神经再生以及功能恢复；鹿茸多肽可抑制辐射诱导大鼠腹部脊髓神经元凋亡，并可抑制辐射诱导的神经母细胞瘤细胞凋亡。鹿茸提取物能促进 SH-SY5Y 神经细胞增殖和分化且对秀丽隐杆线虫帕金森模型具有多巴胺神经保护作用。鹿茸多肽可通过抑制 Tau 过度磷酸化及细胞凋亡，抑制冈田酸诱导的神经细胞损伤。

(8) Regulating central nervous system *Lù róng* extract could improve the learning and memory ability of mice induced with scopolamine and sodium nitrite. *Lù róng* polypeptide could improve the learning and memory impairment of rats induced by scopolamine, which is related to increase of ACh content in brain tissue, decrease of AChE activity and inhibition of excessive oxidative stress. Local administrated with *Lù róng* peptide could promote the regeneration and functional recovery of injured sciatic nerve. *Lù róng* peptide could inhibit radiation-induced apoptosis of abdominal spinal cord neurons and inhibit radiation-induced neuroblastoma cell apoptosis in rats. The extract of *Lù róng* could promote the proliferation and differentiation of SH-SY5Y nerve cells. *Lù róng* polypeptide could prevent neuronal injury induced by Okadaic acid by inhibiting Tau hyperphosphorylation and apoptosis.

9. 影响心血管系统　鹿茸可修复冠状动脉左前降支结扎致心梗大鼠的心肌损伤，改善心功能，促进血管新生。鹿茸多肽可降低心肌缺血损伤模型大鼠的心率。鹿茸精对氯仿诱发的小鼠心室纤颤、氯化钡诱发的大鼠心律失常均有治疗作用。其作用环节有扩张冠脉血管，增加冠脉流量；提高对缺血心肌的能量供应，提高 Ca^{2+}-Mg^{2+}-ATP 酶和 Na^+-K^+-ATP 酶活性；维持再灌注损伤心肌细胞膜和微粒体膜的稳定性。

(9) Effects on cardiovascular system *Lù róng* could repair myocardial injury in rats with myocardial infarction caused by ligation of left anterior descending branch of coronary artery, improve cardiac function and promote angiogenesis. *Lù róng* polypeptide could reduce the heart rate of the rat model of myocardial ischemic injury. The potential mechanisms are as follows. ①Dilating coronary vessels. ②Increasing coronary flow. ③Increasing energy supply to ischemic myocardium. ④Increasing the activities of Ca^{2+}-Mg^{2+}-ATP and Na^+-K^+-ATP enzymes. ⑤Maintaining the stability of myocardial cell membrane and microsomal membrane in reperfusion injury.

10. 抗肝损伤　鹿茸粉可抑制 CCl_4、APAP、乙醇等导致的肝损伤，改善肝脏超微结构损伤，降低血清中 ALT 和 AST 活性等。鹿茸水提物、鹿茸多肽可改善 CCl_4 所致肝损伤，作用机制可能与抗氧化自由基、抗炎有关。

(10) Hepatoprotection *Lù róng* powder could inhibit liver injury caused by CCl_4, APAP or alcohol. *Lù róng* could alleviate liver ultrastructure damage, and reduce the activities of serum alanine transaminase (ALT) and aspartate transaminase (AST). *Lù róng* water extract and *Lù róng* polypeptide could improve the liver injury induced by CCl_4, and the mechanism may be related to antioxidant free radicals and anti-inflammation.

11. 其他作用　鹿茸提取物可降低四氧嘧啶致糖尿病小鼠血糖、血脂水平，改善过度氧化应激反应。鹿茸多糖在免疫功能低下的机体内可激活免疫机制杀伤肿瘤细胞，促进抗肿瘤免疫应答。鹿茸多糖对应激性胃溃疡及结扎幽门引起的胃溃疡有抑制作用，其抗溃疡作用主要是促进前列腺素 E_2（PGE_2）的合成。

(11) Other effects *Lù róng* extract could reduce the levels of blood glucose and blood lipids in alloxan-induced diabetic mice and improve the reaction of excessive oxidative stress. In addition, *Lù róng* polysaccharides could activate the immune system against tumor cells and promote anti-tumor immune response. *Lù róng* polysaccharide has an inhibitory effect on stress gastric ulcer and gastric ulcer caused by ligation of gastric pylorus, and its anti-ulcer effect is mainly related to promoting the synthesis of prostaglandin E_2 (PGE_2).

【不良反应 / Adverse effects】

部分患者使用鹿茸后出现消化系统不良反应，可见上腹部疼痛不适、恶心等。鹿茸精注射可见过敏反应。

Adverse digestive system reactions may occur, including epigastric pain, discomfort, nausea and etc. Allergic reaction can be seen in injection of pantocrine.

淫羊藿 ┊ *Yín yáng huò* (*Herba Epimedii*)

【来源 / Origin】

本品为小檗科植物淫羊藿（*Epimedium brevicornum* Maxim.）、箭叶淫羊藿（*Epimedium sagittatum* Maxim.）或柔毛淫羊藿（*Epimedium pubescens* Maxim）、朝鲜淫羊藿（*Epimedium koreanum* Nalcai.）等的全草。主要产于陕西、甘肃、山西、湖北、四川等地。夏秋二季采收地上部分，晒干，切碎生用或以羊脂油炙用。

Yín yáng huò is the dried leaf of *Epimedium brevicorum* Maxim., *Epimedium sagittatum* Maxim., *Epimedium pubescens* Maxim., and *Epimedium koreanum* Nakai., family of Berberridaceae. It is widely cultivated in Shaanxi province, Gansu province, Shanxi province, Hubei province and Sichuan province, etc., and harvested in spring and autumn. Cutting it into pieces after drying in the sun and is directly used or baked with mutton fat for Chinese medicinal preparation.

【化学成分 / Chemical ingredients】

主要有效成分为黄酮类成分，如淫羊藿苷（icariin）、去氢甲基淫羊藿苷（β-anhydroicaritine）、异槲皮素（isoquercetin）、金丝桃苷（hyperoside）、去氧甲基淫羊藿苷（des-O-methylicariine）等。还含有淫羊藿多糖、生物碱、木脂素及微量元素锌、锰等。

The main active components of *Yín yáng huò* are flavonoids, such as icariin, β-anhydroicaritine, isoquercetin, hyperoside and des-O-methylicariine. The others are polysaccharide, alkaloid, lignans, some trace elements (Zn, Mn), etc.

【药性与功效 / Chinese medicine properties】

味辛、甘，性温，归肝、肾经。具有补肾壮阳、祛风除湿的功效。主治男子肾阳虚脱导致的阳痿遗精、尿频、筋骨痿软、风湿痹痛、筋骨不利及肢体麻木。

In Chinese medicine theory, *Yín yáng huò* has the nature of pungeng, sweet and warm. It can enter the meridians of liver and kidney. *Yín yáng huò* can tonify kidney-Yang, expel wind and remove dampness. Clinically it can be used for impotence, seminal emission, frequent micturition, flaccidity of extremities, rheumatic paralysis and pain, stiffness of muscle and joint, numbness of limb due to kidney-Yang deficiency.

【药理作用 / Pharmacological effects】

1. 促进性腺功能　淫羊藿具有雄性激素样作用。淫羊藿水煎液可升高雄性小鼠血浆睾酮的含量，增加前列腺、精囊腺的重量；能有效修复大鼠睾丸间质细胞损伤，支持睾丸精曲小管上皮正常生精。淫羊藿还具有雌性激素样作用，能提高雌性动物垂体对促性腺激素释放激素的反应性，提高卵巢对黄体生成素的反应性，刺激小鼠卵巢、子宫的发育，提高血清中雌二醇、黄体生成素、卵泡刺激素的水平。淫羊藿苷和淫羊藿多糖是其性激素样作用的主要活性成分。

(1) Sex hormone-like effects　*Yín yáng huò* has androgen-like effects. *Yín yáng huò* decoction

can increase the level of testosterone in plasma and the weight of prostate gland and seminal vesicle in male mice. It can effectively repair the testicular mesenchymal cells injury and maintain the normal spermatogenesis of testiculariferous tubules epithelium in rats. *Yín yáng huò* also has estrogen-like effects. It can enhance the responsiveness of pituitary to gonadotropin releasing hormone (GnRH) and the responsiveness of ovary to luteinizing hormone, stimulate the development of ovary and uterus, and increase the levels of estradiol, LH and follicle-stimulating hormone (FSH) in serum of female mice. Icariin and icariin polysaccharide are the main active components of its sex hormone-like effects.

2. 促进骨代谢　淫羊藿提取物可以拮抗长期应用醋酸泼尼松所致的大鼠骨质疏松，能促进骨形成，增加骨小梁面积及骨密度。淫羊藿总黄酮可促进大鼠骨Ⅰ型胶原蛋白合成、抑制其水解吸收，提高大鼠骨密度；增加维A酸致骨质疏松大鼠的股骨钙、磷含量和骨密度；增加去卵巢大鼠股骨钙、磷含量和股骨重量。淫羊藿总黄酮通过影响成骨细胞增殖、分化和矿化促进骨形成，减少破骨细胞数目，减弱破骨细胞吸收功能而发挥防治骨质疏松作用。

(2) Promoting bone growth　*Yín yáng huò* extract can antagonize the osteoporosis caused by long-term application of prednisone acetate in rats, promote bone formation, and increase the bone trabecular area and bone density. *Yín yáng huò* flavonoids can promote the synthesis of Ⅰ type collagen protein in bone, inhibit the hydrolysis and absorption of collagen protein, and improve the bone density of rats. *Yín yáng huò* flavonoids can increase the level of calcium and phosphorus, and bone density of osteoporosis rats caused by retinoic acid. *Yín yáng huò* flavonoids also can increase the content of calcium and phosphorus, and the weight of femur of ovariectomized rats. The mechanisms of *Yín yáng huò* flavonoids on osteoporosis include: promoting bone formation by affecting proliferation, differentiation and mineralization of osteoblasts, reducing the number of osteoclasts and the absorption of osteoclasts.

3. 增强免疫系统功能　淫羊藿对免疫细胞、免疫因子及免疫器官均有调节作用，主要成分为淫羊藿多糖和淫羊藿苷。淫羊藿多糖和淫羊藿苷能促进小鼠胸腺和脾脏细胞产生白细胞介素-2，提高巨噬细胞吞噬能力，恢复环磷酰胺损伤小鼠腹腔巨噬细胞吞噬能力。淫羊藿多糖能促进小鼠T淋巴细胞的增殖和产生抑制性T淋巴细胞。淫羊藿苷可增加T淋巴细胞数量，增强CoA诱导的小鼠T淋巴细胞的增殖转化率，减少抑制性T淋巴细胞产生。淫羊藿多糖通过增加脾脏抗体生成细胞数，促进浆细胞产生抗体，促进体液免疫应答和增强免疫记忆功能。淫羊藿总黄酮可以增加正常小鼠血清溶血素水平、脾脏抗体形成细胞数量，提高植物血凝素（PHA）刺激的淋巴细胞转化反应和腹腔巨噬细胞吞噬功能；也可以增加氢化可的松和羟基脲致免疫低下小鼠胸腺指数、脾脏指数及血清溶血素水平。

(3) Regulating immune system function　*Yín yáng huò* can regulate immune cells, immune factors and immune organs. *Yín yáng huò* polysaccharide and icariin are mainly active components. Icariin and icariin can promote the production of IL-2 in thymus and spleen cells of mice, improve the phagocytosis of macrophages, and restore the phagocytosis of macrophages in abdomen of mice injuried by cyclophosphamide. *Yín yáng huò* polysaccharides can promote T lymphocyte proliferation and inhibitory T cells production. Icariin increase the number of T lymphocytes and the proliferation and conversion rate of T cells in mice induced by CoA, but decreased the production of inhibitory T cells. *Yín yáng huò* polysaccharides increase the number of antibody forming cell in spleen and promote plasma cells to produce antibodies, which can promote humoral immune response and enhance immune memory. The total flavonoids of *Yín yáng huò* can increase the hemolysin level in serum and the number of antibody-forming cells in spleen of normal mice, and increase the lymphocyte transformation response and the phagocytosis of macrophages in mice stimulated by PHA. *Yín yáng huò* flavonoids can also increase the thymus index, spleen index and serum hemolysin levels in immunodeficiency mice induced by hydrocortisone and hydroxyurea.

4. 抗炎　淫羊藿总黄酮对醋酸诱导的小鼠腹腔毛细血管通透性增强、巴豆油致小鼠耳肿胀和大鼠肉芽组织增生、角叉菜胶诱导的大鼠足趾肿胀、佐剂性关节炎大鼠的足肿胀均有显著抑制作用。其抗炎作用可能与降低炎症渗出物中前列腺素 E 和丙二醛含量、提高小鼠红细胞过氧化氢酶活性有关。

(4) Anti-inflammation　*Yín yáng huò* flavonoids had significant inhibitory effects on capillary permeability in mice induced by acetic acid, ear swelling of mice induced by croton oil, granulation proliferation in rats induced by cotton ball, paw edema of rat induced by carrageenan and adjuvant arthritis. The anti-inflammation of *Yín yáng huò* is related to the decrease of prostaglanin E and malondialdehyde level, the increse of catalase activity in inflammatory exudate.

5. 对心血管系统的影响

(5) Effects on cardiovascular system functions

（1）对心脏的影响　淫羊藿提取物可减小冠状动脉结扎致犬急性心肌缺血的缺血面积，降低血清中磷酸激酶、LDH 水平及游离脂肪酸、LPO 含量，提高 SOD 和 GSH-Px 活性。淫羊藿总皂苷可对抗异丙肾上腺素、垂体后叶素所致急性心肌缺血大鼠的心电图改变，降低血清肌酸激酶和 LDH 水平。淫羊藿苷可提高异丙肾上腺素诱导的原代培养乳鼠心肌细胞存活率，改善线粒体的膜电位，降低心肌细胞的凋亡率。

1) Anti-myocardial ischemia and anti-arrhythmia　*Yín yáng huò* extract can reduce the area of acute myocardial ischemia in dogs caused by coronary artery ligation, which can reduce the levels of CPK, LDH, free fatty acid and LPO, and increase the activity of SOD and GSH-Px in serum. *Yín yáng huò* saponins can resist the changes of electrocardiogram, and reduce the serum CK and LDH levels in acute myocardial ischemia rats caused by isoproterenol or pituitrin. Icariin can improve the membrane potential of mitochondria, reduce the apoptosis rate of myocardial cells and increase the survival rate of primary culture rat myocardium cells induced by isoproterenol.

淫羊藿水提液和醇浸出液可增强戊巴比妥钠致心衰动物的心肌收缩力。淫羊藿水提物还可对抗氯化钡和乌头碱诱发的大鼠心律失常及肾上腺素诱发的豚鼠心律失常，明显缩短其持续时间，减少室性期前收缩和室性心动过速。提示其抗心律失常作用与阻断 β 受体、阻断 Na^+ 和 Ca^{2+} 内流有关。

Yín yáng huò water extract and alcohol extract can enhance the myocardial contractility of heart failure animals induced by pentobarbital sodium. *Yín yáng huò* water extract can also alleviate the arrhythmia in rats induced by $BaCl_2$ or aconitine and arrhythmia in guinea pigs induced by adrenaline, which can obviously shorten the duration of arrhythmia, reduce the ventricular premature beat and ventricular tachycardia. The antiarrhythmia effects of *Yín yáng huò* are related to blocking β receptor and reducing intracelluar Na^+ and Ca^{2+} concentration.

（2）对血管的作用　淫羊藿总黄酮对正常大鼠和应激性高血压大鼠平均动脉压均有降低作用。腹腔注射淫羊藿苷可降低自发性高血压大鼠的血压。淫羊藿苷具有阻断血管平滑肌上的受体操纵型 Ca^{2+} 通道和电压依赖型 Ca^{2+} 通道的作用，从而扩张血管，降低血压。

2) Dilating blood vessels　*Yín yáng huò* flavonoids can decrease the mean arterial blood pressure in normal rats and hypertensive rats induced by stress. Intraperitoneal injection of icariin can reduce the blood pressure of spontaneously hypertensive rats. Icariin blocks receptor-dependent Ca^{2+} channels and voltage-dependent Ca^{2+} channels on vascular smooth muscle, leads to vasodilation and reducing blood pressure.

6. 对血液系统的影响

(6) Effects on hematological function

（1）促进造血功能 淫羊藿苷可增强小鼠脾淋巴细胞产生集落刺激因子（CFS）样活性，促进骨髓造血并刺激成熟；还可协同诱导生成 IL-2、IL-3、IL-6。

1) Promoting hematopoietic function Icariin can enhance colony stimulating factor (CFS) -like activity of mouse spleen lymphocytes, which can promote hematopoiesis of bone marrow and stimulate maturation. It can also synergistically promote interleukins (IL-2, IL-3, IL-6) production.

（2）改善血液流变学，抗血栓形成 淫羊藿总黄酮灌胃能显著降低家兔全血黏度和红细胞聚集指数，抑制 ADP 诱导的家兔血小板聚集以及抑制家兔体外血栓形成。

2) Improving hemorheology, anti-thrombosis Total flavonoids of *Yín yáng huò* administered orally can reduce the blood viscosity and erythro-agglutation index in rabbit, and inhibit platelet aggregation induced by ADP and thrombosis *in vitro*.

7. 其他作用
淫羊藿还有降血糖、降血脂、抗肿瘤、改善学习记忆等作用，主要活性成分为淫羊藿黄酮、多糖及淫羊藿苷。

(7) Other effects
Yín yáng huò also has the effects of lower blood glucose, lower blood lipid, anti-tumor, improving learning and memory, etc. The main active ingredients are flavonoids of *Yín yáng huò*, polysaccharides of *Yín yáng huò and* Icariin.

【不良反应 / Adverse effects】

曾有患者长期服用淫羊藿叶煎剂发生肝损伤，出现腹胀、纳差、乏力、皮肤瘙痒等症状的报道。

There has been reported that the long-term administration with *Yín yáng huò* decoction in a patient cause liver injury, which showed the abdominal distention, poor appetite, fatigue, and itchy skin.

冬虫夏草 ¦ *Dōng chóng xià cǎo* (Cordyceps)

【来源 / Origin】

本品为麦角菌科真菌冬虫夏草菌［*Cordyceps sinensis*（Berk.）Sacc.］寄生在蝙蝠蛾科昆虫幼虫上的子座及幼虫尸体的复合体。主要分布于西藏、四川、青海、甘肃等地。夏至前后，在积雪尚未融化时采集。在虫体潮湿未干时，除去泥土和膜皮，晒干或黄酒喷使平直，微火烘干，生用。

Dōng chóng xià cǎo is the dried stroma and sporophore of *Cordyceps sinensis* (Berk.) Sacc., family of Clavicipitaceae, which parasitized in the larva of *Hepialus varians Staudinger*, family of Hepialidae. It is widely cultivated in Xizang Autonomous region, Sichuan province, Qinghai province and Gansu province, etc., and harvested in summer solstice, before the snow melted. Dried in the sun after removing the soil and outer skin or dried by slight fire after making it flat by spraying rice mice, directly used for Chinese medicinal preparation.

【化学成分 / Chemical ingredients】

含虫草酸（cordycepic acid)、虫草素（cordycepin)、虫草多糖等。还含有粗蛋白、脂肪、D-甘露醇、碳水化合物、麦角甾醇、腺苷及多种氨基酸和维生素。

Dōng chóng xià cǎo mainly contains cordycepic acid, cordycepin and cordycepic polysaccharides. The others are proteins, fat, D-mannitol, carbohydrate, ergosterol, adenosine, amino acid, vitamin, etc.

【药性与功效 / Chinese medicine properties】

味甘，性温，归肾、肺经。具有补肺益肾、止血化痰的功效。主治久咳虚喘、劳嗽咯血、阳痿遗精、腰膝酸痛等症。

In Chinese medicine theory, *Dōng chóng xià cǎo* has the nature of sweet, warm. It can enter the meridians of lung and kidney. *Dōng chóng xià cǎo* can tonify lung, replenish kidney, stop bleeding and resolve phlegm. Clinically it can be used for chronic cough, deficiency-type dyspnea, hemoptysis, impotence, seminal emission, aching pain in waist and knee.

【药理作用 / **Pharmacological effects**】

1. **性激素样作用** 冬虫夏草水煎液可增加家兔睾丸重量指数及精子数，增加雄性大鼠血浆睾酮含量及包皮腺、精囊腺和前列腺的重量。雌性大鼠灌服冬虫夏草细粉可增加受孕百分率和产子数。

(1) **Sex hormone-like effects** *Dōng chóng xià cǎo* decoction can increase the testis index and the number of sperm in rabbits, also increase the content of testosterone in plasma and the weight of preputial gland, seminal vesicle and prostate in the normal male rats. Oral administration of *Dōng chóng xià cǎo* powder increase the percentage of conception and the number of offspring.

2. **对免疫系统的作用** 冬虫夏草水煎液可增加小鼠脾脏重量，对抗泼尼松龙、环磷酰胺所致的小鼠脾脏重量减轻；提高小鼠抗体形成细胞数和血清 IgM 水平，对抗环磷酰胺的免疫抑制作用；抑制红斑狼疮小鼠抗体产生，延长存活时间；抑制 BALB/c 纯系小鼠脾细胞对 Con A 或 LPS 诱导的淋巴细胞增殖，抑制 IL-1 和 IL-2 的产生；减低同种异型抗原诱导的迟发型超敏反应及混合淋巴细胞反应，延长小鼠同种异体移植皮片的存活时间。虫草多糖能提高小鼠腹腔巨噬细胞的吞噬率及吞噬指数，对抗可的松引起的吞噬功能下降；剂量依赖性地促进 Con A 或 LPS 诱导的小鼠脾脏淋巴细胞转化，促进 Con A 诱导 IL-2 生成。高浓度几乎完全抑制 PHA 诱导的健康人外周血淋巴细胞产生 IL-2 和 γ-TNF。

(2) **Regulating immune system function** *Dōng chóng xià cǎo* decoction can increase the spleen weight of mice, antagonize the reduction of the spleen weight in mice caused by prednisolone and cyclophosphamide. increase the number of antibody forming cells and the level of IgM in serum of mice, which can antagonize the immunosuppression of cyclophosphamide; inhibit the production of antibody and prolong the survival time in mice with lupus erythematosus; inhibit the proliferation of lymphocyte in spleen, inhibit the production of IL-1 and IL-2 in BALB/c mice induced by Con A or LPS; reduce the delayed-type hypersensitivity and mixed lymphocyte reaction induced by alloantigen, which prolong the survival time of heterodermic graft. *Dōng chóng xià cǎo* polysaccharides can increase the phagocytic percentage and phagocytic index of peritoneal macrophages in mice, and prevent the decrease of phagocytic function caused by cortisone; promote the lymphocyte transformation of mouse spleen induced by Con A or LPS in a dose-dependent manner, and promote the production of IL-2 induced by Con A. High concentration of *Dōng chóng xià cǎo* polysaccharides almost completely inhibit the production of IL-2 and γ - TNF in peripheral blood lymphocytes of healthy people induced by PHA.

3. **平喘** 冬虫夏草水提液能明显扩张离体豚鼠支气管，增强肾上腺素的扩张支气管作用，也能对抗乙酰胆碱引起的豚鼠哮喘。冬虫夏草菌粉能减轻慢性阻塞性肺病（COPD）小鼠气道炎症反应，改善肺通气功能。

(3) **Anti-asthma** The water extract of *Dōng chóng xià cǎo* can obviously dilate the isolated bronchus from guinea pig, enhance the dilation of the bronchus induced by adrenaline and resist the asthma of guinea pig caused by acetylcholine. The powder of *Dōng chóng xià cǎo* can inhibit inflammation in airway and improve ventilatory function of chronic obstructive pulmonary diseases (COPD) mice.

4. **促进造血功能** 冬虫夏草水煎醇沉液的结晶物对造血干细胞、骨髓红系祖细胞、成纤维祖细胞和粒单系祖细胞的增殖有促进作用，可对抗三尖杉对造血功能的损害。

(4) Improving hematopoietic function   The crystal prepared from water-extraction and alcohol-precipitation liquid of *Dōng chóng xià cǎo* can promote the proliferation of hematopoietic stem cells, erythroid progenitor cells, fibroblast progenitor cells and granulocyte-monophyletic progenitor cells. It also alleviate the damage of hematopoietic function induced by cephalotaxus cuspidata.

5. **对肾脏功能的影响**   冬虫夏草能降低肾脏大部分切除（5/6）所致慢性肾功能不全大鼠的死亡率，改善贫血状况，降低血清尿素氮和肌酐水平，促进 IL-2 产生，增加脾淋巴细胞转化率，延缓肾功能不全的进展。冬虫夏草水提液还能减轻庆大霉素和环孢素 A 引起的急性肾衰竭大鼠的肾小管损伤。冬虫夏草改善肾功能的机制包括稳定肾小管上皮细胞溶酶体膜，防止溶酶体破坏；促进肾小管内皮细胞生长因子的合成释放，加速肾小管组织修复；保护细胞膜 Na^+-K^+- ATP 酶功能、降低 LDH 活性、减少脂质过氧化损伤等。

(5) Nephroprotection   *Dōng chóng xià cǎo* can reduce the mortality of chronic renal insufficiency rats caused by 5/6 nephrectomy, improve anemia, reduce the level of urea nitrogen and creatinine in serum, promote the production of IL-2, increase the transformation rate of spleen lymphocyte, and delay the progress of renal insufficiency. The water extract of *Dōng chóng xià cǎo* can also reduce the renal tubular damage of acute renal failure rats caused by gentamicin and cyclosporine A. The main mechanisms of its nephroprotection include: stabilizing lysosomal membrane of renal tubular epithelial cells and preventing lysosomal destruction; promoting synthesis and release of renal tubular endothelial cell growth factor; accelerating repairment of renal tubular tissue, protecting Na^+- K^+-ATPase function of cell membrane, decreasing LDH activity and lipid peroxidation damage, etc.

6. **延缓衰老**   冬虫夏草水提液能降低小鼠心肌及肝脏中脂质过氧化物的含量，提高小鼠肝组织 SOD 活性，减缓 D–半乳糖诱导的小鼠衰老。冬虫夏草菌丝体还能显著抑制大鼠和小鼠脑内 MAO-B 活性。

(6) Anti-aging   The water extract of *Dōng chóng xià cǎo* can also reduce the content of lipid peroxides in the heart and liver, increase the activity of SOD in the liver tissue , and alleviate the aging characteristics of mice induced by D-galactose. *Dōng chóng xià cǎo* mycelium can also significantly inhibit the activity of MAO-B in the brain of rats and mice.

7. **抗肿瘤**   冬虫夏草水提物对 Lewis 肺癌的原发灶生长和自发性肺转移均有抑制作用。冬虫夏草中多种成分具有抗肿瘤作用，虫草多糖能抑制小鼠肉瘤 S_{180}、人白血病细胞 U_{937} 的增殖；虫草素能抑制小鼠体内 B_{16} 黑色素瘤细胞的增殖和生长；虫草酸能抑制小鼠艾氏腹水癌、鼻咽癌的发展。冬虫夏草抗肿瘤作用与其直接抑制肿瘤细胞增殖和调节机体免疫功能平衡的间接作用有密切关系。

(7) Anti-tumor   The water extract of *Dōng chóng xià cǎo* can inhibit the primary focus growth and spontaneous lung metastasis of Lewis lung cancer mice. *Dōng chóng xià cǎo* polysaccharide can inhibit the proliferation of sarcoma S_{180} and U_{937} leukemia cells in mice. Cordycepin can inhibit the proliferation and growth of B_{16} melanoma cells in mice. Cordycepic acid can inhibit the development of Ehrlich ascites carcinoma and nasopharyngeal carcinoma in mice. The anti-tumor effect of *Dōng chóng xià cǎo* is closely related to its direct inhibition of tumor cell proliferation and indirect regulation of immune function balance.

8. **降血糖**   虫草多糖、人工虫草碱提取物可降低正常小鼠、四氧嘧啶及链脲佐菌素诱发糖尿病小鼠的血糖。人工虫草多糖还改善糖尿病小鼠的糖耐量和胰岛素抵抗指数，增强胰岛素受体敏感性。

(8) Reducing blood glucose   *Dōng chóng xià cǎo* polysaccharide and alkaloid of artificial cultured

Dōng chóng xià cǎo can reduce the blood glucose of normal mice and diabetic mice induced by alloxan and streptozotocin. *Dōng chóng xià cǎo* polysaccharide also increase glucose tolerance, insulin resistance index, and insulin receptor sensitivity in diabetic mice.

9. 保肝 冬虫夏草可减轻四氯化碳诱导的大鼠肝纤维化程度，抑制肝内储脂细胞的增殖和转化，减轻狄氏间隙胶原纤维沉积。虫草菌丝可减少肝内Ⅰ型胶原、Ⅲ型胶原的沉积和胶原总量。

(9) Hepatoprotection *Dōng chóng xià cǎo* can reduce the degree of liver fibrosis of rats induced by CCl_4, inhibit the proliferation and transformation of fat-storing cells, and reduce the deposition of disse diastem collagen fibers. *Dōng chóng xià cǎo* mycelium can reduce the deposition of type Ⅰ and type Ⅲ collagen and the total amount of collagen in the liver.

10. 其他作用 冬虫夏草还具有抑制红斑狼疮、减轻器官移植排斥反应、抗疲劳等作用。

(10) Other effects *Dōng chóng xià cǎo* also has inhibitory effects on lupus erythematosus, allograft rejection and fatigue.

【**不良反应 / Adverse effects**】

冬虫夏草的不良反应报道主要以过敏反应为主，表现为皮肤黏膜损害，或伴有呼吸、心血管系统的症状。此外，也有患者出现闭经、肾功能不全、脘腹胀满、抑制胃肠排空等不良反应。

The main adverse effects of *Dōng chóng xià cǎo* are allergy, the syndroms are the damage of skin and mucous or with the dysfunction of respiratory and cardiovascular system. In addition, amenorrhoea, renal insufficiency, or indigestion occasionally occured in some individuals.

（方 芳 董世芬 汪 宁）

题库

第二十章 收涩药
Chapter 20 Astringent medicines

学习目标｜Objectives

1. **掌握** 收涩药的主要药理作用；五味子、山茱萸与功效相关的药理作用及药效物质基础。

2. **了解** 滑脱证的主要病理表现。

1. **Must know** The main pharmacological effects of astringent medicines; the efficacies related pharmacological effects, mechanism of action, and material basis of of *Wǔ wèi zǐ* and *Shān zhū yú*.

2. **Desirable to know** The clinical manifestations of the efflux desertion syndrome.

第一节 概述
Section 1 Overview

PPT

　　凡以收敛固涩为主要功效，主治滑脱证的药物，称为收涩药。本类药物大多味酸涩，性温或平，主入肺、脾、肾、大肠经。收涩药通常具有敛汗、止泻、固精、缩尿、止血、止带和止咳等功效，可用于气血津液滑脱耗散之证。常用药有五味子、山茱萸、麻黄根、乌梅、诃子、石榴皮、肉豆蔻、赤石脂、禹余粮、覆盆子、桑螵蛸、罂粟壳等。

　　Medicines which exert astringent and convergent effects and are applied to treat syndrome of efflux desertion are called astringent medicines. The astringent medicines are commonly sour and astringent in flavor, warm or neutral in nature, entering the lung, spleen, kidney and large intestine meridians. Astringent medicines generally have the functions of restraining perspiration, preventing diarrhea, solidifying essence, reducing urine, stopping bleeding, stopping leucorrhoea and relieving cough, etc. They can be used to treat syndrome of efflux desertion of Qi, blood and body fluid. The commonly medicines include *Wǔ wèi zǐ*, *Shān zhū yú*, *Má huáng gēn*, *Wū méi*, *Hē zǐ*, *Shí liú pí*, *Ròu dòu kòu*, *Chì shí zhǐ*, *Yú yú liáng*, *Fù pén zǐ*, *Sāng piāo xiāo*, *Yīng sù qiào*, etc.

　　气血津液是营养人体的重要物质，既不断被消耗，又不断得到补充，维持相对平衡，以保持人体功能正常。气血津液一旦消耗过度，正气虚亏，则致滑脱不禁，甚至可以危及生命。中医学认为，滑脱证主要为久病或体虚使正气不固、脏腑功能衰退所致。如气虚自汗、阴虚盗汗、脾肾阳虚致久泻；肾虚致遗精、滑精、遗尿、尿频，冲任不固致崩漏下血；肺肾虚损则致久咳虚喘。

Qi, blood and body fluid are the important material of nutrition for human body, which are consumed and get complement ceaselessly maintaining relative balance to keep human body normal function. Once the consumption of Qi, blood and body fluid is excessive, healthy Qi will be deficiency and threaten life. In Chinese medicine theory , the syndrome of efflux desertion is mainly caused by chronic disease or weak health which leads to unconsolidation of healthy Qi, or due to deficiency of bowel and visceral functions, such as Qi deficiency with spontaneous sweating, Yin deficiency with night sweating, enduring diarrhea caused by spleen-kidney Yang deficiency, metrorrhagia and metrostaxis caused by deficiency of the thoroughfare and conception vessels, enduring cough and panting caused by lung-kidney deficiency, and spermatorrhea, seminal efflux, enuresis, frequent urination caused by kidney deficiency.

西医学认为，滑脱证主要是机体各系统和器官功能衰退所致。临床可见多汗、腹泻、痢疾、遗精、遗尿、尿频、子宫出血、咳喘等症状。故滑脱证与西医学中自主神经功能紊乱、慢性结肠炎、肠易激综合征、克罗恩病、结肠癌、肠结核、脂肪泻、糖尿病性腹泻、痢疾、遗尿症、尿崩症、尿道综合征、功能性子宫出血、哮喘等的症状表现相似。现代药理研究表明，收涩药治疗滑脱证的作用与下列药理作用有关。

In western medicine, efflux desertion syndrome is mainly induced by functional decline of system and organ. Clinical manifestations include hyperhidrosis, diarrhea, dysentery, spermatorrhea, enuresis, urinary frequency, uterine blood, cough and asthma. The efflux desertion syndrome is associated with various diseases including autonomic nervous disorders, chronic colitis, irritable bowel syndrome, Crohn's disease, colon cancer, intestinal tuberculosis, fat diarrhea, diabetic diarrhea, dysentery, enuresis, diabetes insipidus, urethral syndrome, functional uterine bleeding, asthma, etc. The actions of constraining sweat, checking diarrhea, suppressing cough and anti-pathogeny microorganism are the mainly basis for astringent and convergent efficacy.

1. **收敛**　收涩药中多数药物含有大量鞣质，与创面、黏膜、溃疡面等部位接触后，可沉淀或凝固局部蛋白质，在组织表面形成致密的保护层，以减少体液和血浆损失及减轻创面刺激，预防感染，并促进其愈合。此外，鞣质和有机酸等可收缩微血管，鞣质还能促进血液中蛋白质凝固，堵塞小血管，有助于局部止血。鞣质与汗腺、消化腺、生殖器官等分泌细胞中的蛋白质结合，使腺体表面细胞蛋白质变性或凝固，从而改变细胞功能，使腺体分泌减少，保持黏膜干燥。

(1) Protective effects on wound and mucosa　The herbs in this chapter usually contain tannin and organic acids. These components can coagulate or precipitate part of proteins when they are applied on ulcerative surface or wound, and form a compact protective layer on the damaged tissue surface to reduce loss of body fluid and plasma, which can help to relieve wound irritation and accelerate wound healing. Furthermore, tannin and organic acids can cause capillary contraction. Tannin can promote protein agglutination, which will block capillary and facilitate local hemostasis. In addition, tannin is able to bind to the membrane proteins of sweat gland, digestive gland and reproductive organ, finally leading to decrease of the gland secretion.

2. **止泻**　收涩药止泻作用涉及多个环节。五味子、石榴皮、乌梅、诃子、金樱子、肉豆蔻、赤石脂、禹余粮等含有大量鞣质，能与蛋白质结合在肠黏膜表面形成保护层，可减轻肠内容物对神经丛的刺激；赤石脂、禹余粮口服后能吸附于胃肠黏膜起保护作用，还能吸附细菌、毒素及其代谢产物，减轻其对肠黏膜的刺激；乌梅、五倍子、石榴皮等对多种肠道致病菌有抑制作用，通过消除肠道感染而止泻；罂粟壳所含吗啡可提高胃肠道及其括约肌张力，减少消化液分泌，抑制排便反射。

(2) **Anti-diarrhea** The astringent medicines exert checking diarrhea effects through several ways. For example, *Wǔ wei zǐ, Hē zǐ, Shí líu pí, Ròu dòu kòu, Chì shí zhǐ* and *Yú yǔ liáng* all contain large amount of tannin, which can coagulate proteins of intestinal mucosa to form a protective layer and relieve harmful substance caused irritation to the nerve plexus in intestinal wall. The active ingredients of *Chì shí zhǐ* and *Yú yǔ liǎng* can be absorbed by gastrointestinal mucous to prevent it from being stimulated by bacteria and their metabolite, which helps to check diarrhea. All of these effects of tannin can slow down peristalsis of intestines and check diarrhea. Furthermore, *Wū méi, Wǔ bèi zǐ*, and *Shí líu pí* can check diarrhea through inhibiting bacteria growth. *Yīng sù qiào* contains a small amount of morphine, which can increase muscle tension in digestive tract, reduce gastric juice secretion, suppress defecation reflex and finally help to stop diarrhea.

3. **镇咳** 五倍子、五味子、罂粟壳等均具有镇咳功效。罂粟壳所含生物碱能抑制咳嗽中枢和咳嗽反射而镇咳；五味子及其乙醚提取物可明显减少氨水刺激引起的动物咳嗽次数。

(3) **Cough suppression** *Wǔ bèi zǐ, Wǔ wei zǐ* and *Yīng sù qiào* all can suppress cough. Alkaloids in *Yīng sù qiào* are able to depress cough reflex. Moreover, both *Wǔ wei zǐ* and its ether extract can reduce frequency of cough induced by ammonia water in animal experiments.

4. **抗病原微生物** 收涩药所含的鞣质及有机酸均具有抗菌活性，如五味子、山茱萸、石榴皮、乌梅等，对金黄色葡萄球菌、链球菌、伤寒杆菌、痢疾杆菌、铜绿假单胞菌、真菌或部分寄生虫等有抑制或杀灭作用。

(4) **Anti-microorganisms** Tannin and organic acids contained in astringent medicines have antibacterial activity in different degree. For example, tannin and organic acid isolated from *Wǔ wei zǐ, Shān zhū yú* and *Wū méi* can inhibit the growth of *staphylococcus aureus, streptococcus, salmonella typhi, dysentery bacillus, pseudomonas aeruginosa*. They are capable of restraining or sterilizing part of funguses and parasites as well.

5. **其他作用** 收涩药还具有止血、保肝等药理作用。如山茱萸对子宫出血、月经过多具有较好的止血作用；五倍子对便血痔血具有较好的止血作用；五味子、乌梅、诃子等具有保肝作用。

(5) **Other effects** Some astringent medicines have blood-stanching and liver safeguarding abilities. For example, *Shān zhū yú* can be used to relieve uterine bleeding and profuse menstruation. *Wǔ bèi zǐ* can be used to treat bloody stool and bleeding hemorrhoids. Others like *Wǔ wei zǐ, Wū méi* and *Hē zǐ* have liver safeguarding ability.

常用收涩药的主要药理作用见表 20-1。

The main pharmacological effects of commonly used astringent medicines are summarized in Table 20-1.

表 20-1 常用收涩药的主要药理作用

药物	收敛	止泻	抗病原微生物	其他药理作用
五味子	+	+	+	镇静、催眠、保肝、抗溃疡、祛痰、镇咳、改善心功能、免疫调节
山茱萸	+	−	+	保肝、降血糖、抗氧化、抗衰老、免疫调节、强心、抗休克、抗炎、镇痛
乌梅	+	+	+	抗过敏、抗肿瘤、抗氧化
肉豆蔻	+	+	+	促进胃肠功能、抗氧化、抗炎
五倍子	+	+	+	抗氧化、降血糖、抑制胃酸分泌
罂粟壳	+	+	−	镇痛、镇静、镇咳、呼吸抑制

注："+"表示有明确作用；"−"表示无作用，或未查阅到相关研究文献

第二节　常用药

Section 2　Commonly used medicines

PPT

微课

五味子 ┊ *Wǔ wèi zǐ (Fructus Schisandrae Chinensis Galla Chinensis)*

【来源 / Origin】

本品为木兰科植物五味子 [*Schisandra chinensis* (Turcz.) Baill.] 的干燥成熟果实。主要分布于黑龙江、辽宁、吉林、河北等地，习称"北五味子"。秋季采收，晒干或蒸后晒干，去除果梗和杂质。

Wǔ wèi zǐ is the dry ripe fruit of *Schisandra Chinensis* (Turcz.) Baill. The plant is mainly cultivated in Heilongjiang province, Jilin province, Liaoning province and Hebei province in China. Thus, *Wǔ wèi zǐ* is traditionally called *Běi wǔ wèi zǐ*. Harvested in autumn, dried or steamed to remove stems and impurities.

【化学成分 / Chemical ingredients】

主要含木脂素（18.1%~19.2%）、挥发油（约 3%）和多糖（59.9%）。木脂素中主要有效成分为五味子素、五味子甲素、五味子乙素、五味子丙素、五味子醇甲、五味子醇乙、五味子酯甲、五味子酯乙及戈米辛 A 等。五味子挥发油主要成分为萜类化合物，包括单萜类、含氧单萜类、倍半萜类、含氧倍半萜类和少量醇、酸等含氧化合物，其中以倍半萜类为主。此外，五味子还含有机酸、维生素、脂肪油和鞣质等成分。

Wǔ wèi zǐ mainly contains lignin (18.1%~19.2%), volatile oil (3%) and polysaccharide (59.9%). The Lignins from *Wǔ wèi zǐ* mainly include schisandrin, schisandrin A, schisandrin B, schisandrin C, schisandrol A, schisandrol B, schisantherin A, schisantherin B, and gomisin D, etc. Volatile oils in *Wǔ wèi zǐ* are mainly terpenoids including monoterpenes, oxygenated monoterpenes, sesquiterpenes, oxygenated sesquiterpenes and some oxygenated compounds including alcohols or acids. Sesquiterpenes are the most abundant among these ingredients. In addition, *Wǔ wèi zǐ* also contains organic acids, vitamins, fatty oils and tannins.

【药性与功效 / Chinese medicine properties】

味酸、甘，性温，归肺、心、肾经。具有收敛固涩、益气生津、补肾宁心的功效。主治久咳虚喘、梦遗滑精、遗尿尿频、久泻不止、自汗盗汗、津伤口渴、内热消渴、心悸失眠等证。

In Chinese medicine theory, *Wǔ wèi zǐ* has the nature of sour, sweet and warm. It can enter the meridians of liver, heart and kidney. *Wǔ wèi zǐ* is capable to induce astringency and convergence, boost Qi and engender liquid, tonify kidney and tranquilize mind. Accordingly, *Wǔ wèi zǐ* can be applied to treat deficiency-type dyspnea and chronic cough, spontaneous seminal emission and nocturnal emission, enuresis and frequent urination, chronic diarrhea, spontaneous sweat and night sweat, fluid consumption and thirst, consumptive thirst and internal heat and palpitation and insomnia.

【药理作用 / Pharmacological activities】

1. **镇静、催眠**　五味子水提取物能明显延长戊巴比妥钠诱导小鼠睡眠的时间，减少小鼠自发性活动，并可协同氯丙嗪及利血平抑制自主活动。五味子水煎液能明显延长大鼠睡眠时间，增加戊巴比妥钠致小鼠睡眠发生率和睡眠时间。五味子甲素、五味子丙素、五味子醇乙和五味子酯乙是五味子镇静、催眠的主要有效成分。

(1) Tranquilization and hypnotic effects The ethanol or water extracts of *Wǔ wèi zǐ* can prolong the sleep time of mice induced by pentobarbital sodium, reduce spontaneous activity in mice, exert cooperative action with chlorpromazine and reserpine to inhibit autonomous activity of mice. Water decoction of *Wǔ wèi zǐ* can increase the incidence of sleep and extend sleeping time in mice caused by sodium pentobarbital. Schisandrin A, schisandrin C, schisandrol B, and schisantherin B are the main tranquilizing and hypnotic components in *Wǔ wèi zǐ*.

2. 保肝　五味子及五味子乙醇提取物、五味子乙素等对化学毒物所致动物急慢性肝损伤有保护作用，能降低血清 ALT 活性，减轻肝细胞坏死，防止脂肪变性，抗纤维化。人工合成五味子丙素的中间产物联苯双酯已被用于临床治疗肝炎，具有降酶和改善肝功能作用。木脂素是其保肝的主要物质基础。五味子保肝作用机制可能有以下环节。①抗脂质过氧化：五味子可提高肝细胞胞质内超氧化物歧化酶（SOD）和过氧化氢酶（CAT）活性，提高肝脏谷胱甘肽抗氧化系统作用，减轻氧自由基对肝细胞的损害，抑制 CCl_4 引起的肝微粒体脂质过氧化，减少肝内 MDA 的生成，提高肝细胞的存活率。②促进肝细胞修复和再生：五味子可促进肝细胞内蛋白质和糖原的生物合成，加速肝细胞的修复与再生。③增强肝脏解毒功能：五味子甲素、乙素、丙素等多种成分可增强肝细胞微粒体细胞色素 P450 活性，促进肝药酶的合成，从而增强肝脏的解毒功能。④促进胆汁分泌：五味子多糖可促进胆汁分泌，加速有毒物质的排泄，有利于保护肝脏。⑤减轻炎症反应：五味子具有肾上腺皮质激素样作用，能减轻肝细胞炎症反应。⑥稳定细胞结构：五味子乙素能维持大鼠肝细胞膜在氧化性损伤状态下的稳定性，保护细胞膜结构完整和功能正常。

(2) Hepatoprotection Ethanol extracts of *Wǔ wèi zǐ* protects hepatocytes from injury induced by chemical agents, such as CCl_4, thioacetamide (TAA) and paracetamol. It can reduce serum glutamatepyruvate transaminase (ALT) level, alleviate necrosis of hepatocytes, and prevent hepatic cells form hepatic steatosis and fibrosis. Bifendate, an intermediate product of schisandrin C, has been used to treat hepatitis, which has the function of reducing enzyme and improving liver function. Lignin is the main effective component of protecting liver effect of *Wǔ wèi zǐ*. The hepatoprotection of *Wǔ wèi zǐ* may be associated to the following mechanisms. ①Anti-lipid peroxidation: *Wǔ wèi zǐ* is able to increase superoxide dismutase (SOD), catalase (CAT) and glutathione peroxidase (GSH-Px) activity in liver, decrease the production of malondialdehyde (MDA) in hepatocytes and suppress lipid peroxidation triggered by CCl_4, thus to improve the survival rate of hepatocytes. ②Promote hepatocytes regeneration and repairment: *Wǔ wèi zǐ* can stimulate the protein production and glycogenesis to accelerate hepatocytes regeneration and repairment. ③Enhance liver detoxication property: many components of *Wǔ wèi zǐ* increase the activity of P450 in hepatocytes and promote drug-metabolizing enzyme synthesis, resulting in improving detoxication property. ④Promote bile secretion: schisandra polysaccharide can promote bile secretion, accelerate the excretion of toxic substances, which is conducive to protecting the liver. ⑤Anti-inflammatory: *Wǔ wèi zǐ* has adrenal cortical hormone-like function and it reduces inflammatory responses of hepatocytes. ⑥Stabilizing cell structure: schisandrin B is able to increase hepatocyte survival under oxidative damage status through maintaining cell membrane integrated and function normal.

3. 抗胃溃疡　五味子甲素可抑制水浸应激性、幽门结扎、阿司匹林、组胺等所致胃溃疡模型大鼠的胃液分泌，降低胃液酸度，促进溃疡愈合。五味子有效成分五味子醇乙、五味子甲素可抑制大鼠应激性溃疡。

(3) Anti-gastric ulcer Schisandrin A is able to inhibit gastric secretion and decrease acidity of gastric juice in gastric ulcer model rats induced by water-immersion stress, pylorus ligation, aspirin or histamine. Schisandrin A and schisandrol B can alleviate gastric ulcer in rats induced by stress.

4. 止泻　五味子能明显降低腹泻小鼠稀便率、腹泻指数，五味子甲素可抑制小鼠胃肠推进，五味子提取物可缓解伊立替康所致腹泻。

(4) Anti-diarrhea　*Wǔ wèi zǐ* is capable to reduce the rate of loose stools and the diarrhea index in mice. Schisandrin A is capable to inhibit the gastrointestinal propulsion of mice and extract of *Wǔ wèi zǐ* can alleviate diarrhea caused by irinotecan.

5. 祛痰、镇咳　五味子水煎液具有祛痰和镇咳作用。五味子乙醇提取物能提高慢性支气管炎小鼠支气管上皮细胞内核 RNA 含量，增强支气管上皮细胞功能；五味子素能增强家兔和大鼠的呼吸功能，并能对抗吗啡的呼吸抑制作用。

(5) Suppressing cough and eliminating phlegm　Water decoction of *Wǔ wèi zǐ* have the ability to suppress cough and eliminate phlegm. The ethanol extract can increase RNA level of bronchial epithelial cells to improve its function in mice with chronic bronchitis. Schisandrin can enhance the respiratory function of rats and rabbits, and suppress the respiratory inhibition of morphine.

6. 影响心血管系统　五味子可抑制心脏收缩、减慢心率、降低心肌耗氧量；五味子粉能增强家兔心血管功能、扩张血管、降低血压、增加心肌细胞内 RNA 含量、提高三磷酸腺苷 (ATP)、碱性磷酸酶 (ALP) 活性，从而加强心肌细胞的能量代谢，改善心肌的营养和功能；五味子素能增加豚鼠离体心脏及麻醉犬冠脉流量。五味子提取液对动物缺氧及急性心肌缺血损伤有较强的保护作用。

(6) The effects on cardiovascular system　*Wǔ wèi zǐ* have the ability to inhibit heart contraction, slow heart rate, and reduce oxygen consumption in the myocardium. *Wǔ wèi zǐ* powder can enhance cardiovascular function, dilate blood vessels, lower blood pressure, increase the content of RNA in myocardial cells, improve the activity of adenosine triphosphate (ATP) and alkaline phosphatase (ALP), so as to strengthen the energy metabolism of myocardial cells and improve the nutrition and function of myocardial. Schisandrin is able to increase the coronary artery flow of isolated guinea pigs heart and in anesthetized dogs. Schisandra extract has a strong protective effect on animal hypoxia and acute myocardial ischemic injury.

7. 调节免疫功能　五味子油乳剂可促进淋巴细胞 DNA 合成，使淋巴母细胞生成增多。五味子多糖能对抗环磷酰胺所致小鼠外周血白细胞减少，增加小鼠胸腺和脾脏重量，显著提高腹腔巨噬细胞的吞噬率和吞噬指数，促进溶血素及溶血空斑形成，促进淋巴细胞转化。五味子酚能保护脾淋巴细胞免受氧自由基的损伤。

(7) The effects on immune system　*Wǔ wèi zǐ* oil emulsion can enhance the DNA generation to promote lymphoblast proliferation. In mouse experiments, polysaccharides contained in *Wǔ wèi zǐ* can antagonize the reduction of peripheral blood leukocytes induced by cyclophosphamide in mice, and increase the weight of thymus and spleen, raise the phagocytic index of peritoneal macrophage, promote the formation of hemolytic plaque and hemolysin, and promote lymphocyte transformation. In addition, schisanhenol protects lymphocytes from damage induced by oxygen free radicals.

【不良反应 / Adverse effects】

口服五味子乙醚提取物后，胃部有烧灼感、泛酸及胃痛，并有呃逆、困倦、肠鸣等不良反应。五味子酸偶有过敏反应。

Oral administration of ethyl ether extracts of *Wǔ wèi zǐ* may lead to burning sensation in stomach, acid regurgitation, hiccough, sleepy and borborygmus. Fructus schisandrae acids also cause allergic reaction occasionally.

山茱萸 ┊ *Shān zhū yú* (Corni Fructus Corni Fructus)

【来源 / Origin】

本品为山茱萸科植物山茱萸 (*Cornus officinalis* Sieb. et Zucc.) 的干燥成熟果肉。主要分布于浙江、陕西和河南等地。秋末冬初采收，文火烘沸、水烫后，除去果核，干燥。

Shān zhū yú is the dry fruit pulp of *Cornus officinalis* Sieb. et Zucc. The plant is widely cultivated in Zhejiang province, Shaanxi province, and Henan province in China. Harvested at the end of autumn and early winter. After simmering in boiling water, the core is removed and dried.

【化学成分 / Chemical ingredients】

主要含有环烯醚萜类、三萜类、鞣质和有机酸等化学成分，其中环烯醚萜类是其主要成分。环烯醚萜类成分包括山茱萸苷（即马鞭草苷）、莫诺苷、马钱子苷（即番木鳖苷）、獐牙菜苷、山茱萸新苷等；三萜类主要包括齐墩果酸和熊果酸；鞣质类成分包括喜树鞣质 A、喜树鞣质 B 等；有机酸类成分主要有没食子酸、苹果酸、酒石酸、原儿茶酸、对羟基桂皮酸等。此外，山茱萸还含有黄酮、多糖和维生素等成分。

Shān zhū yú mainly contains iridoid glycosides, triterpenoids, tannins and organic acids. Iridoid glycosides are the main constituents of *Shān zhū yú*. The iridoid glycosides mainly include cornin, morroniside, loganin, sweroside and cornuside. The triterpenoids contain oleanolic acid and ursolic acid. The tannins mainly include camptothin A、B, etc. Organic acids include gallic acid, malic acid and tartaric acid, etc. In addition, *Shān zhū yú* contains flavonoids, polysaccharides and vitamins.

【药性与功效 / Chinese medicine properties】

味酸、涩，性微温，归肝、肾经。具有补益肝肾、收涩固脱的功效。用于治疗眩晕耳鸣、腰膝酸痛、阳痿遗精、遗尿尿频、崩漏带下、大汗虚脱、内热消渴等证。

In Chinese medicine theory, *Shān zhū yú* has the nature of sour, astringent and slightly warm. It can enter the meridians of liver and kindey. *Shān zhū yú* can nourish liver and kidney and astringe essence and secure consolidation. Accordingly, it can be used for dizziness and tinnitus, lumbus and knees aching，impotence and nocturnal emission，enuresis and frequent urination，metrorrhagia and metrostaxis, leukorrheal diseases, profuse sweating and collapse, consumptive thirst and internal heat, etc.

【药理作用 / Pharmacological effects】

1. 保肝　山茱萸有效降低四氯化碳（CCl_4）所致的急性肝损伤动物血清谷草转氨酶（AST）与谷丙转氨酶（ALT）活性，减轻肝细胞变性坏死。山茱萸所含獐牙菜苷能抗肝细胞损伤，促进肝细胞恢复。

(1) **Hepatoprotection**　*Shān zhū yú* reduces the serum glutamic-pyruvic transaminase (ALT) and glutamic oxalacetic transaminase (AST) levels in rats with acute CCl_4 induced liver injury. Sweroside, one of the active components in *Shān zhū yú*, can reduce hepatic cells damage and promote hepatic cells recovery.

2. 降血糖　环烯醚萜类（主要为马钱子苷和莫诺苷）和三萜酸类（主要为熊果酸和齐墩果酸）成分是山茱萸降糖作用的主要物质基础。山茱萸降血糖作用与提高糖耐量、保护胰岛 B 细胞或促进受损 B 细胞的修复、增加肝糖原合成有关。山茱萸醇提取物能够降低肾上腺素、四氧嘧啶及链脲佐菌素（STZ）诱导糖尿病大鼠模型血糖水平，并能降低高血糖动物的血液黏度，抑制血小板聚集。山茱萸环烯醚萜总苷能显著减少糖尿病血管并发症，其可能是通过抑制氧化应激来保护肾小球系膜细胞免受糖化终产物的损害。

(2) **Anti-diabetes**　The iridoids (including marcitin and monoside) and triterpenoids (including

ursolic acid and oleanolic acid) are the main material bases for the hypoglycemic effect of *Shān zhū yú*, which is related to increasing glucose tolerance, protecting the B cells of pancreas from damage and promoting liver glycogen synthesis. Ethanol extract of *Shān zhū yú* is able to lower blood sugar level in diabetic rats induced by adrenaline, alloxan or streptozotocin, decrease the blood viscosity and inhibit platelet aggregation as well. Iridoid glycosides of *Shān zhū yú* can significantly reduce diabetic vascular complications and diabetic nephropathy due to protecting mesangial cells from the damage of glycation end products by inhibiting oxidative stress.

3. **抗氧化、抗衰老** 山茱萸水煎液、山茱萸多糖可提高大鼠红细胞中 SOD 的活力，降低血清脂质过氧化物 (LPO) 含量。山茱萸多糖、熊果酸、马钱子苷可提高衰老小鼠血清 SOD、过氧化氢酶、谷胱甘肽过氧化物酶活性，降低肝、脑组织的过氧化脂质含量。

(3) Anti-oxidation and anti-aging The water decoction and polysaccharide of *Shān zhū yú* can enhance the activity of SOD in erythrocytes and decrease the serumal lipid peroxidation (LPO) level in rat. In addition, polysaccharide ursolic acid and syringin in *Shān zhū yú* can increase the activities of serumal SOD, CAT and GSH-Px, as well as reduce the level of LPO in liver and brain tissues.

4. **调节免疫** 山茱萸可升高小鼠血清免疫球蛋白 G（IgG）和免疫球蛋白 M（IgM）的含量。山茱萸多糖可提高大鼠淋巴细胞转化率，促进溶血空斑形成，激活自然杀伤（NK）细胞，提高巨噬细胞活性，促进白细胞介素 –1（IL-1）、白细胞介素 –2（IL-2）、肿瘤坏死因子（TNF）和干扰素 –γ（IFN-γ）的分泌。另一方面，山茱萸总苷能抑制淋巴细胞转化，抑制淋巴因子激活的杀伤细胞（LAK）的增殖和 IL-2 的产生，能对抗动物器官移植后产生的排斥反应。

(4) Immunoregulation *Shān zhū yú* can increase the content of IgG and IgM in serum of mice. Polysaccharides from *Shān zhū yú* increase lymphocyte transformation rate, enhance formation of hemolytic plaque, activate natural killer (NK) cells and macrophages, and promote interleukin 1 (IL-1), interleukin 1 (IL-2), tumor necrosis factor (TNF) and interferon-γ (IFN-γ) secretion in rat model. On the other hand, total glycosides of *Shān zhū yú* inhibit lymphocyte transformation, lymphokine-activated killer (LAK) cells proliferation and IL-2 secretion both *in vitro* and *in vivo*. They can also relieve immunological rejection of organ transplantation.

5. **强心、抗休克** 山茱萸注射液静脉给药可改善心功能，增加心肌收缩力和心输出量，提高心脏工作效率。山茱萸注射液能对抗家兔、大鼠晚期失血性休克，升高血压，增加肾脏血流量，延长动物存活时间。

(5) Cardiotonic and anti-shock effects Intravenous administration of *Shān zhū yú* injection can improve cardiac function, increase myocardial contractility and cardiac output, and improve cardiac efficiency. *Shān zhū yú* injection is able to suppress terminal hemorrhagic shock, increase blood pressure and blood flow to the kidneys, thus to prolong animal survival.

6. **抗炎、镇痛** 山茱萸水煎剂能抑制醋酸诱发的小鼠腹腔毛细血管通透性增高，能显著抑制二甲苯所致小鼠耳肿胀和蛋清、角叉菜胶所致大鼠足肿胀，降低大鼠肾上腺内维生素 C 的含量。其抗炎机制与增强垂体–肾上腺皮质功能有关。山茱萸环烯醚萜总苷可抑制佐剂关节炎大鼠血浆中前列腺素 E_2 (PGE_2) 的产生，发挥抗炎和镇痛作用。

(6) Anti-inflammation and analgesia Water decoction of *Shān zhū yú* can inhibit the increase of peritoneal capillary permeability caused by acetic acid in mice model. It also inhibits mouse ear swelling induced by dimethylbenzene and foot swelling caused by albumen or carrageen in rats. Moreover, it decreases vitamin C concentration in rat adrenal gland. Its anti-inflammatory mechanism relates with enhancing the pituitary-adrenal function. The total iridoid glycosides is capable to suppress the production of prostaglandin E_2 (PGE_2) in serum rat serum adjuvant arthritis to help inhibiting inflammatory and pain.

（肖洪贺　汪　宁）